Anaesthesia Databook

A CLINICAL PRACTICE COMPENDIUM

*To Chris, without whom the writing of this book would
not have been possible, and in memory of the late
H. Stuart Winsey—an anaesthetist's surgeon.*

For Churchill Livingstone

Publisher: Geoffrey Nuttall
Project Editor: Lowri Daniels
Copy Editor: Joanna Smith
Design: Design Resources Unit/Charles Simpson
Production Controller: Mark Sanderson
Sales Promotion Executive: Caroline Boyd

Anaesthesia Databook

A CLINICAL PRACTICE COMPENDIUM

Rosemary A. Mason

MB ChB DObst RCOG FRCA
Consultant Anaesthetist,
Swansea N.H.S. Trust,
Singleton Hospital,
Swansea,
UK

SECOND EDITION

CHURCHILL LIVINGSTONE
EDINBURGH LONDON MADRID MELBOURNE NEW YORK AND TOKYO 1994

CHURCHILL LIVINGSTONE
Medical Division of Longman Group UK Limited

Distributed in the United States of America by Churchill
Livingstone Inc., 650 Avenue of the Americas, New York,
N.Y. 10011, and by associated companies, branches and
representatives throughout the world.

First edition 1990
Second edition 1994

ISBN 0 443 04763 4

British Library Cataloguing in Publication Data
A catalogue record for this book is available from the
British Library.

Library of Congress Cataloging in Publication Data
A catalog record for this book is available from the Library
of Congress.

The
publisher's
policy is to use
**paper manufactured
from sustainable forests**

Produced by Longman Publishers Singapore (Pte) Ltd
Printed in Singapore

Contents

Preface to the second edition

Responses to the first edition have been gratifying. As ever, differing individuals have found differing sections to be helpful, therefore changes inevitably will not be to everyone's satisfaction.

Overwhelmingly, the sections on 'Medical disorders and anaesthetic problems' and 'Perioperative emergency conditions' have proved to be the most popular. These have been thoroughly updated and expanded and more than thirty new topics added. My sentiments accord with those who wished that the book could be reduced to pocket size, but attempts at this have been a total failure, even after abandoning the two sections on drugs.

Some medical topics have only been mentioned in one or two anaesthetic papers and, as yet, have not gained sufficient importance to be included as a full entry in Section 1. I have grouped these together as 'Rare and unusual syndromes'. Anaesthetic problems generated by the patient (automatic implantable cardioverter-defibrillators) or those inherent in a new procedure (anaesthesia for magnetic resonance imaging) now find a place in an expanded 'Miscellaneous' section.

My original concerns about the increasing complexity of anaesthesia and the difficulties of dealing with its interaction with intricate medical problems are becoming regularly more apparent. Even though it still does not fit the pocket, I hope that this book can ward off some problems and ease the predicament in others.

Swansea 1994   R.A.M.

Preface to the first edition

Year by year, both the scope and complexity of anaesthesia increase. Frequently, and often at short notice, decisions on patient management are required, in which the role of the anaesthetist may be critical. For this advice to be soundly based, it may be necessary not only to evaluate the appropriateness of a variety of possible anaesthetic techniques, but also to draw together widely disparate pieces of medical knowledge. At a time of increasing specialization, this is and will become progressively more difficult.

I have felt that there are few texts written which lie between the standard textbook and the specialist monograph and which are specifically for the experienced anaesthetist facing awkward problems. My aim therefore has been to attempt to produce a relatively advanced practical reference system for the trained anaesthetist.

This is not a book for beginners. There is no discussion of basic principles or techniques. The information has been collated from a wide range of sources and the bibliography at the end of each topic not only covers the quoted references but also will often provide a guide to more extensive reading. No attempt has been made to provide a didactic manual and, where conflicting opinions exist, these have been recorded so that a balanced judgement can be made in the light of particular circumstances.

To compress the large amount of information into a book of reasonably compact size has meant the adoption of a tight and somewhat indigestible style of writing. However it is envisaged that it will be consulted for specific clinical problems rather than read in continuity.

It is unusual nowadays for a book covering many topics to be written by a single author. However, I wished to develop a systematic and unified approach, and it does reflect my personal view on the integration of both medicine in general and anaesthesia.

I hope that this book's niche will prove to be the briefcase or the back of the car and that it might provide a little help in times of crisis!

Swansea 1990

R.A.M.

Introduction

This book is laid out as a reference system rather than as a descriptive text. Each section reviews a major consideration in anaesthesia though, where necessary, certain subjects are cross-referenced between differing sections. Where possible, a standardized approach to each topic is taken, and there is a full terminal index.

Section 1

Covers a range of medical conditions which may present anaesthetic problems. The information, including the bibliography, is self-contained except where cross-references are indicated. Each section describes systematically the preoperative abnormalities, anaesthetic problems and management.

Unlike a standard medical textbook, the space allocated to a particular condition is not necessarily proportional to its frequency of occurrence. Thus, a rare disease producing potentially serious anaesthetic complications may be considered in much more detail than a common condition with fewer associated problems.

Section 2

Reviews emergency conditions which may present for the first time in the perioperative period. Inevitably there is some overlap of information with that in Section 1.

Section 3

Deals with miscellaneous problems including those inherent in new procedures and those posed by the patient himself. Anaesthesia for patients with automatic implantable cardioverter-defibrillators, surgery in Jehovah's Witnesses, management of patients with cervical spine injuries, management and training for awake fibreoptic intubation, laser surgery of the airway, and problems of anaesthesia for magnetic resonance imaging as well as cardiopulmonary resuscitation, brain death and organ donor management are covered.

Section 4

Rare and unusual syndromes. A number of syndromes that have only one, or at the most two references in the anaesthetic literature and were not considered to warrant the detail devoted to subjects in Section 1. The salient features are briefly described, as are the reported anaesthetic problems and relevant references.

Normal values

Appendix
Useful addresses and telephone numbers.

Acknowledgements

The responsibility for the accuracy of the contents of this book remains with myself. However, I owe a large debt of gratitude to my friends and colleagues, who were not only a continuing source of advice and encouragement, but laboured hard to reduce errors to a minimum.

DR S A D Al-Ismail MB ChB MRCP MRCPath
Consultant Haematologist, West Glamorgan Health Authority, Swansea, South Wales, UK

Dr A C Ames BSc MB BS FRCPath
Consultant Chemical Pathologist, West Glamorgan Health Authority, Swansea, South Wales, UK

Dr J C Mason MA D Phil BM BCh MRCP
Consultant Renal and General Physician, Portsmouth Health District, Portsmouth, England, UK

Mr M C Mason BSc BM BCh FRCS
Consultant Surgeon, West Glamorgan Health Authority, Swansea, South Wales, UK

List of abbreviations

ACE	Angiotensin-converting enzyme
AChE	Acetylcholinesterase
ACTH	Adrenocorticotrophic hormone
ADH	Antidiuretic hormone
AF	Atrial fibrillation
AIDS	Acquired immune deficiency syndrome
AIP	Acute intermittent porphyria
ALA	d-Aminolaevulinic acid (synthase)
AMP	Adenosine monophosphate
APTT	Activated partial thromboplastin time
APUD	Amine precursor uptake and decarboxylation
ARDS	Adult respiratory distress syndrome
ASD	Atrial septal defect
AV	Atrioventricular
A-V	Arteriovenous
AVP	Arginine vasopressin
AZT	Zidovudine ('Retrovir')
BBB	Bundle branch block
b.d.	Twice per day
BG	Blood glucose
BMR	Basal metabolic rate
BP	Blood pressure
b.p.m.	Beats per minute
C1	First component of complement
C2	Second component of complement
C4	Fourth component of complement
CABG	Coronary artery bypass graft
CAPD	Continuous ambulatory peritoneal dialysis
ChE	Cholinesterase
CNS	Central nervous system
CPAP	Continuous positive airway pressure
CPB	Cardiopulmonary bypass
CK	Creatine kinase
CPR	Cardiopulmonary resuscitation
CRF	Corticotrophin-releasing factor
CVP	Central venous pressure
CXR	Chest X-ray

DDC	3,5-Dicarbethoxy-1,4-dihydrocolidine
DDAVP	Desmopressin (1-desamino-8-D-arginine vasopressin)
DIC	Disseminated intravascular coagulopathy
DMD	Duchenne muscular dystrophy
DNA	Desoxyribose nucleic acid
DVI	Digital vascular imaging
DVT	Deep venous thrombosis
EBV	Epstein–Barr virus
ECG	Electrocardiogram
ECM	External cardiac massage
ECMO	Extracorporeal membranous oxygenation
EEC	European Economic Community
EMG	Electromyogram
EMLA	Eutectic mixture of local anaesthetics (cream)
ENT	Ear nose and throat
ETCO2	End tidal carbon dioxide
ETT	Endotracheal tube
E_1f	Fluoride-resistant gene
FBG	Fasting blood glucose
FDA	Food and Drugs Administration (USA)
FDF	Fibrin degradation products
FEV1	Forced expiratory volume in the first second of expiration
FFP	Fresh frozen plasma
FGF	Fresh gas flow
FIO_2	Fractional inspired oxygen
FRC	Functional residual capacity
FSH	Follicle stimulating hormone
G	Gauge
GABA	Gamma amino butyric acid
GFR	Glomerular filtration rate
GH	Growth hormone
GIK	Glucose, insulin, potassium (infusion)
GTT	Glucose tolerance test
G6PD	Glucose-6-phosphate dehydrogenase
HAV	Hepatitis A virus
HBV	Hepatitis B virus
HBcAg	Hepatitis B core antigen
HBeAg	Hepatitis B e antigen
HBsAg	Hepatitis B surface antigen
Hb	Haemoglobin
HbA	Normal adult haemoglobin

HbAS	Sickle cell trait
HbA2	Haemoglobin A2
HbC	Haemoglobin C
HbCO	Carboxyhaemoglobin
HbF	Fetal haemoglobin
HbS	Sickle cell haemoglobin
HbSC	Sickle cell C disease
HbSS	Homozygous sickle cell anaemia
HbThal	Thalassaemia haemoglobin
HC	Hereditary coproporphyria
HELLP	Haemolysis Elevated Liver enzymes and Low Platelet count (syndrome)
HGPRT	Hypoxanthine guanine phosphoribosyl transferase
HIV	Human immunodeficiency virus
HOCM	Hypertrophic obstructive cardiomyopathy
ICP	Intracranial pressure
IDD	Insulin-dependent diabetes
IgE	Immunoglobulin E
IgG	Immunoglobulin G
IgM	Immunoglobulin M
i.m.	Intramuscular
INR	International normalized ratio
IPPV	Intermittent positive-pressure ventilation
IQ	Intelligence quotient
ISI	International sensitivity index
ITU	Intensive therapy unit
iu	International units
i.v.	Intravenous
J	Joule
JVP	Jugular venous pulse
kPa	Kilopascal
KCCT	Kaolin cephalin clotting time
l	Litre
L	Length
LA	Local anaesthesia
LAP	Left atrial pressure
LBBB	Left bundle branch block
LFTs	Liver function tests
LSCS	Lower segment Caesarean section
LSD	Lysergic acid diethylamide
LT	Leukotrienes
LVEDP	Left ventricular end diastolic pressure

LVF	Left ventricular failure
MAC	Minimal alveolar concentration
MAO	Monoamine oxidase
MAOI	Monoamine oxidase inhibitor
MAP	Mean arterial pressure
MCV	Mean corpuscular volume
MEN	Multiple endocrine neoplasia
MH	Malignant hyperthermia
MHE	Malignant hyperthermia equivocal result, consider as MHS
MHN	Malignant hyperthermia non-susceptible from proven MH pedigree
MHS	Malignant hyperthermia susceptible
mIBG	*Meta*-iodobenzylguanidine
mmHg	Millimetres of mercury
MMR	Masseter muscle rigidity
MPS	Mucopolysaccharidosis
MRI	Magnetic resonance imaging
MS	Multiple sclerosis
MSH	Melanocyte-stimulating hormone
MV	Minute volume
MVP	Mitral valve prolapse
MVV	Minute volume ventilation
N	Normal
NAB	Nasally assisted breathing
NANBV	Non-A non-B virus (hepatitis)
NIDD	Non-insulin-dependent diabetes
NMS	Neuroleptic malignant syndrome
NPO	Neurogenic pulmonary oedema
NSAID	Non-steroidal anti-inflammatory drug
OD	Outside diameter
$PaCO_2$	Arterial partial pressure of carbon dioxide
PAH	Pregnancy-aggravated hypertension
PAN	Polyarteritis nodosa
PaO_2	Arterial partial pressure of oxygen
PAP	Pulmonary artery pressure
PAWP	Pulmonary artery wedge pressure
PCP	Pulmonary capillary pressure
PCV	Packed cell volume
PCWP	Pulmonary capillary wedge pressure
PDA	Patent ductus arteriosus

PE	Pulmonary embolism
PEEP	Positive end expiratory pressure
PEFR	Peak expiratory flow rate
PIH	Pregnancy-induced hypertension
P mitrale	A prolonged bifid P wave on ECG indicating left atrial enlargement
PP	Pancreatic polypeptide
P pulmonale	A taller than normal P wave on ECG indicating right atrial hypertrophy
PPF	Plasma protein fraction
PPH	Primary pulmonary hypertension
PT	Prothrombin time
PTH	Parathormone
PVC	Polyvinyl chloride
PVR	Pulmonary vascular resistance
q.d.s.	Four times per day
Q-Tc	Corrected QT interval
RAP	Right atrial pressure
RBBB	Right bundle branch block
RBC	Red blood corpuscle
RDS	Respiratory distress syndrome
RF	Radio frequency
RLF	Retrolental fibroplasia
RR	Respiratory rate
R-R variation	Variations in the intervals between two consecutive R waves (ECG)
RSR1	An initial upward deflection (R) is followed by a downward deflection (S) followed by a second upward deflection (R1) on ECG lead VI
RVEDP	Right ventricular end diastolic pressure
SAP	Systemic arterial pressure
SBE	Subacute bacterial endocarditis
SIADH	Syndrome of inappropriate antidiuretic hormone
SIDS	Sudden infant death syndrome
SLE	Systemic lupus erythematosus
SVC	Superior vena cava
SVT	Supraventricular tachycardia
t	Tesla (10 000 gauss)
T3	Tri-iodothyronine
T4	Thyroxine
TCAD	Tricyclic antidepressant

TCT	Thrombin clotting time
t.d.s.	Three times per day
TIA	Transient ischaemic attack
TRH	Thyrotrophin-releasing hormone
TSH	Thyroid-stimulating hormone
TURP	Transurethral resection of the prostate
TV	Tidal volume
u	Unit
UK	United Kingdom
VC	Vital capacity
VF	Ventricular fibrillation
VIP	Vasoactive intestinal peptide
VP	Variegate porphyria
VSD	Ventricular septal defect
VT	Ventricular tachycardia
vWd	von Willebrand's disease
vWF:Ag	von Willebrand factor
WCC	White cell count
WPW	Wolff–Parkinson–White syndrome

Medical disorders and anaesthetic problems

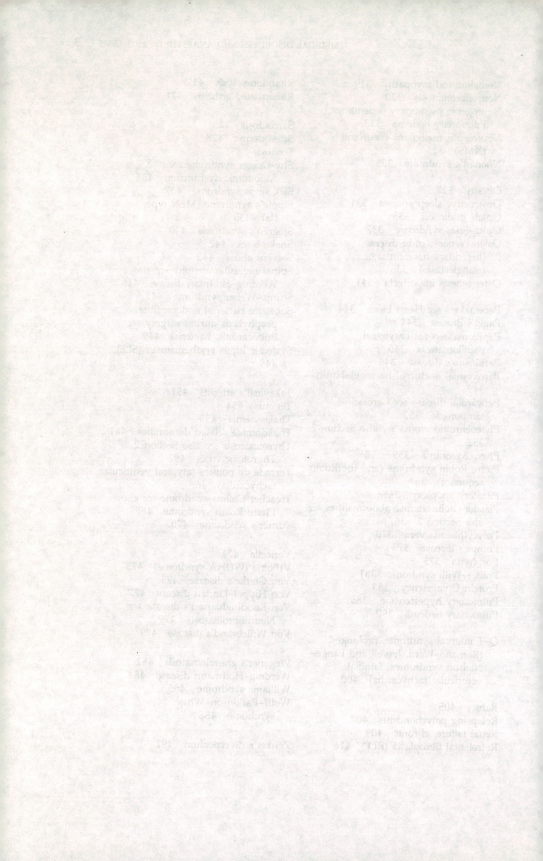

1

Medical Disorders and Anaesthetic Problems

ACHALASIA OF THE OESOPHAGUS

A chronic, progressive motor disorder of the oesophagus associated with degenerative changes in the myenteric ganglia and vagal nuclei. There are three components: a failure of the lower oesophageal sphincter to relax with an increased resting sphincter pressure resulting in a functional obstruction; an absence of sequential peristalsis in response to a bolus of food; and finally a dilated, contorted oesophagus. Overspill may produce bronchopulmonary complications, and 5–10% of patients ultimately develop carcinoma of the oesophagus. Nitrates and calcium channel blockers given before meals sometimes produce symptomatic improvement, but the mainstay of treatment is oesophageal dilatation or surgical myotomy.

Preoperative abnormalities

1. Symptoms include dysphagia, retrosternal pain, regurgitation and weight loss. In young people the condition may be misdiagnosed as anorexia nervosa or asthma (Creagh-Barry et al 1988).
2. Respiratory complications, which may be attributed to asthma or chronic bronchitis, are secondary to overspill of undigested material. Nocturnal coughing occurs in 30% and bronchopulmonary complications in 10% of patients. Aspiration of larger volumes may result in lobar collapse, bronchiectasis or lung abscess.
3. Rarely, may present with a cervical mass and acute upper respiratory tract obstruction, necessitating urgent intervention.
4. Diagnosis can be made on barium swallow, manometric studies and endoscopy. Occasionally, acute dilatation may be seen on CXR, in which case, abnormal flow-volume curves will indicate variable intrathoracic tracheal obstruction.

Anaesthetic problems

1. A predisposition to regurgitation and pulmonary aspiration in the perioperative period.
2. Upper airway obstruction or respiratory failure. Rarely, acute dilatation of the oesophagus may result in upper airway obstruction

(Travis et al 1981, Westbrook 1992). One patient developed acute respiratory failure 8 days after surgery for a fractured neck of femur. The diagnosis was made on CXR, which showed an air-containing cavity along the right upper heart border (Kendall & Lin 1991). The opening pressure of the cricopharyngeus muscle from above is much lower than that from below, therefore progressive dilatation of the upper oesophagus may occur, particularly with air swallowing or IPPV.

3. Acute thoracic inlet obstruction with stridor, deep cyanosis of the face and hypotension occurred during recovery from anaesthesia after gynaecological surgery (McLean et al 1976). Passage of the tracheal tube beyond the dilated oesophagus was achieved with difficulty. In a second, less severe case, neck swelling and venous engorgement was precipitated by coughing or straining (King & Strickland 1979).

4. If acute airway obstruction is present, sudden decompression of the oesophagus may cause the pharynx to flood with food and fluid.

Management

1. If anaesthesia is required, precautions must be taken to reduce the risk of aspiration of gastric contents. The dilated oesophagus must be emptied and decompressed. This needs a period of prolonged starvation, possibly with washouts of the oesophagus, although the need for this has been challenged. A rapid sequence induction should be undertaken, and tracheal extubation performed in the awake patient. Recovery should take place in the lateral position.

2. Sublingual isosorbide dinitrate 5 mg and nifedipine 20 mg have both been shown to reduce basal lower oesophageal sphincter pressure, 10 minutes after administration. Isosorbide produces the greater decrease and is more effective than nifedipine in reducing symptoms (Gelfond et al 1982).

3. Management of acute upper airway obstruction secondary to tracheal compression has been reported using:
   a. Sublingual glyceryl nitrate (Westbrook 1992).
   b. Passage of a naso-oesophageal tube (Zikk et al 1989).
   c. Transcutaneous needle puncture (Evans et al 1982).
   d. Tracheal intubation (Becker & Castell 1989).
   e. Rigid oesophagoscopy (Carlsson-Norlander 1987).
   f. Emergency tracheostomy (Barr & MacDonald 1989).

BIBLIOGRAPHY
Barr G D, MacDonald I 1989 Management of achalasia and laryngotracheal compression. Journal of Laryngology and Otology 103: 713–714
Becker D J, Castell D O 1989 Acute airway obstruction in achalasia. Possible role of defective belch reflex. Gastroenterology 97: 1323–1326
Carlsson-Norlander B 1987 Acute upper airway obstruction in a patient with achalasia. Archives of Otolaryngology and Head and Neck Surgery 113: 885–887

Creagh-Barry P, Parsons J, Pattison C W 1988 Achalasia and anaesthesia, a case report. Anaesthesia and Intensive Care 16: 371–373

Evans C R, Cawood R, Dronfield M W et al 1982 Achalasia: presentation with stridor and a new form of treatment. British Medical Journal 285: 1704

Gelfond M, Rozen P, Gilat T 1982 Isosorbide dinitrate and nifedipine treatment of achalasia: a clinical, manometric and radionuclide evaluation. Gastroenterology 83: 963–969

Kendall A P, Lin E 1991 Respiratory failure as a presentation of achalasia of the oesophagus. Anaesthesia 46: 1039–1040

King D M, Strickland B 1979 An unusual cause of thoracic inlet obstruction. British Journal of Radiology 52: 910–913

McLean R D W, Stewart C J, Whyte D G C 1976 Acute thoracic inlet obstruction in achalasia of the oesophagus. Thorax 31: 456–459

Travis K W, Saini V K, O'Sullivan P T 1981 Upper-airway obstruction and achalasia of the oesophagus. Anesthesiology 54: 87–88

Westbrook J L 1992 Oesophageal achalasia causing respiratory obstruction. Anaesthesia 47: 38–40

Zikk D, Rapoport Y, Halperin D et al 1989 Acute airway obstruction and achalasia of the esophagus. Annals of Otology, Rhinology and Laryngology 98: 641–643

ACHONDROPLASIA

A type of dwarfism inherited as an autosomal dominant. Cartilage formation at the epiphyses is defective. Bones dependent on cartilage proliferation are thus shortened, whereas periosteal and membranous bones are unaffected. Head and trunk size are normal, but the extremities shortened. Anaesthesia may be required for spinal or cranial surgery, limb lengthening and Caesarean section.

Preoperative abnormalities

1. Individuals are less than 1.4 m tall and of normal intelligence. Hands and feet are short, and the fingers are of equal length. The forehead protrudes, the nose is flattened, the mandible and tongue are large, but the maxilla is short. There is severe lumbar lordosis, a reduced symphysis pubis to xiphoid distance, and often kyphoscoliosis with reduced anterioposterior diameter of the thorax. The pelvis is small.

2. Spinal canal and foramen magnum stenosis is common and spinal cord compression may occur at any level and result in neurological deficits. The foramen magnum is small at birth and growth rate is impaired. Recent studies have shown deficits in children to be more common than was previously thought. Anaesthesia may be required for suboccipital craniectomy, laminectomy or ventriculoperitoneal shunts.

3. Although fertility is low, pregnancy does occur. As a result of the skeletal problems, the fetus remains high, in an intra-abdominal position. This may result in severe respiratory embarrassment in the later stages of pregnancy. The baby is, however, of near normal size, making Caesarean section mandatory.

Anaesthetic problems

1. The larynx is smaller than normal, and its size is related to patient weight rather than to age (Mayhew et al 1986). Upper airway obstruction has been reported, in association with adenotonsillar hypertrophy and pharyngeal hypoplasia. Mask ventilation may be difficult because of the facial structure. Intubation problems can result from premature fusion of the bones at the base of the skull and limited mobility of the cervical vertebrae (Lauri et al 1988). However, in a series of 36 patients (Mayhew et a1 1986), no intubation difficulty was experienced.

2. Intravenous access may be difficult, particularly in the infant, because of lax skin and subcutaneous tissues.

3. Technical problems using automatic blood pressure monitoring may be encountered since it can be difficult to match the cuff size to a short, fat arm. McArthur (1992) found that excessive arterial pressures were recorded by indirect methods when compared with direct arterial monitoring.

4. Abnormal respiratory function may be central or peripheral in origin. Sleep apnoea and hypoxaemia, which may be improved after brainstem decompression, is probably secondary to foramen magnum stenosis. Hypotonia of the upper airway muscles is common in the infant and may contribute to airway obstruction during sleep (Berkowitz et al 1990). Studies of lung volumes in adults show that the vital capacity is reduced out of proportion to that which would be expected if limb sizes were normal, but that the lungs and airways are functionally normal (Stokes et al 1990).

5. Technical difficulties may be experienced during regional anaesthesia as a consequence of the skeletal defects (Walts et al 1975). The narrow spinal canal and reduced extradural space increase the risk of accidental dural puncture and the production of an extensive extradural block. Since neurological problems also often develop spontaneously during the third and fourth decades, regional blockade should be approached with circumspection.
Initial clinical symptoms of thoracolumbar involvement are lower limb motor weakness and low back pain. Sensory and sphincter disturbances occur less frequently.

6. Neurosurgical operations. Twenty-four patients with achondroplasia undergoing craniectomies were reviewed (Mayhew et al 1986). Out of 16 patients whose surgery was performed in the sitting position, nine had some degree of air embolism, whereas only one operated on in the prone position had such a problem. The air was usually successfully aspirated, and no patient died. Six other major complications occurred; two patients had C1 – level spinal cord infarctions, two had brachial plexus palsies, and one was accidentally extubated. The sixth patient, after developing severe

oedema of the tongue, required tracheostomy. The cause was thought to be extreme flexion of the neck producing venous thrombosis (Mayhew et al 1985).

7. Anaesthesia for Caesarean section may compound all of these problems. In the later stages of pregnancy, the supine position can be associated with severe aortocaval compression and respiratory embarrassment. Successful anaesthetics using both general and extradural techniques have been described (Cohen 1980). However, even if the technical difficulties of regional anaesthesia are overcome, it should be remembered that small doses of local anaesthetic given extradurally can produce extensive, and sometimes patchy, neural blockade. In one patient, bupivacaine 0.5% 12 ml produced a block from C5 to S4 (Brimacombe & Caunt 1990), and in a second, 5 ml only was required for Caesarean section (Wardall & Frame 1990). Problems were not encountered in all patients and Carstoniu et al (1992) emphasize that extradural analgesia should not be denied should the need for it arise.

Management

1. Possible intubation difficulties should be considered when the patient is assessed. A range of tracheal tubes, of sizes smaller than normal, should be available. Mayhew et al (1986) have suggested that size should be based on age, according to the formula:

$$\text{Tube size (i.d. in mm)} = \frac{[\text{age (year)} + 16]}{4}$$

2. Particular care is needed when positioning the patient for surgery. Upper limbs should be well supported, and extreme neck flexion avoided.

3. During neurosurgical procedures performed in the sitting position, it has been suggested that great care should be taken to avoid air embolus (Katz & Mayhew 1985, Mayhew et al 1986). However, no patient died in the series presented. In addition, the prone position may be associated with heavy blood loss, and does not guarantee freedom from air embolism. Whatever position is chosen, air embolism must be anticipated, diagnosed and treated early.

4. If respiratory function is compromised in late pregnancy, blood gases should be estimated before Caesarean section. During the performance of an extradural block, doses should be fractionated and adequate time allowed between increments of local anaesthetic.

5. In labour, aortocaval compression must be prevented.

BIBLIOGRAPHY
Berkowitz I D, Raja S N, Bender K S et al 1990 Dwarfs: pathophysiology and anesthetic implications. Anesthesiology 73: 739–759
Brimacombe J R, Caunt J A 1990 Anaesthesia in a gravid achondroplastic dwarf. Anaesthesia 45: 132–134

Carstoniu J, Yee I, Halpern S 1992 Epidural anaesthesia for Caesarean section in an achondroplastic dwarf. Canadian Journal of Anaesthesia 39: 708–711

Cohen S E 1980 Anesthesia for Caesarean section in achondroplastic dwarfs. Anesthesiology 52: 264–266

Katz J, Mayhew J F 1985 Air embolism in the achondroplastic dwarf. Anesthesiology 63: 205–207

Lauri A, Marri M, Galli C et al 1988 Anaesthesia in achondroplastic dwarves. Basic Life Sciences 48: 167–174

Mayhew J F, Miner M, Katz J 1985 Macroglossia in a 16 month old child following a craniotomy. Anesthesiology 62: 683–684

Mayhew J F, Katz J, Miner M et al 1986 Anaesthesia for the achondroplastic dwarf. Canadian Anaesthetists' Society Journal 33: 216–221

McArthur R D A 1992 Obstetric anaesthesia in an achondroplastic dwarf at a regional hospital. Anaesthesia and Intensive Care 20: 376–378

Stokes D C, Wohl M E, Wise R A et al 1990. The lungs and airways in achondroplasia. Do little people have little lungs? Chest 98: 145–152

Walts L F, Finerman G, Wyatt G M 1975 Anaesthesia for dwarfs and other patients of pathological small stature. Canadian Anaesthetists' Society Journal 22: 703–709

Wardall G J, Frame W T 1990 Extradural anaesthesia for Caesarean section in achondroplasia. British Journal of Anaesthesia 64: 367–370

ACROMEGALY

A rare, chronic disease of insidious onset which usually presents in middle life. An increased secretion of growth hormone, most commonly by an adenoma of the eosinophil cells of the pituitary, results in an overgrowth of bone, connective tissue and viscera. Death from respiratory causes is three times more common than that in the general population. This is usually secondary to airway obstruction and, less often, in association with CNS dysfunction (Murrant & Gatland 1990). Treatment includes trans-sphenoidal hypophysectomy, bromocriptine and the long-acting somatostatin analogue, octreotide (Klibanski & Zervas 1991), which may cause gall stones.

Preoperative abnormalities

1. The head, tongue, jaw, hands and feet are enlarged. Facial features are coarse, and the voice husky.
2. Kyphoscoliosis, muscular weakness, nerve entrapment syndromes, hypertension, acromegalic heart disease (10%), goitre, diabetes mellitus (10–20%), diabetes insipidus, hypercalcaemia, and visual field defects may be present.
3. There is a greatly increased incidence of colonic cancer (8%), skin tags and colonic polyps (46%) when compared with the normal population (Melmed 1990).
4. Patients with active disease have an increase in total lung capacity, but evidence of small airway narrowing (Harrison et al 1978). Abnormalities of lung function are increasingly likely when the disease has been present for more than 8 years. However, upper

airway obstruction is also common and may be secondary to pharyngeal soft tissue hypertrophy, thickening of the glottis and supraglottis or reduced mobility of the vocal cords.

5. Muscle weakness may occur.
6. Enlargement of the sella turcica may be evident on skull X-ray in 90% of cases.

Anaesthetic problems

1. Extrathoracic airway obstruction occurs in 30–50% of acromegalics (Murrant & Gatland 1990, Trotman-Dickenson et al 1991). Upper airway obstruction is particularly common in men and results in nocturnal hypoxaemia. Four types of perioperative airway problem may present (Southwick & Katz 1979):
   a. Difficulty in obtaining an airtight fit with the mask.
   b. Difficulty in visualizing the larynx – often because of massive hypertrophy of the pharyngeal mucosa.
   c. Difficulty in passing a tracheal tube as a result of mucosal thickening, glottic stenosis, fixation or palsy of the vocal cords.
   d. Postintubation, or postoperative obstruction. After trans-sphenoidal hypophysectomy, packing of the nose may predispose to upper airway obstruction and pulmonary oedema (Singelyn & Scholtes 1988).
   Extensive calcification (chondrocalcinosis) of the larynx may also occur (Edge & Whitwam 1981), and decreased cricoid width has been reported (Hassan et al 1976).

2. Increased daytime somnolence and sleep apnoea have been described, and both are more likely to occur in active disease (Hart et al 1985). Treatment does not necessarily cure the problem. Central depression of respiration may be compounded by the residual effects of anaesthetic drugs and result in severe postoperative hypoxia, hypercarbia or respiratory arrest (Kitahata 1971, Ovassapian et al 1981). Sudden deaths, which sometimes occur on return to the ward, may be explicable by a combination of these factors and respiratory obstruction.

3. Hypertension and ischaemic heart disease are frequently present. In a controlled study of cardiac arrhythmias, complex ventricular arrhythmias were found in 48% of acromegalics as opposed to 12% in normal subjects (Kahaly et al 1992a). Left ventricular muscle mass was increased secondary to concentric ventricular hypertrophy and was related to the duration of the disease, rather than to its severity (Kahaly et al 1992b).

4. Acute pulmonary oedema may occur secondary to upper airway obstruction (Goldhill et al 1982).

5. Impaired ulnar artery circulation was reported in 5 out of 10 acromegalic patients undergoing hypophysectomy (Campkin 1980). However, this observation has not been confirmed by others.

Losasso et al (1990) inserted 51 radial artery cannulae into such patients without performing Allen's test. None had subsequent ischaemic complications.

Management

1. Airway problems must be anticipated in advance, and a careful history should be directed towards this. X-rays of the neck may indicate overgrowth of pharyngeal tissue, glottic stenosis or chondrocalcinosis. Indirect laryngoscopy may be helpful. Airway abnormalities in acromegaly may be classified (Southwick & Katz 1979) as:

   a. No involvement.

   b. Hypertrophied nasal and pharyngeal mucosa, but normal cords.

   c. Glottic stenosis or vocal cord paresis.

   d. Combination of both (b) and (c).

   In the presence of either (c) or (d), and especially if there is sleep apnoea, elective tracheostomy should be considered (Murrant & Gatland 1990). Intubation, using a fibreoptic bronchoscope, has been claimed to obviate the need for tracheostomy (Venus 1980, Ovassapian et al 1981, Messick et al 1982). However, one patient in whom tracheostomy was avoided required emergency reintubation on three occasions in the postoperative period – twice for airway obstruction and once for respiratory arrest (Ovassapian et al 1981). Fibreoptic techniques may have transformed the management of difficult intubation as such, but in acromegalics the airway problems are not restricted to the intraoperative period, nor are they solely of a technical nature.

2. Postoperatively, acromegalics should be admitted to an area of high dependency, where cardiac rhythm and respiration can be carefully monitored. If nasal packing is required, it has been suggested that 18-gauge suction catheters, cut to sufficient length to pass beyond the base of the tongue, be inserted into each nostril prior to the packing (Singelyn & Scholtes 1988).

BIBLIOGRAPHY

Campkin T V 1980 Radial artery cannulation. Potential hazards in patients with acromegaly. Anaesthesia 35: 1008–1009

Edge W G, Whitwam J G I 1981 Chondrocalcinosis and difficult intubation in acromegaly. Anaesthesia 36: 677–680

Goldhill D R, Dalgleish J G, Lake R H N 1982 Respiratory problems and acromegaly. Anaesthesia 37: 1200–1203

Harrison B D W, Millhouse K A, Harrington M et al 1978 Lung function in aeromegaly. Quarterly Journal of Medicine 47: 517–532

Hart T B, Radow S K, Blackard W G et al 1985 Sleep apnea in active acromegaly. Archives of Internal Medicine 145: 865–868

Hassan S Z, Matz G J, Lawrence A M et al 1976 Laryngeal stenosis in acromegaly: a possible cause of airway difficulties associated with anesthesia. Anesthesia and Analgesia 55: 57–60

Kahaly G, Olshausen K V, Mohr-Kahaly S et al 1992a Arrhythmia profile in acromegaly. European Heart Journal 13: 51–56

Kahaly G, Stover C, Beyer J et al 1992b Relation of endocrine and cardiac findings in acromegalics. Journal of Endocrinological Investigation 15: 13–18

Kitahata L M 1971 Airway difficulties associated with anaesthesia in acromegaly. British Journal of Anaesthesia 43: 1187–1190

Klibanski A, Zervas N T 1991 Diagnosis and management of hormone secreting pituitary adenomas. New England Journal of Medicine 324: 822–831

Losasso T, Dietz N M, Muzzi D A 1990 Acromegaly and radial artery cannulation. Anesthesia and Analgesia 71: 204

Melmed S 1990 Acromegaly. New England Journal of Medicine 322: 966–977

Messick J M, Cucchiara R F, Faust R J 1982 Airway management in patients with acromegaly. Anesthesiology 56: 157

Murrant N J, Gatland D J 1990 Respiratory problems in acromegaly. Journal of Laryngology and Otology 104: 52–55

Ovassapian A, Doka J C, Romsa D E 1981 Acromegaly – use of fiberoptic laryngoscopy to avoid tracheostomy. Anesthesiology 54: 429–430

Singelyn F J, Scholtes J L 1988 Airway obstruction in acromegaly. Anaesthesia and Intensive Care 16: 491–492

Southwick J P Katz J 1979 Unusual airway difficulty in the acromegalic patient – indications for tracheostomy. Anesthesiology 51: 72–73

Trotman-Dickenson B, Weetman A P, Hughes J M B 1991 Upper airflow obstruction and pulmonary function in acromegaly: relationship to disease activity. Quarterly Journal of Medicine 79: 527–538.

Venus B 1980 Acromegalic patient-indication for fiberoptic bronchoscopy but not tracheostomy. Anesthesiology 52: 100–101.

ADDICTION
(see also ALCOHOLISM, AMPHETAMINE ABUSE, COCAINE ABUSE, LSD ABUSE, OPIATE ADDICIION, SOLVENT ABUSE)

The incidence of drug addiction is increasing. In addition, new drugs are being used and hence new complications reported. Anaesthesia may be required for addicts in either an acute or a chronic state of intoxication. Alternatively, the anaesthetist is increasingly involved in resuscitation and treatment of patients suffering toxic side effects of drugs or drug cocktails. Hazards exist not only for the patient, but for staff in the hospital. Accidental rupture of drug packages concealed in body cavities may result in severe acute absorption or intestinal obstruction.

Individual drugs are dealt with separately in the text, but the following comments are generally applicable.

Anaesthetic problems

1. Difficulties in obtaining an accurate history.
2. Problems associated with chronic abuse.
3. Problems of withdrawal syndrome during a period of illness.
4. Difficulties with venepuncture.
5. Associated malnutrition and liver disease.
6. Problems of acute toxicity. The possibility exists that the patient may inject a drug into his infusion.
7. Increased risk of hepatitis B and HIV, septicaemia, bacterial endocarditis and tetanus in intravenous drug users.

8. Rhabdomyolysis, and occasionally acute renal failure, may be associated with the consumption of cocaine.
9. During pregnancy there is increased maternal and fetal morbidity and mortality.
10. Problems of resuscitation from overdose of drug or drug cocktails.
11. Problems of mixing drugs and contamination with other substances.
12. 'Ecstasy' (3,4-methylenedioxymethamphetamine, MDMA) and 'Eve' (3,4-methylenedioxyethamphetamine, MDEA), sometimes in combination with other substances, have been associated with a syndrome of convulsions, hyperthermia, hyperkalaemia, rhabdomyolysis and disseminated intravascular coagulation.

General management

1. In general, drugs should not be withdrawn in the perioperative period.
2. Patients should be treated as if they were infected with hepatitis B virus.
3. An addiction centre may provide information and advice.

BIBLIOGRAPHY

Caldwell T B 1990 Anesthesia for patients with behavioral and environmental disorders. In: Anesthesia and uncommon diseases. W B Saunders, Philadelphia

DHSS 1991 Drug misuse and dependence. Guidelines on clinical management. HMSO, London

Gerada C, Farrell M 1990 Management of the pregnant opiate user. British Journal of Hospital Medicine 43: 138–141

McCammon R L 1987 Anesthesia for the chemically dependent patient. Anesthesia and Analgesia Review Course Lectures 47–55.

McGoldrick K E 1980 Anesthetic implications of drug abuse. Anesthesiology Review 7: 12–17

Wood P R, Soni N 1989 Anaesthesia and substance abuse. Anaesthesia 44: 672–680

ADDISON'S DISEASE
(ADRENOCORTICAL INSUFFICIENCY) (See also Section 2)

Chronic adrenocortical insufficiency results from a variety of causes. In the commonest form (idiopathic), adrenal autoantibodies are found, and other endocrine deficiencies may be demonstrated. Tuberculosis, secondary carcinoma and amyloidosis are other causes. In patients with adenocarcinoma, adrenal metastases are not uncommon (Ihde et al 1990), but clinically apparent disease occurs only after a 90% loss of adrenocortical tissue. In the majority of patients, Addison's disease will present in a chronic form, and therefore may be difficult to diagnose. However, hyponatraemia and hyperkalaemia in the absence of renal failure should immediately suggest the diagnosis (Waise & Young 1989). Cardiovascular collapse from classical acute adrenocortical failure is only rarely seen. However, since surgery and anaesthesia are both potent stress factors which require an increased steroid output, this deficiency may become apparent under these circumstances.

Acute adrenocortical insufficiency following sudden withdrawal of long-term steroid therapy, is always a potential problem (Weatherill & Spence 1984) and hypothalamic–pituitary axis suppression may persist for a year after stopping treatment.

Preoperative abnormalities

1. Addison's disease can present with weight loss, weakness, infertility, emotional instability, abdominal pain, diarrhoea, hyperpigmentation of skin and mucous membranes (particularly lips, skin creases, elbows and knees) and intractable hiccups.
2. In mild cases there may be a normochromic, normocytic anaemia, leucocytosis, eosinophilia and a low normal plasma cortisol.
3. In severe cases, steroid hormones may be undetectable in the blood. The characteristic metabolic changes of hyponatraemia, hyperkalaemia, hypoglycaemia, hypercalcaemia and an elevated urea will be present. ECG may be of low voltage with flattening of ST segments. Hypotension, cardiovascular collapse, confusion or even coma, may occur.
4. In the cancer patient, symptoms of anorexia, nausea, orthostatic hypotension and confusion may be attributed to the malignancy itself, or to its treatment. CT scan may show bilateral enlargement of the adrenal glands (Kung et al 1990).

Anaesthetic problems

1. A previously undiagnosed Addisonian crisis may be a rare cause of cardiovascular collapse (see Section 2) during or after surgery and anaesthesia (Salam & Davies 1974, Smith & Byrne 1981, Hertzberg & Schulman 1985, Huiras et al 1989), or pregnancy (Seaward et al 1989). Resuscitation may be required in the accident and emergency department (Frederick et al 1991), on the ITU (Dorin & Kearns 1988) or during treatment of malignancies (Kung et al 1990).

   In the majority of these cases, the diagnosis was made only in retrospect, saline, glucose and steroids having formed part of the general resuscitation of the collapsed patient. Subsequent confirmation of this diagnosis in such patients is potentially hazardous, since withdrawal of the exogenous steroids to test . adrenocortical function may put the patient at risk. The author knows of a case in which collapse first occurred during anaesthesia for investigation of infertility. Resuscitation with steroids and antibiotics was successful but during the later investigation to exclude Addison's disease, steroids were withdrawn, and sudden death followed. Postmortem examination showed adrenal tuberculosis. This danger can be minimized by the administration of dexamethasone, which does not interfere with plasma cortisol estimation (see below).

2. Drugs given during anaesthesia may modify a patient's response to stress.

Etomidate can adversely affect pituitary–adrenal function (Owen & Spence 1984). Increased death rates from infection were reported in patients having intravenous etomidate for sedation in intensive care. Prolonged infusions were shown to produce reversible suppression of adrenocortical response, as a result of mitochondrial enzyme inhibition. One patient with alveolar proteinosis, who had received two bolus doses of etomidate within 18 hours, developed cardiovascular instability and was subsequently found to have low serum cortisol levels (McGrady & Wright 1989). The effect and clinical significance of a single dose of etomidate, or an infusion limited to the duration of anaesthesia alone, is subject to debate (Owen & Spence 1984, Yeoman et al 1984, Boidin 1986).

3. Respiratory muscle weakness, including that of the diaphragm, may occur. This improves on treatment of the condition (Mier et al 1988).

Management

1. If the diagnosis is suspected preoperatively, and some adrenal reserve remains, the plasma corticosteroids will tend to be in the low normal range. A cortisol value of >600 nmol/l excludes Addison's disease, but a low normal does not prove it. Therefore, for confirmation, a stimulation test will be required. If time permits, ACTH should also be estimated. An ACTH >200 pg/ml, together with a plasma cortisol of <275 nmol/l under stress situations, should establish the diagnosis.

Short tetracosactrin test

0.900 a.m. 10 ml heparinized blood for plasma cortisol estimation. Tetracosactrin 250 µg given i.m. or i.v.

09.30 a.m. Blood taken for plasma cortisol and aldosterone levels.

Results

Normal: Base-line >200 nmol/l. At 30 minutes an increase of at least 300 nmol/l above this.

Addison's: Low base-line. At 30 minutes, a less than 160 nmol/l increase in response to stimulation.

Normally, no steroids should be administered for 3 days prior to this test. However, if steroids have been given under emergency circumstances, then they should be changed to dexamethasone 0.5 mg b.d. 24 hours before the test starts. Dexamethasone does not register in plasma cortisol assays. An ACTH assay will demonstrate an inappropriate high level (>200 pg/ml) in primary adrenocortical insufficiency.

2. Treatment of an Addisonian crisis

This should precede confirmation of the diagnosis, since any delay may prove fatal.

a. Infuse 0.9% saline 1 litre rapidly, then more slowly.

b. Hydrocortisone (hemisuccinate or sodium phosphate) 100 mg i.v. immediately, then 6-hourly.

c. Correct hypoglycaemia, if present.

3. Maintenance therapy for Addison's disease

Normal production of cortisol is 15–20 mg/day but hypoadrenal patients require twice this amount. Although replacement has traditionally been given twice daily, there is evidence that a thrice-daily regimen gives better plasma cortisol levels and improvement in wellbeing (Groves et al 1988).

a. Hydrocortisone 10 mg three times a day, or prednisolone 2.5 mg three times a day.

b. Fludrocortisone acetate 0.1–0.2 mg daily is required for primary, but not for secondary hypoadrenalism.

Equivalent dosages for a given glucocorticoid effect:

Hydrocortisone	100 mg
Cortisone	130 mg
Prednisolone	25 mg
Prednisone	25 mg
Methylprednisolone	20 mg
Betamethasone	4 mg
Triamcinolone	25 mg
Dexamethasone	4 mg

Drugs with mineralocorticoid effects:

Hydrocortisone	weak
Cortisone	weak
Fludrocortisone	strong

4. Patients should wear a 'Medi-alert' bracelet.

5. Increases in replacement therapy may be required to cope with minor or major stress. For minor stress, 50–100 mg hydrocortisone daily should be tapered off after 5–10 days. Under conditions of major stress, 100–300 mg cortisol acetate i.v. daily, withdrawing over 2 weeks once the stress factors have been removed.

BIBLIOGRAPHY

Boidin M P 1986 Can etomidate cause an Addisonian crisis? Acta Anaesthesiologica Belgica 37: 165–170

Dorin R I, Kearns P J 1988 High output circulatory failure in acute adrenal insufficiency. Critical Care Medicine 16: 296–297

Frederick R, Brown C, Renusch J et al 1991 Addisonian crisis: emergency presentation of primary adrenal insufficiency (clinical conference). Annals of Emergency Medicine 20: 802–806

Groves R W, Toms G C, Houghton B J et al 1988 Corticosteroid replacement therapy: twice or thrice daily? Journal of the Royal Society of Medicine 81: 514–516

Hertzberg L B, Schulman M S 1985 Acute adrenal insufficiency in patient with appendicitis during anaesthesia. Anesthesiology 62: 517–519

Huiras C M, Pehling G B, Caplan R H 1989 Adrenal insufficiency after operative removal of apparently nonfunctioning adrenal adenoma. Journal of the American Medical Association 261: 894–989

Ihde J K, Turnbull A D, Bajorunas D R 1990 Adrenal insufficiency in the cancer patient: implications for the surgeon. British Journal of Surgery 77: 1335–1337

Kung A W C, Pun K K, Lam K et al 1990 Addisonian crisis as presenting feature in malignancies. Cancer 65: 177–179

McGrady E M, Wright I H 1989 Cardiovascular instability following bolus dose of etomidate. Anaesthesia 44: 404–405

Mier A, Laroche C, Wass J et al 1988 Respiratory weakness in Addison's disease. British Medical Journal 297: 457–458

Owen H, Spence A A 1984 Etomidate. British Journal of Anaesthesia 56: 555–557

Salam A A, Davies D M 1974 Acute adrenal insufficiency during surgery. British Journal of Anaesthesia 46: 619–622

Seaward P G, Guidozzi F, Sonnendecker E W 1989 Addisonian crisis in pregnancy. Case report. British Journal of Obstetrics and Gynaecology 96: 1348–1350

Smith M G, Byrne A J 1981 An Addisonian crisis complicating anaesthesia. Anaesthesia 36: 681–684

Waise A, Young R J 1989 Pitfalls in the management of acute adrenocortical insufficiency: discussion paper. Journal of the Royal Society of Medicine 82: 741–742

Weatherill D, Spence A A 1984 Anaesthesia for disorders of the adrenal cortex. British Journal of Anaesthesia 56: 741–749

Yeoman P M, Fellows I W, Byrne A J et al 1984 The effect of anaesthetic induction using etomidate upon pituitary-adrenocortical function. British Journal of Anaesthesia 56: 1291–1292

AIDS
(ACQUIRED IMMUNE DEFICIENCY SYNDROME)

A spectrum of disease thought to be caused by infection with a human T-lymphotropic retrovirus, HIV. This may lead to a chronic condition of lymphadenopathy, fever, weight loss and diarrhoea, or to a state of cellular immune deficiency and the development of unusual malignancies or opportunistic infections. It is most common in the homosexual and drug-taking communities, but is found in haemophiliac patients who have received infected blood products prior to antibody screening and heat treatment of Factor VIII concentrates. Some individuals may be carriers, but the full significance of this state and its natural history is not yet known. The virus is transmitted by body fluids, particularly blood and semen, but it would appear that a breach in either skin or mucosa is necessary for infection to occur. Saliva or airborne transmission when the mucosa is intact, has not yet been demonstrated, but neither has it been disproved. It is probably less infectious than hepatitis B, and present surveys indicate that the risks to health workers are low unless accidental inoculation has occurred (Lee & Soni 1986). However, the recent appearance of this potentially fatal disease has meant that epidemiological studies are, as yet, incomplete. The most recent literature should be consulted. For the USA, prevalence varied from 0.32% to 23.6% (Gerberding et al 1990). Guidelines for anaesthetists have been produced by the Association of Anaesthetists (1992).

An increasing problem concerns the management of children with HIV, most of whom will have contracted the disease in utero (Schwartz et al 1991). Although not all infants of HIV-positive mothers will become infected, it should be assumed that they are. Clinical evidence of the disease will be apparent in 50% by the age of 12 months, and in 80% by 3 years. In the hospital environment, strict asepsis in dealing with them is necessary because of their immune deficient state. However, segregation is not necessary, since the risk of transmission of infection under ordinary circumstances is negligible. These individuals are often living in institutional care and may need psychological and emotional support. In the USA, an initial presentation to the ITU was common, and the diagnosis of HIV was considered in any child with acute respiratory, CVS or CNS symptoms. Serious ethical dilemmas are posed in the management of HIV-related respiratory failure and in the issue of confidentiality.

Preoperative abnormalities

1. The patient may either be HIV antibody positive, or show signs of the disease.
2. The neurological manifestations include dementia, peripheral neuropathy, radiculopathy and cranial nerve palsies. Five AIDS patients, one of whom died, had vasovagal episodes associated with lung biopsy. Subsequent investigation suggested a diagnosis of autonomic dysfunction (Craddock et al 1987).
3. The commonest opportunistic infection is *Pneumocystis carinii* pneumonia, but candidal, tuberculous and viral pneumonias occur. Up to 85% of patients will develop *Pneumocystis* pneumonia at some time, and acute infections carry a mortality of 9–35% (Thomas et al 1990). Treatment is with pentamidine either nebulized or intravenously. Pentamidine is also used for primary and secondary prophylaxis. Corticosteroids may prevent the early deterioration of oxygenation in *Pneumocystis* pneumonia (Consensus Statement) and has been recommended when Pao_2 <70 mmHg.
4. Destructive adrenal lesions have been reported, but clinical evidence of Addison's disease is scanty (Hilton et al 1988).
5. Side effects of treatment with antiviral agents may be severe. Zidovudine (Retrovir, AZT) has contributed to increased survival (Moore et al 1991) but it may cause megaloblastic anaemia and neutropenia. It is theoretically possible that interaction with nitrous oxide could occur (Phillips & Spence 1987). Neurological complications of the drug may be difficult to distinguish from those of the disease.

6. Increasing numbers of children are becoming infected and the pattern of the disease is slightly different from that seen in adults. Lung disease is the commonest cause of morbidity and mortality, and infection with *Pneumocystis* carries a worse prognosis. Lymphoid interstitial pneumonitis can develop with chronic lung disease. Cardiac abnormalities occur in 90% (Lipschultz et al 1989). Most children have neurological abnormalities, including autonomic neuropathy. General problems comprise recurrent infections, anaemia and lymphadenopathy. Interventional procedures may involve CVP insertion, gastrostomy, and lung and liver biopsies.

Anaesthetic problems

1. The problems of anaesthesia in the presence of lung disease.
2. Autonomic neuropathy may cause cardiovascular instability.
3. The possibility of transmission of the virus to healthcare workers exists, although this was thought to be rare (Greene 1986a). It is most likely to occur as a consequence of needlestick injuries. The incidence of seroconversion following needle puncture from an HIV-positive patient is calculated to be 0.5. Eight health care workers who had either received a needlestick injury or who had suffered from dermatitis (Weiss 1985), and five surgeons in whom there was massive exposure of skin or mucous membranes to blood (Gazzard & Wastell 1990) were reported as being HIV positive. However, more recent studies suggest that the risk to anaesthetists is not trivial in areas where the infection rate is high. Buergler et al (1992) postulated that the three factors which determined occupational risk for HIV were: the risk of needlestick injury per year, the risk of seroconversion should injury occur, and the prevalence of HIV in the particular population served by the hospital. Their occupational risk calculations for USA anaesthetists, based on existing figures, was 0.05% for a low prevalence area, increasing to 4.5% in a high prevalence area.
4. The problems of disposal of contaminated material and the sterilization of equipment.
5. About 20% of patients with AIDS develop parapareses associated with vacuolar degeneration of the spinal cord, and as many as one-third develop encephalitis (Greene 1986b). The advisability of spinal and extradural anaesthesia has therefore been questioned.
6. The safety or otherwise of treating an HIV-seropositive patient with an extradural blood patch, should postdural puncture headache occur.
7. An increasing number of children are presenting with HIV infection. The pattern of the disease differs from that in adults and they should not be segregated from other children. Appropriate consent to treatment may be difficult to obtain.

Management

1. The same precautions should be taken as for hepatitis B (See Association of Anaesthetists 1992). Gown, gloves, mask and eye protection should be worn during anaesthesia. Blood spillage should be avoided. Disposal of needles in a tough disposal bin, without resheathing, is crucial. They should not be passed from one person to another. Care should be taken not to spread blood, sputum or saliva during tracheal intubation and extubation. In San Francisco, the problems of identifying each individual HIV carrier has prompted such precautions to be employed for all patients (Arden 1988).

    In the UK, the wearing of gloves as a minimum, is being recommended for all anaesthetics (Association of Anaesthetists 1988, Editorial 1990). However in 1991, a survey revealed that less than 16% of UK anaesthetists routinely followed this advice (O'Donnell & Asbury 1992a). The use of double gloves, with or without reinforcement of the distal phalanges by application of adhesive tape directly to the gloves, has been suggested (Paglia & Sommer 1989). Double gloving may reduce the occupational risk of HIV by an average of 80% (Matta et al 1988, Buergler et al 1992).

2. Equipment should be disposable or sterilizable. The virus is destroyed by both heat and chemicals. Reusable equipment should be scrubbed with detergent solution and decontaminated by soaking in glutaraldehyde or sodium hypochlorite solution. Nursing staff should wear goggles during cleaning of equipment. Steam or gas sterilization is also reported to be effective (Arden 1988).

    a. Ventilators. Although HIV infection is not airborne, the use of disposable circuitry and bacterial filters is advisable.

    b. Blood gas machines. The introducer port should be syringed through with 1% sodium hypochlorite and left for 5 minutes. This is followed by two wash cycles and recalibration.

    c. Surfaces. Should be cleaned with sodium hypochlorite.

3. To reduce risk to laboratory personnel, only urgent laboratory investigations likely to influence management should be requested. Sterilization of any instrument used for the analysis of contaminated blood is mandatory.

4. In view of the poor prognosis, the wisdom of instituting IPPV for respiratory failure should be considered carefully.

5. Before administering regional anaesthesia, a neurological assessment should be performed. Local anaesthetic techniques may be contraindicated if parapareses are already present.

6. A follow-up of six patients 6-24 months after having been given autologous extradural blood patch following dural puncture headache did not show any CNS morbidity which could be attributed to the procedure (Tom et al 1992).

7. Response to occupational exposure. If accidental inoculation of infected blood occurs, it has been suggested that zidovudine should be given prophylactically as soon as possible, preferably within one hour. There is however little evidence to support or refute this practice (Jeffries 1991), and the risk of toxicity is unknown (Smart 1990). Any prophylaxis is best organized through the occupational health department because counselling and follow-up will be necessary.

BIBLIOGRAPHY

Arden J 1988 Managing patients with AIDS – update. Anesthesiology 68: 164–165

Association of Anaesthetists 1988 AIDS and hepatitis B. Guidelines for anaesthetists. Association of Anaesthetists, London

Association of Anaesthetists 1992 HIV and other blood borne viruses; guidance for anaesthetists. Association of Anaesthetists, London

Buergler J M, Kim R, Thisted R A et al 1992 Risk of human immunodeficiency virus in surgeons, anesthesiologists and medical students. Anesthesia and Analgesia 75: 118–124

Consensus statement (1990) on the use of corticosteroids as adjunctive therapy for pneumocystis pneumonia in the acquired immunodeficiency syndrome. New England Journal of Medicine 323: 1500–1504

Craddock C, Pasvol G, Bull R et al 1987 Cardiorespiratory arrest and autonomic neuropathy in AIDS. Lancet 2: 16–18

Editorial 1990 Occupational infection among anaesthetists. Lancet 336: 1103

Gazzard B G, Wastell C 1990 HIV and surgeons. British Medical Journal 301: 1003–1004

Gerberding J L, Littell C, Tarkington A et al 1990 Risk of exposure of surgical personnel to patient's blood during surgery at San Francisco's General Hospital. New England Journal of Medicine 322: 1788–1793

Greene E R 1986a AIDS: an overview for anesthesiologists. Anesthesia and Analgesia 65; 1054–1058

Greene E R 1986b Spinal and epidural anesthesia in patients with the acquired immunodeficiency syndrome. Anesthesia and Analgesia 65: 1090–1091

Hilton C T, Harrington P T, Prasad C et al 1988 Adrenal insufficiency in the acquired immunodeficiency syndrome. Southern Medical Journal 81: 1493–1495

Jeffries D J 1991 Zidovudine after occupational exposure to HIV. Hospitals should be able to give it within an hour. British Medical Journal 302: 1349–1351

Lee K G, Soni N 1986 AIDS and anaesthesia. Anaesthesia 41: 1011–1016

Lipschultz S E, Chanock S, Sanders S P et al 1989 Cardiovascular manifestations of human immunodeficiency virus infection in infants and children. American Journal of Cardiology 1989 63: 1489–1497

Matta H, Thompson A M, Rainey J B 1988 Does wearing two pairs of gloves protect operating theatre staff from skin contamination? British Medical Journal 297: 597–598

Moore R D, Hidalgo J, Sugland B W et al 1991 Zidovudine and the natural history of the acquired immunodeficiency syndrome. New England Journal of Medicine 324: 1412–1416

O'Donnell N G, Asbury A J 1992a The occupational hazard of human immunodeficiency virus and hepatitis. I. Perceived risks and preventive measures adopted by anaesthetists: a postal survey. Anaesthesia 47: 923–928

O'Donnell N G, Asbury A J 1992b The occupational hazard of human immunodeficiency virus and hepatitis B virus. II. Effect of grade, age, sex and region of employment on perceived risks and preventive measures adopted by anaesthetists. Anaesthesia 47: 929–935

Paglia S L, Sommer R M 1989 AIDS infection protection – reinforced gloves. Anesthesia and Analgesia 69: 407

Phillips A J, Spence A A 1987 Zidovudine and the anaesthetist. Anaesthesia 42: 799–800

Schwartz D, Schwartz T, Cooper E et al 1991 Anaesthesia and the child with HIV infection. Canadian Journal of Anaesthesia 38: 626–633

Smart N G 1990 Occupational exposure to HIV and zidovudine chemoprophylaxis. Anaesthesia 45: 989–990

Thomas S, O'Doherty M, Bateman N 1990 Pneumocystis carinii pneumonia. Aerosolised pentamidine gives effective prophylaxis. British Medical Journal 300: 211–212

Tom D J, Gulevich S J, Shapiro H M et al 1992 Epidural blood patch in the HIV-positive patient: a review of clinical experience. Anesthesiology 76: 943–947

Weiss S H 1985 HTLV-III infections among health care workers. Association with needle stick injuries. Journal of the American Medical Association 254: 2089–2093

AIR EMBOLISM
(SEE SECTION 2)

ALCOHOLISM

Alcoholism has been defined as excessive drinking which results in impairment of both the subject's health and social activities. If surgical treatment is required, three main problems must be considered:

1. The effect of the numerous metabolic and endocrine changes which occur in longstanding alcoholics.
2. Whether or not there is also acute alcohol toxicity.
3. The problems of alcohol withdrawal, which can occur at any time between 8 hours and 5 days after abstention.

Preoperative abnormalities

1. Haematological effects. The MCV exceeds 93 fl in 85% of heavy drinkers. Bone marrow depression can occur, and if liver function is impaired there may be coagulation defects.
2. Biochemical. Blood alcohol levels:
   80 mg/dl – legal limit for driving (UK).
   200 mg/dl – severe intoxication.
   >400 mg/dl – stupor.
   >500 mg/dl – frequently fatal.
   Electrolyte disturbances, particularly hypokalaemia, may exacerbate delirium tremens.
3. Liver function. Gamma-glutamyltransferase and the aminotransaminases may be abnormal and the albumin low. Plasma cholinesterase activity is normal unless hepatic damage is severe. There may be impaired glucose tolerance after alcohol, followed by hypoglycaemia occurring between 6 and 24 hours after acute ingestion.
4. Cardiac disease. A dilated cardiomyopathy may occur, and can be associated with dyspnoea, heart failure, conduction defects, bifid T waves, digitalis-like ST segments and arrhythmias.

5. Central nervous system effects of Wernicke's encephalopathy (Reuler et al 1985), ocular abnormalities, (horizontal nystagmus, lateral rectus paralysis), ataxia and a global confusional state. Korsakoff's psychosis (retrograde and anterograde amnesia, confabulation) and epileptic fits.
6. A peripheral neuropathy may be produced by the combined effect of alcohol and malnutrition.
7. The individual's immune response and leucocyte function are affected by alcohol and it should be considered an immune suppressive drug (McGregor 1986). In acute alcoholism, there is interference with primary responses to a new antigen and poor control of bacterial infection.

Anaesthetic problems

1. Acute alcohol toxicity and electrolyte imbalance.
2. Coagulation abnormalities.
3. Possible presence of a full stomach and delayed gastric emptying.
4. Delirium tremens or lesser withdrawal symptoms. Increased adrenaline and noradrenaline concentrations are found when long-term drinking is suddenly stopped.
5. Impaired liver metabolism and cirrhosis.
6. Decreased adrenocortical response to stress.
7. Malnutrition and vitamin deficiencies.
8. Dilated cardiomyopathy and arrhythmias. Heavy drinking increases the risk of cardiac arrhythmias, particularly idiopathic atrial fibrillation, whether or not heart disease is present (Koskinen & Kupari 1992).
9. The presence of, or bleeding from, oesophageal varices (Cello et al 1986).
10. Peripheral or autonomic neuropathy.
11. Morbidity was increased, and the length of stay in hospital after hysterectomy was doubled, in heavy drinkers when compared with moderate and light drinkers (Fielding et al 1992). Complications included wound infection, cystitis, pneumonia and vaginal abscess. These accord with similar studies on men undergoing colonic and prostatic surgery, and may result from interference with the immune system (McGregor 1986).

Management

1. If acute alcohol toxicity is present, then surgery should be delayed if possible (Bruce 1983). Alcohol levels above 250 mg/dl increase surgical morbidity. Correction of dehydration should be tempered by the knowledge that diuresis occurs mainly while the blood alcohol level is rising. Beware of fluid overload. Hypokalaemia may precipitate delirium tremens. Hypoglycaemia may occur 6–24 hours

after intake. If i.v, glucose is required, thiamine should be given concurrently. Alcohol-related cardiac arrhythmias usually stop spontaneously within 24–48 hours.

2. An i.v. preparation of vitamins B and C, such as Parentrovite, is given. Prevention of hypoglycaemia has been stressed (Naidu & Brock-Utne 1988) and the concomitant use of thiamine 100 mg i.v. to prevent Wernicke's encephalopathy has been suggested (Mayes 1989).

3. Coagulation abnormalities, if present, should be treated with vitamin K1, fresh frozen plasma or platelets.

4. Thiopentone is avoided if a cardiomyopathy is present or there is hypoalbuminaemia (see Cardiomyopathy, dilated). Atracurium is the neuromuscular blocker of choice if liver function is impaired. Postoperative jaundice frequently occurs several days after surgery, irrespective of the anaesthetic agent used, and results from defective processing of old red blood cells by an impaired liver. The use of halothane is therefore best avoided. A more rational choice would be either erflurane or isoflurane, since they undergo less liver metabolism.

5. Analgesics should be used with caution, and only for pain. Dependence can readily occur.

6. Alcohol withdrawal can be treated with alcohol or chlormethiazole infusions, or benzodiazepines i.v.
   a. Alcohol may be appropriate when surgery is actually required during the phase of withdrawal symptoms. A preoperative infusion of 8% ethanol in isotonic saline, at a rate of 0.5 g/kg, is given over a 15-minute period (Edwards 1985).
   b. Chlormethiazole edisylate 0.8% soln, 320–800 mg (40–100 ml) over 5-10 minutes, then the rate is adjusted.
   Note: Chlormethiazole is dangerous in severe liver disease, or when a patient is acutely intoxicated with alcohol. Severe respiratory depression can result from the combination (McInnes 1987).
   c. Delirium tremens can be treated with midazolam 2.5 mg, using additional increments up to a maximum of 10 mg. Diazepam is used in increments up to a total dose of 20 mg.

7. An existing peripheral neuropathy is a contraindication to regional anaesthesia.

8. In the presence' of cirrhosis, gastrointestinal bleeding may precipitate hepatic failure. Nasogastric tubes should be inserted cautiously in case oesophageal varices are present.

9. Consideration should be given to a period of alcohol withdrawal before elective surgery.

BIBLIOGRAPHY
Bruce D L 1983 Alcoholism and anesthesia. Anesthesia and Analgesia 62: 84–96

Cello J P, Crass R A, Grendell J H et al 1986 Management of the patient with
    hemorrhaging esophageal varices. Journal of the American Medical Association
    256: 1480–1484
Edwards R 1985 Anaesthesia and alcohol. British Medical Journal 291: 423–424
Edwards R, Mosher V B 1980 Alcohol abuse, anaesthesia and intensive care.
    Anaesthesia 35: 474–489
Fielding C, Jensen I M, Tonnesen H 1992 Influence of alcohol intake on postoperative
    morbidity after hysterectomy. American Journal of Obstetrics and Gynecology 166:
    667–670
Koskinen P, Kupari M 1992 Alcohol and cardiac arrhythmias. British Medical Journal
    304: 1394–1395
McGregor R R 1986 Alcohol and immune defense. Journal of the American Medical
    Association 256: 1474–1479
McInnes G T 1987 Chlormethiazole and alcohol. British Medical Journal 294: 592
Mayes G A 1989 Thiamine for prevention of Wernicke's encephalopathy: a reminder.
    Anesthesia and Analgesia 69: 407–408
Naidu R, Brock-Utne J G 1988 Generalised convulsions following regional anesthesia
    – a pertinent lesson. Anesthesia and Analgesia 67: 1192–1193
Reuler J B, Giraud D E, Cooney T G 1985 Wernicke's encephalopathy. New England
    Journal of Medicine 312: 1035–1039

ALDOSTERONISM, PRIMARY
(see CONN'S SYNDROME)

ALVEOLAR PROTEINOSIS

A lung condition in which protein, phospholipid, cholesterol and free
fatty acids accumulate within the alveolar spaces, possibly secondary to a
failure of surfactant to be reprocessed by type II alveolar cells.
Clinically it is difficult to distinguish from interstitial lung disease, and
must therefore be diagnosed on lung biopsy or bronchial lavage. The
only successful treatment is whole-lung lavage with saline to wash out
the intra-alveolar phospholipids. This results in symptomatic and
functional improvement in about 80% of patients. The diagnosis is often
made late, and if delayed until hypoxia ensues, the prognosis is poor.
Infection may supervene and the situation be made worse by
inappropriate treatment with corticosteroids.

Preoperative abnormalities

1. Symptoms include a dry cough and breathlessness at rest, which is
   even worse on exercise, chest pain, fever and weight loss. Wheezing
   is usually absent, but there are fine inspiratory crepitations. Finger
   clubbing may be present.
2. CXR shows diffuse nodular infiltration of both lung fields, especially
   in the perihilar regions.
3. Lung function tests indicate a restrictive ventilatory defect. In a
   series of 10 patients, before bronchial lavage, the VC varied
   between 33–86%, total lung capacity 35–89% and transfer factor

16–74% of the predicted values (Du Bois et al 1983). Arterial blood gases often showed hypoxia (in one patient as low as 3.7 kPa) and sometimes hypocapnoea.

4. Smokers or ex-smokers are most often affected.
5. Opportunistic infections, such as nocardiosis, may be superimposed (Pascual et al 1989).
6. The diagnosis may be delayed because the condition is mistaken for interstitial lung disease or sarcoidosis.
7. Definitive diagnosis is made on electron microscopy of sputum, bronchial washings or lung biopsy.

Anaesthetic problems

1. Anaesthesia is required for bronchial lavage, during which significant reductions in arterial oxygen saturation may be a problem (Bradfield & Maynard 1979). Gas exchange and haemodynamic parameters have been studied (Cohen & Eisenkraft 1990, Aguinaga et al 1991). When the lung is filled with saline, an improvement in Pao_2 occurs. On emptying the lung, the Pao_2 decreases, but increases in cardiac output result in oxygen delivery being unchanged.
2. Since there are increases in intrathoracic pressure and marked fluctuations in cardiac output, bronchial lavage may be stressful to a patient whose myocardium is compromised.
3. The procedure is lengthy (up to 2 hours) and hypoxia is sometimes severe.
4. Technical problems include malposition of the double-lumen tube, underinflation of the cuff resulting in spill over of fluid into the inflated lung, and overinflation of the cuff such that it is difficult to drain the fluid (Busque 1977).
5. One patient with alveolar proteinosis, who had received two bolus doses of etomidate within 18 hours, developed cardiovascular instability and was subsequently found to have low serum cortisol levels (McGrady & Wright 1989).

Management

1. Whole lung lavage is now the treatment of choice and usually results in considerable improvement in oxygenation (Selecky et al 1977, Du Bois et al 1983). Alveolar proteinosis did not recur during a follow-up period of 8.8 years in one-third of the patients (Prakash et al 1987). Bronchial lavage is performed after isolation of one lung with a double-lumen tube. This side is filled with isotonic saline at 37°C until a volume equal to the FRC has been introduced. The lung is then washed with 0.5–1 l at a time until washings are clear, or until 40 l has been used. Vigorous manual or mechanical chest percussion during lavage increases the efficiency of the technique

(McKenzie et al 1989). Bronchial suction and manual ventilation is performed, and finally an ordinary tracheal tube is inserted and IPPV instituted for 2–4 hours. Additional safeguards for proper positioning of the double-lumen tube and cuff inflation include: the use of a fibre-optic bronchoscope to check the position of tube and an airway leak detector to ensure that the two lungs have been separated (Spragg et al 1982). Lavage may need to be repeated at 2–3 day intervals. A technique for children uses a bronchoscopically positioned bronchial tube, whilst ventilation of the opposite lung is maintained via a modified nasal airway (McKenzie et al 1989).

2. Oxygenation is monitored with pulse oximetry or arterial blood gases.

3. Cardiopulmonary bypass has occasionally been used in the presence of severe hypoxia, (Freedman et al 1981, Lippman et al 1977).

BIBLIOGRAPHY

Aguinaga M A, Santos P, Renes E et al 1991 Hemodynamic changes during whole bronchoalveolar lavage in two cases of pulmonary alveolar proteinosis. Intensive Care Medicine 17: 421–423

Bradfield H G C, Maynard J P 1979 Pulmonary lavage in a case of alveolar proteinosis: the value of continuous display oxygen-haemoglobin saturation using ear-oximetry. Anaesthesia 34: 1032–1034

Busque L 1977 Pulmonary lavage in the treatment of alveolar proteinosis. Canadian Anaesthetists' Society Journal 24: 380–388

Cohen E, Eisenkraft J B 1990 Bronchopulmonary lavage: effects on oxygenation and hemodynamics. Journal of Cardiothoracic Anesthesia 4: 609–615

Du Bois R M, McAllister W A C, Branthwaite M A 1983 Alveolar proteinosis: diagnosis and treatment over a 10-year period. Thorax 38: 360–363

Freedman A P, Petias A, Johnston R F et al 1981 Alveolar proteinosis lung lavage using partial cardiopulmonary bypass. Thorax 36: 543–545

Lippman M, Mok M S, Wasserman K 1977 Anesthetic management for children with alveolar proteinosis using extracorporeal circulation. British Journal of Anaesthesia 49: 173–176

McGrady E M, Wright I H 1989 Cardiovascular instability following bolus dose of etomidate. Anaesthesia 44: 404–405

McKenzie B, Wood R E, Bailey A 1989 Airway management for unilateral lung lavage in children. Anesthesiology 70: 550–553

Pascual J, Aguinaga G, Vidal R et al 1989 Alveolar proteinosis and nocardiosis: a patient treated by bronchopulmonary lavage. Postgraduate Medical Journal 65: 674–677

Prakash U B S, Bahram S S, Carpenter H A et al 1987 Pulmonary alveolar phospholipoproteinosis: experience with 34 cases and a review. Mayo Clinic Proceedings 62: 499–518

Selecky P A, Wasserman K, Benfield J R et al 1977 The clinical and physiological effect of whole-lung lavage in pulmonary alveolar proteinosis: a ten-year experience. Annals of Thoracic Surgery 24: 451–461

Spragg R G, Benumof J L, Alfery D D 1982 New methods for the performance of unilateral lung lavage. Anesthesiology 57: 535–538.

AMNIOTIC FLUID EMBOLISM
(see Section 2)

AMPHETAMINE ABUSE

Amphetamines are sympathomimetic amines, which, in the initial stages of intoxication, elevate the mood and increase alertness, thus reducing the need for sleep. They act both directly and indirectly on the sympathetic nervous system, via the peripheral nerve endings. Catecholamines are released within the CNS, and catecholamine re-uptake by adrenergic nerve endings is prevented. Tolerance readily occurs. A number of synthetic amines, which share structural similarities to methamphetamine, are being used for their ability to produce euphoria and sociability. These include 3,4-methylenedioxy-methamphetamine (MDMA, 'Ecstasy') and 3,4-methylenedioxy-ethamphetamine (MDEA, 'Eve'). Deaths have occurred (Dowling et al 1987) and a syndrome resembling MH, of convulsions, hyperthermia, hyperkalaemia and rhabdomyolysis, observed (Brown & Osterloh 1987, Singarajah & Lavies 1992, Tehan et al 1993). Serotoninergic mechanisms may cause increased heat production which is exacerbated by high ambient temperatures. This could account for the occurrence of this syndrome at 'rave' parties, where it is used as a 'dance drug' (Henry 1992). Amphetamine abusers often misuse other drugs, and frequently street preparations are contaminated with other substances. The anaesthetist may be involved in anaesthesia for the acute or chronic abuser, for patients acutely intoxicated who injure themselves, or for resuscitation and intensive care of those who present with convulsions, hyperthermia and rhabdomyolysis.

Preoperative abnormalities

1. The patient may be suffering from acute toxicity. Initially, signs of irritability, with tremor, dilated pupils and sweating may be displayed. Increasing doses cause tachycardia, fever and mild hypertension, with agitation and confusion. Delirium, rising blood pressure, hyperthermia and the onset of arrhythmias, precede convulsions, coma and death. There have been several reports of reactions to MDMA or MDEA in which rhabdomyolysis and hyperkalaemia are associated with convulsions and hyperthermia, producing a syndrome which resembles MH (Singarajah & Lavies 1992, Tehan et al 1993). Disseminated intravascular coagulation (Chadwick et al 1991) and renal failure have also been reported (Fahal et al 1992).
2. In chronic abuse there may be marked tolerance.
3. The long-term effects of MDMA are not yet fully known but may include psychiatric disturbances and hepatic damage.

Anaesthetic problems

1. Patients who are chronic amphetamine abusers or who have acute toxicity may require anaesthesia. Intracranial hypertension was reported in a young girl who required elevation of a skull fracture (Michel & Adams 1979). Individuals who smuggle drugs by 'body-packing' may need surgical intervention because of the risk of fatal toxicity (Watson et al 1991).

2. Studies on dogs have shown that MAC values for halothane were altered by both acute and chronic amphetamine intake. Acute intoxication resulted in an increased MAC for halothane (Johnston et al 1972), and duration of anaesthesia and time to ambulation were reduced. In contrast, chronic abuse for 7 days decreased the MAC for halothane, and dogs subjected to chronic abuse had a poor response to indirectly acting sympathetic agents.

3. Hazards during pregnancy, particularly during Caesarean section in chronic amphetamine abusers, have been reported. In one patient, a longstanding heroin and amphetamine abuser, extradural anaesthesia was established with lignocaine 2% 10 ml (Samuels et al 1979). Alter transfer to theatre, two successive doses of 12 ml and 6 ml of chloroprocaine 3% did not extend the block, and it was assumed that the catheter had become displaced. General anaesthesia was induced with thiopentone 200 mg and suxamethonium. Cardiac arrest occurred soon after surgery began. Resuscitation with adrenaline, bicarbonate and isoprenaline proved successful. On recovery, the patient admitted to taking amphetamines just prior to admission. The authors postulated that chronic users of amphetamines do not respond to stress and may develop a type of autonomic dysfunction. Another patient, also a chronic amphetamine abuser, developed hypotension, tachycardia and peripheral vasoconstriction intraoperatively, for which 500 ml colloid and 1300 ml crystalloid was given (Smith & Gutsche 1980). After extubation, pulmonary oedema developed and IPPV, with PEEP, was required for 8 hours. Her rapid recovery was felt to be consistent with the diagnosis of hydrostatic pulmonary oedema, rather than gastric inhalation or septicaemia. A third patient who had taken amphetamine in late pregnancy, presented with convulsions, agitation, hypertension and proteinuria. This was misdiagnosed as eclampsia and a Caesarean section performed (Elliott & Rees 1990).

4. Arrhythmias may occur, particularly in the presence of agents which sensitize the heart to the effects of catecholamines (McGoldrick 1980).

5. There may be delayed recovery from anaesthesia (McCammon 1986).

Management

1. A careful history should be taken in an attempt to establish the presence of acute or chronic abuse. Denial or concealment is common (Samuels et al 1979, Michel & Adams 1979). Urinary estimations of amphetamines and their metabolites can be performed, but this facility is not usually available in the acute situation. In addition, samples may not have been taken at a sufficiently early stage because such a diagnosis had not been considered.

2. EGG, core temperature and blood pressure should be monitored from the induction of anaesthesia. Benzodiazepines are reported as being suitable for use in the chronic abuser (Caldwell 1990).

3. Acute intoxication. Rehydration may be required when toxicity is present, particularly in those who are pyrexial. In cases of acute intoxication, chlorpromazine has been recommended. The use of dantrolene in the treatment of rhabdomyolysis and hyperthermia has been reported (Singarajah & Lavies 1992, Tehan et al 1993).

4. The management of hypertension may require the use of alpha adrenoceptor blockers. Because of its longer action, diazoxide 300 mg (or 5 mg/kg) may be more appropriate than phentolamine (Caldwell 1981).

5. Halothane should be avoided in the presence of amphetamines.

6. Direct acting vasopressors are recommended to treat hypotension in the chronic abuser (Johnston et al 1972).

BIBLIOGRAPHY

Brown C, Osterloh J 1987 Multiple severe complications from recreational ingestion of MDMA ('Ecstasy'). Journal of the American Medical Association 258: 780–781

Caldwell T B 1990 Anesthesia for patients with behavioral and environmental disorders. In: Anesthesia and uncommon diseases. W B Saunders Philadelphia

Chadwick I S, Curry P D, Linsley A et al 1991 3,4-methylenedioxymethamphetamine (MDMA), a fatality associated with hyperthermia and coagulopathy. Journal of the Royal Society of Medicine 84: 371

Dowling G P, McDonough E T, Bost R O 1987 'Eve' and 'Ecstasy'. A report of five deaths associated with the use of MDEA and MDMA. Journal of the American Medical Association 257: 1615–1617

Elliott R H, Rees G B 1990 Amphetamine ingestion presenting as eclampsia. Canadian Journal of Anaesthesia 37: 130–133

Fahal I H, Sallomi D F, Yaqoob M et al 1992 Acute renal failure after ecstasy. British Medical Journal 305: 29

Hennry J A 1992 Ecstasy and the dance of death. Severe reactions are unpredictable. British Medlical Journal 305: 5–6

Johnston R R, Way W L, Miller R D 1972 Alteration of anaesthetic requirements by amphetamine. Anesthesiology 36: 357–363

McCammon R L 1986 Anesthesia for the chemically dependent patient. Anesthesia Research Society Review Course Lectures 47–55

McGoldrick K E 1980 Anesthetic implications of drug abuse. Anesthesiology Review 7: 12–17

Michel R, Adams A P 1979 Acute amphetamine abuse. Problems during general anaesthesia for neurosurgery. Anaesthesia 34: 1016–1019

Samuels S I, Maze A, Albright G 1979 Cardiac arrest during Cesarean section in a chronic amphetamine abuser. Anesthesia and Analgesia 58: 528–530

Singarajah C, Lavies N G 1992 An overdose of ecstasy. A role for dantrolene. Anaesthesia 47: 686–687

Smith D S, Gutsche B B 1980 Amphetamine abuse and obstetrical anesthesia. Anesthesia and Analgesia 59: 710–711

Tehan B, Harden R, Bodenham A 1993 Hyperthermia associated with 3,4-methylenedioxyethamphetamine ('Eve'). Anaesthesia. In press

Watson C J E, Johnston P S, Thomson H J 1991 Body-packing with amphetamines – an indication for surgery. Journal of the Royal Society of Medicine 84: 311–312

AMYLOIDOSIS

Amyloidosis is a general term for a variety of different disease processes involving the deposition of fibrillary material in tissues. This is formed of protein subunits sharing a common beta-pleated sheet structure, but derived from proteins of great chemical diversity. These fibrils are resistant to normal proteolytic digestion and share a common histochemical staining property to Congo red. In the light of advances in the understanding of the structural chemistry of amyloid, the old terms primary and secondary have been replaced (Glenner 1980).

1. Immunocytic (including myeloma-associated) amyloidosis predominantly involves mesenchymal tissue. This results in neuropathies, carpal tunnel syndrome, macroglossia, a restrictive cardiomyopathy (90% of cases), skin, gut and kidney lesions.
2. Reactive amyloidosis can occur in association with chronic infective, inflammatory and neoplastic disorders. In a survey of 64 patients, the underlying disorder was an arthropathy (42), infectious disease (11), inflammatory bowel disease (6) and others (5). The more common include rheumatoid arthritis, tuberculosis, Still's, Crohn's and Hodgkin's diseases, ankylosing spondylitis and renal cell carcinoma. Parenchymal tissue tends to be primarily involved, particularly in the kidneys, liver, spleen and thyroid. In more than 50% of cases the heart is affected, but less severely so than in the immunocytic form. Amyloid deposition, particularly involving joints, bones and tendons may occur in patients on long-term dialysis (Editorial 1991)

Preoperative abnormalities

1. Cardiac involvement may present with a digitalis-resistant heart failure, arrhythmias and conduction defects.
2. Unusual skin lesions, bullae or non-thrombocytopenic purpura feature in 40% of cases with the immunocytic disease. Macroglossia is common. Neurological lesions may affect any type of nerve, including those of the autonomic system.
3. The reactive form may present with the nephrotic syndrome, renal failure, hepatosplenomegaly, adrenal failure or lung disease.
4. Bleeding occurs frequently, although coagulation studies may be normal. Three types of abnormalities have been described (Mizutani

& Ward 1990): abnormalities of platelet function, increased vessel fragility secondary to amyloid infiltration of the blood vessels (Yood et al 1983), and defects in coagulation and fibrinolysis. Qualitative and quantitative defects in Factors IX and X have been described and there may be defects in the interactions between platelets and the vessel walls. In a series of 100 patients, 41 had one or more bleeding episodes, three of which resulted in death.

5. Amyloidosis should be suspected when a patient presents with multiple organ involvement. Confirmation is by biopsy of an affected organ but rectal biopsy is diagnostic in 90% of cases of systemic amyloid.

6. Anaesthesia may be required for biopsies or for incidental surgery. Although heart transplantation has been undertaken for cardiac amyloid, recent studies suggest that it is inappropriate, because progression of the systemic disease reduces long-term survival (Hosenpud et al 1991)

Anaesthetic problems

1. Cardiac failure or arrhythmias may produce hypotension during anaesthesia. Resistant heart failure developed after general anaesthesia for cystoscopy in a patient who had unusual skin petechiae. The diagnosis of amyloidosis was made subsequently, and death occurred on the 15th postoperative day (Welch 1982).

2. Macroglossia, common in the immunocytic form, may pose difficulties with intubation and potential postoperative airway obstruction.

3. Extreme fragility of the skin may occur and ecchymoses of the mucosae, eyelids, face, neck and axillary folds may be seen. In one patient, haemorrhagic rashes and frank bleeding was seen at all the sites where ECG electrodes and adhesive tape had been placed (Dixon 1987).

4. There have been several reports of bleeding during surgery, or bleeding which resulted in surgical investigation being required. A patient with small bowel obstruction in whom there was mild prolongation of the bleeding time rapidly developed large haematomas and required 10 units of platelets and 4 units of FFP. Subsequently, Factor IX and X levels were found to be 70% of normal (Mizutani & Ward 1990). Routine coagulation studies are unreliable predictors of the likelihood of bleeding. Of 41 patients with amyloid who had bled, only 20% had an abnormal prothrombin time. Bleeding can follow mild trauma and may require surgical intervention. The gastrointestinal tract was the source in 18, a further eight bled after diagnostic procedures, and three had haematuria. Coagulation tests were normal in all eight who bled after diagnostic procedures (Yood et al 1983).

5. In the reactive form, the additional problems are those of the primary associated disease, e.g. rheumatoid arthritis. Most have proteinuria or renal insufficiency.

6. Occasionally, the larynx is affected, but almost invariably this is a localized form of amyloidosis. Hoarseness was found to be the most common symptom and the false vocal cords was the most likely site to be affected (Lewis et al 1992). Tracheal amyloidosis may also occur either concurrently or subsequently. Urgent tracheal intubation, followed by tracheostomy, was required for laser resection of localized subglottic amyloidosis (Woo et al 1990).

Management

1. The diagnosis should be suspected in a patient who has multiple organ involvement, especially in the presence of a disease known to be associated with the reactive form.

2. Careful assessment of the heart, lungs, and liver for impairment of function is important. Anaesthetic management should be directed appropriately.

3. Difficulties in intubation should be anticipated in the presence of macroglossia. Postoperatively, the patient should be nursed in an intensive recovery area. Treatment of laryngeal amyloid should be as for any upper airway lesion causing obstructive symptoms.

4. Coagulation studies should be performed but, even when these are normal, haemorrhage should be anticipated. A normal result does not guarantee that haemorrhage will not occur.

BIBLIOGRAPHY

Dixon J 1987 Primary amyloidosis and skin damage. Anaesthesia 42: 218

Editorial 1991 Dialysis amyloidosis. Lancet 338: 349–350

Gertz M A, Kyle R A 1991 Secondary systemic amyloidosis: response and survival in 64 patients. Medicine 70: 246–256

Glenner G G 1980 Amyloid deposits and amyloidosis New England Journal of Medicine 302: 1283–1292, 1333–1343

Hosenpud J D, DeMarco T, Frazier O H et al 1991 Progression of systemic disease and reduced long-term survival in patients with cardiac amyloidosis undergoing heart transplantation. Circulation 84 (Suppl III): 338–343

Lewis J E, Olsen K D, Kurtin P J, Kyle R A 1992 Laryngeal amyloidosis: a clinicopathologic and immunohistochemical review. Otolaryngology and Head and Neck Surgery 106: 372–377

Mizutani A R, Ward C F 1990 Amyloidosis-associated bleeding diathesis in the surgical patient. Canadian Journal of Anaesthesia 37: 910–912

Welch D B 1982 Anaesthesia and amyloidosis. Anaesthesia 37: 63–66

Woo K S, Van Hasselt C A, Waldron J 1990 Laser resection of localized subglottic amyloidosis. Journal of Otolaryngology 19: 337–338

Yood R A, Skinner M, Rubinow A et al 1983 Bleeding manifestations in 100 patients with amyloidosis. Journal of the American Medical Association 249: 1322–1324

AMYOTROPHIC LATERAL SCLEROSIS
(see MOTOR NEURONE DISEASE)

ANKYLOSING SPONDYLITIS

An inflammatory arthropathy of insidious onset with systemic involvement. Granulation tissue infiltrates the bony insertions of ligaments and joint capsules, and the disease progresses variably to fibrosis, ossification and ankylosis. The primary sites of involvement are the sacroiliac joints and the spine, but 50% of patients will have extraspinal joint involvement at some time. Since it is a systemic disorder a proportion of the patients will develop non-articular manifestations of the inflammatory process.

Preoperative abnormalities

1. Bone and joints
   a. The inflammatory process usually begins at the sacroiliac joints and spreads upwards to involve the spine and costovertebral joints. A limitation of chest expansion to 2.5 cm or less is one of the criteria contributing to the clinical diagnosis. Ossification of interspinous ligaments and the formation of bony bridges between vertebrae occur in the lumbar spine, whilst cervical spine involvement varies from a degree of limitation of movement of the neck, to complete ankylosis. Those with advanced disease have an increased risk of sustaining a cervical fracture; 36% of this group have evidence of a previous occult cervical spine fracture. The majority of lesions involve the disc spaces of C5–C7, although sometimes a vertebral body is involved.
   b. Temporomandibular joint involvement is thought to cause limited mouth opening in 10% of patients, but in longstanding disease the incidence may be as high as 30–40%. Sometimes this progresses to complete ankylosis.
   c. Cricoarytenoid arthritis occurs rarely. Dyspnoea, hoarseness and vocal cord fixation may be present.
2. Non-articular disease
   a. Systemic effects include fatigue, weight loss, fever, a high ESR and hypochromic anaemia.
   b. 35% of patients have uveitis, and 85% of male patients have prostatitis, at some stage of the disease.
   c. Cardiovascular complications have been reported in 3.5% of patients with a 15-year history, and in 10% of patients who have had the disease for 30 years. Scarring of the adventitia and

fibrous proliferation of the intima of the aorta and the valve cusps produce aortitis and aortic insufficiency, and occasionally mitral valve disease. Purkinje tissue involvement may result in conduction defects. Occasionally, patients present with complete heart block and yet have minimal skeletal symptoms (Bergfeldt et al 1982).

d. Pulmonary disease may occur. Upper lobe fibrosis is a well-recognized complication. The seriousness of any pulmonary complication will be accentuated by the limited chest expansion.

e. Neurological effects are protean. Spinal cord compression, cauda equina syndrome, focal epilepsy, vertebrobasilar insufficiency and peripheral nerve lesions have all been described. In addition, there is an increased risk of mild trauma causing cervical fractures (Murray & Persellin 1981).

Anaesthetic problems

1. Cervical spine involvement may increase the difficulties of intubation. Forcible neck movements in the presence of neuromuscular blockade should be avoided because of the possible risk of cervical fracture, or vertebrobasilar insufficiency. Quadriparesis and dislocation of C6 vertebra became apparent after emergency tracheal intubation of a patient who had collapsed at work (Salathe & Johr 1989). The role of resuscitation manoeuvres in the generation of the lesion was unclear, but tracheal intubation was thought to have contributed. Death from a retropharyngeal abscess, the result of repeated attempts at blind intubation, has been recorded (Hill 1980).

2. The position in which the neck becomes fixed in longstanding disease may preclude the performance of a tracheostomy. Flexion deformity may be such that no structure below the thyroid cartilage is palpable.

3. Patients with vertebrobasilar insufficiency should be treated with caution. The author has encountered a patient who had syncope during cervical spine screening whenever extension of the neck was attempted. Presumably, bony encroachment of the vertebral artery canal had compromised blood flow. The radiologist thought that general anaesthesia was inadvisable, and limited abdominal surgery was performed after a difficult spinal anaesthetic (see Management 4). However, the patient had a respiratory arrest one week later and died after unsuccessful cardiopulmonary resuscitation.

4. Temporomandibular joint involvement may add to intubation difficulties. Ankylosis of this joint, further complicated by massive haematemesis, has been described (Sinclair & Mason 1984).

5. Respiratory problems and limited chest wall expansion increase the pulmonary complication rate and hence the need for postoperative IPPV.
6. Aortic valve disease and conduction defects can occur.
7. Spinal anaesthesia is technically difficult because of joint ankylosis.
8. If intubation is predicted to be difficult, lumbar and caudal extradural anaesthesia may be contraindicated. Difficulties in intubation are common because the relative youth of some severely affected patients means that they often have their own teeth. Technical difficulties may also increase the risk of complications. Convulsions secondary to accidental intraosseous injection of bupivacaine 20 ml during an attempted caudal block (Weber 1985), and a spinal haematoma following extradural analgesia (Gustafsson et al 1988) are recorded.
9. There is a high incidence of gastrointestinal bleeding following treatment with non-steroidal anti-inflammatory agents.
10. External cardiac massage is ineffective in patients with a rigid chest wall.

Management

1. Neck movements should be assessed with radiological screening in flexion and extension. If there is limitation of movement, and the patient has a full set of teeth, intubation difficulties should be anticipated. Wittmann & Ring (1986), who reported hip replacement in eight spondylitics, emphasized the value of indirect laryngoscopy to predict difficult intubation. Conventional intubation failed in both patients in whom preoperative indirect laryngoscopy using a spatula and a dental mirror could not demonstrate the larynx. In such patients, awake intubation is the safest course of action. A fibreoptic bronchoscope has been used to perform nasal intubation in a patient whose upper lip was pressed against her chest wall (Ovassapian et al 1983). In this particular case, tracheostomy would have been impossible. However, in some circumstances, for example, surgery for active haematemesis, preliminary tracheostomy under local anaesthesia may be the technique of choice (Sinclair & Mason 1984). In patients in whom intubation is potentially difficult, lumbar and caudal extradural anaesthesia may be contraindicated.
2. A preoperative ECG is mandatory in patients with longstanding disease because of the risk of conduction defects. Cardiovascular complications should be treated as appropriate.
3. A cervical support should be used during anaesthesia, especially if there are signs of vertebrobasilar insufficiency. Should this problem be severe, general anaesthesia may be contraindicated.
4. If general anaesthesia is contraindicated, spinal anaesthesia may be possible using radiological control, a 19-gauge needle and the assistance of an orthopaedic drill or hammer.

5. After major surgery, a short period of postoperative IPPV may be required to anticipate possible lung problems, and admission to an ITU is advisable.

BIBLIOGRAPHY

Bergfeldt L, Edhag O, Vedin L et al 1982 Ankylosing spondylitis. An important cause of severe disturbances of the cardiac conduction system. American Journal of Medicine 73: 187–191

Gustafsson H, Rutberg H, Bengtsson M 1988 Spinal haematoma following epidural analgesia. Anaesthesia 43: 220–222

Hill C M 1980 Death following dental clearance in a patient suffering from ankylosing spondylitis. British Journal of Oral Surgery 18: 73–76

Murray G C, Persellin R H 1981 Cervical fracture complicating ankylosing spondylitis. American Journal of Medicine 70: 1033–1041

Ovassapian A, Land P, Schafer M F et al 1983 Anesthetic management for surgical corrections of severe flexion deformity of the cervical spine. Anesthesiology 58: 370–372

Salathe M, Johr M 1989 Unexpected cervical fractures: a common problem in ankylosing spondylitis. Anesthesiology 70: 869–870

Sinclair J R, Mason R A 1984 Ankylosing spondylitis. The case for awake intubation. Anaesthesia 39: 3–11

Weber S 1985 Caudal anaesthesia complicated by intraosseous injection in a patient with ankylosing spondylitis. Anesthesiology 63: 716–717

Wittmann F W, Ring P A 1986 Anaesthesia in hip replacement in ankylosing spondylitis. Journal of the Royal Society of Medicine 79: 457–459

AORTIC REGURGITATION
(INCOMPETENCE)

Regurgitation of blood from the aorta into the left ventricle during diastole may result from aortic cusp distortion (rheumatic heart disease), cusp perforation (bacterial endocarditis) or dilatation of the aortic ring (Marfan's syndrome, aortic dissection, connective tissue diseases, etc.).

The volume of blood regurgitated depends on the extent of the incompetence, the aortic/left ventricular pressure gradient during diastole, and the diastolic filling time. The regurgitated volume is added to that entering from the left atrium, so that both left ventricular hypertrophy and dilatation occur. Left ventricular volume overload occurs in a ventricle which is initially distensible, and in some cases the stroke volume may be increased to more than 20 l/min. Later the myocardium becomes stiffer, the LVEDP increases, premature mitral valve closure may occur and cardiac failure finally supervenes. Symptoms may appear late in the disease, and do not correlate well with the severity of regurgitation or the degree of myocardial depression. Severe aortic regurgitation carries a poor prognosis (Turina et al 1987).

Acute lesions, usually in association with endocarditis, may occasionally occur. In these cases of rapid onset, the haemodynamic situation is very different from that in the chronic disease, and many of the signs associated with the chronic lesion are absent. Hence the presentation and treatment of the two forms is different.

Preoperative abnormalities

1. Symptoms do not correlate well with signs. Initially, reduced exercise tolerance and dyspnoea occur. Later there are signs of congestive cardiac failure. Chest pain may occur in advanced disease, when diastolic coronary artery flow is impaired and coronary flow may be limited to systole.
2. The signs are a large volume, rapid upstroke, collapsing pulse (high systolic, low diastolic), a precordial left ventricular impulse and an early diastolic murmur, maximum on expiration, at the left sternal edge.
3. Increasing left ventricular hypertrophy and cavity dilatation can lead to gross cardiomegaly on CXR, and increased left ventricular voltages with repolarization abnormalities on ECG.
4. The left ventricle is initially compliant, with a large stroke volume and a low LVEDP. Finally, when myocardial structural changes take place, the ejection fraction falls and failure occurs, with signs of increased pulmonary venous pressure, a third heart sound and pulmonary inspiratory crackles.
5. In acute aortic regurgitation, there is a normal-sized left ventricle. Pulmonary oedema is usually the presenting feature.

Anaesthetic problems

These largely depend upon the severity of the regurgitation, and the presence or absence of myocardial failure. In mild or moderate regurgitation there are usually no problems. In the severe case, risks may be high. Anaesthesia can acutely disturb compensatory mechanisms. Factors which oppose these compensatory mechanisms may produce pulmonary oedema, reduced forward cardiac output and myocardial ischaemia.

1. There are significant pathophysiological differences between acute and chronic aortic regurgitation.

   In chronic disease, compensation is accomplished by hypertrophy and dilatation of the left ventricle, and a reduction in systemic vascular resistance. A tachycardia prevents overdistension of the ventricle in diastole. Initially, the left ventricle is compliant, and left ventricular filling pressures alter relatively little with volume changes. In these cases, vasoconstriction is likely to increase the regurgitant volume.

   In acute lesions, however, the normal-sized left ventricle has only a limited capacity for distension, and life-threatening pulmonary oedema occurs early. Compensation for the fall in stroke volume and cardiac output is in part achieved by peripheral vasoconstriction and tachycardia. In such cases, the effect of anaesthetic techniques which produce peripheral vasodilatation is potentially disastrous. A death occurred during extradural anaesthesia for Caesarean section, in a patient who presented with previously undiagnosed aortic regurgitation, systolic and diastolic hypertension and increasing cardiac failure (Alderson 1987). Acute aortic regurgitation, which produced sudden cardiac failure in a young woman with rheumatoid arthritis and required urgent valve replacement, has also been described (Camilleri et al 1991).

2. A bradycardia is disadvantageous. It allows overdistension of the ventricles, an increase in left atrial pressure and pulmonary congestion.

3. Inhalation agents may intensify myocardial depression.

Management

1. Mild or moderate chronic aortic regurgitation requires a careful anaesthetic, avoiding volume depletion, myocardial depression and bradycardia. Antibiotic prophylaxis should be given. Both regional and general anaesthesia are well tolerated.

2. If there is evidence of decompensation, a detailed cardiological assessment is required. In addition, the differentiation of acute from chronic aortic regurgitation is crucial for the management of the severe case. In either case, there may be sensitivity to changes in systemic vascular resistance.

3. Agents which depress myocardial contractility are avoided.

4. Bradycardia is prevented and a fairly fast heart rate maintained. Pancuronium has been suggested as a suitable agent for producing a mild tachycardia.

5. With severe disease, haemodynamic monitoring is essential. This will enable the effects of drug and fluid therapy to be monitored closely. The response to acute events cannot always be predicted. In the case of chronic aortic regurgitation, vasodilators and, sometimes, inotropic agents may be required. The use of extradural anaesthesia, or a drug with mild alpha adrenoceptor blocking effects, such as droperidol, has been recommended to reduce afterload. Adequate preload must first be achieved.

   In acute aortic regurgitation, however, techniques which produce an uncontrolled fall in systemic vascular resistance must be avoided.

6. Catastrophic pulmonary oedema requires intensive therapy. A dilating inotrope such as dobutamine, a reduction of left atrial pressure with diuretics and vasodilators such as glyceryl trinitrate or nitroprusside, and IPPV, may all be required (Stone et al 1980).

BIBLIOGRAPHY
Alderson J D 1987 Cardiovascular collapse following epidural anaesthesia for Caesarean section in a patient with aortic incompetence. Anaesthesia 42: 643–645
Camilleri J P, Douglas-Jones A G, Pritchard M H 1991 Rapidly progressive aortic valve incompetence in a patient with rheumatoid arthritis. British Journal of Rheumatology 30: 379–381
Stone J G, Hoar P F, Calabro J R et al 1980 Afterload reduction and preload

augmentation improve the anesthetic management of patients with cardiac failure and valvular regurgitation. Anesthesia and Analgesia 59: 737–742

Turina J, Hess O, Sepulchri F et al 1987 Spontaneous course of aortic valve disease. European Heart Journal 8: 471–483

AORTIC STENOSIS

Aortic stenosis may be valvular, subaortic or supravalvular. The normal area of the valve is 3 cm^2. Symptoms and signs appear when the area is reduced to about 0.8 cm^2. The long-term prognosis depends upon the degree of stenosis;

<0.7 cm^2:   severe
0.7–1.5 cm^2:   moderate
>1.5 cm^2:   mild.

Unlike hypertension, in which the resistance to left ventricular function is variable and depends upon the state of the peripheral vasculature, the resistance to ejection of blood by the left ventricle in aortic stenosis is fixed. A pressure gradient across the valve of >50 mmHg is considered to be severe, and <20 mmHg mild. These gradients are increased by tachycardia and exercise. In order to overcome the obstruction, left ventricular hypertrophy occurs and this is associated with a loss of compliance, and without an increase in cavity size. Stroke volume is therefore limited. Ventricular dilatation only occurs in the late stages, or when the valve becomes incompetent.

The dangerous feature of this condition is that signs and symptoms appear late in the disease. Once they occur, the prognosis is poor. However, even those with moderate disease are at risk, and those with valve areas from 0.7–1.2 cm^2 are at significant risk, of developing complications, particularly if there is a subnormal ejection fraction (Kennedy et al 1991). In a study of the natural history of aortic stenosis, 21% (66 patients) in the moderate group died in the short term from causes attributed to aortic stenosis. In older patients, coronary artery disease may contribute to symptoms and cardiac dysfunction. Aortic stenosis may be one feature of a variety of inherited conditions; for example, supravalvular stenososis is associated with Williams syndrome (Larson & Warner 1989).

Preoperative abnormalities

1. The onset of symptoms occurs relatively late in the disease and includes dyspnoea, intolerance of exertion, angina and syncope. LVEDP is increased, and the occurrence of pulmonary oedema on exertion may be the first sign of decompensation. Even in haemodynamically severe disease, patients may be asymptomatic or only mildly symptomatic (Turina et al 1987).

2. The pulse is slow rising and of decreased amplitude. A pulse pressure of <30 mmHg reflects severe disease. Conversely, if the systolic blood pressure is >180 mmHg, the disease is not significant.
3. An ejection systolic murmur, maximal at the base and radiating into the right side of the neck.
4. CXR initially shows normal cardiac size. Left atrial enlargement and dilatation of the aortic root may be seen later.
5. In the presence of significant stenosis, the ECG usually, but not invariably, shows left ventricular hypertrophy. The diagnosis should be considered in elderly patients with LVF. In failure, when the cardiac output is low, the murmur is soft or absent.
6. Sudden death may occur. Severe ventricular arrhythmias may be linked to dysfunction of the left ventricle, and conduction abnormalities may also occur.
7. The diagnosis is rapidly made by echocardiography, and Doppler studies give the pressure gradients.

Anaesthetic problems
Significant aortic stenosis (a systolic ejection murmur of at least grade II–VI) in patients more than 40 years old was identified as a risk factor for life-threatening and fatal cardiac complications in non-cardiac surgical procedures (Goldman et al 1977). In symptomatic aortic stenosis, a number of factors will alter the haemodynamic state and disturb compensatory mechanisms. One or more of the following problems may result:

1. Myocardial ischaemia. The hypertrophied myocardium is extremely vulnerable to ischaemia. Prolonged tachycardia, hypotension or hypovolaemia may produce myocardial insufficiency. At low heart rates there is an inability to increase stroke volume. Myocardial ischaemia, following cardiac catheterization, was responsible for the death of three children with Williams syndrome and supravalvular aortic stenosis (Conway et al 1990).
2. Decreases in cardiac output or cardiovascular collapse. Precipitated by hypovolaemia, myocardial depressants, bradycardias, peripheral vasodilatation and atrial arrhythmias.
3. Pulmonary oedema. Interference with atrial function by arrhythmias or fluid overload causes cardiac decompensation.
4. Decreased cerebral blood flow.
5. Resuscitation from a state of asystole is difficult. Following asystolic cardiac arrest, the prognosis is poor.

Management
Management of the symptomatic patient requires careful monitoring with the insertion of an arterial line and CVP. Some authors recommend PAP in addition. All anaesthetic drugs must be given with caution, and

therapeutic manoeuvres, such as fluid loading and treatment of adverse heart rates, must be performed with particular care, to avoid wide swings in cardiovascular pressures and myocardial oxygen supply.

1. If the condition is symptomatic, cardiological advice should be obtained. Aortic valve replacement or a balloon valvuloplasty may be more important than the proposed operation. In young patients, particularly those with congenital stenosis, balloon valvuloplasty may be preferable because it delays the necessity for long-term anticoagulation (Hall & Kirk 1992). In older patients, any improvement produced is usually short-lived and the complication rate, in particular the incidence of aortic regurgitation, is high.
2. Control of heart rate. Slow rhythms are treated with atropine and atrial arrhythmias are prevented. Atrial fibrillation with decompensation may be an indication for cardioversion.
3. Prevention of hypotension. Induction must be slow. High concentrations of myocardial depressants, such as halothane and enflurane, are avoided, and the vascular volume maintained. The exact method of anaesthesia is probably less important than the care with which it is administered and the patient monitored. The use of a Swan-Ganz catheter to monitor absorption of irrigating fluid has been described (Toft & Knudsen 1991). In the presence of outflow obstruction, a regional technique is probably less controllable than a general anaesthetic. However, opinions vary. Inotropes may be needed.
4. Precordial ECG lead is observed for evidence of myocardial ischaemia.
5. Prophylaxis against bacterial endocarditis.
6. Should cardiac arrest occur, effective cardiac massage can only be obtained after opening the chest.

BIBLIOGRAPHY

Conway E E Jr, Noonan J, Marion R W et al 1990 Myocardial infarction leading to sudden death in the Williams syndrome: report of three cases. Journal of Pediatrics 117: 593–595
Goldman L, Caldera D L 1977 Multifactorial index of cardiac risk in non cardiac surgical procedures. New England Journal of Medicine 297: 845–850
Hall R, Kirk R 1992 Balloon dilatation of heart valves. British Medical Journal 305: 487–488
Kennedy K D, Nishimura R A, Holmes D R et al 1991 Natural history of moderate aortic stenosis. Journal of the American College of Cardiologists 17: 313–319
Larson J S, Warner M A 1989 Williams syndrome: an uncommon cause of supravalvular aortic stenosis in a child. Journal of Cardiovascular Anesthesia 3: 337–340
Toft P, Knudsen F 1991 Prevention of the TURP syndrome by using the Swan-Ganz catheter in a patient with severe aortic stenosis. (English Abstract.) Ugeskr-Laeger 153: 3487–3494
Turina J, Hess O, Sepulchri F et al 1987 Spontaneous course of aortic valve disease. European Heart Journal 8: 471–483

APUDOMAS

A group of tumours of neuroectodermal origin, whose cells have common cytochemical characteristics. The name arises from their ability to handle certain amines (Amine Precursor Uptake and Decarboxylation). They can secrete a wide variety of peptides or amine products, a number of which have anaesthetic significance. In addition, but less frequently, bleeding or compression effects of the tumour may necessitate emergency surgery (Philippe 1992).

This section enumerates the differing types of tumour, the normal and ectopic hormones which have been attributed to them, and some of their actions (Whitwam .1977, Bouloux 1987, Weatherill 1988). For specific syndromes reported as having anaesthetic significance, see under the individual names.

Tumour	Normal hormones	Some ectopic hormones
Bronchial carcinoid and oat cell carcinoma	(5-HT)	ACTH, ADH, MSH, VIP, glucagon, calcitonin, insulin, prolactin, GH
Chemodectoma	Noradrenaline, dopamine	Calcitonin, ACTH
Ganglioneuro-blastoma		Noradrenaline, VIP
Gastrointestinal carcinoid	Gastrin, VIP, glucagon enteroglucagon	ADH, ACTH, MSH
Islet cell adenoma	Insulin, glucagon, PP	ACTH, MSH, ADH, VIP
Paraganglioma	(Adrenaline, noradrenaline, 5-HT)	ACTN, MSH, VIP
Phaeochromocytoma	Adrenaline, dopamine, noradrenaline,	ACTH, insulin
Pituitary adenoma	GH, prolactin. LH, ACTH, MSH	
Thymoma		Calcitonin, ACTH
Thyroid medullary carcinoma	Calcitonin (5HT)	ACTH, MSH, insulin

Hormones:	abbreviations and actions
ACTH:	Adrenocorticotrophic hormone – hypokalaemic alkalosis, oedema, pigmentation, diabetes.
ADH:	Antidiuretic hormone – water retention, hyponatraemia leading to confusion and fits.
Adrenaline:	Intermittent hypertension, headache, sweating and palpitations.
Calcitonin:	Regulates plasma calcium; decreases bone resorption, increases renal calcium and phosphate excretion. Increased calcitonin secretion in thyroid medullary carcinoma, but plasma calcium usually normal.
Gastrin:	Gross gastric acid hypersecretion, peptic ulceration.
Glucagon:	Hyperglycaemia unresponsive to insulin, weight loss, migratory skin rash, anaemia.
GH:	Growth hormone – acromegaly, hypertension, impaired glucose tolerance.

5-HT:	5-hydroxytryptamine – diarrhoea, intermittent hypertension and tachycardia, hyperglycaemia, possible flushing.
Insulin:	Hypoglycaemic attacks. Often diagnosed as fits, faints, hysteria, drunkenness.
LH:	Luteinizing hormone – ovulatory control and spermatogenesis.
MSH:	Melanocyte stimulating hormone – pigmentation.
Noradrenaline:	Sustained hypertension, headache, sweating and palpitations.
PP:	Pancreatic polypeptide – inhibits pancreatic exocrine secretion, relaxes gall bladder.
Prolactin:	Amenorrhoea, galactorrhoea and infertility.
VIP:	Vasoactive intestinal peptide – watery diarrhoea, hypokalaemia and hypotension.

BIBLIOGRAPHY

Bouloux P-M 1987 Multiple endocrine neoplasia. Surgery 1: 1180–1185

Philippe J 1992 APUDomas: acute complications and their medical management. Baillieres Clinical Endocrinology and Metabolism 6(1): 217–228

Vasen H F, van der Feltz M, Raue F et al 1992 The natural course of multiple endocrine neoplasia type IIb. A study of 18 cases. Archives of Internal Medicine 152: 1250–1252

Weatherill D 1988 Anaesthesia, APUDomas and multiple endocrine neoplasia. Surgery 60: 1437–1439

Whitwam J G 1977 APUD cells and the apudomas. A concept relevant to anaesthesia and endocrinology. Anaesthesia 32: 879–888

ARTHROGRYPOSIS MULTIPLEX CONGENITA
(AMC)

Not a distinct entity but, rather, a symptom complex, in which there is congenital but non-progressive stiffness and deformity of joints, most probably associated with immobility of limbs in utero (Dubovitz 1978). The primary cause may be neurogenic, myopathic, an abnormality of joints or connective tissue, or restrictive, secondary to oligohydramnios. In a pathological study of 21 fatal cases, 11 were myogenic (10 congenital muscular dystrophy) in origin (Quinn et al 1991). One case occurred after the mother had received tubocurarine in the tenth week of pregnancy for the treatment of tetanus. It is suggested that those cases of neurogenic origin may be associated with degeneration of anterior horn cell columns. Those in the neurogenic group have a number of congenital abnormalities in association. Birth fractures are common (Thompson & Bilenker 1985) and patients may present for orthopaedic, ENT and oral surgical procedures.

Preoperative abnormalities

1. The joint rigidity is fibrous, not bony, and most marked in distal joints. Frequently, the arms are rotated internally and the hips externally, sometimes with dislocation. Talipes and flexion deformities of the wrists are common. Both contractures and muscle atrophy occur secondary to immobility. Although the postural deformities are similar, the underlying lesion, and hence the individual prognosis, is very different.
2. The face is expressionless, with drooling of saliva. Some patients have micrognathia, high arched palate, temporomandibular joint involvement and trismus.
3. A number of other congenital abnormalities, including those of the cardiovascular, respiratory, nervous and genitourinary systems have been reported.
4. About 20% of patients have ENT complications (Cohen & Isaacs 1976). It has been postulated that the primary CNS pathology results in dysfunction of the tongue, palate, pharynx and larynx. Dysphagia, aspiration, and airway obstruction have been reported.
5. EMG and muscle biopsy will distinguish neuropathic from myopathic and dystrophic conditions.

Anaesthetic problems

1. Patients are prone to recurrent aspiration pneumonitis (Laureano & Rybak 1990) secondary to dysphagia and poor control of pharyngeal and laryngeal reflexes.
2. Severe deformities may cause difficulties in tracheal intubation. Temporomandibular joint involvement (Heffez et al 1985), micrognathia, high arched palate and trismus have been reported.
3. Hypermetabolic responses to anaesthesia have occurred. Some authors have therefore suggested that AMC is associated with an increased incidence of MH. The evidence has been largely anecdotal. In only one case were the MH criteria convincing (Baudendistel et al 1984) The likelihood of this association was also challenged in a review of 67 patients with arthrogryposis who had undergone a total of 398 anaesthetics (Baines et al 1986). No evidence could be found that an MH episode had occurred in any of them, although the temperature was not always recorded. Hopkins et al (1991) reported two cases of hypermetabolic reactions in AMC which were distinct from MH and independent of the anaesthetic agents used. However, it is possible for two rare conditions such as AMC and MH to be present coincidentally in the same patient.
4. Pregnancy is rare. During Caesarean section, extradural anaesthesia failed and was followed by moderate difficulty in tracheal intubation (Quance 1988).

Management

1. Elucidation of the cause of the condition may be helpful, if only for the future resolution of anaesthetic risk factors. Conduction studies and ENG may assist in this.

2. If dysphagia and recurrent aspiration pneumonitis are features, gastrostomy and tracheostomy may be required (Cohen & Isaacs 1976).

3. The presence of maxillofacial abnormalities could warn of the possibility of difficult tracheal intubation.

4. During general anaesthesia the patient should be observed and specifically monitored for signs of a hypermetabolic response. Should this occur, it will respond to active Cooling (Hopkins et al 1991). Since the risk of MH is unproven, it is suggested that the use of halothane in these patients is justified, particularly if alternative agents may place the child at an even greater risk (Baines et al 1986). A child with an arthrogryposis of myopathic origin requiring a pyelolithotomy, and whose serum CK was 880 iu/l, had an uneventful anaesthetic when ketamine and pancuronium were used (Oberoi et al 1987)

BIBLIOGRAPHY

Baines D B, Douglas I D, Overton J H 1986 Anaesthesia for patients with arthrogryposis multiplex congenita. What is the risk of malignant hyperpyrexia? Anaesthesia and Intensive Care 14: 370–372

Baudendistel L, Goudsouzian N, Cote C et al 1984 End-idal CO_2 monitoring. Its use in the diagnosis and management of malignant hyperthermia. Anaesthesia 39: 1000–1003

Cohen S R, Isaacs H 1976 Otolaryngological manifestations of arthrogryposis multiplex congenita. Annals of Otology, Rhinology and Laryngology 85: 484–490

Dubovitrz V 1978 Arthrogryposis multiplex congenita. In: Muscle disorders in childhood. W B Saunders, Philadelphia

Heffez L, Doku H C, O'Donnell J P 1985 Arthrogryposis multiplex congenita involving the temporomandibular joint. Journal of Oral and Maxillofacial Surgery 43: 539–542

Hopkins P M, Ellis F R, Halsall P J 1991 Hypermetabolism in arthrogryposis multiplex congenita. Anaesthesia 46: 374–375

Laureano A N, Rybak L P 1990 Severe otolaryngologic manifestations of arthrogryposis multiplex congenita. Annals of Otology, Rhinology and Laryngology 99: 94–97

Oberoi G S, Kaul H L, Gill I S et al 1987 Anaesthesia in arthrogryposis multiplex congenita: case report. Canadian Journal of Anaesthesia 34: 288–290

Quance D R 1988 Anaesthetic management of an obstetrical patient with arthrogryposis multiplex congenita. Canadian Journal of Anaesthesia 35: 612–614

Quinn CM, Wigglesworth J S, Heckmatt J 1991 Lethal arthrogryposis multiplex congenita: a pathological study of 21 cases. Histopathology 19: 155–162

Thompson G H, Bilenker R M 1985 Comprehensive management of arthrogryposis multiplex congenita: Clinical Orthopedics 194: 6–14

ASTHMA

A condition of hyper-reactivity of the tracheobronchial tree, in which a number of exogenous and endogenous stimuli can produce reversible airway obstruction. Histamine and the leukotrienes (LT) are thought to be the most active chemical mediators, while acetylcholine may contribute via a disturbance in autonomic balance (Galant 1987). As obstruction worsens, increasingly smaller airways are affected. Expiration is prolonged, residual volume and functional residual capacity are increased, whilst vital capacity, inspiratory capacity and expiratory reserve volume are reduced. Widespread ventilation perfusion inequalities may occur to produce hypoxia, at a time when the work of breathing is considerably increased. In addition to bronchospasm, pathological inflammatory changes include oedema of the bronchial mucosa, secretion of mucus and epithelial desquamation.

For more detailed descriptions see Hirshman & Bergman (1990), Cottam & Eason (1991) and Hirshman (1991).

Preoperative abnormalities

1. There may be a history of wheezing, dyspnoea, cough, and sputum production. The chest may be hyper-resonant and the breath sounds diminished, with prolonged expiration and an audible wheeze. In particularly severe cases the wheeze disappears.

2. Therapy in asthma can be aimed at blocking airway reflexes, relaxing smooth muscle, inhibiting the release of inflammatory mediators and increasing beta adrenoceptor tone.

   An increasing appreciation of the role of the inflammatory component in asthma has led to a change of emphasis in drug therapy for long-term treatment (Barnes 1989, Guidelines 1990). For the chronic state, emphasis is now placed on the early introduction of regular inhaled anti-inflammatory drugs such as corticosteroids (beclomethasone dipropionate or budesonide), sodium cromoglycate and nedocromil sodium. Since the onset of action of these drugs is slow, long-term therapy is required.

   Bronchodilators are primarily indicated for short-term relief of bronchospasm, acute asthma attacks and the prevention of exercise-induced asthma. The main bronchoclilators are, in decreasing order of effectiveness: beta$_2$ adrenoceptor agonists, theophylline derivatives and anticholinergics. The use of the aerosol form of bronchoactive drugs reduces systemic side effects. In addition, bronchodilators given by inhalation act more rapidly than oral, and equally as fast as intravenous preparations.

3. CXR may show an increase in bronchovascular markings and hyperinflation and, in the later stages, some degree of emphysema. In the acute asthmatic a CXR is essential to exclude pneumothorax.

4. An FEV_1 of less than 1 litre, or an FEV_1/VC ratio of less than 40% and an increased $PaCO_2$, may all indicate the need for postoperative IPPV. A PEFR of less than 120 l/min and an MVV of less than 50% of the predicted level also indicate severe obstruction.
5. There may be an improvement in pulmonary function tests and blood gases after administration of bronchodilators.
6. Studies of near-fatal episodes of asthma on arrival in hospital suggest that these were secondary to asphyxia as a consequence of under- rather than overtreatment of the asthma by beta adrenoceptor agonists, as had previously been suggested (Molfino et al 1991).

Anaesthetic problems

1. The inflammatory component is particularly significant for the patient needing anaesthesia (Hirshman & Bergman 1990). The effect of reflex increases in airway tone depends upon the initial calibre of the airway. If inflammation causing mucosal oedema and secretion of mucus is present, then reflex bronchospasm may have profound effects on airway resistance. An apparently asymptomatic patient who has inflamed airways may thus develop complete airway closure after tracheal intubation, despite having had no audible wheeze on preoperative examination.
2. There is an increased sensitivity to airway manipulations during light anaesthesia. Tracheal intubation may produce acute bronchospasm. In a computer-aided incidence study of 136 929 anaesthetics, it was found that bronchospasm was usually triggered by mechanical stimuli (Olsson 1987).
3. Cardiac arrhythmias can occur more frequently in the presence of hypoxia and acidosis, or following the overuse of sympathomimetic agents. Sudden spontaneous deaths in asthmatics have been attributed to the combination of nebulized high-dose $beta_2$ agonists and long-acting theophylline derivatives, although doubt has been cast on this theory (Molfino et al 1991).
4. Halothane can interact with aminophylline to produce serious arrhythmias, even when theophylline levels are within the therapeutic range. This combination was suggested to have been the cause of ventricular fibrillation (Stirt & Sternick 1982) and ventricular tachycardia (Roizen & Stevens 1978). The xanthines are beta adrenoceptor stimulators which release noracrenaline and inhibit the breakdown of cyclic AMP.
5. Inhalational agents may aggravate ventilation perfusion inequalities and increase hypoxia, by reducing hypoxic pulmonary vasoconstriction.
6. Perioperative steroid cover is advisable if steroids have been used within the previous year.

7. In severe cases, postoperative IPPV may be required. It does, however, carry a high risk of complications such as pneumothorax, cardiac arrhythmias, pneumonia and heart failure.
8. An increased incidence of postoperative pulmonary complications.

Management

1. Elective surgery should not take place in the presence of infection or untreated bronchospasm. Preoperative preparation will include physiotherapy, bronchodilators, antibiotics and corticosteroid cover if these drugs have been used within the previous 12 months. A short course of corticosteroids is also indicated before surgery if inflammation is present (Hirshman & Bergman 1990). In severe cases it is important to assess the likelihood of the need for IPPV in the postoperative period.
2. Anxiety may be a significant feature in the asthmatic patient. Care and understanding should be shown at the preoperative visit, and a sedative premedication, such as an antihistamine, is advantageous. The potential seriousness of this disease must not be underestimated.
3. Despite having a drying effect on secretions, atropine may be desirable for a smooth induction. It can also improve dilatation in the larger bronchi by blocking vagal constrictor effects. Although pethicine has been promoted as a bronchodilator, it has recently been shown to be a more common cause of histamine release than morphine. Even when bronchospasm is absent, some form of preoperative bronchodilator therapy is advisable. Beta adrenoceptor blockers are contraindicated, since even those with a primarily cardiac action can aggravate airway obstruction.
4. The choice of induction agent is controversial. Bronchoconstriction can arise from the drug itself or directly from tracheal intubation. Even when attacks are infrequent, tracheal intubation is one of the commonest causes of intraoperative bronchospasm in patients who have any history of asthma. The carina is particularly sensitive to stimulation. Thiopentone may affect the airways in a variable, dose-related manner. There is evidence that airway reflexes are depressed at high, but not at low doses. There are no particular contraindications to the use of benzodiazepines, etomidate or propofol. However, since none of these depresses airway reflexes, it is wise to deepen anaesthesia before intubation. There is experimental evidence that reflex bronchospasm is prevented by i.v. lignocaine (1 mg/kg), but not that resulting from the release of allergic mediators (Downes et al 1980). In humans, the cough reflex in response to tracheal instillation of sterile water was suppressed by lignocaine 1.5 mg/kg (Nishino et al 1990). Thus the use of i.v. lignocaine (1–1.5 mg/kg) before induction has been recommended.

Topical lignocaine is not effective and may actually induce bronchoconstriction in asthmatic patients (McAlpine & Thomson 1989).

5. Ketamine has been recommended as a suitable induction agent for emergency anaesthesia in asthmatics when a rapid sequence induction is required (Hirshman et al 1979). A comparison with thiopentone in dogs showed it to have a protective effect against bronchospasm, which was abolished by beta adrenoceptor blockers.

6. Halothane, enflurane and isoflurane are all effective at reversing antigen-induced bronchospasm (Hirshman et al 1982). However, halothane sensitizes the heart to the effect of exogenous and endogenous catecholamines. It also interacts with aminophylline to produce arrhythmias, even when theophylline levels are within the therapeutic range. The choice of isoflurane or enflurane may therefore be more appropriate. However, in severe asthma, inhalational agents may exacerbate ventilation perfusion inequalities and increase hypoxia, by reducing hypoxic pulmonary vasoconstriction.

7. Neuromuscular blockers. Atracurium constricts peripheral airways in doses that produce significant cardiovascular effects and probably results from the release of histamine acting on H_1 receptors (Mehr et al 1992). The peak effects occur 3 minutes after a dose of 0.5 mg/kg. Thus, if the use of atracurium is essential it should be given in low or divided doses, possibly With a H_1, receptor antagonist administered beforehand.

8. Regional anaesthesia may be used for surgery or during labour. A retrospective study of asthmatic parturients (Ramanathan et al 1990) and a prospective study of suitable patients undergoing surgery (Tanaka et al 1991) showed that extradural anaesthesia could be safely administered, even during acute exacerbations of asthma.

9. Treatment of acute bronchospasm.
   a. If this occurs following tracheal intubation, the easiest initial manoeuvre is to try to deepen the anaesthetic using an inhalation agent.
   b. If there is complete airway closure, adrenaline 1 in 10 000 should be given in divided doses, 1–10 ml. This may need to be repeated.
   c. Salbutamol infusion, 5 µg/min (5 ml of 1 mg/ml solution added to 500 ml 0.9% saline to give a final concentration of 10 µg/ml).
   d. Ketamine in subanaesthetic doses (bolus dose 0.75 mg/kg, infusion of 0.15 mg/kg per h) has been used to treat intractable bronchospasm in two patients (Sarma 1992).
   e. Residual bronchospasm can be treated with aminophylline, 5 mg/kg over a period of 10–15 minutes. If necessary, an infusion of 0.5 mg/kg per h, is started. However, the narrow margin between therapeutic and toxic levels of theophylline means that

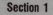
the dug is being used decreasingly. If aminophylline is used, plasma theophylline levels must be estimated if treatment is prolonged for more than 24 hours. The therapeutic range is 10–20 mg/l but toxic effects such as fits, arrhythmias and cardiac arrest have been described with plasma levels as low as 25 mg/l. Extreme caution is necessary if the patient has already been taking sustained-release theophylline preparations.

10. Indications for IPPV in asthmatics.
    a Distress and exhaustion.
    b. Deterioration in arterial blood gases. Pao_2 >6.7 kPa or $Paoc_2$ <6.7 kPa, and increasing metabolic acidosis.
    c. Cardiac arrhythmias or hypotension.
    d. Acute crises such as cardiorespiratory arrest, decreased conscious level due to sedatives, or a collapsed lung.

11. Technique of IPPV in asthmatics. Inotropes should be available at intubation because acute circulatory collapse may accompany the initiation of IPPV. Patients should be underventilated and therefore neuromuscular blockers may be required. Provided that life-threatening hypoxia is avoided, it is unnecessary to aim for normal blood gases. Care should be taken to prevent hyperinflation.

BIBLIOGRAPHY

Barnes P J 1989 A new approach to the treatment of asthma. New England Journal of Medicine 321: 1517–1527

Cottam S, Eason J 1991 The intensive care management of acute asthma. In: Anaesthesia review 8. Churchill Livingstone Edinburgh

Downes H, Gerber N, Hirshman C A 1980 I.v. lignocaine in reflex and allergic bronchoconstriction. British Journal of Anaesthesia 52: 873–878

Galant S P 1987 Anaesthesia and asthma. In: Anaesthesia review 4. Churchill Livingstone, Edinburgh

Guidelines for the management of asthma in adults 1990. Statement by the British Thoracic Society, Research Unit of the Royal College of Physicians, King's Fund Centre, National Asthma Campaign. I – Chronic persistent asthma in adults. British Medical Journal 301: 651-653, II – Acute severe asthma in adults. British Medical Journal 301: 797–800

Hirshman C A 1991 Perioperative management of the asthmatic patient. Canadian Journal of Anaesthesia 38: R26–38

Hirshman C A, Bergman N A 1990 Factors influencing intrapulmonary airway calibre during anaesthesia. British Journal of Anaesthesia 65: 30–42

Hirshman C A, Downes H, Farbood A et al 1979 Ketamine block of bronchospasm in experimental canine asthma. British Journal of Anaesthesia 51: 713–718

Hirshman C, Edelstein G, Peetz S et al 1982 Mechanisms of action of inhalational agents on airways. Anesthesiology 56: 107–111

Kingston H G G Hirshman C A 1984 Perioperative management of the patient with asthma. Anesthesia and Analgesia 63: 844–855

McAlpine L G, Thomson N C 1989 Lidocaine-induced bronchoconstriction in asthmatic patients. Relation to histamine airway responsiveness and effect of preservatives. Chest 96: 1012–1015

Mehr E H, Hirshman C A, Lindeman K S 1992 Mechanism of action of atracurium in airway constriction. Anesthesiology 76: 448–454

Molfino N A, Nannini L J, Martelli A N et al 1991 Respiratory arrest in near-fatal asthma. New England Journal of Medicine 324; 285–288

Nishino T, Hiraga K, Sugimori K 1990 Effects of i.v. lignocaine on airway reflexes elicited by irritation of the tracheal mucosa in humans anaesthetised with enflurane. British Journal of Anaesthesia 64: 682–687

Olsson G L 1987 Bronchospasm during anaesthesia. A computer-aided incidence study of 136,929 patients. Acta Anaesthesiologica Scandinavica 31: 244–252

Ramanathan J, Osborne B, Sibai B 1990 Epidural anesthesia in asthmatic parturients. Anesthesia and Analgesia 70: S317

Roizen M F, Stevens W C 1978 Multiform ventricular tachycardia due to the interaction of aminophylline and halothane. Anesthesia and Analgesia 57: 738–741

Sarma V J 1992 Use of ketamine in acute severe asthma. Acta Anaesthesiologica Scandinavica 36: 106–107

Stirt J A, Sternick C S 1982 Aminophylline and anesthesia. Anesthesiology 57: 252–253

Tanaka K, Shono S, Watnabe R, Dan K 1991 Epidural anesthesia and analgesia is safe for patients with asthma – a survey of 383 patients. Anesthesia and Analgesia 72: S292

ATHLETIC HEART SYNDROME

A name given to certain cardiac and ECG changes found in some high performance athletes, and which most probably represent physiological adaptations of the heart and cardiovascular system to the demands of the sport. The changes depend upon the nature of the demand: endurance (isotonic or dynamic) athletes such as marathon runners have chronic volume overload because of sustained increases in cardiac output (as much as seven-fold), whereas weight lifters (isometric or static athletes) experience transient episodes of enormous pressure overload. Both have cardiac enlargement. However, the former have increases in left ventricular end-diastolic volume (from 120 ml in an untrained person to 220 ml in a resting athlete) and stroke volume (up to 170 ml during exercise) with proportionate increases in ventricular wall thickness. Isometric athletes develop massive increases in wall thickness, to withstand the huge aortic pressures, without increases in ventricular end-diastolic diameter (Huston et al 1985).

In either case, when cardiac abnormalities occur, the main problem is to differentiate these from pathological heart disease, in particular, hypertrophic obstructive cardiomyopathy (HOCM). This is increasingly recognized as an important cause of sudden death in young people, a number of whom have a family history (Editorial 1992).

The cardiovascular changes which prepare athletes for exercise may be disadvantageous during anaesthesia and surgery. In a study of normotensive athletes with cardiac hypertrophy impairment of cardiopulmonary receptor reflexes was found (Giannattasio et al 1990). This indicates a potential lack of response to haemorrhage and orthostatic stress by means of a tachycardia.

Preoperative abnormalities

1. Physical examination may show a resting bradycardia and displaced left ventricular impulse. Mid-systolic murmurs may be heard in up

to 50% of dynamic athletes and third and fourth heart sounds are common.

2. CXR often shows an increased cardiothoracic ratio, a globular heart and increased pulmonary vascularity.

3. ECG changes. Certain rhythm disturbances are more frequent than in the general population but the patients are usually of an age group, and a degree of fitness, which would not routinely justify a preoperative ECG. However, an unduly slow, and sometimes irregular pulse may lead an observant physician to perform one. The ECG may show large voltages and tall T waves, with both dilatation and hypertrophy of the left ventricle. A sinus bradycardia will be found in the majority of athletes. There may be a range of depolarization abnormalities including wandering atrial pacemaker, first- and second-degree heart block, right bundle branch block or ST-segment abnormalities (Pedoe 1983). Occasionally third-degree heart block has been reported.

4. Endurance athletes have poor tolerance to orthostatic stress. Echocardiographic investigations suggest that the cause is mechanical rather than autonomic in origin (Levine et al 1991). In endurance athletes, a greater effective left ventricular chamber compliance and distensibilty was found compared with non-athletes. This resulted in a steeper slope to the Starling curve, which relates left ventricular filling pressure to stroke volume.

Anaesthetic problems

1. General anaesthesia. There have been reports of fit young patients presenting with unexpected episodes of arrhythmias or conduction defects during general anaesthesia (Bullock & Hall 1985, Abdulatif et al 1987). In these cases, neither event was serious and the major problem was one of diagnosis.

2. Whilst reduced heart rate responses to baroreceptor stimulation may favour cardiovascular function during exercise, it may be disadvantageous during haemorrhagic or orthostatic stress, when pronounced tachycardia is an important component in the maintenance of stable cardiovascular haemodynamics (Giannattasio et al 1990).

3. Regional anaesthesia. One athlete had two periods of asystole and unconsciousness, from which he was resuscitated with atropine, 25 minutes after induction of spinal anaesthesia (Kreutz & Mazuzan 1990). Subsequent ECG showed resting sinus bradycardia, left ventricular hypertrophy and ST-segment abnormalities. This may be related to the known intolerance to orthostatic stress.

4. In the first week after athletic competition, endurance athletes can have elevated heart-specific serum CK-MB enzyme levels. Thus, caution must be exercised in the interpretation of such

investigations. However, athletes are not immune from heart disease, and sudden death during exercise has been caused by previously undiagnosed cardiomyopathies (Editorial 1992).

Management

1. When unexpected arrhythmias occur in young, apparently fit patients, the first problem is to exclude causes such as hypercarbia, hypotoxia, inhalational agents, the response to surgical stimuli and the use of vasoconstrictors. The second is to be aware of rarer causes of arrhythmias, such as malignant hyperthermia, solvent abuse, ankylosing spondylitis, sarcoidosis, mitral valve prolapse and cardiomyopathies.
2. If these pathological abnormalities have been excluded, then treatment is not necessarily indicated. Earlier reports suggested that patients with 'athlete's heart' remain haemodynamically stable during anaesthesia, and that conduction defects respond to atropine. However, not all arrhythmias during anaesthesia are benign and if serious conduction defects occur they should be treated expeditiously.
3. Care should be taken not to subject athletes to sudden orthostatic stress such as the upright position, particularly when performing spinal or extradural anaesthesia.
4. It is equally essential that such patients are not labelled as having a pathological cardiac condition. If doubt persists, referral to a cardiologist who is known to be aware of the condition is advised. Extensive invasive investigations will not usually be appropriate, but echocardiography will usually discriminate between athlete's heart and HOCM. Echocardiography in athletes may demonstrate an increase in left ventricular wall and cavity size by as much as 20% above the normal for the size of patient. Unlike patients with coronary artery disease, these individuals should not show progressive abnormalities with exercise ECGs

BIBLIOGRAPHY

Abdulatif M, Fahkry M, Naguib M et al 1987 Multiple electrocardiographic anomalies during anaesthesia in an athlete. Canadian Journal of Anaesthesia 34: 284–287

Bullock R E, Hall R J C 1985 Athletic dysrhythmias. A case report. Anaesthesia 40: 647–650

Editorial 1992 Sporting hearts. Lancet 340: 1132–1133

Giannattasio C, Seravalle G, Bolla G B et al 1990 Cardiopulmonary receptor reflexes in normotensive athletes with cardiac hypertrophy. Circulation 82: 1222–1229

Huston T P, Puffer J C, Rodney W M 1985 The athletic heart: syndrome. New England Journal of Medicine 313: 24–32

Kreutz J M, Mazuzan J E 1990 Sudden asystole in a marathon runner: the athletic heart syndrome and its anesthetic implications. Anesthesiology 73: 1266–1268

Levine B D, Lane L, Buckey J C et al 1991 Left ventricular pressure-volume and Frank-Starling relations in endurance athletes. Circulation 84: 1016–1023

Pedoe D T 1983 Sports injuries. Cardiological problems. British Journal of Hospital Medicine 29: 213–220

AUTONOMIC FAILURE

Failure, or dysfunction, of the autonomic nervous system is being increasingly recognized as a complication of a number of disease processes. In familial dysautonomia (Riley–Day syndrome), there is a decrease in all the neuronal populations, as well as a decrease in synthesis of noradrenaline. Dysfunction may be secondary to diabetes, Guillain–Barré syndrome, Parkinson's disease, Shy–Drager syndrome, tetanus, AIDS, postcerebrovascular states, alpha-adrenoceptor blocking drugs, and the peripheral neuropathy of amyloid disease. Occasionally, an acute autonomic neuropathy, of sudden onset, can occur in young people (Hart & Kanter 1990). Sympathetic or parasympathetic systems, or the functions of both, may be affected. Gastroparesis and syncope are the commonest presenting signs, and the cerebrospinal fluid protein level may be increased.

Autonomic dysfunction can be central or peripheral in origin, and may affect sympathetic or parasympathetic nerves. Whilst autonomic failure will produce widespread disturbance of organ function, it is the cardiovascular and respiratory effects which are of particular concern to the anaesthetist.

Preoperative abnormalities

1. Patients exhibit orthostatic hypotension, and an inability, in response to stress, to produce the normal pressor response which depends on reflex vasoconstriction and tachycardia. There is reversal of the usual diurnal pattern of blood pressure and also of that normally produced by postural changes. A number of clinical features of autonomic dysfunction have been described:

   a. Postural hypotension. The blood pressure increases when in the supine position at night, and decreases on standing. A decrease in the systolic blood pressure of 30 mmHg on standing is significant.

   b. Abnormal blood pressure response to the Valsalva manoeuvre. This manoeuvre involves taking a maximum inspiration, blowing into a tube connected to a mercury manometer, and elevating the mercury level to 40 mmHg for 10 seconds. A slow blow-off valve in the system requires the subject to blow continuously to maintain the pressure. Four phases of response are described in normal individuals:

      i. A rapid increase in arterial pressure immediately after the onset of straining, as the intrathoracic pressure is added to systemic arterial pressure.

ii. A decrease in blood pressure, with an associated tachycardia secondary to diminished venous return. Some restoration in pressure occurs later in this phase.

iii. Following the release in straining, there is a sudden brief reduction in pressure.

iv. Finally there is a terminal elevation of pressure above control values, associated with a bradycardia. The release of the Valsalva manoeuvre restores venous pressure and cardiac output at a time when the peripheral vessels are still constricted. The arterial pressure increases above normal, the baroreceptors are stimulated, and a bradycardia occurs until the pressure returns to its normal value.

Since a patient with autonomic failure cannot respond with vasoconstriction, the blood pressure continues to fall during the Valsalva manoeuvre. There is no overshoot in blood pressure when the straining is released, with a gradual return to normal. No tachycardia or bradycardia occurs. In clinical practice this has been difficult to demonstrate without direct arterial monitoring (Brown 1987). However a technique, in which a pulse oximeter is linked to a chart recorder has been described, to show this (Broome & Mason 1988).

2. The R–R variation on the ECG is lost, and there are no heart rate changes on taking six deep breaths.

3. Fluid and electrolyte homeostasis is disturbed, resulting in a failure to concentrate urine at night. There is a nocturnal diuresis and sodium loss (Watson 1987).

Anaesthetic problems

1. Hypotension. Blood pressure is extremely sensitive to changes in extracellular fluid volume, and hypotension may occur on induction of anaesthesia. In a prospective study of 17 diabetic patients having eye surgery, 35% required vasopressors compared with 5% of non-diabetic controls. They were required more often in those with the poorest autonomic function (Burgos et al 1989). Tracheal intubation produces less of a pressor response than is seen in normal patients and, in fact, the first few minutes after tracheal intubation is the period of highest risk for hypotension and bradycardia.

2. Arrhythmias, bradycardias and unexpected cardiac arrest have been described. Atropine-induced heart rate was found to be significantly lower in diabetics than in non-diabetics (Tsueda et al 1991).

3. Respiratory arrest and diminished sensitivity to hypoxia and hypercarbia have been reported (Page & Watkins 1978).

4. The response to catecholamines is variable (Stirt et al 1982). In central dysfunction, the response to indirect-acting catecholamines is normal, and there is no sensitivity to those acting directly. With

peripheral dysfunction, there may be lesser response to indirect-acting catecholamines, but an exaggerated (denervation hypersensitivity) response to those acting directly.

Management

For the problems of the individual diseases, see Diabetes, Familial dysautonomia, Shy-Drager syndrome, Guillain-Barre syndrome, Tetanus, AIDS etc. It is important to realize that autonomic dysfunction exists to varying degrees. It is not an all-or-none phenomenon (Ewing & Clarke 1986).

1. Good management lies in the anticipation of possible problems, close patient monitoring, and the minimization of cardiovascular changes by judicious fluid and drug therapy.
2. ECG and blood pressure should be monitored from the outset of the anaesthetic.
3. All drugs should be given with caution. Hypotension may require a fluid load and intropic agents.
4. The patient's lungs should be ventilated, or respiration closely monitored, particularly in the postoperative period.

BIBLIOGRAPHY
Broome I J, Mason R A 1988 Use of a pulse oximeter for the identification of autonomic dysfunction. Anaesthesia 43: 833–836
Brown M J 1987 The measurement of autonomic function in clinical practice. Journal of the Royal College of Physicians 21: 206–209
Burgos L G, Ebert T J, Asiddao C et al 1989 Increased intraoperative cardiovascular lability in diabetics with autonomic neuropathy. Anesthesiology 70: 591–597
Ewing D J, Clarke B F 1986 Autonomic neuropathy: its diagnosis and prognosis. Clinics in Endocrinology and Metabolism 15: 855–888
Hart R G, Kanter M C 1990 Acute autonomic neuropathy. Two cases and a clinical review. Archives of Internal Medicine 150: 2373–2376
Page M McB, Watkins P J 1978 Cardiorespiratory arrest and diabetic autonomic neuropathy. Lancet 1: 14–16
Stirt J A, Frantz R A, Gunz E F et al 1982 Anesthesia, catecholamines and hemodynamics in autonomic dysfunction. Anesthesia and Analgesia 61: 701–704
Tsueda K, Huang K C, Dumont $ W et al 1991 Cardiac sympathetic tone in anaesthetised diabetics. Canadian Journal of Anaesthesia 38: 20–23
Watson R D S 1987 Treating postural hypotension. British Medical Journal 294: 390–391

BUDD-CHIARI SYNDROME

A syndrome caused by obstruction to the hepatic venous outflow. It may be secondary to haematological disorders, malignancy, oral contraceptives, heart failure or constrictive pericarditis. The site of the obstruction may be anywhere from the inferior vena cava to the smaller hepatic veins. The condition may be acute or chronic. Acute Budd–Chiari syndrome with hepatocyte necrosis may require urgent portosystemic decompressive surgery. Untreated hepatic venous thrombosis Usually results in progressive liver failure and death. Medical treatment is of little help, therefore surgery may be required for shunt procedures or liver transplantation (Gupta et al 1986, Klein et al 1990).

Preoperative abnormalities

1. Ascites and hepatomegaly will be present in the majority of cases. Abdominal pain, splenic enlargement, jaundice or bleeding from oesophageal varices may also occur. If the vena cava is involved there will be dependent oedema.
2. Liver function abnormalities depend on the site and severity of the obstruction. Liver biopsy may show outflow obstruction, hepatic necrosis and fibrosis.
3. Aetiological factors include polycythaemia, paroxysmal nocturnal haemoglobinuria, protein C deficiency, myeloproliferative disorders and mechanical factors such as webs and tumours.
4. Treatment is aimed at the preservation of liver function and includes thrombolysis, angioplasty, portacaval shunt, mesoatrial shunt and liver transplant (Henderson et al 1990).

Anaesthetic problems

1. Hepatic function may be compromised
2. Surgery may be required for portacaval or mesoatrial shunt or liver transplant. This has been described in a patient with paroxysmal nocturnal haemoglobinuria (Taylor et al 1987).
3. Postpartum Budd-Chiari syndrome may occur in association with prolonged hypercoagulability, in spite of high-dose anticoagulant treatment (Ilan et al 1990).

Management

1. Haematological examination is important because, in the absence of mechanical causes for hepatic vein thrombosis, there is a high incidence of underlying haematological abnormalities (Boughton 1991); these include myeloproliferative disorders, paroxysmal nocturnal haemoglobinuria, systemic lupus erythematosus and antithrombin III deficiency.
2. Assessment of liver function, including coagulation studies.
3. Low-dose heparin infusion from the first postoperative day has been recommended (Henderson et al 1990), with subsequent low-dose aspirin and l0ng-term anticoagulation to reduce the risks of graft thrombosis.

BIBLIOGRAPHY
Boughton B J 1991 Hepatic and portal vein thrombosis. Closely associated with chronic myeloproliferative disorder. British Medical Journal 302: 192–193
Gupta S, Blumgart L H, Hodgson H J F 1986 Budd-Chiari syndrome: Long-term

survival and factors affecting mortality. Quarterly Journal of Medicine 60: 781–791

Henderson J M, Warren W D, Millikan W J et al 1990 Surgical options, hematologic evaluation, and pathologic changes in Budd-Chiari syndrome. American Journal of Surgery 159: 41–48

Ilan Y, Oren R, Shouval D 1990 Postpartum Budd-Chiari syndrome with prolonged hypercoagulability state. American Journal of Obstetrics and Gynecology 162: 1164–1165

Klein A S, Sitzmann J V, Coleman J et al 1990 Current management of the Budd-Chiari syndrome. Annals of Surgery 212: 144–149

Taylor M B, Whitwam J C, Worsley A 1987 Paroxysmal nocturnal haemoglobinuria. Perioperative management of a patient with Budd-Chiari syndrome. Anaesthesia 42: 639–642

BUERGER'S DISEASE

A type of occlusive peripheral vascular disease which, until recently, predominantly affected young men. Some changes in the disease spectrum are being observed (Olin et al 1990). An increasing number of women, more common involvement of the upper extremity and its occurrence in older patients are being reported. There is a strong association with smoking. The disease primarily affects small vessels of the feet, legs and hands, and is exacerbated by vasospasm. The aetiology is not fully understood but there may be an irnmunological component. Abnormal responses to type I and III collagen have been demonstrated. The intense inflammation of the early stages progresses to fibrous encasement of the whole neurovascular bundle.

Preoperative abnormalities

1. Raynaud's disease, non-healing ulcers or gangrene of the feet may occur, even in the presence of femoral and popliteal pulses. The hands may be similarly affected. Frequently there is preceding or accompanying phlebitis.
2. Peripheral pulses are reduced or absent. Allen's test may show a poor collateral circulation to the hand.
3. Patients may be improved by stopping smoking and sympathectomy.

Anaesthetic problems

1. Intra-arterial cannulation for blood pressure monitoring is not usually recommended, and indirect Doppler methods are advised. However, in major procedures there may be over-riding indications for direct pressure measurements.
2. Analgesia may be needed for peripheral ischaemia.

Management

1. Axillary artery pressure monitoring in a patient with Buerger's disease and an intracranial aneurysm has been described (Yacoub et al 1987). A continuous axillary brachial plexus block was established prior to cannulation of the axillary artery with a 20-G catheter. Care was taken to maintain the patient's core temperature with a warming blanket, and there was minimal reduction in arterial pressure during clipping of the aneurysm.
2. Continuous local anaesthesia via a silastic catheter inserted in the region of the median nerve for pain relief has been reported (Saddler & Crosse 1988).

BIBLIOGRAPHY

Olin J W, Young J R, Graor R A et al 1990 The changing clinical spectrum of thromboangiitis obliterans. Circulation 82 (suppl IV): 3–8

Saddler J M, Crosse M M 1988 Ischaemic pain in Buerger's disease Anaesthesia 43: 305–306

Yacoub O F, Bacaling J H, Kelly M 1987 Monitoring of axillary arterial pressure in a patient with Buerger's disease requiring clipping of an intracerebral aneurysm. British Journal of Anaesthesia 59: 1059–1062

Section 1

Burns

BURNS

For the anaesthetist who is only occasionally involved in the management of patients with thermal injury, two particular aspects are likely to be of concern:

1. The immediate resuscitation of the patient before transfer to a specialist unit (Ellis & Rylah 1990).
2. The surgical treatment of a previously burned patient at some time after the original incident

Presenting problems

1. Loss of water, solutes and albumin from the damaged area. The amount will depend upon the area and thickness burned and the time since injury.
2. Airway and lung problems. These may consist of:
   a. Heat injury to the upper respiratory tract with possible mucosal oedema.
   b. Systemic carbon monoxide poisoning, which may be fatal.
   c. Cyanide poisoning.
   d. Chemical damage to the lungs from acid smoke constituents.
   e. Sepsis.
3. Provision of adequate analgesia and sedation, in the presence of altered pharmacodynamics.
4. The stress response to burns. Levels of circulating catecholamines and cortisol are raised and the metabolic rate is increased. There is a

high incidence of acute gastric erosions and stress ulcers, which develop within the first 72 hours.

5. Vasoactive mediators, released from the burn, increase vascular permeability and cause cell membrane defects which contribute to intracellular swelling. They may also be involved in the development of the respiratory distress syndrome, which can present as late as the fourth day.

6. Bacterial invasion of the burned tissue.

7. Anaesthesia for surgery at some time after the burn incident, with particular reference to the altered response to neuromuscular blocking agents.

Management

1. Resuscitation.

Initially, assessment is directed to the extent and thickness of the burns, in order to calculate colloid and crystalloid replacement. The aim is to maintain cardiac output and renal blood flow, but to minimize oedema of burned and non-burned tissue. In general, fluid replacement is required for burns of >15% in adults and of >10% for children. Established protocols are available and should be used. Disagreement still exists as to whether colloid or crystalloid should be used. A mixture is probably appropriate (Brown 1985). An estimate of the percentage area burned can be calculated by knowing the approximate normal distribution of surface area: thorax 18%, abdomen 18%, legs 18% each, arms 9% each, and the head 9%. This distribution differs in children and particularly in babies. A number of methods of calculation have been recommended. In the absence of an established protocol, the following may act as a guide prior to transfer.

A = Colloid   1 ml × % burns × wt in kg
B = Crystalloid   1 ml × % burns × cvt in kg
C = Metabolic water requirements 1000 ml, or more if needed

For the first day of burn give:

2A + 8 + C (half of which should be given in the first 8 hours, the other half in the next 16 hours)

The colloid may be albumin solution, Haemaccel or Gelofusine. The aim is to maintain a normal Hct and a urine output of greater than 50 ml per hour, a pulse of <120/min and a sodium excretion of >30 mmol/l.

2. Respiratory problems.

a. If heat injury has occurred, fibreoptic bronchoscopy may be indicated to establish its extent. Occasionally, laryngeal oedema occurs.

b. Carbon monoxide combines with haemoglobin to form carboxyhaemoglobin (HbCO). The affinity of carbon monoxide for haemoglobin is such that a concentration of 0.1% can reduce the oxygen carrying capacity by 50%, and the oxygen dissociation curve is shifted to the left. On admission, 100% oxygen is given and HbCO estimated (Armstrong 1985).

c. Some fatalities have been noted to have high blood cyanide levels which, although difficult to measure in the acute situation, have been reported to correlate well with HbCO levels. If the latter is increased, cyanide poisoning should be considered.

d. Smoke contains carbon particles, gases and vapours which may cause chemical damage to the alveoli. Respiratory parameters, including blood gases, require close monitoring since deterioration may indicate the onset of pulmonary oedema or acute ARDS. An increasing respiratory rate, a Pao_2 of <11 kPa on 40% O_2, and a shunt of greater than 15% are indicators of the need for tracheal intubation and PEEP. Tracheostomy should be avoided if possible. Steroids are ineffective and may increase morbidity and mortality.

3. Pain relief is a problem both in the acute stage and later, during changes of dressings.

   a. Opiates may be required acutely before transfer. Although initial studies on burned patients have indicated no difference in the pharmacokinetics of morphine when compared with normal subjects, the narcotic requirements are generally increased (Martyn 1986). Fears of addiction are theoretical. A large survey in the USA did not reveal a single case.
   Intravenous analgesia is required initially, and patient controlled analgesia has been shown to be safe and effective (Choiniere et al 1992).

   b. Self-administration of Entonox is useful for dressings, analgesia beginning after 20 seconds, with a peak effect between 40 seconds and 2 minutes.

   c. Low-dose ketamine. This has been suggested for short-term pain relief. The use of ketamine 0.1% solution in 5% dextrose, by slow i.v. infusion and adjusted according to effect (Ito & Ichiyanagi 1974), or as an i.m. dose of 0.5 mg/kg (Grant et al 1981), has been reported.

4. Antacids and cimetidine 5–6 mg/kg 6 hourly, or ranitidine, are given in the first 24 hours.

5. Subsequent surgery.

   a. Suxamethonium is well known to release massive amounts of potassium in burned patients from the 20th to 60th day. There is now evidence that this response may last for up to 2 years. It is suggested that, following burns, instead of being present only at the motor end-plates, acetylcholine receptors spread throughout the whole muscle. Since suxamethonium is structurally similar to acetylcholine, then potassium is released from the whole membrane (Demling 1985). However, studies on children have also shown that extreme sensitivity to the effects of small doses of suxamethonium may occur between day 4 and 12 following the burn (Brown & Bell 1987). In addition, resistance to non-depolarizing relaxants has been noted and larger than normal doses may have to be used. A number of mechanisms may be responsible. Neuromuscular monitoring of these patients is essential.

b. The use of alfentanil (1.24 μ/kg per min) and propofol (100 μ/kg per min) infusions has been reported (Reyneke et al 1989). It was found that alfentanil needed to be discontinued 15 minutes before the propofol to avoid respiratory depression.

BIBLIOGRAPHY

Armstrong R F 1985 Burns and the inhalation injury. In: Anaesthesia review 3. Churchill Livingstone, Edinburgh

Brown J M 1985 Thermal injury. In: Recent advances in anaesthesia 15. Churchill Livingstone, Edinburgh

Brown T C K, Bell B 1987 Electromyographic responses to small doses of suxamethonium in children after burns. British Journal of Anaesthesia 59: 1017–1021

Choiniere M, Grenier R, Paquette C 1992 Patient-controlled analgesia: a double-blind study in bum patients. Anaesthesia 47: 467–472

Demling R H 1985 Burns. New England Journal of Medicine 313: 1389–1398

Ellis A, Rylah T A 1990 Transfer of the thermally injured patient. British Journal of Hospital Medicine 44: 20–211

Grant I 5, Nimmo W 5, Clements J A 1981 Pharmacolunehcs and Analgesic effects of i.m. and oral ketamine. British Journal of Anaesthesia 53: 805–810

Ito Y, Ichiyanagi K 1974 Postoperative pain relief with ketamine infusion. Anaesthesia 29: 222–229

Martyn J 1986 Clinical pharmacology and drug therapy in the burned patient. Anesthesiology 65: 67–75

Reyneke C J, James M F M, Johnson R 1989 Alfentanil and propofol infusions for surgery in the burned patient. British Journal of Anaesthesia 63: 418–422

CARCINOID SYNDROME
(see also Section 2)

Carcinoids are gastrointestinal tumours which arise from the fore-, mid- and hindgut. Mid-gut tumours are the commonest, 36–46% occurring in the appendix. Less than 25% of tumours produce the carcinoid syndrome, and the symptoms are probably proportional to the amount of secreting tissue present. Serotonin (5-hydroxytryptamine) and the bradylunins are the commonest hormones produced. More recently the role of the tachykinins (neuropeptides which include substance P, neurokinin A and neuropeptide K) has become apparent. Elevated plasma tachykinin levels have been found in nearly 80% of carcinoid tumours.

The majority of patients with the syndrome have liver metastases. Exceptions to this are the tumours from which the venous blood passes directly into the systemic circulation (e.g. bronchial and ovarian). In most cases, the liver inactivates the hormones, and no symptoms are produced.

The advent of somatostatin analogues has dramatically improved the medical control of carcinoid symptoms and the management of the perioperative period (Editorial 1989, Wynick & Bloom 1991). Five patients treated with octreotide, prepared for surgery or embolization, showed decreased basal and provoked release of 5-HT and had no intraoperative complications. Two patients who had not initially been given octreotide, developed severe crises on induction of anaesthesia which responded to i.v. octreotide (Ahlman et al 1988). The crises correlated well with extremely high levels of 5-HT in the arterial blood. The main therapeutic indications are: failure to control symptoms with surgery or other drugs, unfitness of the patient for surgery, and as prophylaxis during surgery or investigative procedures (Woods et al 1990).

Preoperative abnormalities

1. Serotonin can cause diarrhoea, hypertension and tachycardia, mild hyperglycaemia, hypoproteinaemia and possibly flushing.
2. Bradykinin, if secreted, causes flushing, hypotension, bronchospasm and increased capillary permeability. The latter results in oedema and loss of electrolytes from the vascular compartment. A careful history may help to indicate whether or not significant amounts of bradykinins are being secreted.
3. The tachykinins cause vasodilatation and possibly play a role in bronchospasm and fibrosis of the cardiac valves.
4. Other vasoactive peptides such as histamine and prostaglandins may be involved, but their part in the syndrome has not been elucidated.
5. Preoperative investigations should include the urinary 5-hydroxyindole acetic acid levels which will be increased, and blood glucose which may be elevated. Liver scan and LFTs may be abnormal, with raised liver enzyme levels and hypoproteinaemia.
6. In some cases there may be tricuspid or pulmonary valve disease secondary to chronic serotonin secretion.
7. Pharmacological treatment may involve inhibitors of 5-HT synthesis, peripheral 5-HT antagonists and inhibitors of 5-HT release (Saini & Waxman 1991).

Anaesthetic problems

A small number of patients with carcinoid syndrome have developed serious cardiovascular complications during anaesthesia. These may be due to secretion of hormones by the tumour, provoked by mechanical, biochemical or pharmacological stimuli. Symptoms are proportional to the amount and nature of the hormone produced, and certainly the prognosis has been found to be related to the level of 5-HIAA excreted at the time of diagnosis. This is poor if excretion is greater than 1000 µg/24 hours (Coupe et al 1990). Flush, hyperperistalsis and bronchoconstriction resulted in prolonged postoperative problems after cardiac valve replacement. The use of octreotide improved these (Lundin et al 1990). General anaesthesia is not always implicated. A fatal acute crisis occurred immediately after fine-needle liver biopsy of liver metastases (Bissonnette et al 1990) and a non-fatal one after bronchial biopsy (Sukamaran et al 1982). Both of these procedures were performed under local anaesthesia.

1. Serotonin is invariably produced, and if secreted in excess during anaesthesia is thought to cause hyperkinetic states of hypertension and tachycardia (Casthely et al 1986, Hughes & Hodkinson 1989), certain types of flushing, and prolonged recovery.
2. Bradykinins may or may not be secreted. Their possible effects include hypotension (Marsh et al 1987) secondary to both vasodilatation and increased capillary permeability, flushing and bronchospasm (Miller et al 1980). The bradykinin effects seem to be the most life-threatening.
3. Tachykinins (substance P, neurokinin A and neuropeptide K). These primarily cause vasodilatation, but in some cases they may be associated with flushing. However, in other patients, the flush may occur in the absence of a detectable increase in circulating tachykinins.
4. Other vasoactive substances, such as prostaglandins and histamine, may be secreted but their significance is still not clear.

Management

1. Treatment of heart failure and hypoproteinaemia, if present.
2. Adequate preparation both for surgery and investigative radiological or bronchoscopic procedures.
3. Drugs used to block the release of mediators from the tumour, or to block the actions of the mediators. The mainstay of treatment is now the somatostatin analogue, octreotide. However, most authors still report the supplementary use of other drugs with antiserotonin and antibradykinin properties.
    a. Somatostatin analogues have been found to inhibit the release of active mediators from carcinoid tumours. Octreotide (Sandostatin, Sandoz SMS 201–995) has been used both prophylactically as a preparation for surgery (Roy et al 1987, Watson et al 1990), and for emergency treatment of a carcinoid crisis (Marsh et al 1987, Lundin et al 1990).

Preoperative: octreotide 100 μg s.c., b.d. or t.d.s. prior to surgery.
Intraoperative: octreotide 50–100 μg i.v. to heat a carcinoid crisis

b. Specific antiserotonin therapy.

Cyproheptadine is a non-specific antihistamine. Ketanserin is a selective antagonist at 5-HT2 receptors, alpha-1 adrenoceptors and H1, histamine receptors.

Preoperative:

EITHER   cyproheptadine 4 mg t.d.s. for 3 days and 4 mg with the premedication.

OR   ketanserin 40 mg b.d. for 3 days (if available).

Intraoperative:

In attempts to treat hypertension and tachycardia arising during anaesthesia, a variety of antiserotoninergic drugs have been used. These have included methotrimeprazine 2.5 mg i.v. (Mason & Steane 1976), cyproheptadine 1 mg i.v. (Solares et al 1987), ketanserin 10 mg given over a period of 3 minutes and then an infusion of 3 mg/h (Fischler et al 1983, Hughes & Hodkinson 1989). The choice is often governed by the availability of the particular drug.

c. Specific antibradykinin therapy. Now largely historical, but has included aprotinin (an infusion of 200 000 kiu, set up 1 hour before surgery and continued 4-hourly) and corticosteroids.
Reports of their effectiveness in treating complications have been mixed and octreotide has now replaced specific antibradykinin therapy.

d. The role of histamine is uncertain. Flushing in a patient with a gastric carcinoid was blocked by a combination of H1, and H2 antagonists (Roberts et al 1979).

4. Anaesthetic drugs. Morphine should be avoided because of histamine release. Suxamethonium fasciculations may increase intra-abdominal pressure and release tumour hormones. D-tubocurarine and alcuronium cause undesirable hypotension. Pancuronium or vecuronium are probably the most appropriate neuromuscular blockers.

5. Vasopressors of the catecholamine type, or those which act by the release of catecholamines, may activate tumour kallilkrein, which is the inactive precursor of bradykinin. However, the successful use of adrenaline has been reported following cardiopulmonary bypass, when the hypotension was thought not to have been carcinoid in origin (Hamid & Harris 1992).

6. Regional anaesthesia does not block the effect of the hormones on the receptors, and hypotension may precipitate a bradykininergic crisis. Uneventful extradural anaesthesia for transurethral resection of the prostate has, however, been reported in a patient treated with octreotide and other antihormonal drugs (Monteith & Roaseg 1990).

BIBLIOGRAPHY

Ahlman H, Ahlund L, Dahlstrom A et al 1988 SMS 201–995 and provocation tests in preparation of patients with carcinoids for surgery or hepatic arterial embolization. Anesthesia and Analgesia 67: 1142–1148

Bissonnette R T, Gibney R G, Berry B R et al 1990 Fatal carcinoid crisis after percutaneous fine-needle biopsy of hepatic metastasis: case report and review of the literature. Radiology 174: 751–752

Casthely P A, Jablons M, Griepp R B et al 1986 Ketanserin in the preoperative and intraoperative management of a patient with carcinoid tumour undergoing tricuspid valve replacement. Anesthesia and Analgesia 65: 809–811

Coupe M, Levi S, Ellis M et al 1989 Therapy for symptoms in the carcinoid syndrome. Quarterly Journal of Medicine 73: 1021–1036

Editorial 1989 Octreotide. Lancet ii: 541–542

Fischler M, Dentan M, Westerman M N et al 1983 Prophylactic use of ketanserin in a patient with carcinoid syndrome. British Journal of Anaesthesia 55: 920

Hamid S K, Harris D N F 1992 Hypotension following valve replacement surgery in carcinoid heart disease. Anaesthesia 47: 490–492

Hughes E W, Hodldnson B P 1989 Carcinoid syndrome: the combined use of ketanserin and octreotide in the management of an acute crisis during anaesthesia. Anaesthesia and Intensive Care 17: 367–370

Lundin L, Hansson H-E, Landelius J et al 1990 Surgical treatment of carcinoid heart disease. Journal of Thoracic and Cardiovascular Surgery 100: 552–561

Marsh H M, Martin J K, Kvols L K et al 1987 Carcinoid crisis during anaesthesia: successful treatment with a somatostatin analogue. Anesthesiology 66: 89–91

Mason R A, Steane P A 1976 Carcinoid syndrome: its relevance to the anaesthetist. Anaesthesia 31: 228–242

Miller R, Boulukos P A, Warner R RI P 1980 Failure of halothane and ketamine to alleviate carcinoid syndrome-induced bronchospasm during anaesthesia. Anesthesia and Analgesia 59: 621–623

Monteith K, Roaseg O P 1990 Epidural anaesthesia for transurethral resection of the prostate in a patient with the carcinoid syndrome. Canadian Journal of Anaesthesia 37: 349–352

Roberts L J II, Marney S R Jr, Oates J A 1979 Blockade of the flush associated with metastatic gastric carcinoid by combined histamine H1 and H2 receptor antagonists. New England Journal of Medicine 300: 236–238

Roy R C, Carter R F, Wright P D 1987 Somatostatin, anaesthesia and the carcinoid syndrome. Anaesthesia 42: 627–632

Saini A, Waxman J 1991 Management of carcinoid syndrome. Postgraduate Medical Journal 67: 506–508.

Solares G, Blanco E, Pulgar S et al 1987 Carcinoid syndrome and intravenous cyproheptadine. anaesthesia 42: 989–992

Sukumaran M, Wilkinson Z S, Christianson L 1982 Acute carcinoid syndrome: a complication of flexible fibreoptic bronchoscopy. Annals of Thoracic Surgery 34: 702-705

Watson J T, Badner N H, Ali M J 1990 The prophylactic use of octreotide in a patient with ovarian carcinoma and valvular heart disease. Canadian Journal of Anaesthesia 37: 798–800

Woods H F, Bax N D, Ainsworth I 1990 Abdominal carcinoid tumours in Sheffield. Digestion 45: 17–22

Wynick D, Bloom S R 1991 Clinical review 23. The use of long-acting somatostatin analog octreotide in the treatment of gut neuroendocrine tumours. Journal of Clinical Endocrinology and Metabolism 73: 1–3.

CARDIAC TAMPONADE
(see also Section 2)

Can occur when a pericardial effusion (or a collection of blood within the pericardial cavity) restricts, by the effect of external pressure, cardiac filling during diastole. When the pericardium becomes no longer distensible, small volume increases produce a rapid increase in pericardial pressure. There is a fixed decreased diastolic volume of both ventricles. In inspiration, the right ventricle fills at the expense of the left, and the left ventricular stroke volume falls producing pulsus paradoxus, a cardinal sign. A tachycardia and systemic vasoconstriction will initially compensate for the decrease in cardiac output. Signs of respiratory distress then supervene and sudden cardiac arrest may occur. Malignant disease is the cause; infection, trauma, postcardiac surgery, pacemaker or CVP line insertion, intracardiac injection and anticoagulants are others. The long-term prognosis is related to the cause, irrespective of treatment (Markiewicz et al 1986).

Preoperative abnormalities

1. An elevated CVP, rapid low-volume pulse, hypotension, and reflex systemic arterial and venous vasoconstriction. The fixed, low cardiac output may be aggravated by straining at stool, or on the assumption of the supine position. Straining may cause syncope (Keon 1981). In a study of 36 patients, the majority had respiratory distress, jugular venous distension, heart rate >90/min, cardiomegaly and pulsus paradoxus (Markiewicz et al 1986).
2. Pulsus paradoxus. Normally on inspiration there is a slight decrease in systolic blood pressure. In cardiac tamponade this decrease is accentuated, usually to greater than 10 mmHg, and sometimes to in excess of 20 mmHg. Pulsus paradoxus is easily detected by palpation, but may be measured by an auscultation method (Lake 1983). Using a sphygmomanometer, the cuff pressure should first be reduced until the sound is intermittent, then deflation continued until all the beats are heard. The difference between the two pressures is then measured.
3. Respiratory distress occurs, especially when lying down.
4. If the collection of fluid is greater than 250 ml, the CXR may show an enlarged, globular cardiac outline, the left border of which may be straight or even convex. The right cardiophrenic angle will be less than 90°. The lung fields are clear. The diagnosis can be confirmed by echocardiography (Horgan 1987).

Anaesthetic problems

1. Induction of anaesthesia in the presence of cardiac tamponade may be fatal. Abolition of the vasoconstrictor compensation will cause cardiovascular collapse. A fatal cardiac arrest during a halothane induction in a 9-year-old boy who was due to have a cervical node biopsy has been reported (Keon 1981). The patient had a mild degree of respiratory distress, worse in the supine position. Before admission, an episode of loss of consciousness with peripheral

cyanosis had occurred whilst straining at stool. Postmortem examination showed a large malignant lymphoma which enveloped the heart and infiltrated the pericardium. Profound hypotension after induction of anaesthesia in a patient involved in a mountaineering accident was the first sign of tamponade (Cyna et al 1990). Immediate restoration of arterial pressure occurred after incision of the pericardium. An asymptomatic pericardial effusion in a young woman with seropositive rheumatoid arthritis presented with cardiovascular collapse after induction of anaesthesia for abdominal surgery (Bellamy et al 1990). Fenestration of the pericardium decreased the CVP from 24 mmHg to 10 mmHg.

2. Sudden drainage of a chronic cardiac tamponade may cause acute haemodynamic changes and pulmonary oedema (Vandyke et al 1983, Downey et al 1991). This gradually resolves over 24 hours. In one patient a volume of 500 ml of pericardial fluid had been removed. Full haemodynamic monitoring was being undertaken and in both cases there was a sudden increase in pulmonary artery pressure after pericardiocentesis. In cardiac tamponade it is the right, rather than the left, ventricle that is compressed. After release of the tamponade there is sudden overload of the left ventricle while the PVR is still high. Acute dilatation of the thinner walled right ventricle, and temporary mismatch between the outputs of the two ventricles were thought to have been responsible for the pulmonary oedema in these cases.

3. Occasionally, isolated right atrial compression, which may be difficult to diagnose, can occur following cardiac surgery (Skacel et al 1991). A pulmonary artery catheter was in use and normal pressures were found in all chambers except the right atrium. There was also a CVP to right ventricular end-diastolic gradient. The chest was re-explored and right atrial compression from bleeding was found. In this case, the pulmonary artery catheter helped to exclude other causes.

Management

1. Monitor direct arterial and central venous pressures.
2. Minimize the factors which worsen the haemodynamic situation. These are:
   a. An increase in intrathoracic pressure. If IPPV is already being undertaken, for example after cardiac surgery, then PEEP should be avoided. This further reduces cardiac output, especially at slow rates of ventilation (Mattila et al 1984). Otherwise, the maintenance of spontaneous respiration until relief of the tamponade is imminent has been recommended (Moller et al 1979). High-frequency jet ventilation (HFJV) was found to produce less decrease in stroke volume in experimentally-induced

cardiac tamponade than continuous mandatory ventilation (CMV) (Goto et al 1990).
  b. Low intravascular volume. The blood volume must be maintained with i.v. fluids according to the haemodynamic responses.
  c. Decreased myocardial contractility. Dopamine is thought to have a favourable effect on haemodynamics, even in the presence of severe tamponade (Mattila et al 1984). Should general anaesthesia be essential, diazepam has been recommended to prevent the reduction in ventricular filling pressure caused by thiopentone.
3. Relief of tamponade. If possible, needle pericardiocentesis, with or without catheter insertion, should be performed under local anaesthesia (Stanley & Weidauer 1973, Horgan 1987). ECG and radiological screening should be used, with facilities for emergency thoracotomy available. A subxiphoid approach can be used in which the needle enters the angle between the xiphisternum and the left costal margin, and is aimed towards the left shoulder (Cobbe 1980, John & Treasure 1990). A Seldinger technique with insertion of a soft catheter should be used. Continuous gentle aspiration assists identification of the pericardial sac. Safety may be increased by the use of a sterile ECG lead attached to the needle. An alternative apical approach can be made through the fifth intercostal space on the left side. More recently, a technique of percutaneous balloon periocardiotomy has been described. This involves passage of a guidewire into the pericardium via a subxiphoid approach, draining the effusion with a pigtail catheter, then dilating the pericardium with a balloon dilating catheter. The pigtail catheter can be left in situ for 24 hours. This technique may have a place in the management of malignant pericardial effusions, since it carries less risk than open surgery (Keane & Jackson 1992). It has been suggested that, in chronic tamponade, fluid be removed gradually, with close monitoring of haemodynamics to prevent the occurrence of pulmonary oedema (Vandyke et al 1983). Since symptomatic improvement occurs with the removal of the first 50–200 ml of fluid withdrawn, there is no urgency to fully decompress the heart. Other complications include laceration of the ventricular wall or a coronary artery, pneumothorax or perforation of a viscus (John & Treasure 1990).

BIBLIOGRAPHY
Bellamy M C, Natarajan V, Lenz R J 1990 An unusual presentation of cardiac tamponade. Anaesthesia 45: 135–136.
Cobbe S M 1980 Pericardial effusions. British Journal of Hospital Medicine 23: 250–255.
Cyna A M, Rodgers R C, McFarlane H 1990 Hypotension due to unexpected cardiac tamponade. Anaesthesia 45: 140–142
Downey R J, Bessler M, Weissman C 1991 Acute pulmonary oedema following pericardiocentesis for chronic cardiac tamponade secondary to trauma. Critical Care Medicine 19 1323–1325

Goto K, Goto K, Benson K T et al 1990 Efficacy of high-frequency jet ventilation in cardiac tamponade. Anesthesia and Analgesia 70: 375–381

Horgan J H 1987 Cardiac tamponade. British Medical Journal 295: 563

John R M, Treasure T 1990 How to aspirate the pericardium. British Journal of Hospital Medicine 43: 221–223

Keane D, Jackson G 1992 Managing recurrent malignant pericardial effusions. Percutaneous balloon pericardiotomy may have a role. British Medical Journal 305: 729–730

Keon T P 1981 Death on induction of anesthesia for cervical node biopsy. Anesthesiology 55: 471–472

Lake C L 1983 Anesthesia and pericardial disease. Anesthesia and Analgesia 62: 431–443

Markiewicz W, Borovik R, Ecker S 1986 Cardiac tamponade in medical patients; treatment and prognosis in the ethocardiographic era. American Heart Journal 111: 1138–1142

Mattila I, Talkunen O, Mattila P et al 1984 Cardiac tamponade and different modes of ventilation. Acta Anaesthesiologica Scandinavica 28: 236–240

Moller C T, Schoonbee C G, Rosendorff C 1979 Haemodynamics of cardiac tamponade during various modes of ventilation. British Journal of Anaesthesia 51: 409–415

Skacel M, Harrison G A, Verdi I S 1991 A case of isolated right atrial compression following cardiac surgery. The value of pulmonary artery catheterisation. Anaesthesia and intensive Care 19: 114–115

Stanley T H, Weidauer H E 1973 Anesthesia for the patient with cardiac tamponade. Anesthesia and Analgesia 52: 110–114

Vandyke W H, Cure J, Chakko C 5 et al 1983 Pulmonary edema after pericardiocentesis for cardiac tamponade. New England Journal of Medicine 309: 595–596

CARDIOMYOPATHIES

A group of diseases of unknown aetiology, affecting cardiac muscle. There are three main pathophysiological groups, diagnosed by echocardiography (Oakley 1987):

1. Dilated (congestive) cardiomyopathy, in which there is a decrease in contractile force in the left or right ventricle, resulting in systolic failure. It may be associated with a number of conditions including those of toxic (e.g. alcohol), metabolic, neurological and inflammatory origins. Peripartum cardiomyopathy is a dilated form specifically associated with late pregnancy or the first 5 months of the puerperium. A small group remain who have idiopathic dilated cardiomyopathy, and in whom no obvious cause can be found (Caforio et al 1990).

2. Hypertrophic (obstructive) cardiomyopathy (HOCM) is an autosomal dominant inherited condition in which there is often massive ventricular hypertrophy and impaired diastolic function.

3. In restrictive cardiomyopathy (Wilmshurst & Katritsis 1990) there is a loss of ventricular distensibility, which can be secondary to either endocardial or myocardial problems. There is a restriction to diastolic filling, resembling constrictive pericarditis. This is a rare form of cardiomyopathy.

Preoperative abnormalities

1. Dilated cardiomyopathy (Johnson & Palacios 1982).
   There is a marked reduction in ejection fraction (often <0.4 when heart failure supervenes). The heart becomes dilated and there is often increased peripheral resistance to compensate. Vasodilators and ACE inhibitors therefore form part of the treatment, which aims to reduce the myocardial work. Systemic embolism can occur, and when arrhythmias (chronic AF or non-sustained ventricular tachycardia) supervene, the patient should be anticoagulated indefinitely. In idiopathic, dilated cardiomyopathy there is a high incidence of sudden death, which suggests an arrhythmic cause (Caforio et al 1990).

2. Hypertrophic cardiomyopathy (HOCM, idiopathic hypertrophic subaortic stenosis).
   The hypertrophy and fibrosis mostly affects the septum, but may involve the whole of the left ventricle. There is resistance to inflow, and therefore diastolic failure is the main problem in advanced disease. The patient may present with dyspnoea, dizziness, syncope, angina or arrhythmias. Sudden death can occur, particularly during physical exercise (Editorial 1992). Whilst sinus rhythm is usual, the late onset of atrial fibrillation is ominous. An apical and left stemal edge systolic murmur may occur. The patient may be on beta adrenoceptor blockers to prevent tachycardias, or calcium channel blockers to improve myocardial relaxation and hence pressure/volume relationships (Lorell et al 1982). Again, the risks of systemic embolism may necessitate anticoagulation.

   The ECG shows left ventricular hypertrophy, and often Q waves and ST- and T-wave changes. CXR usually shows slight cardiomegaly. May occur as part of Noonan's syndrome.

3. Restrictive cardiomyopathy.
   Individual features of this rare condition are extremely variable and depend on the underlying cause. Loss of ventricular distensibility secondary to rigidity imposed by endocardial or myocardial disease is the main feature. One type is associated with marked eosinophilia. In this there is a reduction in the ventricular cavity size and distortion of the AV valves. Again, there are diastolic filling problems, with a picture resembling constrictive pericarditis. The endocardial disease may produce thromboembolic problems.
   Diuretics and vasodilators may be deleterious, and digitalis and beta adrenoceptor blockers should be used cautiously.

Summary

Cardio-myopathy	Primary problem	Presentation	Principal treatment	Avoid
Dilated	Systolic	Heart failure Arrhythmias Systemic embolism	Diuretics Anticoagulants Vasodilators ACE inhibitors	Myocardial depressants
Hypertrophic	Diastolic	Dyspnoea Syncope Angina Arrhythmias	Amiodarone Anticoagulants Beta blockers Ca antagonists	Digoxin Beta stimulators Vasodilators Hypotensives
Restrictive	Diastolic	Eosinophilia Heart failure	Steroids Cytotoxics	Morphine Vasodilators Diureticsy

Anaesthetic problems

In advanced cases of these three disease types, the pathophysiology is extremely variable and the effect of anaesthesia unpredictable. If the diagnosis is known in advance, then expert cardiological assessment is essential. However, in many cases, the condition mimics ischaemic or hypertensive heart disease, or may be unrecognized until an anaesthetic causes decompensation. More detailed advice should be obtained from the bibliography, but a broad outline is described.

1. Dilated cardiomyopathy
   a. Myocardial depressants may precipitate acute cardiac failure. In pregnancy, decompensation usually occurs in association with the periods of maximum haemodynamic change. The peak increase in blood volume (35–40%) and cardiac output (30–40%) occurs in the third trimester. In labour and immediately postpartum there is a further increase in venous return and cardiac output. Thus, peripartum cardiac failure may occur either in late pregnancy (Dodds et al 1991, Lavies & Turner 1989, Brown et al 1992) or at delivery. Three cases of unexpected peripartum cardiomyopathy each presented with acute pulmonary oedema at Caesarean section (Malinow et al 1985, Brown et al 1992). One occurred during spinal anaesthesia, and two after a general anaesthetic. Postoperative echocardiography showed dilated, hypokinetic ventricles, which subsequently returned to normal. The prognosis in the dilated form is, in general, poor but the peripartum disease is variable. Some patients die in the acute phase, some have chronic cardiac problems, whilst others will make a complete recovery but may relapse in subsequent pregnancies (O'Connell et al 1986). If cardiomegaly persists at the onset of the next pregnancy, the mortality may be as high as 60%.
   b. Arrhythmias are common and sudden death can occur. Cardiac arrest followed SVT after induction of anaesthesia in a young man having day-case surgery (Hanson 1989). A mild tachycardia

and infrequent ventricular ectopics had been present on induction, and anaesthesia was induced with thiopentone 600 mg, atropine 1 mg and lignocaine 400 mg. Subsequent investigation showed a dilated cardiomyopathy.

2. Hypertrophic cardiomyopathy (HOCM)

   a. Tachycardias from emotion, exercise and pain, and drugs such as digoxin and beta stimulators, will all increase the outflow tract gradients and may considerably reduce the cardiac output to essential organs, such as the myocardium and brain. Patients are often already on beta adrenoceptor blockers to prevent tachycardias.

   b. Hypotension from blood loss, regional anaesthesia, or vasodilator drugs, cause similar reductions in cardiac output and can exacerbate obstruction. A series of 52 general and four spinal anaesthetics in patients with HOCM was reviewed (Thompson et al 1985). One having a spinal anaesthetic sustained a myocardial infarction and subsequently died. Severe bradycardia and hypotension has been reported in patients with hypertrophic cardiomyopathy during spinal anaesthesia (Baraka et al 1987) and extradural anaesthesia (Loubser et al 1984).

   c. Pregnancy may be associated with increasing shortness of breath which responds to diuretics, and occasionally angina (Oakley et al 1979).

   d. A systolic murmur may be present that increases in intensity when blood loss occurs, and decreases when intravascular volume is increased (Lanier & Prough 1984). These authors believe that HOCM should be considered in any elderly patient who develops a systolic murmur during longstanding hypertension.

   e. Arrhythmias. The patient may already be taking amiodarone for these.

   f. Anticoagulant therapy.

3. Restrictive cardiomyopathy

   a. A fall in intravascular volume will decrease the ventricular filling pressure and accentuate the existing restriction to diastolic filling.

   b. Changes in heart rate in either direction will impair diastolic filling.

   c. Frequently the systolic function is normal. In some cases there is an additional impairment of ventricular function. In these, myocardial depressants may cause cardiovascular collapse.

Management

In advanced cases, careful cardiological assessment is required. The presence of cardiac failure will necessitate the monitoring of direct arterial blood pressure and ventricular filling pressures. Facilities for temporary pacing should be immediately available. The anaesthetist should understand the pathophysiology of the condition and the cardiovascular effects of the drugs and anaesthetic agents used.

1. Dilated cardiomyopathy
   a. Myocardial depressants such as thiopentone, halothane and enflurane should be avoided. A nitrous oxide, oxygen, narcotic, benzodiazepine, relaxant technique is best.
   b. The ECG should be carefully observed for ventricular arrhythmias and heart block, so that treatment can be rapidly instituted.
   c. Regional anaesthesia may be considered for appropriate surgical procedures, provided the filling pressures are well controlled and there is no myocardial ischaemia. An extradural anaesthetic given for hip replacement, to a patient with severe dilated cardiomyopathy caused by alcohol, has been reported (Amaranath et al 1986). PAP was measured, and the only complication was an episode of pulmonary hypertension after insertion of the femoral prosthesis. Extradural anaesthesia has also been used for Caesarean section using an impedence cardiograph for haemodynamic monitoring (Gambling et al 1987). Two episodes of hypotension were treated with ephedrine.
   d. Patients in heart failure require diuretics, and may need dobutamine or dopamine if there is a low perioperative cardiac output state. Occasionally, isoprenaline may be necessary. Sodium nitroprusside can improve cardiac output by reducing the ventricular afterload. Continuous arteriovenous haemofiltration has been used to treat refractory congestive heart failure urgently in preparation for Caesarean section under extradural anaesthesia (Dodds et al 1991).
2. Hypertrophic cardiomyopathy
   The obstruction is dynamic (Maron et al 1987). Management should aim to decrease the obstruction, by decreasing myocardial contractility, and increasing preload and afterload.
   a. A tachycardia from premedication, tracheal intubation, too light anaesthesia, ketamine, or cardiac stimulants, must be avoided. Preoperative beta blockers should be maintained. An infusion of esmolol was used for the management of cerebral aneurysm surgery (Freilich & Jacobs 1990).
   b. Drugs and techniques which cause vasodilatation and hypotension must not be used. An adequate preload should be given and blood loss replaced promptly. An intraoperative diagnosis of hypertrophic cardiomyopathy was made during hip replacement in a patient with a history of hypertension (Lanier & Prough 1984). Blood loss was associated with a sudden increase in intensity of her systolic murmur and the appearance of a systolic click. Postoperative echocardiography confirmed the diagnosis.

Regional anaesthesia is contraindicated. Since isoflurane and morphine produce venodilatation, halothane or enflurane, and opiates such as fentanyl or alfentanil, should be used in preference (Campbell & Bousfield 1992). Isoflurane may be required for neurosurgical procedures (Freilich & Jacobs 1990). In this patient, phenylephrine was used to control the resultant hypotension Provided that the pulse is slow and the vascular volume maintained, halothane will minimize the severity of the obstruction by decreasing the force of ventricular contraction. A propofol infusion has been used for cardiac surgery (Bell & Goodchild 1989).

c. Caesarean section should be managed with general rather than extradural anaesthesia (Oakley et al 1979), and enflurane is preferred to isoflurane (Boccio et al 1986). The routine use of ergometrine has been recommended (Oakley et al 1979), although an infusion of syntocinon will result in less vasodilatation than a bolus dose.

d. Hypotension should be heated by restoring vascular volume. If vasopressors are required, an alpha$_1$ agonist such as phenylephrine (Freilich & Jacobs 1990) or methoxamine is the most suitable.

3. Restrictive cardiomyopathy
Maintenance of the compensatory mechanisms for the impaired diastolic filling are essential.

a. Adequate ventricular filling. Blood volume is maintained, and morphine and isoflurane avoided because of venous dilatation.

b. Adequate heart rate. Pancuronium may be advantageous.

c. Myocardial contractility. In severe disease, fentanyl, ketamine and benzodiazepines should be used rather than thiopentone, halothane and enflurane.

d. Vasodilators and diuretics are avoided.

BIBLIOGRAPHY

Amaranath L, Esfandiari S, Lockrem J et al 1986 Epidural analgesia for total hip replacement in a patient with dilated cardiomyopathy. Canadian Anaesthetists' Society Journal 33: 84–88

Baraka A, Jabbour S, Itani I 1987 Severe bradycardia following epidural anesthesia in a patient with idiopathic hypertrophic subaortic stenosis. Anesthesia and Analgesia 66: 1337–1338

Bell M D, Goodchild C S 1989 Hypertrophic obstructive cardiomyopathy in combination with prolapsing mitral valve. Anaesthesia for surgical correction with propofol. Anaesthesia 44: 409–411

Boccio R V, Chung J H, Harrison D M 1986 Anesthetic management of cesarean section in a patient with idiopathic hypertrophic subaortic stenosis. Anesthesiology 65: 663–665

Brown G, O'Leary M, Douglas I et al 1992 Perioperative management of a severe peripartum cardiomyopathy Anaesthesia and Intensive Care 20: 80–83

Caforio A P L, Stewart J T, McKenna W J 1990 Idiopathic dilated cardiomyopathy. Rational treatment awaits better understanding of pathogenesis. British Medical Journal 300: 890–891

Campbell A M, Bousfield J D 1992 Anaesthesia in a patient with Noonan's syndrome and cardiomyopathy. Anaesthesia 47: 131–133

Dodds T M, Haney M F, Appleton F M 1991 Management of peripartum congestive heart failure using continuous arteriovenous haemofiltration in a patient with myotonic dystrophy. Anesthesiology 75: 907–911

Editorial 1992 Sporting hearts. Lancet 340: 1132–1133

Freilich J D, Jacobs B R 1990 Anesthetic management of cerebral aneurysm resection in a patient with idiopathic hypertrophic subaortic stenosis. Anesthesia and Analgesia 71: 558–560

Gambling D R, Flanagan M L, Huckell V E et al 1987 Anaesthetic management and non-invasive monitoring for Caesarean section in a patient with cardiomyopathy. Canadian Journal of Anaesthesia 34: 505–508

Hanson C W 1989 Asymptomatic cardiomyopathy presenting as cardiac arrest in the day surgical unit. Anesthesiology 71: 982–984

Johnson R A, Palacios I 1982 Dilated cardiomyopathies of the adult. New England Journal of Medicine 307: 1051–1058

Lanier W, Prough D S 1984 Intraoperative diagnosis of hypertrophic obstructive cardiomyopathy. Anesthesiology 60: 61–63

Lavies N G, Turner D A B 1989 Peripartum cardiomyopathy. A rare cause of pulmonary oedema in late pregnancy. Anaesthesia 44: 770–772

Lorell B H, Paulus W J, Grossman W et al 1982 Modification of abnormal left ventricular diastolic properties by nifedipine in patients with hypertrophic cardiomyopathy. Circulation 65: 499–507

Loubser P, Suh K, Cohen S 1984 Adverse effects of spinal anesthesia in a patient with idiopathic hypertrophic subaortic stenosis. Anesthesiology 60: 228–230

Malinow A M, Butterworth J F, Johnson M D 1985 Peripartum cardiomyopathy presenting at Cesarean delivery. Anesthesiology 63: 545–547

Maron B J, Bonow R O, Cannon R O et al 1987 Hypertrophic cardiomyopathy. New England Journal of Medicine 316: 780–790, 844–852

Morrison W L, Petch M C 1991 Peripartum cardiomyopathy. British Journal of Hospital Medicine 17: 693–699

Oakley C M 1987 Cardiomyopathies. In: Weatherall D J, Ledingham J G G, Warrell D A (eds) Oxford textbook of medicine. Oxford Scientific Publications, Oxford

Oakley G D G, McGarry K, Limb D G et al 1979 Management of pregnancy in patients with hypertrophic cardiomyopathy. British Medical Journal 1: 1749– 1750

O'Connell J B, Constanzo-Nordin M R, Subramanian R et al 1986 Peripartum cardiomyopathy: clinical hemodynamic, histologic and prognostic characteristics. Journal of the American College of Cardiology 8: 52–56

Thompson R C, Liberthson R R, Lowenstein E 1985 Perioperative anesthetic risk of noncardiac surgery in hypertrophic obstructive cardiomyopathy. Journal of the American Medical Association 254: 2419–2421

Wilmshurst P T, Katrtsis D 1990 Restrictive cardiomyopathy. British Heart Journal 63: 323–324

CARNITINE PALMITOYL TRANSFERASE DEFICIENCY

An autosomal recessive metabolic myopathy involving an inability to use fatty acids for energy production in muscle. It is characterized by episodes of rhabdomyolysis, myoglobinuria and lipid accumulation. Carnitine palmitoyl transferase (CPT) is present on both sides of the mitochondrial membrane. It converts acyl-CoA to acylcarnitine, to enable it to cross the mitochondrial membrane, and on the inner side it converts it back again. Thus, CPT deficiency impairs the entry of long chain acyl-CoA compounds from the cytosol into mitochondria, with the result that mitochondria are unable to utilize long chain fatty acids for energy production. Muscle requires 50% of its energy from fatty acids and ketone bodies, even at rest. During fasting or exercise, glucose becomes depleted and if fatty acids cannot be used, energy production is reduced, the ATP which is needed to maintain the integrity of the sarcoplasm is depleted and rhabdomyolysis ensues (Kelly et al 1989). A high-fat diet may also cause problems by overloading the system.

An alternative theory is that the disease involves alteration in the regulatory properties of CPT rather than a deficiency (Zierz & Schmitt 1989) and these authors have shown that CPT is abnormally inhibited by malonyl-CoA or by increasing the substrate/product concentration. The enzyme is vulnerable if lipid metabolism is stressed and they suggest that general anaesthetics may precipitate rhabdomyolysis by interfering with the lipid matrix.

Preoperative abnormalities

1. The patient may be totally asymptomatic, or episodes of muscle pains, rigidity and rhabdomyolysis may occur after exercise, with asymptomatic periods between.
2. A fatal attack of rhabdomyolysis and renal failure occurred in a child in association with a severe viral infection (Kelly et al 1989). Investigation of the child and her sister showed the unsuspected abnormality.
3. During an attack, patients are advised to rest, maintain fluid intake and a suitable diet

Anaesthetic problems

1. An adult male given suxamethonium for gastrectomy passed dark brown urine postoperatively, then became oliguric and subsequently developed renal failure (Katsuya et al 1988).
2. Starvation and dehydration may precipitate rhabdomyolysis and myoglobinuria.

Management

1. Give glucose and fluids during periods of starvation.
2. Avoid the use of suxamethonium, in case it precipitates rhabdomyolysis.

BIBLIOGRAPHY
Katsuya H, Misumi M, Ohtani Y et al 1988 Postanesthetic acute renal failure due to carnitine palmityl transferase deficiency. Anesthesiology 68: 945–948
Kelly K 7, Garland J S, Tang T T et al 1989 Fatal rhabdomyolysis following influenza infection in a girl with familial carnitine palmityl transferase deficiency. Pediatrics 84: 312–316
Zierz S, Schmitt U 1989 Inhibition of carnitine palmitoyl transferase by malonyl-CoA in human muscle is influenced by anesthesia. Anesthesiology 70: 373

CAROTID BODY TUMOUR
(see also APUDOMAS)

A tumour of ectodermal origin. One of a group known as the paraganglionomas, which are associated with the sympathetic nervous system. The cells of the carotid body normally act as chemoreceptors, but in common with other APUD cells, can secrete a variety of amines and peptides. Most carotid body tumours are non-functional, but occasionally they secrete noradrenaline, dopamine, calcitonin or ACTH. They may be malignant, may enlarge and invade locally and can metastasize. Surgery is the treatment of choice (Bernard 1992).

Preoperative abnormalities

1. The tumour usually presents as a mass in the neck.
2. Arteriography or DVI is essential to delineate the blood supply.
3. Radioisotope scans may show tumours elsewhere.
4. Clinical signs of catecholamine secretion should be sought. If these are present, definitive biochemical tests may be required. However, endocrine activity is rare.

Anaesthetic problems

1. Those of catecholamine secretion if the tumour is functional. Patients with multiple carotid body tumours, or a family history, often have associated phaeochromocytomas (Campeau & Graves 1991) which are detectable by MIGB scan. Episodes of severe hypertension and tachycardia during anaesthesia for biopsy of undiagnosed neck masses have been recorded (Clarke et al 1976, Newland & Hurlbert 1980). Both patients were found to have increased catecholamine levels, and were treated as for phaeochromocytoma during their subsequent tumour resection.
2. Blood loss may be brisk and heavy.
3. Heparinization is occasionally required.
4. Reflex bradycarcia, and occasionally cardiovascular collapse, secondary to carotid sinus stimulation has been reported (Kraayenbrink & Steven 1985).
5. Postoperative neurological complications are well recognized. They include cranial nerve palsies and cerebrovascular accident (Wright et al 1979).

Management

1. Look for evidence of phaeochromocytoma. If present, management is that of phaeochromocytoma.
2. Embolization of the tumour prior to surgery has been reported to reduce intraoperative blood loss (LaMuraglia et al 1992).

3. The use of nasotracheal intubation improves surgical access (Bernard 1992).
4. Atropine may be required for bradycardias, although this may not protect the patient from cardiovascular collapse even when the carotid sinus is only lightly stimulated. A technique has been proposed (Boyd 1980), in which the dissection to expose the carotid bifurcation is performed in such a manner as to avoid pressure on the sinus. Lignocaine is then irrigated locally, before infiltration with further lignocaine.
5. The surgeon may require to use a nerve stimulator to reduce the risk of nerve injury, in which case complete neuromuscular paralysis should be avoided.

BIBLIOGRAPHY

Bernard R P 1992 Carotid body tumors. American Journal of Surgery 163: 494–496

Boyd C H 1980 Anaesthesia for carotid body tumour resection. Anaesthesia 35: 720

Campeau R J, Graves C 1991 Pheochromocytoma associated with prior carotid body tumors (chemodectomas). Detection with I-131 MIGB. Clinical Nuclear Medicine 17: 511–512

Clarke A D, Matheson H, Boddie HG 1976 Removal of catecholamine-secreting chemodectoma. Anaesthesia 31: 1225–1230

Kraayenbrink M A, Steven C M 1985 Anaesthesia for carotid body tumour resection in a patient with the Eisenmenger syndrome. Anaesthesia 40: 1194–1197

LaMuraglia G M, Fabian R L, Brewster D C et al 1992 The current surgical management of carotid body paraganglionomas. Journal of Vascular Surgery 15: 1038–1044

Newland M C, Hurlbert B J 1980 Chemodectoma diagnosed hypertension and tachycardia during anesthesia. Anesthesia and Analgesia 59: 388–390

Wright D J, Pandya A, Noel F 1979 Anaesthesia for carotid body tumour resection. Anaesthesia 34: 806–808

CENTRAL CORE DISEASE

A nonprogressive congenital myopathy, usually inherited as autosomal dominant. Pathological abnormalities of the sarcoplasmic reticulum and the t-tubules have been shown (Hayashi et al 1989). There is a strong association with malignant hyperthermia and genetic studies suggest that the gene responsible is situated on chromosome 19 close to the MH gene (Haan et al 1990). Surgery may be required for correction of hip or other orthopaedic deformities.

Preoperative abnormalities

1. Infantile or childhood hypotonia and proximal muscle weakness. Although in general the myopathy is mild and nonprogressive, wide variations in the clinical picture are seen. The myopathy is clinically undetectable in some patients but in a small number it is severe.
2. Deep tendon reflexes may be reduced or absent.
3. Orthopaedic abnormalities include congenital dislocation or subluxation of the hip (probably secondary to muscle weakness), pes

planus and joint hypermobility (Gamble et al 1988). Scoliosis and patellar dislocation have also been seen. Patients are prone to develop joint contractures.

4. An increased incidence of mitral valve prolapse has been reported (Shuaib et al 1987).
5. The diagnosis is made on muscle biopsy; type 1 fibres show 'cores' within the fibres which have a deficiency of mitochondria.

Anaesthetic problems

1. Patients with central core disease appear to be susceptible to malignant hyperthermia (Frank et al 1980, Brownell 1988) and one death has occurred. Status epilepticus, hyperthermia of 42°C and a pH of 7.1 developed in a patient 4 hours after resection of a meningioma. Suxamethonium was given for subsequent evacuation of a blood clot. Myoglobinuria and renal failure developed during the following day and death ensued (Prescott et al 1992). Histological examination of muscle showed central core disease. Sevoflurane was the triggering agent in one patient who had a non-fatal episode of MH which responded to dantrolene (Otsuka et al 1991). Harriman (1986) has shown that seven out of eight patients with central core disease were susceptible to malignant hyperthermia on in-vitro contracture testing. Another study confirmed that 11 patients from four families were found to be susceptible (Shuaib et al 1987).

Management

1. Assessment of severity of the myopathy.
2. All patients with central core disease should be considered at risk for malignant hyperthermia unless in-vitro contracture tests show that the particular patient is free from the trait (Shuaib et al 1987).
3. Investigate for mitral valve prolapse.

BIBLIOGRAPHY

Brownell A K N 1988 Malignant hyperthermia: relationship to other diseases. British Journal of Anaesthesia 60: 303–308
Editorial 1988 Central core disease. Lancet 1: 866
Frank J P Harati Y, Butler I J et al 1980 Central core disease and malignant hyperthermia syndrome. Annals of Neurology 7: 11–17
Gamble J G, Rinsky L A, Lee J H 1988 Orthopaedic aspects of central core disease. Journal of Bone and Joint Surgery (A) 70: 1061–1066
Haan E A, Freemantle C J, McCure J A et al 1990 Assignment of the gene for central core disease to chromosome 19. Human Genetics 86: 187–190
Harriman D G F 1986 The definition of normal muscle and of malignant hyperthermia and the association of myopathies with the malignant hyperthermia trait. Muscle and Nerve 9 (suppl 1): 222
Hayashi K, Miller R G, Brownell R G 1989 Central core disease: ultrastructure of the sarcoplasmic reticulum and T-tubules. Muscle and Nerve 12: 95–102
Otsuka H, Komura Y, Mayumi T et al 1991 Malignant hyperthermia during

sevoflurane anesthesia in a child with central core disease. Anesthesiology 75: 699–701
Prescott R J, Roberts S P, Williams G 1992 Malignant hyperpyrexia: a rare cause of postoperative death. Journal of Clinical Pathology 45: 361–363
Shuaib A, Paasuke R T, Brownell K W 1987 Central core disease. Clinical features in 13 patients. Medicine 66: 389–396

C1 ESTERASE INHIBITOR DEFICIENCY
(ACQUIRED)

This may be a familial (see Hereditary angioneurotic oedema) or, less commonly, an acquired disorder involving the complement system. The acquired form is mostly associated with a B-lymphocyte malignancy, and antibodies have been detected against abnormal immunoglobulins present on the malignant B-cells. Reaction between the two causes C1 activation, which in turn produces a secondary reduction in the concentrations of C1, C2 and C4 and a reduced functional activity of C1 esterase inhibitor (Geha et al 1985). This form must be distinguished from the physical forms of angioedema which occur in response to food, drugs or insect bites, or in association with connective tissue disorders. A number of patients have developed angioedema in response to treatment with ACE inhibitors, particularly enalapril and captopril (Barna & Frable 1990).

Preoperative abnormalities

1. Intermittent attacks of angioneurotic oedema which can involve any part of the body, and result from extravasation of intravascular fluid and protein into subcutaneous and mucosal structures (Gelfand et al 1979).
2. As with hereditary angioneurotic oedema there is a low level of C1 esterase inhibitor, and sometimes life-threatening episodes of oedema of the upper airway may develop in response to stress or local trauma, particularly dental treatment (Frigas 1989). However, attacks of oedema may occur without any obvious reason and recurrent abdominal pain may be the presenting feature.
3. As with the hereditary form, adrenaline, antihistamines and steroids are known to be ineffective as prophylaxis and treatment for these attacks.
4. The two conditions may be distinguished by the fact that in the acquired form the onset is late, no family history is elicited, and no complement abnormalities are found in the patient's blood relatives. The underlying malignancy may already have been diagnosed.
5. Differentiation can now be made on measurement of the C1q subunit of C1; patients with acquired deficiency have a decreased level of C1q compared with those with the hereditary form, in whom the C1 level is normal (Alsenz et al 1987).

Anaesthetic problems

1. Tracheal intubation and manipulation of the upper airway may precipitate local angioneurotic oedema for which treatment with adrenaline, steroids and antihistamines are ineffective. Angioedema may also occur after dental extractions.
2. Although tranexamic acid has been recommended to prevent attacks in both forms, venous thrombosis has been reported after its prophylactic use during surgery in the acquired disease (Razis et al 1986).

Management

1. Danazol is a progestogen derivative which probably increases the hepatic synthesis of C1 esterase inhibitor. Its prophylactic value in the acquired and hereditary disorders has been reported (Razis et al 1986). Danazol 200 mg t.d.s should be given preoperatively, but may take several days to become effective. Alternatively, stanozolol 0.5–8 mg/day can also be used (Frigas 1989). The lower levels will be required for maintenance, whilst higher levels may be needed in the initial stages.
2. Tranexamic acid should probably be avoided in the acquired form, especially in the presence of a thrombocytosis.
3. The preoperative prophylactic use of fresh frozen plasma, and C1 inhibitor concentrate has been reported (Plenderleith et al 1988). Purified C1 esterase inhibitor can be obtained from Immuno Limited (Rye Lane, Dunton Green, Sevenoaks, Kent TN14 5HB, UK)

BIBLIOGRAPHY
Alsenz J, Bork K, Loos M 1987 Autoantibody-mediated acquired deficiency of C1 inhibitor. New England Journal of Medicine 316: 1360–1366
Barna J S, Frable M A 1990 Life-threatening angioedema. Otolaryngology and Head and Neck Surgery 103: 795–798
Frigas E 1989 Angioedema with acquired deficiency of the C1 inhibitor: a constellation of syndromes. Mayo Clinic Proceedings 64: 1269–1275
Geha R S, Quinti I, Austen K F et al 1985 Acquired C1 inhibitor deficiency associated with anti-idiotypic antibody to monoclonal immunoglobulins. New England Journal of Medicine 312: 534–540
Gelfand J A, Boss G R, Conley C L et al 1979 Acquired C1 esterase inhibitor deficiency and angioedema: a review. Medicine 58: 321–328
Plenderleith J L, Algie T, Whaley K 1988 Acquired C1 esterase inhibitor deficiency. Anaesthesia 43: 246–247
Razis P A, Coulson I H, Gould T R et al 1986 Acquired C1 esterase inhibitor deficiency. Anaesthesia 41: 838–840

CHARCOT-MARIE-TOOTH DISEASE
(CMT; PERONEAL MUSCULAR ATROPHY)

An autosomal dominant, chronic, peripheral motor and sensory neuropathy of childhood. Anaesthesia is most commonly required for orthopaedic procedures, muscle or nerve biopsies.

Preoperative abnormalities

1. Distal muscle weakness and wasting with a sensory ataxia, initially producing walking difficulties in the second decade. Later there may be involvement of the hand and forearm with distal muscle atrophy.
2. A mild glove–and–stocking sensory loss.
3. Orthopaedic abnormalities include high pedal arches, club feet and foot drop.
4. Respiratory problems may be more common than previously thought. In a study of patients with respiratory symptoms, a correlation was found between proximal upper limb involvement and respiratory muscle dysfunction (Nathanson et al 1989). Diaphragmatic weakness has been noted (Laroche et al 1988). If respiratory insufficiency occurs, it is usually secondary to restrictive lung disease and only appears late in the disease.
5. Although cardiac involvement has been suggested, a study of 12 patients with CMT disease showed that cardiomyopathy was no more frequent than in unaffected relatives (Dyck et al 1987).
6. The kidney is sometimes involved (Paul et al 1990).
7. Diagnosis is made on abnormal nerve conduction velocities and sural nerve biopsy.

Anaesthetic problems

1. Exacerbations of the disease may occur in pregnancy. Respiratory failure following Caesarean section has necessitated prolonged IPPV (Brian et al 1987). In patients with respiratory complications, increasing support may be required. A 26-year-old with a tracheostomy, who was receiving IPPV at night, had to increase her periods of ventilatory support towards term (Byrne et al 1992).
2. Although postoperative respiratory complications are thought to be rare, a perioperative death after spinal fusion secondary to restrictive lung disease and pneumonia has been reported (Antognini 1992).
3. There is a possibility that suxamethonium may precipitate hyperkalaemia, although its apparently uneventful use has been reported in 41 patients in one series (Antognini 1992), and two out of seven in another (Greenberg & Parker 1992).

Management

1. Assessment of respiratory function, particularly in those patients with upper limb involvement.
2. Cautious use of neuromuscular blockers, especially in the more severely affected patients.

BIBLIOGRAPHY
Antognini J F 1992 Anaesthesia for Charcot-Marie-Tooth disease: a review of 86 cases. Canadian Journal of Anaesthesia 39: 398–400

Brian J E, Boyles G D, Quirk J G, Clark R B 1987 Anesthetic management for
  Cesarean section of a patient with Charcot–Marie–Tooth disease. Anesthesiology
  66: 410–412
Byrne D L, Chappatte O A, Spencer G T et al 1992 Pregnancy complicated by
  Charcot–Marie–Tooth disease, requiring intermittent ventilation. British Journal of
  Obstetrics and Gynaecology 99: 79–80
Dyck P J, Swanson C J, Nishimura R A et al 1987 Cardiomyopathy in patients with
  hereditary motor and sensory neuropathy. Mayo Clinic Proceedings 62: 672–675
Greenberg R S, Parker S D 1992 Anesthetic management for the child with Charcot–
  Marie–Tooth disease. Anesthesia and Analgesia 74: 305–307
Laroche C M, Carroll N, Moxham J 1988 Diaphragmatic weakness in Charcot–Marie–
  Tooth disease. Thorax 43: 478–479
Nathanson B N, Yu D-G, Chan C K 1989 Respiratory muscle weakness in Charcot–
  Marie–Tooth disease. A field study. Archives of Internal Medicine 149: 1389–1391
Paul M D, Fernandez D, Pryse-Phillips W et al 1990 Charcot–Marie–Tooth disease and
  nephropathy in a mother and daughter with a review of the literature. Nephron
  54: 80–85
Roelofse J A, Shipton E A 1985 Anaesthesia for abdominal hysterectomy in Charcot–
  Marie–Tooth disease. A case report. South African Medical Journal 67: 605–606

CHARGE ASSOCIATION

An association of congenital abnormalities characterized by Coloboma of
the eye, Heart disease, Atresia of the choanae, Retarded growth
development and/or central nervous system abnormalities, Genital
hypoplasia in males, Ear anomalies and/or deafness. Diagnosis is made
on the presence of at least four of these criteria. A retrospective study of
50 patients showed that apart from choanal atresia and cleft lip and
palate, 56% of patients had some other upper airway abnormality (Stack &
Wyse 1991). Muscular hypotonia is common. Anaesthesia may be
required for choanal atresia repair, cardiac surgery, tracheo-oesophageal
fistula, ear surgery, Nissen's fundoplication and tracheostomy. Treatment
requires a multidisciplinary approach.

Preoperative abnormalities

1. In an analysis of 50 patients, more than 90% had colobomata, 56%
   had choanal atresia, 84% had congenital heart disease, 96% males
   had external genital abnormalities, and 100% had ear abnormalities.
   Of those who were old enough to assess, 76% had developmental
   delay (Blake et al 1990).
2. Other abnormalities included facial palsy, renal abnormalities,
   tracheo-oesophageal fistula and laryngeal malformations.

Anaesthetic problems

1. An increased risk of airway obstruction, so that tracheal intubation
   or tracheostomy may be required in early life (Coniglio et al 1988).
   Fifty six per cent had choanal atresia or stenosis, 40% micrognathia,
   8% laryngomalacia, 6% subglottic stenosis, and 8% had other upper

airway abnormalities. A tendency for the airway to collapse during light anaesthesia probably results from laryngomalacia (Stack & Wyse 1991).

2. Tracheal intubation difficulties were recorded in 25% of those patients with micrognathia, and intubation problems appeared to increase with increasing age.
3. Patients require multiple anaesthetics and there was a high postoperative mortality.
4. Feeding difficulties and a high incidence of gastro-oesophageal reflux (50%). Postoperative deaths were frequently associated with pulmonary aspiration.
5. Congenital heart disease, predominantly conotruncal abnormalities or patent ductus arteriosus. About 60% of these will require surgery.

Management

1. Careful preoperative assessment for upper airway abnormalities and cardiac disease.
2. A range of sizes of tracheal tube should be available.
3. If micrognathia is present, a gaseous induction may be advisable.
4. Tracheostomy may be required for long-term management.
5. Precautions should be taken against aspiration of gastric contents.

BIBLIOGRAPHY
Blake K D, Russell-Eggitt I M, Morgan D W et al 1990 Who's in CHARGE? Multidisciplinary management of patients with CHARGE association. Archives of Diseases in Children 65: 217–223
Coniglio J U, Manzione J V, Hengerer A S 1988 Anatomic findings and management of choanal atresia and the CHARGE association. Annals of Otology, Rhinology and Laryngology 97: 448–453
Stack C G, Wyse R K H 1991 Incidence and management of airway problems in the CHARGE association. Anaesthesia 46: 582–584

CHERUBISM

A benign, familial condition, transmitted as an autosomal dominant, which may present during childhood with progressive mandibular, and sometimes maxillary enlargement. It usually regresses spontaneously during adolescence (Katz et al 1992), but sometimes facial or incidental surgery is required before this.

Preoperative abnormalities

1. Bilateral swelling usually starts at the age of 2–4 years. The mandible, and sometimes the maxilla, is involved. X-ray shows multilocular cysts expanding the bone, leaving only a thin layer of cortex. Progression of the lesions slows down towards puberty and sometimes they completely regress. The lower eyelids may become

retracted so that a rim of sclera is exposed below the iris and orbital compression may occur. (Marck & Kudryk 1992).
2. Speech, deglutition and mastication may be affected in gross cases.
3. There may be dental abnormalities and premature loss of teeth.

Anaesthetic problems

1. Intubation difficulties have been encountered. Visualization of the vocal cords was made impossible by mandibular enlargement displacing the area of soft tissue bounded by the mandible (Maydew & Berry 1985).
2. A limited range of jaw movements may contribute to intubation difficulties (Faircloth et al 1991).
3. Surgery for gross deformities may be associated with considerable blood loss, and postoperative IPPV may be required (Kaugers et al 1992).

Management

1. Difficult intubation should be anticipated. An awake intubation technique is the safest. If this is refused, a spontaneously breathing technique should be used for induction. Facilities for an immediate tracheostomy must be available.
2. Postoperative IPPV, and occasionally tracheostomy, may be required.

BIBLIOGRAPHY
Faircloth W J Jr, Edwards R C, Farhood V W 1991 Cherubism involving a mother and daughter: case reports and review of the literature. Journal of Oral and Maxillofacial Surgery 49: 535–542
Katz J O, Dunlap C L, Ennis R L 1992 Cherubism: report of a case showing regression without treatment. Journal of Oral and Maxillofacial Surgery 50: 301–303
Kaugars G E, Niamtu J, Svirsky J A 1992 Cherubism: diagnosis, treatment, and comparison with central giant cell granulomas and giant cell tumors. Oral Surgery, Oral Medicine, Oral Pathology 73: 369–374
Maydew R P, Berry F A 1985 Cherubism with difficult laryngoscopy and tracheal intubation. Anesthesiology 62: 810–812
Marck P A, Kudryk W H 1992 Cherubism. Journal of Otolaryngology 21: 84–87

CHRISTMAS DISEASE (HAEMOPHILIA B)
(SEE HAEMOPHILIA A)

COARCTATION OF THE AORTA, ADULT

A congenital narrowing of the aorta which may be pre- or post-ductal. The pre-ductal form is usually a long narrow segment and associated with other cardiac defects. This type usually presents with heart failure before the age of one year and requires treatment in a paediatric cardiac surgical unit. It will not be considered further here. The post-ductal form, however, is often asymptomatic and the patient may present in later life for surgery of some other condition, or for correction of the coarctation itself (Branthwaite 1980). Even after corrective surgery, however, abnormalities can continue (Moskowitz et al 1990). Those who have undergone repair show persistent alterations in left ventricular function and left ventricular mass together with resting gradients between the arm and leg. There is a higher incidence than normal of ischaemic heart disease and sudden death.

Preoperative abnormalities

1. There may be moderate hypertension, the arm blood pressure being higher than that in the leg. If the left subclavian arises at or below the constriction, there may be an absent or reduced left radial pulse. Should both radial and femoral pulses be felt together, the small volume and delay of the femoral pulse will be obvious.
2. Collateral circulation develops in the internal mammary, intercostal and subscapular arteries. The latter may be seen if the scapula is illuminated from the side.
3. A systolic murmur is usually heard along the left sternal edge radiating up into the neck. There may be a bicuspid aortic valve and some aortic regurgitation.
4. CXR may show notching of the undersides of the ribs secondary to intercostal artery dilatation. There may be pre- and post-stenotic dilatation of the aorta.
5. Occasionally, cerebral berry aneurysms coexist with coarctation. In such cases, the high arterial pressure increases the risk of subarachnoid haemorrhage.
6. There is a 25–50% incidence of bicuspid aortic valve.
7. Unusually, angina or left ventricular failure may present late in untreated adult coarctation. Other factors are often contributory.

Anaesthetic problems

If, before elective surgery, a previously undiagnosed coarctation is found, treatment of the coarctation may be considered to be the priority. Even if coarctation has been treated, the possibility of residual cardiovascular abnormalities should be considered since there is an increased incidence of premature death compared with the normal population (Bobby et al 1991). Causes include aneurysms (cerebral, at the operative site, other parts of the aorta and intercostal arteries), hypertension, myocardial infarction and cardiac failure (Editorial 1991).

1. Upper body hypertension. The control of arterial pressure, both above and below the lesion, may be a problem during resection of the coarctation. The less severe the coarctation and the fewer the collaterals, the greater the increase in blood pressure on cross

clamping the aorta is likely to be. This hypertension responds poorly to hypotensive agents since there is little variable systemic resistance available proximal to the coarctation.

Hypertension occurred in a 16-year-old during anaesthesia with halothane, and before aortic clamping (Wilkinson & Clark 1982). It was resistant to sodium nitroprusside and other vasodilators and may have been due to involvement of the renin-angiotensin system. Preoperative treatment with an angiotensin I converting enzyme inhibitor, such as captopril, might be appropriate.

2. Any operation in the area of the dilated collateral vessels may result in heavy bleeding, especially when the chest is opened.
3. Hypoperfusion of the spinal cord may cause paraplegia, and is more likely to present a problem in those patients with few collaterals. Induced hypotension employed for clipping of cerebral aneurysm may compromise spinal cord perfusion (Goodie & Rigg 1991).
4. Susceptibility to bacterial endocarditis.
5. If there are left subclavian abnormalities, the left arm cannot be used for blood pressure monitoring.
6. Postoperative hypertension (for more than 12 hours), associated with high plasma noradrenaline levels as a result of sympathetic overactivity. The magnitude of the increase has been found to relate to the preoperative level of the pressure gradient across the coarctation (Benedict et al 1978). This hypertension can cause bleeding, aortic dilatation or intracranial haemorrhage. Plasma noradrenaline levels may still be significantly increased 6 months postoperatively.
7. Some adults also have aortic incompetence. Acute LVF and cardiac arrest occurred immediately after correction of a coarctation in one patient with severe aortic incompetence. This was thought to be secondary to an acute decrease in coronary perfusion. (Rufilanchas et al 1977).

Management

1. Antihypertensive therapy should be used until the day of operation. Beta adrenoceptor blockers may reduce the hypertensive response to tracheal intubation. Angiotensin converting enzyme inhibitors may be appropriate.
2. Prophylaxis for endocarditis should be given.
3. Resection of coarctation.
   a. Cannulation of the right radial artery, and insertion of an internal jugular venous line are required. Aortic pressure measurement distal to the lesion is more difficult, but can be monitored via a needle inserted by the surgeon (Fisher & Benedict 1977), or by femoral arterial cannulation using a Seldinger technique (Branthwaite 1980).

    b. Moderate induced hypotension is required to reduce bleeding. However, a mean arterial pressure of less than 50 mmHg is not only difficult to achieve, but may compromise perfusion to structures, such as the spinal cord, below the lesion. A short-acting drug, such as sodium nitroprusside or trimetaphan, can be tried, so that it can be discontinued just before aortic cross-clamping.

    c. Careful monitoring to detect and to vigorously treat postoperative hypertension (usually within 72 hours) is needed. A combination of alpha and beta blockade may be required.

4. Other surgery. During clipping of an intracranial aneurysm, the femoral artery pressure was closely observed during induced hypotension in order to monitor spinal cord perfusion (Goodie & Rigg 1991). A mean distal aortic pressure in excess of 50 mmHg has been suggested as adequate for spinal cord perfusion.

BIBLIOGRAPHY

Benedict C R, Grahame-Smith D G, Fisher A 1978 Changes in plasma catecholamines and dopamine beta-hydroxylase after corrective surgery for coarctation of the aorta. Circulation 57: 598–602

Bobby J J, Emami J M, Farmer R D T et al 1991 Operative survival and 40 year follow-up of surgical repair of aortic coarctation. British Heart Journal 65: 271–276

Branthwaite M 1980 Coarctation of the aorta. In: Branthwaite M (ed) Anaesthesia for cardiac surgery and allied procedures. Blackwell Scientific Publications, Oxford

Editorial 1991 Coarctation repair – the first forty years. Lancet 338: 546–547

Fisher A, Benedict C R 1977 Adult coarctation of the aorta: anaesthesia and postoperative management. Anaesthesia 32: 533–538

Goodie D B, Rigg D L 1991 Controlled hypotension for cerebral aneurysm surgery in the presence of severe aortic coarctation. British Journal of Anaesthesia 67: 329–331

Moskowitz W B, Schieken R M, Mosteller M et al 1990 Altered systolic and diastolic function in children after 'successful' repair of coarction of the aorta. American Heart Journal 120: 103–109

Rufilanchas J J, Villagra F, Maronas J M et al 1977 Coarctation of the aorta and severe aortic insufficiency: what to repair first? American Journal of Surgery 134: 428–430

Wilkinson C, Clark H 1982 Refractory hypertension during coarctectomy. Anesthesiology 57: 540–542

COCAINE ABUSE

Cocaine is an alkaloid present in the shrub, *Erythroxylon coca*. It has an onset of action of about 11 minutes and a half-life of 78 minutes and produces CNS stimulation, euphoria and hallucinations. As a sympathetic stimulant, it acts by preventing the uptake of catecholamines into sympathetic nerve endings. In addition, it may release catecholamines from body stores. Whilst there is evidence that it has been used as a euphoriant in the Central Amazon from as early as the ninth century, the last 20 years has seen a notable increase in its use. It has been said to produce emotional, but not physical dependence. However, more recently, the use of chemically modified forms ('paste', 'crack' and 'freebase') for inhalation or smoking, has resulted in higher blood concentrations. These appear to be producing physical dependence. The consumption of cocaine for recreational purposes has been more prevalent in the USA than in the UK. However, the greatly increased production and illicit trade from South America is beginning to change this (Gossop 1987).

Toxic effects of cocaine are marked. A series of 68 deaths associated with its illicit use has been reported in Florida (Wetli & Wright 1979). Analysis of the cases showed that the effect after intravenous use included immediate respiratory collapse and death, or death after up to 3 hours in coma. After nasal or oral ingestion, a delay of up to an hour occurred before convulsions and death. Average blood levels were highest in those with oral intake (average 0.92 mg/dl), lowest in those after i.v. (0.3 mg/dl) and intermediate after use of the nasal route (0.44 mg/dl). Oral ingestion is an uncommon route for those seeking euphoria. The majority of deaths were deliberate, or accidental when packages of cocaine which were swallowed for concealment ('body packing'), burst in the gut. That cocaine is potentially dangerous even when given non-intravenously, has been confirmed (Isner et al 1986). Seven patients had acute cardiac events which bore a temporal relationship to intranasal cocaine use. These included myocardial infarction, ventricular tachycardia and fibrillation, myocarditis, and two sudden deaths. Existing heart disease was not a prerequisite. Large doses of cocaine were not essential, and convulsions did not necessarily occur before cardiac toxicity. A further 19 case reports were analyzed. Cocaine is frequently taken in combination with other drugs. Drug mixtures include 'speedballs' (a combination of heroin laced with cocaine). Anaesthetists may be involved with anaesthesia for chronic users, or in the resuscitation of those with acute toxicity.

Presenting problems

1. The cardiovascular effects of cocaine are biphasic. An initial increase in blood pressure and a tachycardia, secondary to sympathetic stimulation, precedes the pronounced depression of the CNS. Sweating, vomiting and restlessness may occur. Sympathetic vasoconstriction may be intense, with increased metabolism, hyperthermia, hypoxia and convulsions. Ventricular fibrillation or asystole has occurred with doses as low as 30 mg. Tachycardia and hypertension have also been reported during anaesthesia when a patient injected two 'speedballs' into his infusion just before surgery (Samuels et al 1991).

2. Toxic doses produce an initial tachypnoea and increased depth of respiration. This may be rapidly followed by central respiratory depression.

3. When taken nasally, the vasoconstrictor effects on the mucosa may eventually lead to nasal ulceration and septal perforation.

4. There have been an increasing number of reports of rhabdomyolysis in association with cocaine abuse, and acute renal failure has occurred (Singhal et al 1989). In a study of cocaine users presenting to an emergency department, 24% had evidence of rhabdomyolysis (Welch et al 1991). One developed multi-organ failure and died.

5. A greatly increased risk of endocarditis in i.v. cocaine users (Burkett Chambers et al 1987).

6. I.v. users have an increased risk of contracting hepatitis B and AIDS.

7. Smoking or inhalation of hot cocaine fumes may cause pulmonary damage, as may the chemicals used in the processing (Gossop 1987).

8. Plasma cholinesterase is essential for the metabolism of cocaine. Individuals with enzyme abnormality or deficiency are therefore at risk from sudden death (Cregler & Mark 1986).

9. Thrombocytopenia is associated with cocaine abuse (Orser 1991). It may be autoimmune in origin. Antibodies to platelets may be common in drug addicts.

10. Organophosphate insecticides have been used to prolong the action of cocaine by inhibiting plasma cholinesterase (Herschman & Aaron 1991). Under these circumstances, recovery from suxamethonium may be delayed.

11. Experimentally, there is evidence that in pregnancy the cardiovascular toxicity of cocaine is increased. Cocaine-induced hypertension in gravid ewes was modified by hydralazine, but this caused profound maternal tachycardia and failed to restore the cocaine-induced reduction in uterine blood flow (Vertommen et al 1992). In the USA, where cocaine abuse is said to be common among parturients, myocardial infarction and cardiovascular instability, which as temporally related to 'crack' use before delivery, has been reported (Liu et al 1992). Maternal death has occurred and the perinatal mortality is increased (Neerhof et al 1989). The incidence of abruptio placenta is almost doubled in these individuals.

Management

1. Beta adrenoceptor blockers have been used to counteract the sympathetic effects of cocaine, but an alpha adrenoceptor blocker, such as phentolamine, should be available in case of severe hypertension. Regimens have included propranolol (1 mg i.v. each minute up to a total of 8 mg) to obtain a decrease in heart rate within 1–3 min (Gay et al 1976). However, it has been suggested that beta blockade alone may exacerbate hypertension by unopposed alpha stimulation (Gay & Loper 1988). Labetalol (20 mg i.v. stat followed by an infusion of 60 mg/h) may be more appropriate. That the beta effects of labetalol are much greater than the alpha effects, must not be overlooked. A bolus of esmolol 20 mg

followed by an esmolol infusion (1%) was used to treat toxicity from adrenaline and cocaine given before nasal polypectomy (Pollan & Tadjziechy 1989).

2. Calcium channel blockers have been used for arrhythmias (Cregler & Mark 1986) and may be more effective than adrenoceptor blockers in the management of cocaine cardiovascular toxicity (Nahas 1991).

3. For the treatment of convulsions, either a benzodiazepine or incremental doses of thiopentone are indicated.
Immediate attention should be paid to oxygenation and control of the airway. A profound metabolic acidosis occurs in association with convulsions, and their immediate control might decrease the cardiac effects of cocaine (Jonsson et al 1983).

4. Restlessness or agitation in the chronic cocaine abuser can be treated with benzodiazepines. Increasing the usual dosage by 50% has been recommended (Gay et al 1976).

5. Phenothiazines are contraindicated because they potentiate cerebral depressant drugs.

6. The platelet count returns to normal 1–6 weeks after termination of drug exposure. Bleeding time is the best indicator of platelet function. If this is normal, no treatment is required.

7. The possibility that rhabdomyolysis might occur should be remembered. Since clinical symptoms do not predict rhabdomyolysis, laboratory evaluation may be necessary. Treatment with mannitol, intravenous fluids and, occasionally, dialysis may be required.

BIBLIOGRAPHY

Burkett Chambers H F, Morris D L, Tauber M G et al 1987 Cocaine use and the risk for endocarditis in intravenous drug users. Annals of Internal Medicine 106: 833–836

Cregler L L, Mark H 1986 Medical complications of cocaine abuse. New England Journal of Medicine 315: 1495–1500

Fleming J A, Byck R, Barash P G 1990 Pharmacology and therapeutic applications of cocaine. Anesthesiology 73: 518–531

Gay G R, Inaba D S, Rappolt R T et al 1976 Cocaine in current perspective. Anesthesia and Analgesia 55: 582–587

Gay G R, Loper K A 1988 Control of cocaine induced hypertension with labetalol. Anesthesia and Analgesia 67: 92

Gossop M 1987 Beware cocaine. British Medical Journal 295: 945

Herschman Z, Aaron C 1991 Prolongation of cocaine effect. Anesthesiology 74: 631–632

Isner J M, Estes N A, Thompson P D et al 1986 Acute cardiac events temporally related to cocaine abuse. New England Journal of Medicine 315: 1438–1443

Jonsson S, O'Meara M, Young J B 1983 Acute cocaine poisoning. Importance of treating seizures and acidosis. American Journal of Medicine 75: 1061–1064

Liu S S, Forrester R M, Murphy G S et al 1992 Anaesthetic management of a parturient with myocardial infarction related to cocaine use. Canadian Journal of Anaesthesia 39: 858–861

Nahas G G 1991 Treatment of cocaine-induced cardiovascular toxicity. Anesthesiology 75: 544

Neerhof M G, Macgregor S N, Retzky S S et al 1989 Cocaine abuse during pregnancy: peripartum prevalence and perinatal outcome. American Journal of Obstetrics and Gynecology 161: 633–638

Orser B 1991 Thrombocytopenia and cocaine abuse. Anesthesiology 74: 195–196

Pollan S, Tadjziechy M 1989 Esmolol in the management of epinephrine- and cocaine-induced cardiovascular toxicity. Anesthesia and Analgesia 69: 663–664

Samuels J, Schwalbe S S, Marx G F 1991 Speedballs: a new cause of intraoperative tachycardia and hypertension. Anesthesia and Analgesia 72: 397–398

Singhal P, Horowitz B, Quinones M C et al 1989 Acute renal failure following cocaine abuse. Nephron 52: 76–78

Vertommen J D, Hughes S C, Rosen M A et al 1992 Hydralazine does not restore uterine blood flow during cocaine-induced hypertension in the pregnant ewe. Anesthesiology 76: 580–587

Welch R D, Todd K, Krause G S 1991 Incidence of cocaine-associated rhabdomyolysis. Annals of Emergency Medicine 20: 154–157

Wetli C V, Wright R K 1979 Death caused by recreational cocaine use. Journal of the American Medical Association 241: 2519–2522

CONN'S SYNDROME (PRIMARY ALDOSTERONISM)

Excess aldosterone production may be caused by an adrenal adenoma, adrenal hyperplasia or a carcinoma. Aldosterone is a mineralocorticoid secreted by the zona glomerulosa of the adrenal cortex. It promotes sodium reabsorption and potassium exchange, mainly in the renal tubules, but to a lesser extent in the intestine, and salivary and sweat glands. The final stage of aldosterone secretion is controlled by the renin-angiotensin system. Activation of this system occurs in response to sodium or water depletion.

Primary aldosteronism should be suspected if spontaneous hypokalaemia occurs in association with hypertension (Young et al 1990).

Preoperative abnormalities

1. The main features are hypertension, hypokalaemia and alkalosis. Symptoms, should they occur, are usually secondary to the hypokalaemia and may include muscle weakness, polyuria, polydipsia and tetany. A patient who presented with a flaccid quadriparesis had the condition reversed by a potassium infusion (Gangat et al 1976).
2. Urinary potassium is high despite a low total body potassium, and the serum sodium may be in the upper range of normal or be slightly elevated.
3. Plasma renin levels are low and plasma aldosterone is elevated.
4. Tumours must be distinguished from bilateral adrenal hyperplasia, with radionuclide imaging or, occasionally, adrenal vein sampling. In adrenal hyperplasia, surgery is inappropriate.
5. The ECG may show mild left ventricular hypertrophy, prolonged ST segment T-wave flattening and U waves.
6. Glucose tolerance may be abnormal in up to 50% of patients.

Anaesthetic problems

1. Low total body and plasma potassium levels cause muscle weakness and increased sensitivity to non-depolarizing muscle relaxants. Intraoperative arrhythmias may also be produced. A patient in whom tonic muscle contractions occurred during induction and whose subsequent potassium balance studies suggested that the potassium stores had been depleted by 30–40% has been described (Gangat et al 1976).
2. Hypertension and sodium retention. Hypertensive peaks may occur at intubation.

Management

1. Hypertension must be controlled preoperatively. An aldosterone antagonist, such as spironolactone 100 mg t.d.s, should be included since this improves both the hypertension and potassium loss.
2. A potassium infusion is required both pre- and intraoperatively. Total body potassium is depleted, and ECG and plasma potassium levels are both unreliable guides (Gangat et al 1976).
3. Preoperative beta adrenoceptor blockers may reduce the hypertension on intubation (Shipton & Hugo 1982).
4. Normocapnoea should be maintained to prevent potassium returning to the cells (Weatherill & Spence 1984). An initial period of postoperative ventilation may be required to counteract the compensatory respiratory acidosis.
5. Following removal of the tumour, the reversal of the electrolyte abnormalities occurs earlier than the correction of hypertension.
6. Glucocorticoid replacement should not be required if the other adrenal is intact.

BIBLIOGRAPHY

Gangat Y, Triner L, Baer L et al 1976 Primary aldosteronism with uncommon complications. Anesthesiology 45: 542–544

Matsuki M, Muraoka M, Oyama T 1988 Total spinal anaesthesia for a Jehovah's Witness with primary aldosteronism. Anaesthesia 43: 164–165

Shipton E A, Hugo J M 1982 An aldosterone-producing adrenal cortical adenoma. Anaesthesia 37: 933–936

Weatherill D, Spence A A 1984 Anaesthesia and disorders of the adrenal cortex. British Journal of Anaesthesia 56: 741–749

Young W F, Hogan M J, Klee G G et al 1990 Primary aldosteronism: diagnosis and treatment Mayo Clinic Proceedings 65: 96–110

CREUTZFELDT-JAKOB DISEASE

A transmissible human spongiform encephalopathy which may be classified as a prion (proteinaceous infective particle) disease. Kuru, linked with ritual cannibalism in Papua New Guinea, and Gerstmann-

Straussler–Scheinker disease, usually inherited, are the other two human prion diseases. Four such diseases have been defined as occurring in animals, bovine spongiform encephalopathy having achieved substantial notoriety in the UK (Hughes 1993). All are widespread degenerative diseases of the CNS with long incubation periods but, once manifested, a rapid progression to death. Treatment is to no avail.

Patients of late middle age are usually affected and death typically occurs within 6 months. The infective agent can be isolated from the brain, spinal cord and many other tissues, and can be experimentally transmitted to animals. There is no detectable immune reaction. It is difficult to destroy by either physical or chemical methods. Scientific opinion is moving towards the transmissible proteinaceous particle (prion) theory, but the traditional view of the role of a small virus (virino) has not yet been abandoned (Hughes 1993).

There have been reports involving iatrogenic transmission in two neurosurgical procedures – a corneal graft (MacMurdo et al 1984) and the use of growth hormone from cadaveric pituitaries (Buchanan et al 1991), in the latter cases usually following an incubation period of about 18 months. Patients who have received human growth hormone are now excluded from being blood donors.

Preoperative abnormalities

1. Dementia of rapid onset and mutism in the 50–70 year age group. Cerebellar dysfunction with ataxia, increased tone and sometimes myoclonus, is common. Cortical blindness may occur. Deterioration to decerebrate or decorticate states is usually rapid. Epilepsy can occur.
2. EEG is non-specific but there are often periodic discharges of slow waves and spikes.
3. Diagnosis is usually made on clinical grounds. It can only be confirmed by brain biopsy, but this is now not advised because of the risks of accidental transmission.
4. Treatment is symptomatic and does not affect the outcome. The patient may be taking anticonvulsants.

Anaesthetic problems

1. Any tissue or body fluid should be considered as potentially infectious, although in reality the main danger probably lies in accidental inoculation. However, there is nothing to suggest that routine nursing care carries risk. Barrier nursing is unnecessary.
2. Occasionally patients may have autonomic dysfunction.
3. Rarely, there are abnormalities of liver function.

Management

1. Particular care should be taken during brain biopsies in undiagnosed cases of presenile dementia (du Moulin & Hedley-Whyte 1983). If Creutzfeldt–Jakob is suspected, biopsy is inadvisable. The anaesthetist should wear gowns, gloves and mask. Patients with dementia should not be used as organ donors.
2. Equipment should preferably be disposable. Linen and instruments should be soaked in 1% sodium hypochlorite before being bagged (du Moulin & Hedley-Whyte 1983).
3. The agent is difficult to destroy by physical and chemical means. Experiments have shown that soaking in 1% sodium hypochlorite for 1 hour, autoclaving for 1 hour at 132°C (103.4 kPa) or a combination of these, will inactivate it (Brown et al 1982, Knight 1989). Hands should be washed (not scrubbed) with aqueous povidone iodine if penetration of the skin has occurred. Equipment surfaces should be washed with sodium hypochlorite.

BIBLIOGRAPHY

Brown P. Gibbs C J, Amyx H L et al 1982 Chemical disinfection of Creutzfeldt–Jakob disease virus. New England Journal of Medicine 306: 1279–1282

Buchanan C R, Preece M A, Milner R D G 1991 Mortality, neoplasia, and Creutzfeldt–Jakob disease in patients treated with pituitary growth hormone in the United Kingdom. British Medical Journal 302: 824–828

du Moulin G C, Hedley-Whyte J 1983 Hospital-associated viral infection and the anesthesiologist. Anesthesiology 59: 51–65

Hughes J T 1993 Prion diseases. British Medical Journal 306: 288

Knight R 1989 Creutzfeldt–Jakob disease. British Journal of Hospital Medicine 41: 165–171

MacMurdo S D, Jakymec A J, Bleyaert A L 1984 Precautions in the anesthetic management of a patient with Creutzfeldt–Jakob disease. Anesthesiology 60: 590–592

CRI DU CHAT SYNDROME

A chromosomal abnormality due to a short arm deletion on chromosome 5. It is associated with a number of characteristic features. Most patients die in childhood.

Preoperative abnormalities

1. The infant has microcephaly, micrognathia, hypertelorism, severe mental retardation, epicanthic folds and a cat-like cry.
2. There may be a number of other abnormalities, including congenital heart disease.

Anaesthetic problems

1. Difficulties in intubation have been reported (Yamashita et al 1985). Although the characteristic cry may be partially neurogenic in

origin, a number of upper airway abnormalities have been described. These include a small, narrow larynx, a long floppy epiglottis, and retrognathia.

2. The babies are hypotonic and may be sensitive to non-depolarizing muscle relaxants.
3. A tendency to pulmonary aspiration may lead to chronic respiratory infections.

Management

1. Awake intubation or inhalation induction should be performed.
2. Minimal doses of relaxants, or controlled ventilation without relaxation may be wise.
3. Care with nursing and feeding may reduce aspiration problems.

BIBLIOGRAPHY

Yamashita M, Tanioka F, Taniguchi K et al 1985 Anesthetic consideration in Cri du Chat syndome. A report of three cases. Anesthesiology 63: 201–202

CUSHING'S SYNDROME AND CUSHING'S DISEASE

Cushing's syndrome is the general term used for a disorder caused by excess circulating glucocorticoid. Cushing's disease specifies one of its causes, that of pituitary-dependent adrenal hyperplasia secondary to ACTH secretion. This accounts for about 70–80% cases of Cushing's syndrome. Other important causes are adrenal cortical tumour (5–10%) and ectopic ACTH-producing tumours (5–10%).

Preoperative abnormalities

1. A review of 31 patients with Cushing's disease showed that the commonest clinical features, in order of frequency, were: weakness, thin skin, obesity, easy bruising, hypertension, menstrual disorders, hirsutism, impotence, striae, proximal muscle weakness, oedema, osteoporosis, mental disorders, diabetic GTT, backache, acne, hypokalaemia and fasting hyperglycaemia (Urbanic & George 1981). Fractures occur, and wound healing is poor.
2. Biochemical abnormalities include: hypokalaemic alkalosis, sodium and water retention, hyperglycaemia, lack of diurnal variation in plasma cortisol with its failure to decrease at night, and increased urinary free cortisol.
3. Cushing's syndrome is associated with severe left ventricular hypertrophy with a disproportionate hypertrophy of the interventricular septum (Sugihara et al 1992). The cause is unknown.
4. Patients have an increased incidence of infections.

5. Screening is by overnight dexamethasone test and 24-hour urinary excretion of cortisol (Klibanski & Zervas 1991).
6. Occasionally, patients become pregnant. The commonest complications are hypertension and diabetes (Prihoda & Davis 1991, Aron et al 1990).

Anaesthetic problems

1. Venous access may be difficult due to fragility of veins.
2. Hypertension, with or without heart failure, may be present. Left ventricular hypertrophy, particularly of the interventricular septum is seen (Sugihara et al 1992).
3. Hypokalaemia. There may be severe depletion of potassium stores.
4. Diabetes mellitus.
5. Muscle weakness may contribute to postoperative respiratory failure.
6. An increased risk of deep vein thrombosis.

Management

1. Hypertension and heart failure, if present, must be treated.
2. Diabetes must be controlled.
3. Hypokalaemia requires identification and correction.
4. In florid cases, drug control of adrenocortical function with metyrapone, an 11-beta-hydroxylase inhibitor, may be advisable before operation (Montgomery & Welbourn 1978).
5. Careful positioning of the patient to avoid fractures of osteoporotic bone, is required.
6. Steroids should be maintained during and after surgery (Weatherill & Spence 1984).

BIBLIOGRAPHY

Aron D C, Schnall A M, Sheeler L R 1990 Cushing's syndrome and pregnancy. American Journal of Obstetrics and Gynecology 162: 244–252

Klibanski A, Zervas N T 1991 Diagnosis and management of hormone secreting pituitary adenomas. New England Journal of Medicine 324: 822–831

Montgomery D A D, Welbourn R B 1978 Cushing's syndrome: 20 years after adrenalectomy. British Journal of Surgery 65: 221–223

Prihoda J S, Davis L E 1991 Metabolic emergencies in obstetrics. Obstetrics and Gynecology Clinics of North America 18: 301–318

Sugihara N, Shimizu M, Kita Y et al 1992 Cardiac characteristics and postoperative courses in Cushing's syndrome. American Journal of Cardiology 69: 1475–1480

Urbanic R C, George J M 1981 Cushing's disease – 18 years' experience. Medicine 60: 14–24

Weatherill D, Spence A A 1984 Anaesthesia and disorders of the adrenal cortex. British Journal of Anaesthesia 56: 741–749

CYSTIC FIBROSIS

An autosomal recessive syndrome primarily involving the exocrine glands and producing a variable pattern of the disease. Glandular secretions are relatively concentrated, with excess electrolytes and altered mucus glycoproteins. There is excessive sodium absorption and deficient chloride secretion. This leads to abnormal mucociliary transport, although ciliary function is normal (Rutland & Cole 1981). As a result, gland ducts become blocked. Infection, hyperplasia and hypertrophy tend to result. The patient may develop progressive chronic respiratory problems in childhood, malabsorption, and cirrhosis of the liver. Progressive lung damage can lead to pulmonary hypertension and right heart failure. Advances in the management of the disease has extended life-expectancy, therefore more patients are likely to present for surgery. Pregnancy may occur. Operative mortality has decreased dramatically during the last 20 years. In a review of 77 patients undergoing 126 procedures, of which 86% were operations directly related to the disease itself, no evidence was produced that anaesthesia had any deleterious effect on lung function (Lamberty & Rubin 1985). Lung transplantation is one method of treatment for advanced disease. Some improvement in sputum viscosity and elasticity has been shown using nebulized amiloride, a potassium–sparing diuretic, which blocks sodium uptake and increases the water content of sputum (Knowles et al 1990). Studies are being undertaken on the effects of nebulized DNase to reduce sputum viscosity by lysis of neutrophil DNA. The effect of extracellular nucleotides on induction of chloride secretion in nasal mucosa is also being assessed (Knowles et al 1991). Recently, the gene responsible for cystic fibrosis has been identified and sequenced.

Preoperative abnormalities

1. Sweat test. High sodium (>60 mmol/l in infants; >65 mmol/l suggestive and >90 mmol/l diagnostic in children), and high chloride levels.
2. Viscous secretions, defective mucociliary transport and altered lung mechanics produce severe chest infections. Bronchiectasis, pulmonary fibrosis and emphysema follow. Bronchopulmonary aspergillosis, aspergilloma and haemoptysis are other complications.
3. Pneumothorax, which is difficult to treat, is common in adults (Spector & Stern 1989). A study of 243 adults showed that 46 (18.9%) had at least one pneumothorax, from which 7 had died (Penketh et al 1982). This complication is much less frequent in children (2–7%).
4. Nasal polyps and sinusitis occur in 10–15% of cases.
5. Pulmonary hypertension, secondary to hypoxia, may develop in advanced lung disease. Cor pulmonale finally supervenes.
6. A certain number of adults develop abnormal liver function, proceeding to portal hypertension, oesophageal varices and cirrhosis.
7. Pancreatic insufficiency occurs in 80–90% of patients. Malabsorption, hypoproteinaemia and low body weight result.

Prothrombin time may be prolonged due to loss of fat–soluble vitamins.

8. Distal intestinal obstruction syndrome is the commonest gastrointestinal complication. This can usually be managed medically (Smith & Stableforth 1992). Gallstones, peptic ulceration and oesophageal reflux occur more commonly than in the normal population.

Anaesthetic problems

1. Despite the improvement in prognosis, when lung disease is severe, the mortality is increased.
2. Gaseous induction is both slow, because of low ventilation perfusion ratios, and stormy.
3. The tracheal tube is easily blocked by secretions.
4. There is a high incidence of perioperative respiratory complications. These include pneumothorax, pneumonia, airway obstruction, atelectasis, respiratory failure and arrest.
5. Bronchoscopy and lung washout is associated with episodes of profound hypoxia (Harnik et al 1983).
6. Periods of oxygen desaturation during sleep may occur postoperatively.
7. Nasal polyps can cause airway obstruction.
8. There is a high sodium loss, especially when hot.
9. With aggressive treatment and increased survival, some patients are becoming pregnant (Canny et al 1991). A survey of 38 pregnancies in 25 patients, showed it to be well tolerated in most patients. However, these patients had generally less severe disease since half had no pancreatic insufficiency. In other series, mother and fetus fared less well. Maternal complications include pulmonary, liver, cardiac and pancreatic insufficiency. Recurrent infections may require continuous antibiotics and oxygen supplementation. Parenteral nutrition may be necessary. Twelve per cent of patients died within 6 months and 18% within 2 years of their pregnancy. This death rate was no more than that expected in equivalent non-pregnant patients (Cohen et al 1980). Those with lower clinical (Schwachman-Kulczycki) scores were more likely to deteriorate or die (Palmer et al 1983). There may be poor fetal nutrition and oxygen delivery (Valenzuela et al 1988) and an increased perinatal mortality.

Management

1. Respiratory and cardiovascular function must be carefully assessed.
2. Regular, intensive physiotherapy is mandatory. This includes postural drainage, percussion and forced expiration, and encouragement to take exercise.

3. Infections, especially with *Pseudomonas aeruginosa*, require i.v. treatment with an aminoglycoside (tobramycin) and a beta lactam (azlocillin) combination. However, the most appropriate drug depends upon culture and sensitivity. There is increasing use of regular nebulized antibiotics given via high–powered air compressors.

4. Nebulized steroid and bronchodilator drugs will reduce bronchospasm in the presence of asthma.

5. Parenteral vitamin K will be needed if the prothrombin time is prolonged.

6. Local anaesthesia should be employed if possible. Laparoscopic cholecystectomy under continuous extradural anaesthesia in a 30–40° sitting position has been reported (Edelman 1991).

7. Sedative premedication should be avoided. Anti-sialogogues may be used if essential, but preferably immediately before induction.

8. Inhalational induction can be stormy, and should be avoided.

9. All patients require tracheal intubation to facilitate aspiration of secretions, oxygenation and ventilation.

10. Anaesthetic gases must be humidified and tracheal secretions aspirated regularly during surgery. The viscidity of secretions is reduced by keeping the patient well hydrated, but not overloaded.

11. The role of bronchial washouts in the management of cystic fibrosis is controversial. Supporters include Harnik et al (1983). Repeated aliquots of up to 20 ml 5% acetylcysteine in saline were instilled into the main divisions of the bronchial tree, to a total volume of 200–300 ml, over a period of 20–30 minutes. Concomitant monitoring with a transcutaneous oxygen analyzer enabled oxygenation to be restored before dangerous hypoxia occurred.

12. Pneumothorax in the adult, treated by simple drainage, is associated with a high incidence of recurrence (Penketh et al 1982). A persistent leak for 7 days has been suggested as an indication for surgical intervention. Subsequently it has been found that recurrence of a pneumothorax within 6 months of surgery indicates an extremely poor prognosis (Robinson & Branthwaite 1984).

13. Haemoptysis requires location of the bleeding point with fibreoptic or rigid bronchoscopy. Life-threatening haemoptysis has been treated using desmopressin 4 μg followed by vasopressin 20 u over 15 minutes then an infusion of 0.2 u/min for 36 hours (Bilton et al 1990). More invasive therapy includes embolization of the appropriate bronchial artery, bronchial artery ligation or lobectomy. Many adults are, however, not fit enough for major surgery.

14. Lung transplantation may be considered in patients with progressive disease (Smyth et al 1991). After an analysis of serial investigations to study prediction of mortality in 673 patients, Kerem et al (1992) concluded that patients should be considered as candidates for lung

transplantation when the FEV_1 decreased to below 30% of the predicted value.

15. If pregnancy occurs and the patient does not accept termination of pregnancy, a team representing the different disciplines must be assembled at an early stage. Assessment of activity, physical findings, nutrition and CXR should be undertaken (Palmer et al 1983).

BIBLIOGRAPHY

Bilton D, Webb A K, Foster H et al 1990 Life threatening haemoptysis in cystic fibrosis: an alternative therapeutic approach. Thorax 45: 975–976

Canny G J, Corey M, Livingstone R A et al 1991 Pregnancy and cystic fibrosis. Obstetrics and Gynecology 77: 850–853

Cohen L F, Sant' Agnese P A, Friedlander J 1980 Cystic fibrosis and pregnancy. A national survey. Lancet 2: 842–844

Edelrnan D S 1991 Laparoscopic cholecystectomy under continuous epidural anesthesia in patients with cystic fibrosis. American Journal of Diseases of Children 145: 723–734

Elbom J S, Shale D J 1990 Lung injury in Cystic fibrosis. Thorax 45: 970–973

Harnik E, Kulczycki L, Gomes M N 1983 Transcutaneous oxygen monitoring during bronchoscopy and washout for cystic fibrosis. Anesthesia and Analgesia 62: 357–362

Kerem E, Reisman J, Corey M et al 1992 Prediction of mortality in patients with cystic fibrosis. New England Journal of Medicine 326: 1187–1191

Knowles M R, Church N L, Waltner W E et al 1990 A pilot study of aerosolized amiloride for the treatment of lung disease in cystic fibrosis. New England Journal of Medicine 322: 1189–1194

Knowles M R, Clarke L L, Boucher R C 1991 Activation by extracellular nucleotides of chloride secretion in the airway epithelia of patients with cystic fibrosis. New England Journal of Medicine 325: 533–538

Lamberty J M, Rubin B K 1985 The management of anaesthesia for patients with cystic fibrosis. Anaesthesia 40: 448–459

Palmer J, Dillon-Baker C, Tecklin J S et al 1983 Pregnancy in patients with cystic fibrosis. Annals of Internal Medicine 99: 596–600

Penketh A, Knight R K, Hodson M E et al 1982 Management of pneumothorax in adults with cystic fibrosis. Thorax 37: 850–853

Robinson D A, Branthwaite M A 1984 Pleural surgery in patients with cystic fibrosis. Anaesthesia 39: 655–659

Rutland J, Cole P J 1981 Nasal mucociliary clearance and ciliary beat frequency in cystic fibrosis compared with sinusitis and bronchiectasis. Thorax 36: 654–658

Smith D L, Stableforth D G 1992 Cystic fibrosis. British Journal of Hospital Medicine 48: 717–723

Smyth R L, Higginbottam T, Scott J et al 1991 The current state of lung transplantation for cystic fibrosis. Thorax 46: 213–216

Spector M L, Stern R C 1989 Pneumothorax in cystic fibrosis: a 26-year experience. Annals of Thoracic Surgery 47: 204–207

Valenzuela G J, Comunale F L, Davidson B H et al 1988 Clinical management of patients with cystic fibrosis and pulmonary insufficienry. American Journal of Obstetrics.and Gynecology 159: 1181–1183

CYSTIC HYGROMA OR LYMPHANGIOMA

A spectrum of rare developmental anomalies of the lymphatic system consisting of sequestrations of lymphatic tissue which fail to join up with the venous system. They are endothelially-lined, thin-walled lymphatic cysts which penetrate and canalise, their spread depending upon the space available for expansion. Fifty per cent are present at birth and 80% before the age of 2 years. Surgery is the treatment of choice but carries a high morbidity from the disease itself and from the surgery. Recurrence is common even after apparent total resection and usually occurs within the first postoperative year. Mortalities of 2–6% and permanent nerve palsies in 12–33% have been quoted. The postoperative complication rate is high and varies from 19–33% (Hancock et al 1992). Surface CO_2 laser photocoagulation has been used for suitable cases. Rarely, the condition may present in adult life (Scally & Black 1990).

Preoperative abnormalities

1. Lymphangiomas are mostly sited in the head and neck, including the larynx. The shoulder, axilla, arm, chest wall, mediastinum, abdomen, inguinal region and leg can also be involved. In a study of 193 cases, the distribution was: cervical 31.4%, craniofacial 18.9%, extremity 18.9%, intra-abdominal 9.2%, cervico-axillo-thoracic 4.9%, multiple 3.8%, cervicomediastinal 2.2% and intrathoracic 1.6% (Hancock et al 1992).
2. They transilluminate, are multilocular and can range from 1 mm to 20 cm in size. There is no skin attachment but fixation to deep tissues occurs.
3. Those in the head and neck may cause airway obstruction, dysphagia, feeding difficulties and speech problems. If the tongue is involved there may be protrusion beyond the lip margin (Balakrishnan & Bailey 1991): Recurrent enlargement may occur secondary to infection, trauma or bleeding. Suprahyoid lesions are more of a problem than infrahyoid ones and more likely to recur. Any child with tongue or floor of mouth lesions is at risk from sudden airway compromise.
4. Infiltrates vessels and nerves.
5. The lesion may suddenly expand as a result of haemorrhage or infection, particularly in association with either trauma or respiratory tract infection.
6. Recurrence is common, particularly with the suprahyoid lesions.

Anaesthetic problems

1. Airway problems. A survey of 37 cases showed that 41% suffered airway obstruction at some stage. Lymphangiomas of the tongue may suddenly increase in size with trauma and infection. There is a high incidence of respiratory obstruction, and tracheostomy may be required. Surface CO_2 laser coagulation is now used for suitable cases (Balakrishnan & Bailey 1991). Lymphangiomas may also involve the larynx (Cohen & Thompson 1986) and the epiglottis (Weller 1974).

2. Induction, airway maintenance or intubation problems (MacDonald 1966, Scally & Black 1990).
3. Surgery is often prolonged and difficult because the tumour infiltrates and destroys normal dissection planes.
4. Lingual oedema can occur after resection of submandibular lesions. Postoperative swelling of the tongue and floor of mouth may be alarming in the rapidity of its development.
5. Obstructive sleep apnoea and hypoxaemia may occur.
6. Infection is a danger because of the impaired lymphatic drainage.

Management

1. A CT scan or MRI will be required to delineate the anatomical involvement.
2. The patient may need a tracheostomy either pre- or postoperatively. Forty one per cent of children with cystic hygroma involving the neck suffered significant upper airway or feeding problems, and two-thirds of those with airway problems required tracheostomy (Emery et al 1984).
3. May need a feeding gastrostomy.
4. Intralaryngeal tumours may require laser treatment (Cohen & Thompson 1986).
5. Infections will need prompt antibiotic therapy.
6. Sudden swelling in an adult recurrence responded to emergency tracheostomy and corticosteroids (Scally & Black 1990).

BIBLIOGRAPHY

Balakrishnan A, Bailey C M 1991 Lymphangioma of the tongue. A review of pathogenesis, treatment and the use of surface laser photocoagulation. Journal of Laryngology and Otology 105: 924–929
Cohen S R, Thompson J W 1986 Lymphangiomas of the larynx in infants and children. A survey of pediatric lymphangioma. Annals of Otology, Rhinology and Laryngology 95 (suppl): 1–20
Editorial 1990 Cystic hygroma. Lancet 335: 511–512
Emery P J, Bailey C M, Evans J N G 1984 Cystic hygroma of the head and neck. A review of 37 cases. Journal of Laryngology and Otology 98: 613–619
Goodman P, Yeung C S, Batsakis J G 1990 Retropharyngeal lymphangioma presenting in an adult. Otolaryngology, Head and Neck Surgery 103: 476–479
Hancock B J, St-Vil D, Luks F I et al 1992 Complications of lymphangiomas in children. Journal of Pediatric Surgery 27: 220–224
MacDonald D J F 1966 Cystic hygroma. An anaesthetic and surgical problem. Anaesthesia 21: 66–71
Ricciardelli E J, Richardson M A 1991 Cervicofacial cystic hygroma. Patterns of recurrence and management of the difficult case. Archives of Otolaryngology and Head and Neck Surgery. 117: 546–553
Scally C M, Black J H A 1990 Cystic hygroma: massive recurrence in adult life. Journal of Otology and Laryngology 104: 908–910
Weller R M 1974 Anaesthesia for cystic hygroma in a neonate. Anaesthesia 29: 588–594

DEMYELINATING DISEASES

A general term for a group of neurological diseases involving myelin sheath abnormalities. The myelin surrounding an axon may develop normally and then be lost later, to leave the axon itself preserved. Alternatively, there may be some defect in the original formation of myelin as a result of an error of metabolism. The commonest presentation is in multiple sclerosis (MS), the aetiology of which is unknown, but is probably multifactorial.

Susceptibility to MS may be genetically determined. Viral and immune factors are possibly involved. Plaques of demyelination are scattered throughout the nervous system, usually in the optic nerve, brainstem and spinal cord. The peripheral nerves are not involved. Only the problems of multiple sclerosis will be discussed further.

Preparative abnormalities

1. The diagnosis is made on clinical grounds, when neurological lesions are disseminated in both time and space. Consequently the clinical picture is highly variable.
2. The commonest presenting symptoms, in order of frequency, are limb weakness, visual disturbances, paraesthesiae and incoordination. Legs are more commonly involved before the arms, with signs of spasticity and hyper-reflexia. Urinary symptoms may occur.
3. Progression, with remissions and relapses, is very variable. Infection, trauma and stress may be associated with relapses. A small increase in body temperature can cause a definite deterioration in neural function. The relapse rate in the first three months postpartum is three times that of the non-pregnant patient.
4. Pain may be a prominent feature, occurring at any one time in 45% of patients.
5. Mild dementia and dysarthria may appear as the disease progresses.
6. In advanced disease, and sometimes earlier during acute relapses, respiratory complications may occur secondary to a variety of causes. These are, in decreasing order of importance, respiratory muscle weakness, bulbar weakness and central control of breathing (Howard et al 1992).
7. MRI now plays an important part in the diagnosis, and abnormalities in the white matter can be seen in 99% of cases. Gadolinium enhancement seems to reflect areas of inflammation where the blood-brain barrier has broken down. However, there seems to be little relationship between the extent of the lesions seen and the clinical picture.
8. Although high-dose steroids may reduce the duration of a relapse, no long-term therapy has yet been found.

Anaesthetic problems

Reports of anaesthetics given to patients with MS are both numerous and conflicting. Advice about the avoidance of particular drugs or techniques is inconsistent and often based on small numbers of patients. In the event of a relapse, major difficulties exist in the separation of the effects of drugs, surgery, pyrexia or stress. An analysis of 88 general anaesthetics given to 42 patients did not show a relapse rate greater than that which would have been expected to occur spontaneously (Bamford et al 1978).

1. Both experimentally and clinically, an increase in body temperature has been shown to cause a deterioration in nerve conduction and neurological signs.
2. Spinal anaesthesia. A review of the medical literature, and a limited personal experience, led one group to the conclusion that spinal anaesthesia was associated with an increased incidence of neurological complications (Bamford et al 1978).
3. Extradural anaesthesia. A combined experience of 57 extradural anaesthetics in MS patients, without complications, but also regrettably without details, has been claimed by five anaesthetists from four different countries (Crawford et al 1981). Another study showed that extradural analgesia was not associated with a significantly higher incidence of relapses than is seen in women receiving local infiltration for delivery (Bader et al 1988). Temporary neurological deficits have, however, been reported. One patient developed localized paraesthesiae lasting 7 hours and 7 weeks respectively following two epidurals, in consecutive labours (Warren et al 1982). The longer deficit followed a total dose of bupivacaine of 562.5 mg during a 15-hour period. It was surmized that neurotoxicity might have followed the diffusion of the anaesthetic into the dural space. Nothing definite exists in the literature to suggest that patients be denied the benefits of extradural analgesia, should it be considered necessary. However, it has been advised that concentrations of bupivacaine of not greater than 0.25% should be used, since postpartum relapse has been reported with concentrations in excess of this (Bader et al 1988).
4. Local anaesthesia. One thousand procedures performed under local anaesthesia in 98 patients did not significantly increase the relapse rate (Bamford et al 1978). There is, however, evidence that local anaesthetics can cross the blood-brain barrier more readily in MS, and toxicity is more likely to occur.
5. Neuromuscular blockers. Resistance to atracurium, in association with an abnormally high concentration of skeletal muscle acetylcholine receptors, has been reported in a patient with MS and spastic paraparesis (Brett et al 1987).
6. There is an increased incidence of epilepsy in MS patients.

Management

1. It is vital to know, either from the notes or from staff, whether or not the patient is aware of the precise diagnosis. Appropriate discussions will take place with the patient in the light of this knowledge.
2. Elective surgery should not be undertaken in the presence of fever.
3. Spinal anaesthesia should probably be avoided (Bamford et al 1978), although a local anaesthetic and diamorphine given through an intrathecal catheter has been used for sigmoid colectomy in a patient with advanced disease involving paralysis of his intercostal muscles (Leigh et al 1990).
4. If a regional block is required, then extradural anaesthesia is preferable and should not be denied. Accurate documentation of the existing signs and symptoms, and a full discussion with the patient, is essential.
5. The maximal dose of local anaesthetic should be reduced below that normally recommended (Jones & Healy 1980). Techniques which require large doses should not be used.

BIBLIOGRAPHY
Bader A M, Hunt C O, Datta S et al 1988 Anaesthesia for the obstetric patient with multiple sclerosis. Journal of Clinical Anaesthesia 1: 21–24
Bamford C, Sibley W, Laguna J 1978 Anesthesia in multiple sclerosis. Le Journal Canadien des Sciences Neurologiques 5: 41–44
Brett R S, Schmidt J H, Gage J S et al 1987 Measurement of acetylcholine receptor concentration in skeletal muscle from a patient with multiple sclerosis and resistance to atracurium. Anesthesiolog 66: 837–839
Crawford J S, James F M, Nolte H et al 1981 Regional analgesia for patients with chronic neurological disease and similar conditions. Anaesthesia 36: 821
Howard R S, Wiles C M, Hirsch N P et al 1992 Respiratory involvement in multiple sclerosis. Brain 115: 479–494
Jones R M, Healy T E J 1980 Anaesthesia and demyelinating disease. Anaesthesia 35: 879–884
Leigh J, Fearnley S J, Lupprian K G 1990 Intrathecal diamorphine during laparotomy in a patient with advanced multiple sclerosis. Anaesthesia 45: 640–642
Warren T M, Datta S, Ostheimer G W 1982 Lumbar epidural anesthesia in a patient with multiple sclerosis. Anesthesia and Analgesia 61: 1022–1023

DERMATOMYOSITIS/POLYMYOSITIS COMPLEX

A group of autoimmune chronic inflammatory disorders primarily affecting muscle and skin, although there may be multisystem involvement. The related diseases include: primary idiopathic polymyositis, primary idiopathic dermatomyositis, dermatomyositis associated with malignancy, a childhood form of dermatomyositis, and a form of the complex which is associated with other collagen diseases (Bellamy et al 1984).

Preoperative abnormalities

1. In all cases a rash is a presenting feature. A violaceous appearance of the eyelids and upper part of the face is caused by the cutaneous lesions. The rash may also be seen on the knees, knuckles, elbows, and periungually.
2. The inflammatory myopathy may present with muscle aches, tenderness and weakness. This usually involves the legs initially and the arms and limb-girdle muscles subsequently. Contractures and muscle atrophy which may cause respiratory muscle weakness can occur later.
3. An increased risk of malignancy is seen and the mortality rate from cancer is higher than normal.
4. There may be patchy infiltration of the lungs with interstitial fibrosis, peripheral oedema, and soft-tissue calcification.
5. Although all muscle enzyme levels may be elevated, the serum CK is said to be the most sensitive indicator of disease activity. Serum myoglobin may be superior, but is not routinely measured. The patient may be anaemic.
6. Attendance at an ENT department is a common mode of presentation (Metheny 1978). Voice changes, and upper oesophageal dysphagia were the most frequent problems. Laryngo-oesophageal tone is reduced, with dysfunction of the tongue and soft palate. Saliva pools in the pyriform fossa, and regurgitation and aspiration leading to pneumonia may occur. Aspiration pneumonia is a common cause of death.
7. Up to 40% of patients have cardiac problems; these include ECG changes and congestive heart failure (Haupt & Hutchins 1982). Cardiac involvement is associated with a less good prognosis. Necrotizing vasculitis and cardiac involvement may appear in the childhood form.
8. The patient may be on steroids or immunosuppressives.
9. Pregnancy may be associated with fetal loss, particularly in active disease, but reports are contradictory (King & Chow 1985).
10. An abnormal EMG and evidence of a necrotizing inflammatory process on muscle biopsy.

Anaesthetic problems

1. Dermatomyositis is associated with an increased incidence of malignancy (Richardson & Callen 1989, Sigurgeirsson et al 1992).
2. Prolonged neuromuscular blockade after vecuronium has been reported (Flusche et al 1987). The explanation for this is obscure since an inflammatory myopathy should not affect the neuromuscular junction. However, neuromuscular monitoring in two patients receiving atracurium (Ganta et al 1988), one having vecuronium (Saarnivaara 1988) and another having both

suxamethonium and atracurium (Brown et al 1992), did not reveal any abnormal response or sensitivity. An abnormal response to suxamethonium was reported in a young child. Before muscle relaxation occurred, fasciculations were followed by a short period of muscle contraction (Johns et al 1986). However, marked increases in muscle tone following suxamethonium may occur in a percentage of normal patients, so the significance of this is uncertain (Leary et al 1990).

3. Swallowing and vocal cord dysfunction may cause pooling of secretions and aspiration of gastric contents (Metheny 1978). Delayed gastric emptying and uncoordinated peristalsis may increase the risks of inhalation (Plotz et al 1989).

4. Aspiration pneumonia is the commonest pulmonary problem and postoperative respiratory insufficiency may occur.

Management

1. A careful assessment of the systems involved in the disease, and in particular for signs of malignancy.

2. Monitoring of neuromuscular function is essential.

3. In view of the problems with swallowing and pooling of secretions, tracheal intubation has been recommended (Eisele 1981)

BIBLIOGRAPHY

Bellamy N, Kean W F, Buchanan W W 1984 Connective tissue diseases. The dermatopolymyositis complex. Hospital Update 10: 74–76

Brown S, Shupak R C, Patel C et al 1992 Neuromuscular blockade in a patient with active dermatomyositis. Anesthesiology 77: 1031–1033

Caro I 1989 Dermatomyositis as a systemic disease. Medical Clinics of North America 73 (5): 1181–1191

Eisele J H 1990 Connective tissue diseases. In: Katz J, Benumof J, Kadis L (eds) Anesthesia and uncommon diseases. W B Saunders, Philadelphia

Flusche G, Unger-Sargon J, Lambert D H 1987 Prolonged neuromuscular paralysis with vecuronium in a patient with polymyositis. Anesthesia and Analgesia 66: 188–190

Ganta R, Campbell I T, Mostafa S M 1988 Anaesthesia and acute dermatomyositis/polymyositis. British Journal of Anaesthesia 60: 854–858

Haupt H M, Hutchins G M 1982 The heart and cardiac conduction system in polymyositis and dermatomyositis. American Journal of Cardiology 50: 998–1006

Johns R A, Finholt D A, Stirt J A 1986 Anaesthetic management of a child with dermatomyositis. Canadian Anaesthetists' Society Journal 33: 71–74

King C R, Chow S 1985 Dermatomyositis and pregnancy. Obstetrics and Gynecology 66: 589–592

Leary N P, Ellis F R 1990 Masseteric muscle spasm as a normal response to suxamethonium. British Journal of Anaesthesia 64: 488–492

Metheny J A 1978 Dermatomyositis: A vocal and swallowing disease entity. Laryngoscope 88: 147–161

Plotz P H, Dalakas M, Leff R L et al 1989 Current concepts in the idiopathic inflammatory myopathies: polymyositis, dermatositis, and related disorders. Annals of Internal Medicine 111: 143–157

Richardson J B, Callen J P 1989 Dermatomyositis and malignancy. Medical Clinics of North America 73 (5): 1211–1220

Saarnivaara L H M 1988 Anesthesia for a patient with polymyositis undergoing myomectomy of the cricopharyngeal muscle. Anesthesia and Analgesia 67: 701–702

Sigurgeirsson B, Lindelof B, Edhag O et al 1992 Risk of cancer in patients with dermatomyositis or polymyositis. A population based study. New England Journal of Medicine 326: 363–367

Strauss K W, Gonzalez-Buritica H, Khamashta M A et al 1989 Polymyositis-dermatomyositis: a clinical review, Postgraduate Medical Journal 65: 437–443

DIABETES INSIPIDUS

The result of a failure of vasopressin secretion by the posterior part of the pituitary. In the presence of low levels of ADH, the kidney is unable to conserve water, and large volumes of dilute urine are excreted. It may be secondary to pituitary or hypothalamic surgery, head injury, tumour or multiple sclerosis. Diabetes insipidus is also common in brain-dead patients and may prove to be a problem in management of the donor for organ harvesting. Lithium treatment may rarely be associated with a mild diabetes insipidus-like syndrome. Diabetes insipidus appeared two days after chemical meningitis following spinal anaesthesia, thought to be caused by detergent used for washing a reusable glass syringe (Garfield et al 1986).

Preoperative abnormalities

1. Polyuria and polydipsia. The urine volume may reach 24 l/day.
2. Hypovolaemia and hypernatraemia.
3. Urinary osmolality is low (50–100 mosm/kg), and there is an increased plasma osmolality.

Anaesthetic problems

1. If the patient does not increase his fluid intake, there will be dehydration, hypernatraemia and plasma hyperosmolality.
2. Electrolyte imbalance.
3. Severe hypovolaemia associated with diabetes insipidus in cadaveric organ donors will require treatment. If vasopressin is used, and its administration continued until the kindneys are removed, there is an increase in the incidence of tubular necrosis and graft failure in the recipient (Graybar & Tarpey 1987). An analogue, desmopressin, has no vasoconstrictor effects.

Management

1. Desmopressin nasally 10–20 μg b.d., or 0.5–2 μg i.v., increases water reabsorption from the renal tubules.
2. The urine output and serum osmolality is monitored. If the osmolality is >290 mosm/kg, then i.v. fluids and desmopressin are required.

BIBLIOGRAPHY
Garfield J M, Andriole G L, Vetto J T et al 1986 Prolonged diabetes insipidus
    subsequent to an episode of chemical meningitis. Anesthesiology 64: 253-254
Graybar G B, Tarpey M 1987 Kidney transplantation. In: Gelman S (ed) Anesthesia
    and organ transplantation. W B Saunders, Philadelphia

DIABETES MELLITUS

In insulin-dependent diabetes (IDD, type I), the insulin deficiency means that catabolism exceeds anabolism, and in the absence of treatment a state of hyperosmolar ketoacidosis will progress to hypokalaemia, dehydration, coma and death.

In non-insulin-dependent diabetes (NIDD, type II) the pancreas still secretes insulin, but supply may not meet demand and under certain circumstances, such as surgical stress, there is insulin resistance and gluconeogenesis. The metabolic changes produced by surgery will worsen the state of diabetes.

Surgery should not be undertaken in diabetics who are out of control. Conversely, hypoglycaemia may be undetectable, and therefore dangerous, during anaesthesia. The increased insulin requirements must therefore be monitored closely and balanced with a supply of glucose and potassium.

Preoperative abnormalities

1. Diagnosis. A fasting venous or capillary whole blood glucose of >6.7 mmol/l, or a venous plasma level of >7.8 mmol/l. This can then be confirmed with a second FBG or a value after a glucose load. In symptomatic patients a random glucose of 11.1 mmol/l or more is usually diagnostic (Alberti & Hockaday 1987).

2. Metabolic. In the absence of insulin there is increased lipid metabolism with fatty acid release, increased ketone production such that the supply exceeds utilization, and increased gluconeogenesis and glycogenolysis. The net result is acidaemia, ketoacidosis, and hyperglycaemia. This hyperosmolar state leads to polyuria, which in turn causes urinary loss of sodium, potassium, calcium, phosphate and magnesium. The acidosis results in loss of cellular potassium, and the deficiency of insulin prevents cellular uptake of potassium. Sodium is also lost with the urinary excretion of ketoacids.

3. Cardiovascular disease. Large vessel disease leads to atherosclerosis and myocardial disease. The microangiopathy, which affects particularly renal, retinal and digital vessels, appears to be related to the high levels of blood glucose. There is a high mortality from myocardial and peripheral vascular disease.

4. Resistance to infection and wound healing are both impaired.

5. Renal failure is a common complication, and the mortality from renal transplantation is two to four times greater than in non-diabetic patients.

6. Peripheral and autonomic neuropathies, which may be related to high levels of sorbitol, are common. Autonomic neuropathy is more likely to occur in those with poor diabetic control, and symptomatic neuropathy may be exacerbated by pregnancy (Bilous 1990).

7. Limited joint mobility ('stiff joint syndrome'), in which patients are unable to approximate their palms (the 'prayer sign'), is said to occur in 30–40% of insulin-dependent diabetics. The joints of the hands are usually involved early and the skin becomes thick and waxy. There is a positive correlation with microvascular disease and the condition is progressive, ultimately involving all joints. It may be related to abnormal collagen cross-linkages. Lung elasticity may also be reduced.

Anaesthetic problems

1. There is a higher morbidity and mortality in diabetic than in non-diabetic patients. Myocardial disease and infection are chiefly responsible for this.

2. Surgery and stress aggravate diabetes and may be accompanied by some degree of insulin resistance. In addition, insulin resistance occurs with severe infection, obesity, liver disease, steroid therapy and cardiopulmonary bypass.

3. Hypoglycaemia can occur suddenly during anaesthesia. The usual warning signs are absent and brain damage can ensue.

4. Whilst a mild elevation of blood glucose is acceptable during surgery, it should be maintained between 6 and 13 mmol/l. The renal threshold for glucose is 10 mmol/l. At levels greater than this, the glycosuria causes an osmotic diuresis, with loss of water and electrolytes. In addition, hyperglycaemia is associated with impaired wound healing and disordered phagocyte function.

5. Administration of lactate-containing solutions may increase blood glucose, or may exacerbate lactic acidosis when this occurs in hyperglycaemic states.

6. Ketosis may produce insulin resistance and alter the metabolism of anaesthetic agents. It also increases potassium loss from the body. Hypokalaemia may induce cardiac arrhythmias during anaesthesia.

7. Ketoacidosis is associated with gastric atony and ileus, increasing the risk of inhalation of gastric contents.

8. Autonomic neuropathy may be responsible for cardiovascular and respiratory complications during anaesthesia. Five cases were reported in which episodes of cardiorespiratory arrest occurred in association with anaesthesia (Page & Watkins 1978). Episodes of respiratory arrest and loss of consciousness have continued into the second postoperative day (Thomas & Pollard 1989). Autonomic neuropathy could have reduced the respiratory responses to hypoxia and hypercarbia. Certainly, the diabetic heart is more susceptible to hypoxia in the absence of sympathetic drive. In some patients,

prolongation of the QT interval has been associated with sudden death. There is also an impaired ability to respond to stress by vasoconstriction and tachycardia (see Autonomic failure). In a prospective study of 17 diabetic patients having eye surgery, 35% required vasopressors compared with 5% of non-diabetic controls. They were required more often in those with the poorest autonomic function (Burgos et al 1989). The first few minutes after tracheal intubation was the period of highest risk for hypotension and bradycardia. Intubation produced less of a pressor response than is seen in normal patients Atropine-induced heart rate was found to be significantly lower in diabetics than non-diabetics (Tsueda et al 1991).

9. Local anaesthetic procedures are not without problems. Two patients suffered progressive bradycardia and hypotension, which responded to external cardiac massage and adrenaline, 20 minutes after brachial plexus block for the creation of an arteriovenous fistula (Lucas & Tsueda 1990). Although in one patient combined local anaesthetic blood level approached the seizure threshold, it was considerably less than that likely to produce cardiovascular collapse.

10. Difficult intubation is more common in patients with type I diabetes (Salzarulo & Taylor 1986). This may be related to involvement of the atlanto-occipital joint in 'stiff joint syndrome'. A group of type I diabetics have joint contractures and a thick waxy skin associated with rapidly progressive microvascular disease. This accounts for the high incidence of difficult laryngoscopy found in diabetics undergoing renal and pancreatic transplantation (Hogan et al 1988), In a series of 115 diabetics having renal or pancreas transplants, difficult laryngoscopy occurred in about 40%, whereas in 112 non-diabetic patients having renal transplants the incidence was only about 2–3%. Most of the patients with difficulties required blind intubation after several failed attempts, but three were awakened for fibreoptic intubation and two needed emergency tracheostomies. Laryngeal structures tended to be anterior to the line of vision, with only the posterior part of the arytenoids or epiglottis seen.

Management

1. General assessment
   A thorough assessment of the degree of multiorgan involvement by the diabetic process is required. In particular the presence of cardiovascular and renal disease, or autonomic neuropathy (see Autonomic failure) must be determined. If there is autonomic failure, then there should be close respiratory and cardiovascular monitoring throughout the perioperative period. After major surgery, oxygen supplements, ECG and oxygen saturation monitoring should be continued for 48 hours (Thomas & Pollard 1989).

2. If there is physical evidence of 'stiff joint syndrome', then flexion/extension views of the cervical spine may be helpful. The presence of limited atlanto-occipital extension indicates the possible need for awake tracheal intubation. Examination of the ability of the patient to approximate his fingers may reveal the 'palm sign'. A palm print, obtained by inking the dominant hand and placing it, with fingers spread, on white paper, has also been used to predict difficult laryngoscopy (Reissell et al 1990). If only the finger tips were visible, then laryngoscopy was likely to be difficult.

3. Assessment of diabetic control
Includes estimations of FBG levels, glucose test strips and urinalysis. Variations in levels occur dependent on the method of sampling. Whole blood glucose values are 10–15% less than plasma values, and fasting capillary is 7% greater than venous values.

4. Management of diabetes during elective surgery
Traditionally, it was recommended that diabetics be admitted 2–3 days in advance of surgery and appear first on a morning operating list, and that long-acting oral hypoglycaemic agents such as chlorpropamide and glibenclamide be discontinued 2 days in advance, or changed to short-acting ones. Similarly, long-acting insulins should be changed to either actrapid or other short-acting forms. In practice, the anaesthetist is often presented with diabetic patients the evening before operation, none of these conditions having been met! Practical approaches are:

a. Diet controlled and patients with NIDD
   i. Minor surgery. May need no treatment, but the latter should be monitored closely for hypoglycaemia. There is certainly no evidence that GIK is necessary, unless the fasting blood glucose is >13 mmol/l, in which case the GIK regimen should be used,
   ii. Major surgery (or in NIDD patients with a FBG >10 mmol/l on the morning of operation). Treat with an insulin infusion as for IDD.

b. Insulin-dependent diabetics
   Various methods of administering insulin have been described. These include short-acting insulin given subcutaneously 4-hourly, continuously i.v. by syringe pump, or mixed in an infusion with glucose and potassium. Subcutaneous insulin is absorbed erratically in the perioperative period and should not be used.

   A currently accepted method is a glucose/insulin/potassium (GIK) infusion (Alberti & Thomas 1979, Bowen et al 1984). Despite past fears of insulin absorption into the container and tubes, if the first 50 ml are washed through, 75–90% of the insulin is delivered. Should the infusion run too fast or stop, all the constituents are similarly affected. In addition, if the infusion is started when the morning insulin would have been due, the

need for early morning surgery is less urgent. The main disadvantage is the wasted solutions if the insulin dose has to be altered frequently.

Technique
  i. Preoperative FBG should be <13 mmol/l. Cancellation of the proposed surgery should be considered if levels are higher than this. The aim should be to maintain a BG of 5–10 mmol/l.
  ii. Infuse Actrapid 15 u + KCl 10 mmol + 10% glucose 500 ml, at a rate of 100 ml/h.
  iii. Repeat BG in 2–3 hours; if >10 mmol/l, increase insulin to 20 u and check BG in further 2 hours. If <5 mmol/l, then no insulin should be given.
  iv. BG should be measured 2-hourly, and serum potassium twice on the day of infusion.

However, there is still no clear evidence that the GIK regimen is superior to that using one-half to one-third of the patient's normal insulin, given s.c., with i.v. glucose, 5–10 g/h (Hall & Desborough 1988).

An alternative method is to use a syringe pump to administer the insulin, starting at 2–3 u/h, separately from the glucose and potassium. This carries the risk that an imbalance of glucose and insulin may occur if one of the infusions stops.

5. The ketoacidotic diabetic
  a. In young diabetics severe ketoacidosis may cause abdominal pain. If the vomiting starts before the pain, the cause is more likely to be ketoacidosis, whereas pain preceding vomiting is more likely to be surgical.
  b. If severe ketoacidosis is present and conditions permit, surgery should be delayed for 4–5 hours. Without prior control of the diabetes, the mortality is high.
  c. Treatment of severe diabetic ketoacidosis (adult).
    i. Investigations. Glucose, sodium, potassium, urea, serum osmolality, blood gases.
    ii. Monitoring. BP, pulse, respiration, urine output, CVP measurement.
    iii. Rehydration. 0.9% saline 1 line is given in 30 minutes, then 1 litre per hour for 2 hours, followed by 500 ml hourly until a total of 5–7 litres has been given. 500 ml is then infused 2–4-hourly.
      When a BG of 10–14 mmol/l has been achieved, change to 5% glucose 4-hourly.
      If sodium >146 mmol/l then, after the second litre 0.9% saline, substitute sodium chloride 0.18% and glucose 4%
    iv. Insulin therapy. Give 6 u i.v. stat then, using hourly glucose test strips, regulate the rate on a sliding scale.

v. Potassium. Immediately following the first dose of insulin, give potassium chloride 13 mmol/h in the saline. Monitor serum potassium:

K+ <3 mmol/l	give 39 mmol/h
K+ 3–4 mmol/l	give 26 mmol/h
K+ 4–6 mmol/l	give 13 mmol/h
K+ >6 mmol/l	stop potassium

vi. Acidosis pH = <7.0, give sodium bicarbonate 100 mmol and KCl 20 mmol in the first 30 minutes.

pH = 7.0–7.1, give sodium bicarbonate 50 mmol and KCl 10 mmol.

6. Insulin resistance

In a number of circumstances insulin resistance occurs. Normally the ratio of insulin to glucose required is 15 u insulin to 500 ml 10% dextrose. In patients with severe infection, obesity, liver disease, on steroid therapy or undergoing cardiopulmonary bypass, the dose of insulin may have to be increased by up to four times the normal ratio.

7. Impaired conscious level in diabetics

Causes include hypoglycaemia, diabetic ketoacidosis, hyperglycaemic hyperosmolar non-ketotic coma, and lactic acidosis.

Typical laboratory findings are (Alberti & Hockaday 1987):

a. Hypoglycaemia

BG <2 mmol/l

b. Severe diabetic ketoacidosis

BG >15 mmol/l	Ketones + to + + +
Dehydration + + +	Hyperventilation + + +

c. Hyperglycaemic, hyperosmolar, non ketotic coma

BG <15 mmol/l	Ketones 0 to +
Dehydration + + + +	No hyperventilation

d. Lactic acidosis

BG variable	Ketones 0 to +
Dehydration 0 to +	Hyperventilation + + +

Other non-diabetic causes should not be forgotten.

8. Erythromycin, which may act as a motilin agonist, can improve gastric emptying in diabetic gastroparesis (Janssens et al 1990).

BIBLIOGRAPHY

Alberti K G M M 1991 Diabetes and surgery. Anesthesiology 74: 209–211

Alberti K G M M, Hockaday T D R 1987 Diabetes mellitus. In: Weatherall D J, Ledingham J G G, Warrell D A (eds) Oxford Textbook of Medicine. Oxford University Press, Oxford

Alberti K G M M, Thomas D J B 1979 The management of diabetes during surgery. British Journal of Anaesthesia 51: 693–709

Bilous R W 1990 Diabetic autonomic neuropathy. A common complication which rarely causes symptoms. British Medical Journal 301: 565–566

Bowen D J, Daykin A P, Nancekievill M L et al 1984 Insulin-dependent diabetic patients during surgery and labour. Anaesthesia 39: 407–411

Burgos L G, Ebert T J, Asiddao C et al 1989 Increased intraoperative cardiovascular
   lability in diabetics with autonomic neuropathy. Anesthesiology 70: 591–597
Hall G M, Desborough J P 1988 Diabetes and anaesthesia – slow progress.
   Anaesthesia 43: 531–532
Hirsch I B, McGill J B, Cryer P E et al 1991 Perioperative management of surgical
   patients with diabetes mellitus. Anesthesiology 74: 346–359
Hogan K, Rusy D, Springman S R 1988 Difficult laryngoscopy and diabetes mellitus.
   Anesthesia and Analgesia 67: 1162–1165
Janssens J, Peeters T L, Vantrappen G et al 1990 Improvement of gastric emptying in
   diabetic gastroparesis by erythromycin. New England Journal of Medicine 322:
   1028–1031
Lucas L F, Tsueda K 1990 Cardiovascular depression following brachial plexus block
   in two diabetic patients with renal failure. Anesthesiology 73: 1032–1035
Milaskiewicz R M, Hall G M 1992 Diabetes and anaesthesia: the past decade. British
   Journal of Anaesthesia 68: 198–206
Page M McB, Watkins P J 1978 Cardiorespiratory arrest and diabetic autonomic
   neuropathy. Lancet i: 14–16
Reissell E, Orko R, Maunuksela E-L et al 1990 Predictability of difficult laryngoscopy
   in patients with long-term diabetes mellitus. Anesthesia 45: 1024–1027
Salzarulo H H, Taylor L A 1986 Diabetic 'stiff joint syndrome' as a cause of difficult
   endotracheal intubation. Anesthesiology 64: 366–368
Thomas A N, Pollard B J 1989 Renal transplantation and diabetic autonomic
   neuropathy. Canadian Journal of Anaesthesia 36: 590–592
Tsueda K, Huang K C, Dumont S W et al 1991 Cardiac sympathetic tone in
   anaesthetised diabetics. Canadian Journal of Anaesthesia 38: 20–23

DOWN'S SYNDROME

This well-known syndrome with characteristic morphological features
and mental retardation, results from the chromosomal abnormality,
trisomy 21. Mortality is increased at any stage of life, but improved
medical and nursing care means that many more are surviving into
adulthood and may present for surgery. Between 60 and 70% of
patients now survive beyond 10 years of age.

Preoperative abnormalities

1. Cardiac abnormalities occur in 50–60% of patients and are usually
   responsible for the initial mortality in infancy. The commonest
   lesions are septal defects, Fallot's tetralogy and patent ductus
   arteriosus.
2. A defect in the immune system results in an increased incidence of
   infection. Granulocyte abnormalities, decreased adrenal responses
   and defects in cell-mediated immunity have all been identified.
3. Skeletal abnormalities occur. Atlantoaxial instability has only
   recently been recognized as a problem, just at a time when these
   children are being encouraged to participate in gymnastics! In one
   survey, 18% of 85 Down's children had C1/C2 articulation
   abnormalities; 12% had subluxation alone and 6% were associated
   with odontoid peg abnormalities (Semine et al 1978). The cause is
   still uncertain, but poor muscle tone, ligamentous laxity and
   abnormal development of the odontoid peg may act in concert.

4. Biochemical abnormalities have been found and may involve serotonin, catecholamine and amino acid metabolism.
5. Thyroid hypofunction is common in adults. A child with Down's syndrome had a thyrotoxic crisis which mimicked malignant hyperthermia (Peters et al 1981).
6. Sleep-induced ventilatory dysfunction can occur.
7. Institutionalized Down's patients have an increased incidence of hepatitis B antigen.

Anaesthetic problems

The incidence of significant abnormalities is high. In a review of 100 cases of Down's syndrome requiring surgery, 44 patients had lesions requiring cardiac surgery and 41 others had abnormalities or diseases with anaesthetic implications (Kobel et al 1982).

1. Cervical spine abnormalities increase the risk of dislocation of certain cervical vertebrae on intubation, or when the patient is paralyzed with muscle relaxants. Atlantoaxial subluxation and spinal cord compression were discovered in two children after anaesthesia for surgical procedures. In neither case had cervical spine screening been carried out, nor had precautions been taken during intubation (Williams et al 1987, Moore et al 1987). An adult, admitted to ITU for treatment of acute respiratory failure attributed to postoperative pneumonia, was subsequently found to have atlantoaxial subluxation with a sagittal canal diameter in extension of only 2.5 mm (Powell et al 1990). Irreversible neurological damage had occurred.
2. A smaller tracheal tube size is required than would be anticipated for the age of the patient (Kobel et al 1982).
3. Airway and intubation difficulties sometimes occur, due to a combination of anatomical features. These include a large tongue, a small mandible and maxilla, a narrow nasopharynx and irregular teeth.
4. Postoperative stridor after prolonged nasal intubation has been reported (Sherry 1983). Congenital subglottic stenosis occurs occasionally.
5. Obstructive sleep apnoea is common in Down's syndrome (Silverman 1988). Compared with normal children they had an increased incidence of stridor and chest wall recession, a lower baseline oxygen saturation and a greater number of episodes of desaturation to 90% or less (Stebbens et al 1991). Chronic episodes of hypoxia and hypercarbia may lead to pulmonary hypertension and congestive heart failure. Airway patency depends upon both the anatomical structure of the upper respiratory tract, and the normal functioning of the pharyngeal muscles. Abnormalities of either or both may occur.

6. Problems of the associated cardiac disease, which in later life may lead to pulmonary hypertension (Riley & McBride 1991).
7. A higher incidence of atelectasis and pulmonary oedema was reported after surgery for congenital heart disease (Morray et al 1986). Those with Down's syndrome and ventricular septal defects were predisposed to pulmonary vascular obstruction.
8. Posterior arthrodesis of the upper cervical spine carries a high complication rate (Segal et al 1991). These include infection and wound dehiscence, instability at a lower level, neurological sequelae, and postoperative death.

Management

1. Lateral X-rays of the neck in full flexion and extension positions should be taken in an attempt to detect atlantoaxial instability. However, X-rays may be unreliable and Selby et al (1991) found no reliable clinical predictors of subluxation. This may show as an increase in the distance between the posterior surface of the anterior arch of the atlas and the anterior surface of the odontoid process (Hungerford et al 1981). Patients with an atlanto-odontoid interval of 4.5–6.0 mm were asymptomatic, but those in whom the distance exceeded 7 mm had neurological signs. If instability is present, great care should be taken to immobilize the neck during tracheal intubation and muscle relaxation. These changes do not appear to progress with time. A longitudinal study of 141 patients having serial X-ray examinations indicated that significant changes in the atlanto-dens distance did not take place (Pueschel et al 1992), therefore regular screening is not necessary.
2. If significant cardiac disease is present, management must be appropriate to the lesion and endocarditis prophylaxis used as recommended.
3. A tracheal tube should be used which is 1–2 sizes smaller than would be expected from the patient's age.
4. If prolonged nasotracheal intubation is required, steroids should be given before extubation. The child should receive humidification and be observed carefully for signs of stridor. There may be an indication for respiratory stimulants.
5. Close observation is required in the perioperative period to detect episodes of obstructive apnoea. A pulse oximeter may be useful.
6. Loss of locomotor skills or disturbances of gait after surgery should alert staff to the possibility of subluxation and cord compression (Powell et al 1990). In such an event, an urgent neurological opinion should be sought. However, in the absence of neurological signs, non-operative management may be indicated, because of the high complication rate after surgery (Segal et al 1991).

BIBLIOGRAPHY

Bird T M, Strunin L 1984 Anaesthesia for a patient with Down's syndrome and Eisenmenger's complex. Anaesthesia 39: 48–50

Editorial 1989 Atlantoaxial instability in Down's syndrome. Lancet i: 24

Hungerford G D, Akkaraju V, Rawe S E et al 1981 Atlanto-occipital and atlanto-axial dislocations with spinal cord compression in Down's syndrome: a case report and review of the literature. British Journal of Radiology 54: 758–761

Kobel M, Creighton R E, Steward D J 1982 Anaesthetic considerations in Down's syndrome. Canadian Anaesthetists' Society Journal 29: 593–599

Moore R A, McNicholas K W, Warran S P 1987 Atlantoaxial subluxation with symptomatic spinal cord compression in a child with Down's syndrome. Anesthesia and Analgesia 66: 89–90

Morray J P, MacGillivray R, Duker G 1986 Increased perioperative risk following repair of congenital heart disease in Down's syndrome. Anesthesiology 65: 221–224

Peters K R, Nance P, Wingard D W 1981 Malignant hyperthyroidism or malignant hyperthermia? Anesthesia and Analgesia 60: 613–615

Powell J F, Woodcock T, Luscombe F E 1990 Atlanto-axial subluxation in Down's syndrome. Anaesthesia 45: 1049–1051

Pueschel S M, Scola F H, Pezzullo J C 1992 A longitudinal study of atlanto-dens relationships in asymptomatic individuals with Down syndrome. Pediatrics 89: 1194–1198

Riley D P, McBride L J 1991 Ketamine, midazolam and vecuronium infusion. Anaesthesia for Down's syndrome and congenital heart disease. Anaesthesia 46: 122–123

Segal L S, Drummond D S, Zanotti R M et al 1991 Complications of posterior arthrodesis of the cervical spine in patients who have Down syndrome. Journal of Bone and Joint Surgery 73: 1547–1554

Selby K A, Newton R W, Gupta S et al 1991 Clinical predictors and radiological reliability in atlantoaxial subluxation in Down's syndrome. Archives of Diseases in Childhood 66: 876–878

Semine A A, Ertel A N, Goldberg M J et al 1978 Cervical spine instability in children with Down's syndrome. Journal of Bone and Joint Surgery 60-A: 649–652

Sherry K M 1983 Post-extubation stridor in Down's syndrome. British Journal of Anaesthesia 55: 53–55

Silverman M 1988 Airway obstruction and sleep apnoea in Down's syndrome. British Medical Journal 296: 1618–1619

Stebbens V A, Dennis J, Samuels M P et al 1991 Sleep related upper airway obstruction in a cohort with Down's syndrome. Archives of Diseases in Childhood 66: 1333–1338

Williams J P, Somerville G M, Miner M E et al 1987 Atlanto-axial subluxation and trisomy-21: another perioperative complication. Anesthesiology 67: 253–254

DROWNING AND NEAR DROWNING

Drowning is one of the commonest causes of accidental death in young people and is potentially remediable if appropriate treatment is instituted without delay. Early animal experiments led to undue emphasis being placed on the differences between immersion in salt or fresh water, the accompanying osmotic changes and, in fresh water, the possibility of massive haemolysis. In practice, the inhaled volumes are much less than those induced experimentally, the haemolysis is not significant, and in large series of patients reaching hospital the electrolyte and blood values showed no significant difference between the two (Golden 1980). In general, therefore, the management of drowning depends on the clinical state, not the medium. Of more importance is the diagnosis of incidents possibly contributing to the clinical state, such as alcohol intoxication, head and neck or abdominal injury, epilepsy or myocardial infarction.

One of the crucial factors affecting survival from near drowning is the institution of prompt effective CPR at the site of the incident, and prior to hospital admission. Patients who arrive in hospital with fixed, dilated pupils tend to have a poor prognosis. A major exception is the patient in whom hypothermia is a significant feature. In this circumstance, resuscitation should be continued and judgement delayed until rewarming has occurred (Kemp & Sibert 1991). The rapid decrease in temperature on immersion in these cases, rather than the so-called 'diving' reflex, probably protects the brain and may account for the more pronounced protection in children who have a higher surface area to bodyweight ratio.

Recommended review articles include Simcock (1986) and Stuart-Taylor (1990).

Presentation

1. Respiration may be adequate, inadequate or absent. In a review of 130 cases, those with adequate respiration on arrival in hospital had an excellent prognosis (Simcock 1986). However, in hypothermic children, the absence of respiration did not necessarily predict a poor outcome (Kemp & Sibert 1991).

2. A number of features were associated with a poor prognosis. These include: immersion incidents of a duration exceeding 5–9 minutes, arrival in hospital pulseless, in VT or VF, fixed dilated pupils, fits, and a poor Glasgow coma score (Russell 1992). Fits continuing 24 hours after admission also predicted a poor outcome (Kemp & Sibert 1991). Most children with reactive pupils did survive, whereas if the return of pupil reactivity was delayed for 6 hours or more, this was associated with neurological deficit or death. The prognosis also depended on the circumstances of the incident. The study showed that in cold water, even if the patient has dilated pupils, resuscitation should be continued until rewarming occurs. However, when the incident was associated with warm water swimming pools, fixed dilated pupils and coma accurately predicted patients with a bad prognosis (Orlowski 1988).

3. If aspiration of water has occurred, then hypoxia may be present, secondary to washing out of surfactant, and intrapulmonary shunting. However, signs of inhalation may not be immediately evident. Aspiration of gastric contents may occur in up to 25% of victims and secondary infection in up to 40%.

4. Circulatory changes are complex. In the most serious group, asystole or VF may be present. Severe vasoconstriction may make it difficult to determine whether or not there is cardiac output (Modell 1986). In the less severe case there may be hypovolaemia and poor peripheral perfusion.

5. Hypothermia is common. At 26–28°C it may be difficult to reverse VF or asystole. Above 30°C the problem is less urgent. A moderate degree of hypothermia has a cerebral protectant effect.
6. Secondary drowning has been described, in which pulmonary oedema may develop at any time up to 3 days after the event. In children, secondary drowning in salt water has been found to have a worse prognosis than that after fresh-water incidents (Pearn 1980).

Investigations

1. After the initial resuscitation, monitoring of blood gases, CXR and base deficit will indicate whether there is further development, or resolution, of any respiratory complications.
2. ECG may show arrhythmias, especially on rewarming. The CVP will indicate hypovolaemia and urine output helps to guide therapy.
3. Core temperature monitoring.
4. Determinations of haemoglobin, haematocrit, electrolytes and urea levels are required. These will give baseline values in case of subsequent complications, but changes are usually small and rarely need therapy.

Management

1. If there is still no evident cardiac output on admission to hospital, then ECM should be continued until the nature of the cardiac rhythm is established on ECG.
2. An attempt is made to maintain the Pao_2 above 8 kPa with up to 50% oxygen. If this is impossible and there is significant intrapulmonary shunting, IPPV with PEEP will be needed. A nasogastric tube is necessary because fluid may have entered the stomach. Should hypotension result, expansion of the vascular volume will be required.
3. Treatment of any circulatory failure should be monitored with a CVP. Hypovolaemia occurs commonly, particularly in salt-water drowning. Plasma expanders may be required. If crystalloid is needed then dextrose 5% should be used in salt-water drowning, and saline in fresh water. Partial correction of the acidosis is advisable if pH is <7.2.
4. Unless the temperature is less than 30°C in which case serious cardiac arrhythmias may occur, rapid treatment of the hypothermia is unnecessary and possibly dangerous. Sudden vasodilatation may cause hypotension, and increases the hazard of cold acidotic blood returning to the heart. Moderate hypothermia is of positive benefit in reducing hypoxic brain damage, especially in children. Successful resuscitation has been achieved after total immersion for 25 minutes at 4°C in a child (Theilade 1977). However, if the temperature is

below 30°C then warmed peritoneal dialysis should be considered. Cardiopulmonary bypass has been used (Bolte et al 1988).

5. The use of steroids is controversial. Despite this, many authors admit to giving high-dose methylprednisolone, 30 mg/kg for two doses.

6. Antibiotic therapy depends on the likely water pollution. Ampicillin is commonly used prophylactically.

7. It has been suggested that, in the presence of the features associated with a poor prognosis, overenthusiastic treatment should be avoided.

8. Treatment of late complications such as cerebral oedema, pulmonary infection and renal failure.

BIBLIOGRAPHY
Bolte B C, Black P G, Bowers R S 1988 The use of extracorporeal warming in a child submerged for 66 minutes. Journal of the American Medical Association 260: 377–379
Golden F StC 1980 Problems of immersion. British Journal of Hospital Medicine 23: 371–383
Kemp A M, Sibert J R 1991 Outcome in children who nearly drown: a British Isles study. British Medical Journal 302: 931–933
Modell J H 1986 Near drowning. Circulation 74 (suppl IV): 27–28
Orlowski J P 1988 Drowning, near drowning and ice water drowning. Journal of the American Medical Association 260: 390–391.
Pearn J H 1980 Secondary drowning in children. British Medical Journal 281: 1103–1105
Russell R I R 1992 Drowning and near-drowning in children. British Journal of Intensive Care 2: 135–144
Simcock A D 1986 Treatment of near drowning – a review of 130 cases. Anaesthesia 41: 643–648
Stuart-Taylor M C 1990 Management of near-drowning. Hospital Update 16: 419–431
Theilade D 1977 The danger of fatal misjudgement in hypothermia after immersion. Anaesthesia 32: 889–892

DUCHENNE MUSCULAR DYSTROPHY
(DMD)

An X-linked recessive, severe muscular dystrophy which usually presents with proximal lower limb and pelvic muscle weakness. The weakness, which is progressive and varies between muscles, is due to a decrease in the total number of muscle fibres. The young child, on attempting to rise, will use its arms to 'climb' up its own legs. Cardiac muscle disease occurs with characteristic ECG changes and a hypertrophic cardiomyopathy. The condition steadily progresses to involve other muscles until finally death, from respiratory failure (75% of cases), pneumonia or cardiac disease, occurs between the ages of 10 and 20 years.

Anaesthesia in patients with this condition may be hazardous, particularly in the early stages of the disease before the diagnosis has been made. Cardiac arrest during anaesthesia has sometimes been the first indication that a child had a muscular dystrophy (Seay et al 1978).

Preoperative abnormalities

1. Varying degrees of muscle weakness are present, with initial involvement of the thighs and pelvis. The calf muscles are enlarged with fatty tissue (pseudohypertrophy) and if the shoulder girdle is affected there is winging of the scapulae. Relentlessly progressive scoliosis usually occurs after this and may require spinal fusion to improve stability and comfort (Shapiro et al 1992). The child is often obese and eventually becomes confined to a wheelchair.
2. Vital capacity decreases progressively, and when below 700 ml the risk of death is high. Diaphragmatic weakness occurs and blood gases may show hypoventilation and hypoxia in the later stages of the disease.
3. Serum CK levels can be grossly raised, the highest levels often occurring in the early stages of the disease. An EMG will confirm the presence of a myopathy.
4. Clinical signs of a hypertrophic cardiomyopathy, with diastolic failure secondary to left ventricular inflow obstruction, may exist. The ECG shows abnormalities in more than 90% of patients. Characteristic changes are a tall R wave and an RSR1 in lead V1, a deep Q wave in leads V3–6, a prolonged PR interval, and a sinus tachycardia. Echocardiography will demonstrate mitral valve prolapse in 25% of patients. Sudden death can occur.

Anaesthetic problems

Although many apparently uneventful anaesthetics have been given to patients with DMD, a substantial number of individual cases have been reported in which serious complications have occurred. Some have resulted in death. Attempts have been made to quantify the risks of anaesthesia in DMD (Sethna et al 1988, Larsen et al 1989). Most studies have been retrospective. Problems were reported with 16–27% of patients having general anaesthesia for a variety of procedures, whereas those performed under local anaesthesia were uneventful. Complications were usually associated with suxamethonium and halothane, although isoflurane has also been implicated (Chalkiadis & Branch 1990). The precise aetiology of the anaesthetic complications has not always been clear, but they can be broadly divided into respiratory problems, abnormal metabolic responses and cardiac events. The metabolic complications share many of the features seen in MH and it had been thought that DMD was associated with an increased incidence of this condition. This seems to be unlikely. Occasionally, the two conditions have been noted to coexist, but both traits may occur independently (Brownell 1988).

Whilst the respiratory complications usually occurred with advanced disease, as a result of the progressive muscle weakness, this is not necessarily the case with acute cardiac events, which seem more likely to happen in the early stages of the disease.

1. Tachycardia, ventricular fibrillation and cardiac arrest have all been reported during induction of anaesthesia (Genever 1971, Bolthauser et al 1980, Linter et al 1982, Smith & Bush 1985, Buzello & Huttarsch 1988, Chalkiadis & Branch 1990, Shapiro et al 1992). Most reports have concerned the use of suxamethonium, and when biochemical evidence was available, the acute cardiac events seemed mostly to be associated with hyperkalaemia. Cardiac arrest has usually occurred immediately after the administration of suxamethonium but has been reported at any stage, even during the recovery period. Presumably this is because suxamethonium-induced hyperkalaemia persists longer in patients with DMD. In normal individuals given suxamethonium, the increase in plasma potassium levels usually lasts for less than 10 minutes, whereas in DMD it may be significantly prolonged. Serum potassium concentration increased from 3.6 mmol/l to 4.6 mmol/l in a patient given suxamethonium before undergoing tracheal intubation for IPPV (Stephens 1990). Hyperkalaemia may also be precipitated by inhalational agents alone. In one particular case in which cardiac arrest occurred during recovery from anaesthesia with isoflurane, the serum potassium did not return to normal levels until 5 hours after the initial event, despite active treatment (Chalkiadis & Branch 1990). In another case, an increase in temperature and cardiac arrest after 11 minutes of an inhalation induction (assisted ventilation) with halothane alone, has been reported in a child with a serum CK level of 14 000 iu, who was to undergo muscle biopsy (Sethna & Rockoff 1986).

2. Perioperative pyrexia is common and it had been suggested that DMD was associated with an increased incidence of MH (Brownell et al 1983, Rosenberg & Heiman-Patterson 1983, Wang & Stanley 1986). This is now thought to be unlikely. Cases have been reported which have some, and occasionally all, of the clinical features of MH, but few papers present in-vitro or electron microscopic evidence of MH. One reported an abnormal contraction to halothane, but not to caffeine, in muscle taken from a 4-year-old boy with DMD (Rosenberg & Heiman-Patterson 1983). Another showed abnormal responses to both tests in a 5-year-old child, who had suffered cardiac arrest, metabolic acidosis and acute rhabdomyolysis following suxamethonium (Brownell et al 1983). A third paper reported suxamethonium-induced rhabdomyolysis in a 7-week-old child. It was claimed to be the youngest reported child with MH (Wilhoit et al 1989). However, muscle biopsy was diagnostic for DMD and the parents declined MH testing. This claim therefore has to be viewed with considerable scepticism.

   Most authors believe that the two conditions are unrelated, but are both capable of producing common features under anaesthesia. Contracture testing for MH was negative in two children, one with

Becker's muscular dystrophy and the other with DMD (Gronert et al 1992), and these authors considered that the MH-like features seen during anaesthesia were a result of alterations in the muscle membrane secondary to the dystrophy itself. Exposure to volatile agents and suxamethonium might increase membrane permeability, and compensatory hypermetabolism is suggested to result from attempts to re-establish membrane stability and prevent calcium flux.

Whether or not MH and DMD regularly coexist, is debatable. However, from a clinical point of view, in either condition, suxamethonium or halothane may be the triggering agents for a variety of non-specific complications which can occur and are associated with acute disruption of muscle. These include pyrexia, tachycardia, acidosis, hyperkalaemia, asystole, VF, muscle spasm, acute rhabdomyolysis and a high CK level. All of these complications have been reported, either singly, or in various combinations, in some patients with DMD.

3. If asystole or VF should occur, then the cardiomyopathic heart may be resistant to resuscitation measures (Sethna et al 1988).

4. The response to non-depolarizing agents may be abnormal. This cannot be predicted in advance. The stage of the disease and the muscles monitored will presumably have some bearing on this. Cumulative 50% and 90% blocking doses of vecuronium were determined in two 4-year-old boys (Buzello & Huttarsch 1988). Although the authors found no increase in sensitivity to vecuronium, the recovery time from 75% to 25% block of twitch tension was three to nearly six times that of normal.

5. It has been suggested, on theoretical grounds, that the accumulation of acetylcholine at the motor end-plate caused by the administration of neostigmine might trigger rhabdomyolysis (Buzello & Huttarsch 1988). This has not been confirmed clinically.

6. Postoperative respiratory insufficiency. There are a number of reports of 'uneventful' anaesthetics using a barbiturate, suxamethonium and halothane technique, in which delayed respiratory insufficiency occurred from 5 to 36 hours postoperatively (Smith & Bush 1985). Difficulty in swallowing, breathing and clearing secretions all featured in the pattern of deterioration. Despite receiving tracheal intubation and IPPV, a number of the children subsequently had cardiac arrests following which resuscitation failed.

7. Dark urine, in most cases identified as myoglobinuria, has usually been associated with the administration of suxamethonium (Larsen et al 1989). However, isolated myoglobinuria following adenoidectomy was the first indication of DMD in a 5-year-old boy (Rubiano et al 1987).

Management

1. Assessment of respiratory function is helpful, if the child is old enough to cooperate. Diaphragmatic involvement suggests serious impairment. A difference in vital capacity of more than 25% between the erect and supine positions is indicative of diaphragmatic weakness (Heckmatt 1987). In the later stages of DMD, arterial blood gases will show impending respiratory failure. Assessment is particularly important when major elective surgery, such as scoliosis correction, is contemplated (Milne & Rosales 1982, Shapiro et al 1992). It has been suggested that, for scoliosis surgery, the patient should have a VC of at least 20 ml/kg (or 30% of predicted) and an inspiratory capacity of 15 ml/kg.

2. Evidence of cardiac involvement should be sought. This may vary from ECG changes alone to diastolic failure.

3. If advanced disease is present, the wisdom and possible benefits of surgery should be weighed against the risks. If the assessment is misjudged, elective surgery may hasten death, or commit a patient with progressive and ultimately fatal disease to a period of prolonged artificial ventilation.

4. Consideration should be given to the use of a local anaesthetic technique. Larsen et al (1989) in a retrospective review found that no complications occurred in 19 operations performed under local anaesthesia, whereas in 65 cases under general anaesthesia, 18 had complications.

5. Suxamethonium is absolutely contraindicated in patients with DMD since, at present, it does not appear possible to predict which patients might develop hyperkalaemia, cardiac arrest, rigidity, rhabdomyolysis or postoperative respiratory failure. All of these complications have been attributed to its use. Larsen et al (1989) found that nine out of 10 patients given suxamethonium in their series developed complications.

6. In view of the variability of response, neuromuscular monitoring and incremental dosages should be employed when non-depolarizing muscle relaxants are used. Vecuronium has been suggested as being suitable, although there may be a prolonged duration of action. Responses in the peripheral muscles do not always reflect those in respiratory muscles, and the evoked EMG may recover faster than the actual mechanical response (Buzello & Huttarsch 1988).

7. Although many patients have been safely anaesthetized with halothane, its use has been challenged, particularly when the CK levels are very high. The report of cardiac arrest occurring during an inhalational induction with halothane is of concern (Sethna & Rockoff 1986). So also is the critical review condemning the use of halothane in patients with DMD and a high serum CK (Roizen

1987). The cause of the arrest cannot be accurately determined, but it is easy to visualize how a serious arrhythmia might occur in a myopathic heart with a combination of even mild respiratory obstruction, light anaesthesia and halothane. That halothane given alone is capable of producing muscle breakdown, is demonstrated by the report of myoglobinuria following an anaesthetic in which suxamethonium was not used (Rubiano et al 1987).

8. Those authors who have described complications clinically similar to malignant hyperthermia, suggest that a non-MH-triggering anaesthetic should be given to patients with DMD. On the contrary, halothane has been used safely in many cases and it can be argued that it is easier, and hence safer, to use in young children. A propofol infusion has been used in a 10-year-old child with DMD (Ginsburg et al 1991) The serurn CK level was said to be within normal limits, which is somewhat surprising, since the CK is usually considerably elevated in DMD. Whichever technique is chosen, ECG, temperature and ETco$_2$ should be monitored from the start of the anaesthetic and dantrolene must be immediately available.

9. Observation in a high-dependency area for the first 24–48 hours after anaesthesia will assist in the early detection of pulmonary insufficiency. If doubt arises, it is much safer to support respiration until all drugs have been eliminated.

BIBLIOGRAPHY

Brownwell A K W 1988 Malignant hyperthermia: relationship to other diseases. British Journal of Anaesthesia 60: 303–308

Brownell A K W, Paasuke R T, Elash A et al 1983 Malignant hyperthermia in Duchenne muscular dystrophy. Anesthesiology 58: 180–182

Boltshauser E, Steinmann B, Meyer A et al 1980 Anaesthesia-induced rhabdomyolysis in Duchenne's muscular dystrophy. British Journal of Anaesthesia 52: 559

Buzello W, Huttarsch H 1988 Muscle relaxation in patients with Duchenne's muscular dystrophy. British Journal of Anaesthesia 60: 228–231

Chalkiadis G A, Branch K G 1990 Cardiac arrest after isoflurane anaesthesia in a patient with Duchenne's muscular dystrophy. Anaesthesia 45: 22–25

Genever E E 1971 Suxamethonium induced cardiac arrest in unsuspected pseudohypertrophic muscular dystrophy. British Journal of Anaesthesia 43: 984–986

Ginsburg R S, Porterfield K, Lippmann M 1991 Propofol: bolus induction plus continuous infusion in a patient with Duchenne muscular dystrophy. Anesthesiology 75: 376

Gronert G A, Fowler W, Cardinet G H et al 1992 Absence of malignant hyperthermia contractures in Becker–Duchenne dystrophy at age 2. Muscle & Nerve 15: 52–56

Heckmatt J Z 1987 Respiratory care in muscular dystrophy. British Medical Journal 295: 1014–1015

Larsen U T, Juhl B, Hein-Sorensen O et al 1989 Complications during anaesthesia in patients with Duchenne's muscular dystrophy (a retrospective study). Canadian Journal of Anaesthesia 36: 418–422

Linter S P K, Thomas P R, Withington P S et al 1982 Suxamethonium associated hypertonicity and cardiac arrest in unsuspected pseudohypertrophic muscular dystrophy. British Journal of Anaesthesia 54: 1331–1333

Milne B, Rosales J K 1982 Anaesthetic considerations in patients with muscular dystrophy undergoing spinal fusion and Harrington rod insertion. Canadian Anaesthetists' Society Journal 29: 250–254

Roizen M F 1987 Comment. Survey of Anesthesiology 31: 232–233

Rosenberg H, Heiman-Patterson T 1983 Duchenne's muscular dystrophy and malignant hyperthermia: another warning. Anesthesiology 59: 362

Rubiano R, Chang J-L, Carroll J et al 1987 Acute rhabdomyolysis following halothane anesthesia without succinylcholine. Anesthesiology 67: 856–857

Seay A R, Ziter F A, Thompson J A 1978 Cardiac arrest during induction of anaesthesia in Duchenne muscular dystrophy. Journal of Pediatrics 93: 88–90

Sethna N F, Rockoff M A 1986 Cardiac arrest following inhalation induction of anesthesia in a child with Duchenne's muscular dystrophy. Canadian Anaesthetists' Society Journal 33: 799–802

Sethna N F, Rockoff M A, Worthen H M et al 1988 Anesthesia related complications in children with Duchenne muscular dystrophy. Anesthesiology 68: 462–465

Shapiro F, Sethna N, Colan S et al 1992 Spinal fusion in Duchenne muscular dystrophy: a multidisciplinary approach. Muscle & Nerve 15: 604–614

Smith C L, Bush G H 1985 Anaesthesia and progressive muscular dystrophy. British Journal of Anaesthesia 57: 1113–1118

Stephens I D 1990 Succinylcholine and Duchenne's muscular dystrophy. Canadian Journal of Anaesthesia 37: 274

Wang J M, Stanley T H 1986 Duchenne muscular dystrophy and hyperthermia: two case reports. Canadian Anaesthetists' Society Journal 33: 492–497

Wilhoit R D, Brown R E, Bauman L A 1989 Possible malignant hyperthermia in a 7-week-old infant. Anesthesia and Analgesia 68: 688–691

DYSTROPHIA MYOTONICA
(AND OTHER MYOTONIC SYNDROMES)

Dystrophia myotonica, myotonia congenita and paramyotonia are three distinct diseases of autosomal dominant inheritance in which myotonia occurs. Myotonia is a persistence of muscle contraction beyond the duration of the voluntary effort or stimulation. In myotonia congenita (Thomsen's disease), the generalized myotonia is enhanced by cold and resting, but may be improved by exercise. Subjects with paramyotonia have attacks of muscle weakness resembling those in periodic paralysis, to which it is probably closely related. Again, the myotonia is provoked by cold (see Familial periodic paralysis).

Dystrophia myotonica and myotonia congenita will be considered here.

DYSTROPHIA MYOTONICA OR MYOTONIC DYSTROPHY

Dystrophia myotonica is a syndrome in which there is myotonia and dystrophic changes in certain muscles, associated with other clinical features. The site of the abnormality is the muscle fibre, since myotonia may persist after the administration of neuromuscular blocking agents, local anaesthetics, and neural section.

Preoperative abnormalities

1. Usually presents in the third and fourth decades. Myotonia is associated with weakness and muscle wasting. Unlike most other myopathies, it predominantly involves the distal and cranial

muscles. After a handshake, the patient cannot relax his muscles. Percussion myotonia may be demonstrated, particularly in the tongue or thenar eminence. Ocular movements, eye closure, swallowing and chewing may also be affected (Editorial 1987).

2. Dystrophic features dominate the clinical picture as the patient ages, and the weakness is progressive.

3. Frontal baldness, ptosis and facial weakness, cataracts, hypogonadism, cardiomyopathy and conduction abnormalities, and a low IQ, are other features of the condition. There is an increase in serum CK levels. Death may occur in middle age from respiratory or cardiac complications.

4. EMG shows electrical after-discharge.

5. The myotonia may be improved by keeping warm and the use of class I antiarrhythmics such as phenytoin and procainamide (Editorial 1987).

Anaesthetic problems

1. There may be chronic underventilation and respiratory muscle weakness. Vital capacity, expiratory reserve volume, maximum breathing capacity and maximal inspiratory pressure are all markedly reduced, secondary to abnormalities in the respiratory muscles. It has been suggested that central nervous system disease may contribute to the poor respiratory reserve. Somnolence and prolonged apnoea can occur, and respiration is readily depressed by barbiturates, inhalation agents, benzodiazepines and opiates (Aldridge 1985, Harper 1989). However, there may be a wide variation in a patient's response to drugs. This may reflect the state of the disease, as is suggested by two contrasting reports of the use of propofol; one patient showed marked sensitivity to propofol (Speedy 1990), the other did not (White & Smyth 1989, 1990).

2. Branthwaite (1990) pointed out that, in common with other diseases in which there is chest wall restriction, hypoventilation may occur during sleep. Accessory muscle function is lost and, during rapid eye-movement sleep, so is that of the intercostal muscles. The additional presence of diaphragmatic weakness results in hypoventilation, and analgesics and sedatives will depress the arousal response to hypoxia and hypercarbia. Such a mechanism could have accounted for the death of a child after tendon transfer (Brahams 1989, Branthwaite 1990).

3. It may be difficult to prevent myotonia from occurring during surgical manipulation and diathermy, since it is not necessarily abolished by neuromuscular blocking agents, local or regional anaesthesia. Depolarizing agents can produce a prolonged contraction which outlasts the duration of effect. Non-depolarizing drugs may or may not produce relaxation. In one case, masseter spasm and shivering occurred for 4 minutes after the administration

of fentanyl (Paterson et al 1985). Hypothermia, shivering and potassium may all cause generalized myotonia.

4. There may be cardiovascular disease. Arrhythmias, including AF and conduction defects, cardiomyopathy, mitral valve prolapse and heart failure have been reported.
5. Disordered oesophageal contraction may predispose to pulmonary aspiration.
6. There is an increased incidence of postoperative problems (Moore & Moore 1987), particularly pulmonary atelectasis (Tanaka & Tanaka 1991). A 32-year-old man had a stormy course after thymectomy (Mudge et al 1980). Complications included pneumonia, pulmonary emboli and cardiac arrhythmias. Postoperative artificial ventilation may be required (Blumgart et al 1990).
7. Although pregnancy is rare, it may be associated with an increase in myotonic symptoms (Paterson et al 1985). There have been reports of haemorrhage at Caesarean section which has not responded to oxytocics and sometimes necessitated hysterectomy (Blumgart et al 1990). Patients occasionally present for emergency Caesarean section, therefore anaesthesia must be planned in advance (Walpole & Ross 1992).
8. Hypermetabolic events similar to those in patients with MH have occasionally been reported in dystrophia myotonica and myotonia congenita. A group of 44 patients with either myotonias or periodic paralyses underwent in-vitro testing for MH (Lehmann-Horn & Iaizzo 1990). Four with myotonic dystrophy had positive results, although only two had increased resting myoplasmic calcium levels. Suxamethonium also produced muscle contracture in some individuals. It was concluded, not that these patients had a susceptibility to MH (and indeed, neither they nor their families had ever experienced any untoward effects of anaesthesia), but that the standard MH testing procedure lacks specificity.

Management

1. A detailed clinical examination for the distribution of muscle weakness and myotonia.
2. If the respiratory muscles are involved, lung function tests and blood gases will give some indication of the severity of the restrictive lung defect.
3. Arrhythmias should be diagnosed and treated. Occasionally a temporary or permanent pacemaker (Tanaka & Tanaka 1991) may be required.
4. Induction agents should be given in small doses. The anaesthetist should be prepared to treat the apnoea which often follows.
5. The use of suxamethonium should be avoided. Tracheal intubation may be possible using thiopentone or propofol and an inhalational agent alone.

6. Non-depolarizing neuromuscular blockers can be used, but they do not guarantee muscle relaxation. There are conflicting reports concerning the reliability of neostigmine as an antagonist. Incomplete reversal of neuromuscular blockade is common and a second dose of neostigmine may aggravate the paralysis. Uneventful anaesthetics using atracurium and propofol infusions (White & Smyth 1989), vecuronium (Castano & Pares 1987) and atracurium (Nightingale et al 1985) have been described, although myoclonus has been seen following induction with propofol (Bouly et al 1991). Neuromuscular monitoring must be undertaken. If there is any doubt about the return of neuromuscular function, IPPV should be provided until all drugs have been excreted and respiration is adequate.

7. The use of local or regional techniques will avoid some of the problems associated with drugs used for general anaesthesia (Wheeler & James 1979). Successful extradural anaesthesia (Paterson et al 1985), and a combination of spinal and local anaesthesia (Cope & Miller 1986) have been reported in patients for Caesarean section. However, again these techniques will not always guarantee muscle relaxation sufficient for abdominal surgery.

8. A number of measures have been tried in attempts to reduce myotonia. Severe uterine spasm, occurring during Caesarean section under spinal anaesthesia, was relieved by the application of bupivacaine 30 ml 0.5% to the cut surface of the myometrium (Cope & Miller 1986). However, administration of dantrolene failed to produce muscle relaxation in a patient undergoing cholecystectomy (Phillips et al 1984).

9. Measures to prevent pulmonary aspiration, prompt attention to respiratory inadequacy, and the use of antibiotics may all help to prevent the occurrence of pneumonia and lung abscess.

10. The operating theatre should be kept warm and measures taken to avoid shivering.

11. Although there is no evidence that there is any direct relationship between myotonic dystrophy and MH, monitoring ET_{CO_2}, and temperature is advisable.

BIBLIOGRAPHY

Aldridge M 1985 Anaesthetic problems in myotonic dystrophy. British Journal of Anaesthesia 57: 1119–1130

Blumgart C H, Hughes D G, Redfern N 1990 Obstetric anaesthesia in dystrophia myotonica. Anaesthesia 45: 26–29

Bouly A, Nathan N, Feiss P 1991 Propofol in myotonic dystrophy. Anaesthesia 46: 705

Brahams D 1989 Postoperative monitoring in a patient with muscular dystrophy. Lancet ii: 1053–1054

Branthwaite M A 1990 Myotonic dystrophy and respiratory function. Anaesthesia 45: 250

Castano J, Pares N 1987 Anaesthesia for major abdominal surgery in a patient with myotonia dystrophica. British Journal of Anaesthesia 59: 1629–1631

Cope D K, Miller J N 1986 Local and spinal anesthesia for Cesarean section in a
patient with myotonic dystrophy. Anesthesia and Analgesia 65: 687–690

Editorial 1987 Treatment of myotonia. Lancet i: 1242–1243

Harper P S 1989 Postoperative complications in myotonia dystrophica. Lancet ii 1269

Lehmann-Horn F, Iaizzo P A 1990 Are myotonias and periodic paralyses associated
with susceptibility to malignant hyperthemia? British Journal of Anaesthesia 65:
692–697

Moore J K, Moore A P 1987 Postoperative complications of dystrophia myotonica.
Anaesthesia 42: 529–533

Mudge B J, Taylor P B, Vanderspek A F L 1980 Perioperative hazards of myotonic
dystrophy. Anaesthesia 35: 492–495

Nightingale P, Healy T E J, McGuinness K 1985 Dystrophia myotonica and
atracurium. A case report. British Journal of Anaesthesia 57: 1131–1135

Paterson R A, Tousignant M, Skene D S 1985 Caesarean section for twins in a patient
with myotonic dystrophy. Canadian Anaesthetists' Society Journal 32: 418–421

Phillips D C, Ellis F R, Exley K A et al 1984 Dantrolene sodium and dystrophia
myotonica. Anaesthesia 39: 568–573

Speedy H 1990 Exaggerated physiological response to propofol in myotonic dystrophy.
British Journal of Anaesthesia 64: 110–112

Tanaka M, Tanaka Y 1991 Cardiac anaesthesia in a patient with myotonic dystrophy.
Anaesthesia 46: 462–465

Walpole A R, Ross A W 1992 Acute cord prolapse in an obstetric patient with
myotonia dystrophica. Anaesthesia and Intensive Care 20: 526–528

Wheeler A S, James F M 1979 Local anesthesia for laparoscopy in cases of myotonia
dystrophica. Anesthesiology 50: 169

White D A, Smyth D G 1989 Continuous infusion of propofol in dystrophia
myotonica. Canadian Journal of Anaesthesia 36: 200–203

White D A, Smyth D G 1990 Exaggerated physiological responses to propofol in
myotonic dystrophy. British Journal of Anaesthesia 64: 758

MYOTONIA CONGENITA

Congenital myotonic dystrophy occurs in infants of mothers with
myotonic dystrophy. Initially weakness, rather than myotonia, is the
main feature. The symptoms are thought to be associated with
abnormalities of chloride conductance during depolarization (Editorial
1987).

Preoperative abnormalities

1. The infant may present as a 'floppy baby', with generalized
   hypotonia, facial diplegia, feeding difficulties or respiratory
   insufficiency. Myotonia, however, is not a feature.
2. There may be arthrogryposis, a high diaphragm and peripheral
   oedema. Tone and muscle power improve in the first year, but there
   is delayed physical and mental development.
3. Most individuals develop the adult form of the disease before they
   are 10 years old and usually die before the age of 30. Surgery may
   be required for talipes, myringotomy or hernia repair.

Anaesthetic problems

1. Sustained contractions lasting 45 seconds following suxamethonium
   (Anderson & Brown 1989) and hypertonus in two sisters (Heiman-

Patterson et al 1988). Sensitivity to non-depolarizing agents has also been reported.

2. Problems in weaning a patient from the ventilator at the end of surgery (Bray & Inkster 1984).

3. Hypermetabolic events resembling those in patients with MH have occasionally been reported in myotonia congenita and a fatality has occurred. Leg muscle spasms developed 7 hours after an uneventful anaesthetic which was non-triggering for MH had been given to a child with a clinical diagnosis of myotonia congenita (Haberer et al 1989). The condition deteriorated over the next 5 hours, with severe diffuse rigidity, notably of the thorax, slowly increasing pyrexia and metabolic acidosis. A serum CK level of greater than 11 500 iu/l was recorded. Cardiac arrest occurred in the 14th hour, despite treatment with dantrolene, and resuscitation was hampered by the thoracic rigidity.

4. A group of 44 patients with either myotonias or periodic paralyses underwent in-vitro testing for MH (Lehmann-Horn & Iaizzo 1990). None of the six patients with congenital myotonia had positive results, although suxamethonium produced muscle contractures in three, and most showed a small response and slow relaxation after caffeine and halothane. None had family histories of anaesthetic problems. However, muscle rigidity with suxamethonium has been reported in myotonia congenita, and two sisters developed contracture on exposure to halothane whilst the third did not (Heiman-Patterson et al 1988).

Management

1. Assessment and monitoring of neuromuscular function.
2. The use of local anaesthesia in a neonate for hernia repair (Bray & Inkster 1984) and caudal epidural anaesthesia in a two-year-old child for repair of a talipes deformity (Alexander et al 1981) have been reported.
3. ET_{CO_2} and temperature should be monitored.

BIBLIOGRAPHY
Alexander C, Wolf S, Ghia J N 1981 Caudal anesthesia for early onset myotonic dystrophy. Anesthesiology 55: 597–598
Anderson B J, Brown T C K 1989 Congenital myotonic dystrophy in children – a review of ten years' experience. Anaesthesia and Intensive Care 17: 320–324
Anderson B J, Brown T C K 1989 Anaesthesia for a child with congenital myotonic dystrophy. Anaesthesia and Intensive Care 17: 351–354
Bray R J, Inkster J S 1984 Anaesthesia in babies with congenital dystrophia myotonica. Anaesthesia 39: 1007–1011
Editorial 1987 Treatment of myotonia. Lancet i: 1242–1243
Haberer J-P Fabre F, Rose E 1989 Malignant hyperthermia and myotonia congenita (Thomsen's disease). Anaesthesia 44: 166
Heiman-Patterson T, Martino C, Rosenberg H et al 1988 Malignant hyperthermia in myotonia congenita. Neurology 38: 810–812
Lehmann-Horn F, Iaizzo P A 1990 Are myotonias and periodic paralyses associated with susceptibility to malignant hyperthermia? British Journal of Anaesthesia 65: 692–697

EATON-LAMBERT SYNDROME
(LAMBERT–EATON OR MYASTHENIC SYNDROME)

A myasthenia-like disorder secondary to an abnormality of neuromuscular transmission in which weakness and fatiguability often primarily involve the thigh and pelvic muscles. Originally described in association with carcinoma of the lung, cases were subsequently reported in which no carcinoma was found. Both types of Eaton–Lambert syndrome are probably autoimmune in origin, and autoantibodies to voltage-gated calcium channels are thought to be involved. There is a presynaptic abnormality which results in a decrease in the quanta of acetylcholine released by the passage of the nerve impulse, although each quantum released is normal. This contrasts with myasthenia gravis, in which the abnormality involves the postganglionic receptors. Tumour-associated cases are almost exclusively found in association with small-cell carcinoma of the lung. The syndrome sometimes precedes the tumour by as long as 2 years. Tumour therapy may result in improvement of the neurological problem.

Preoperative abnormalities

1. Muscles are fatiguable, as in myasthenia gravis, but the proximal limbs and trunk are initially affected and the external ocular muscles tend to be spared. Although the patient complains of fatiguability, in contrast to myasthenia gravis, the muscle power may actually increase after brief exercise. Lower limb reflexes are reduced or absent, but may be enhanced by prior voluntary contraction. In true myasthenia, reflexes are preserved. Neostigmine produces little or no improvement in the weakness. In a review of 50 cases (O'Neill et al 1988), the main neurological features were: proximal lower limb weakness (100%), reduced or absent tendon reflexes (92%), post-tetanic facilitation (78%), autonomic dysfunction, in particular dryness of the mouth (74%), and mild-to-moderate ptosis (54%).
2. Electrophysiological criteria for diagnosis include a decrease in amplitude of EMG muscle potentials and further decline at low rates of stimulation. In contrast, there is an increase in amplitude of the action potential in response to stimulation at high rates, or following muscle contraction.
3. Patients tend to be older than those with myasthenia.
4. Associated lung carcinomas are usually oat cell in type, and are often small and less aggressive than normal. In a review, half of the patients had a malignancy (O'Neill et al 1988).
5. Some improvement has been noted with guanidine and 4-aminopyridine, which enhances the release of acetylcholine. However, the allowable dose is limited by CNS excitation. More recently 3,4-diaminopyridine, an oral preparation with less CNS effects, has been used (McEvoy et al 1989).

6. Corticosteroids or plasma exchange may result in improvement.
7. Diagnosis may be confirmed by an assay for antibodies (Lennon & Lambert 1989).

Anaesthetic problems

1. Prolonged paralysis can occur after the use of depolarizing or non-depolarizing neuromuscular blockers. In one case this occurred several months in advance of clinical symptoms, although postoperative EMG and serological testing confirmed the diagnosis of Eaton–Lambert syndrome (Small et al 1992). Respiratory failure following anaesthesia may be a presenting feature (O'Neill et al 1988) and reversal with anticholinesterases may be incomplete (Telford & Hollway 1990). An improvement in evoked action potential has been reported after treatment with 4-aminopyridine (Agoston et al 1978) and 3,4-diaminopyridine (Telford & Hollway 1990) which prolongs the activation of the voltage-gated calcium channel at the nerve terminal.
2. Autonomic dysfunction may be a prominent feature (Mamdani et al 1985). Symptoms can include constipation, urinary retention and mouth dryness. Orthostatic hypotension and decreased R–R intervals on ECG may be noted. In such patients, there may be impairment of cardiovascular responses to hypotension.

Management

1. Neuromuscular blockers should, if possible, be avoided. If essential, the effects of small doses should be monitored carefully.
2. A local anaesthetic technique may be appropriate, to avoid the problems associated with general anaesthesia.
3. Respiratory insuffiency should be treated with postoperative IPPV. Sakura et al (1991) described the use of extradural analgesia in a patient undergoing thoracotomy and biopsy for lung carcinoma, and studied the effects on pulmonary function.
4. In the presence of autonomic dysfunction, drugs producing myocardial depression or peripheral vasodilatation should be used with caution.

BIBLIOGRAPHY

Agoston S, van Weerden T, Westra P et al 1978 Effects of 4-aminopyridine in Eaton Lambert syndrome. British Journal of Anaesthesia 50: 383–385
Gracey D P, Southorn P A 1987 Respiratory failure in Lambert-Eaton myasthenic syndrome. Chest 91: 716–718
Lennon V A, Lambert E H 1989 Autoantibodies bind solubilized calcium channel-W-conotoxin complexes from small cell lung carcinoma: a diagnostic aid for Lambert-Eaton myasthenic syndrome. Mayo Clinic Proceedings 64: 1498–1504
McEvoy K M, Windebank A J, Daube J R et al 1989 3,4-diaminopyridine in the treatment of Lambert-Eaton myasthenic syndrome. New England Journal of Medicine 321: 1567–1571.

Mamdani M B, Walsh R L, Rubino F A et al 1985 Autonomic dysfunction and Eaton
    Lambert syndrome. Journal of the Autonomic Nervous System 12: 315–320
O'Neill J H, Murray N M, Newsom-Davies J 1988 The Lambert-Eaton myasthenic
    syndrome: a review of 50 cases. Brain 111: 577–596
Sakura S, Saito Y, Maeda M et al 1991 Epidural analgesia Eaton-Lambert myasthenic
    syndrome. Effects on respiratory function. Anaesthesia 46: 560–562
Small S, Ali H H, Lennon V A et al 1992 Anesthesia for an unsuspected Lambert–
    Eaton myasthenic syndrome with autoantibodies and occult small cell lung
    carcinoma. Anesthesiology 76: 142–144
Telford R J, Hollway T E 1990 The myasthenic syndrome: anaesthesia in a patient
    treated with 3,4-diaminopyridine. British Journal of Anaesthesia 64: 363–366
Wilcox P G, Morrison N J, Anzarut A R et al 1988 Lambert-Eaton myasthenia
    syndrome involving the diaphragm. Chest 93: 604–606

EBSTEIN'S ANOMALY

A rare congenital cardiac abnormality. The septal and posterior cusps of
the tricuspid valve are displaced downwards and are elongated, such
that a varying amount of the right ventricle effectively becomes part of
the atrium. Its wall is thin and it contracts poorly. The remaining
functional part of the right ventricle is therefore small. The foramen
ovale is patent or defective in 80% of cases.

The degree of abnormality of right ventricular function, and the size
of the ASD, are probably the main determinants of the severity of the
condition, which varies considerably. The right ventricular systolic
pressure is low, and the RVEDP is elevated. Tricuspid incompetence can
occur. There may be a right-to-left shunt, with cyanosis on effort, and
pulmonary hypertension and right heart failure may supervene.
However, the natural history of the disease is extremely variable. Fifty
per cent of cases present in infancy with cyanosis and 42% die in the
first 6 weeks of life. In those who survive to adulthood, symptoms may
be precipitated by the onset of arrhythmias, or by pregnancy. A few
patients remain asymptomatic, even as adults, although once symptoms
develop, the severity of disability may increase rapidly (Mair 1992).
Factors predictive of death were examined in a long-term study of
survival (Gentles et al 1992). A cardiothoracic ratio of ≥0.65 was a better
predictor of sudden death than the symptomatic state, and those who
developed atrial fibrillation died within 5 years. It has been suggested
that tricuspid surgery should be undertaken before the cardiothoracic
ratio reaches 0.65.

Preoperative abnormalities

1. There may be dyspnoea and cyanosis at rest or on moderate
   exertion. The patient may be asymptomatic.
2. Episodes of tachyarrhythmias occur in 25% of patients. Some may
   provoke syncopal attacks.
3. ECG can show varying abnormalities, including large peaked P
   waves, a long P–R interval, Wolff–Parkinson–White (WPW)

syndrome, RBBB and right heart strain. Paroxysmal supraventricular tachycardia occurs in 15%, usually because of the presence of WPW syndrome.

4. CXR may show cardiomegaly, with a prominent right heart border and poorly perfused lung fields.
5. Paradoxical systemic embolism and subacute bacterial endocarditis may occur.

Anaesthetic problems

These will depend upon the anatomical abnormality, the degree of right-to-left shunt and the presence or absence of right heart failure.

1. Prolonged anaesthetic induction times, because of pooling of drugs in the large atrial chamber, have been reported (Elsten et al 1981, Halpern et al 1985).
2. The use of intracardiac catheters may be hazardous because they can provoke serious cardiac arrhythmias.
3. Air entering peripheral venous lines or open veins at subatmospheric pressure may cause paradoxical air emboli.
4. Tachycardia is poorly tolerated because of impaired filling of the functionally small right ventricle.
5. Hypotension may increase the right-to-left shunt, if present.
6. Hypoxia causes pulmonary vasoconstriction, which also increases a right-to-left shunt.
7. There is a risk of bacterial endocarditis, especially if a CVP line is in place.
8. Deterioration may occur in pregnancy (Linter & Clarke 1984), or with the onset of arrhythmias. However, a review of 42 pregnancies in 12 women showed that, in the absence of cyanosis or arrhythmias, pregnancy was well tolerated (Donnelly et al 1991). Presumably those females who survive to child-bearing age represent a less severely affected group of patients.

Management

1. The severity of the lesion must be assessed. In the presence of maternal cyanosis or arrhythmias, there should be close monitoring of both mother and fetus.
2. Heart failure and arrhythmias require treatment.
3. Antibiotic prophylaxis against bacterial endocarditis.
4. If a CVP is used for monitoring, its tip should be kept within the superior vena cava. The use of intracardiac catheters should probably be avoided.
5. Anaesthetic techniques should aim to minimize tachycardia and hypotension.
6. Oxygen therapy increases pulmonary vasodilatation.
7. A number of anaesthetic techniques have been reported. To minimize hypotension, a two-catheter extradural technique was used

for vaginal delivery (Linter & Clarke 1984). Caesarean section under general anaesthesia, preceded by fentanyl (Halpern et al 1985) and a neurolept analgesic technique for hysterectomy (Bengtsson et al 1977) have been described.

BIBLIOGRAPHY
Bengtsson I M, Magno R, Wickstrom I 1977 Ebstein's anomaly – anaesthetic problems. British Journal of Anaesthesia 49: 501–503
Donnelly J E, Brown J M, Radford D J 1991 Pregnancy outcome and Ebstein's anomaly. British Heart Journal 66: 368–371
Elsten J L, Kim Y D, Hanowell S T et al 1981 Prolonged induction with exaggerated chamber enlargement in Ebstein's anomaly. Anesthesia and Analgesia 60: 909–910
Gentles T L, Calder A L, Clarkson P M et at 1992 Predictors of long-term survival with Ebstein's anomaly of the tricuspid valve. American Journal of Cardiology 69: 377–381
Halpern S, Gidwaney A, Gates B 1985 Anaesthesia for Caesarean section in a preeclamptic patient with Ebstein's anomaly. Canadian Anaesthetists' Society Journal 32: 244–247
Linter S P K, Clarke K 1984 Caesarean section under extradural analgesia in a patient with Ebstein's anomaly. British Journal of Anaesthesia 56: 203–205
Mair D D 1992 Ebstein's anomaly: natural history and management. Journal of the American College of Cardiology 19: 1047–1048

Section 1

Eclampsia and Severe Pre-Eclampsia (Pregnancy-Induced Hypertension)

ECLAMPSIA AND SEVERE PRE-ECLAMPSIA
(PREGNANCY–INDUCED HYPERTENSION) (see also HELLP SYNDROME)

Pre-eclampsia, or pregnancy-induced hypertension (PIH), is a syndrome of unknown aetiology which is associated with pregnancy. It affects a wide variety of organs and therefore produces diverse manifestations. The main presenting feature is hypertension, with either proteinuria or oedema, or both. Maternal complications include eclampsia, cerebral haemorrhage, cerebral oedema, renal failure and left ventricular failure.

Eclampsia, a cerebral complication, is marked by the onset of convulsions. Cerebral haemorrhage and cerebral oedema are the most frequent causes of death in PIH. Deaths from PIH nearly equal those from eclampsia, and together they are the most important obstetric cause of maternal mortality in the Western world (Redman 1988).

Occasionally an intracranial aneurysm may rupture, or a cerebral A–V malformation bleed, during pregnancy. Their presentations share some of the features of eclampsia and severe PIH – an acute severe headache and neurological signs, with or without a period of unconsciousness. It is crucial that these are distinguished from PIH. It has been suggested that early diagnosis and surgery will improve the morbidity and mortality of these conditions (Giannotta et al 1986).

A small group of patients have been described with the HELLP syndrome which comprises PIH, in association with haemolysis, elevated liver enzymes and a low platelet count.

Section 1

Eclampsia and
Severe
Pre-Eclampsia
(Pregnancy-Induced
Hypertension)

Presentation

1. The definition of PIH includes diastolic hypertension of $\geqslant$90 mmHg (Cunningham & Lindheimer 1992). It has also been recommended that the disappearance of the Korotkoff sound (Phase V) rather than its muffling (Phase IV), be used in its determination. Severe PIH is associated with a BP of 160/110 or more on at least two occasions 6 hours apart, and proteinuria of >5 g in 24 hours (Wright 1983).

2. Whilst PIH is common in the young primiparous patient, there appears to be a subgroup for whom the maternal and fetal risks are particularly high (Connell et al 1987). The patient with PIH at special risk is the older (>25 years), multiparous patient, and particularly the one who develops an impairment in her level of consciousness.

3. The onset of convulsions denotes eclampsia. It may be associated with cerebral haemorrhage or diffuse oedema.

4. The HELLP syndrome may present with bleeding due to thrombocytopenia, a decrease in haemoglobin secondary to haemolysis, and abnormal LFTs (Duffy 1988).

Problems

1. Hypertension, which may be complicated by cerebral oedema, haemorrhage or heart failure. Both PIH and pregnancy-aggravated hypertension are associated with exaggerated pressor responses to accelerated labour, or to noxious stimuli such as tracheal intubation or extubation. The hypertensive response to intubation has provoked cerebral haemorrhage (Fox et al 1977). In a study of patients with PIH undergoing Caesarean section, it has been shown that even in those receiving a conventional antihypertensive regimen, intubation was associated with an average increase in SAP of 54.4 mmHg (Connell et al 1987). In some patients, increases of greater than 70 mmHg occurred. It is recognized that, in normotensive patients, mean arterial pressures exceeding 130–150 mmHg may be associated with a loss of protective cerebral autoregulation (Wright 1983, Richards et al 1986).

2. Impaired renal function which may progress to anuria. Even in mild PIH, the GFR is decreased by 25%.Renal failure accounts for about 10% of deaths from eclampsia.

3. Plasma volume may be decreased by up to 40% in severe cases. Despite sodium and water retention, the CVP is low or normal. This is in part due to increased vascular permeability causing loss of fluid and protein from the circulation. In a study of patients who had pulmonary artery pressure monitoring, variable results were obtained (Mabie et al 1989). However, the general impression was of a high cardiac output state, with an inappropriately high systemic

vascular resistance. The haemodynamic profile suggested that the intravascular volume in PIH is centrally redistributed.

Section 1

Eclampsia and
Severe
Pre-Eclampsia
(Pregnancy-Induced
Hypertension)

4. Maternal systemic blood flow is reduced secondary to vasoconstriction and increased blood viscosity. Diminished placental blood flow results in placental infarction and separation, which leads to decreased fetal growth and sometimes death. Maternal vessels become particularly sensitive to the effects of exogenous catecholamines.

5. A coagulopathy may occur, which is probably consumptive in origin. The number and quality of platelets commonly decrease and the thrombin time becomes prolonged. Prothrombin time, partial thromboplastin time and fibrinogen abnormalities may occur. Significant thrombocytopenia and coagulation abnormalities are usually only encountered in severe PIH (Barker & Callander 1991), and a good correlation between bleeding time and platelet count was found when the platelet count was lower than $100\,000/mm^3$ (Ramanathan et al 1989).

6. Pulmonary oedema, which can be vascular or neurogenic in origin, may produce cyanosis and respiratory distress.

7. Headache, epigastric pain, visual disturbances, hyper-reflexia or cerebral irritability may be warning signs of impending eclampsia. Delayed recovery of consciousness following an eclamptic fit may indicate the occurrence of cerebral oedema or intracranial haemorrhage.

8. Not all fits occurring during pregnancy and labour are the result of eclampsia. Eclamptic fits must be distinguished from those secondary to hyponatraemia associated with the concomitant administration of oxytocics and dextrose-containing fluids, epilepsy, phaeochromocytoma, a ruptured intracranial aneurysm or an A-V malformation, or other intracranial pathology.

9. Pulmonary aspiration and airway obstruction are both more likely to occur in oversedated or unconscious patients.

10. Rarely, severe PIH is associated with haemolysis, abnormal liver function, hepatic damage and thrombocytopenia (see HELLP syndrome) which carries a mortality of up to 24%.

11. Occasionally, pharyngeal or laryngeal oedema may occur unexpectedly, and cause intubation problems (Seager & MacDonald 1980, Brimacombe 1992). One patient developed breathing difficulties after extubation. At laryngoscopy, severe laryngeal oedema was found, despite the vocal cords having been normal at induction of anaesthesia (Rocke & Scoones 1992).

12. Phaeochromocytoma occasionally presents during pregnancy and is associated with a high mortality. The majority of patients have hypertension, and one presented with a convulsion (Harper et al 1989).

Section 1

Eclampsia and
Severe
Pre-Eclampsia
(Pregnancy-Induced
Hypertension)

Management of severe PIH

This is a potentially lethal condition which should be managed in a high-dependency area. Monitoring and treatment requires close cooperation between obstetrician, anaesthetist and paediatrician, whether or not operative delivery is required. General anaesthesia may be particularly hazardous in some patients, and additional precautions should be taken to prevent hypertensive peaks during intubation and extubation.

Management of severe PIH, throughout the peripartum period, should be directed towards:

1. Monitoring
   CVP, ECG, arterial pressure and urine output is monitored, as is neuromuscular function if general anaesthesia is required.
2. Control of maternal blood pressure by arteriolar dilatation.
   A number of methods of controlling blood pressure prior to delivery have been described. The care with which it is monitored and regulated is probably of more importance to maternal and fetal welfare than the exact method of control.
   a. Extradural analgesia. This has the dual therapeutic advantages of providing both vasodilatation and analgesia in PIH. Provided that no coagulation defect is present, it is the method of choice for operative delivery. Platelet count should be $>100 \times 10^9/l$ and prothrombin time and partial thromboplastin time normal.
   b. Hydralazine 5–10 mg increments i.v., or by infusion.
   c. Diazoxide in 30 mg increments to a total of 300 mg i.v.
   d. Magnesium sulphate, which is used more commonly in the USA than in the UK, is both a vasodilator and a sedative. Magnesium sulphate 2 g stat and 2 g/h, via an infusion.
      Magnesium (Mg) levels:

Normal serum	0.7–1.0 mmol/l
Therapeutic anticonvulsant levels	2–3 mmol/l
Loss of patellar reflex	5 mmol/l
Skeletal muscle relaxation	6 mmol/l
Respiratory paralysis	6–7.5 mmol/l
Cardiac asystole	> 12 mmol/l

      Accidental high levels can be treated by Ca gluconate 1 g slowly.
   e. Trimetaphan, as an infusion, has been used for fine control of blood pressure before induction of anaesthesia (Lawes et al 1987).
3. Restoration of vascular volume and vasodilatation
   This should take place synchronously with blood pressure reduction, preferably using plasma protein fraction or a colloid. The CVP should be maintained around 6-8 cmH$_2$O, with reference to the mid-axillary line. Prevention of vasoconstriction and restoration of blood volume has the additional benefit of improving renal function

and uteroplacental blood flow. Fluid administration must be carried out cautiously, since pulmonary oedema is not uncommon in severe PIH and some studies suggest that the CVP may be normal and that there is redistribution of intravascular volume centrally (Mabie et al 1989).

4. Prophylaxis against eclamptic fits. Diazepam, midazolam, magnesium sulphate or chlormethiazole can be used to produce sedation.
5. Protection against acid aspiration syndrome. Sedated patients are particularly at risk.
6. Operative intervention
   Should preferably be performed under extradural anaesthesia. In the very severe case, or if extradural anaesthesia is contraindicated, general anaesthesia may be required but carries additional risks. A careful technique should aim to modulate the hypertensive peaks provoked by intubation and extubation and to prevent sudden uncontrolled reductions in blood pressure. The latter can, however, be produced by either general or regional anaesthesia. It has been suggested that drugs that will help to modify the hypertensive response to intubation should be given before induction. These are given in addition to the preoperative antihypertensive regimen (Lawes et al 1987). As yet, there appears to be no technique which guarantees protection in every patient. The following drugs have been used:
   a. Lignocaine 1 mg/kg i.v., before induction, to reduce haemodynarnic responses (Connell et al 1987). Lignocaine can prevent intracranial hypertension during tracheal suction in comatose head injury patients (Donegan & Bedford 1980).
   b. Practolol in 2 mg increments, to a maximum dose of 0.2 mg/kg, has been found to modify tachycardia in response to intubation if the patient's pulse rate is >120/min (Connell et al 1987). Higher doses than this should not be used as heart rate responses may be impaired in the event of haemorrhage.
   c. An additional bolus of trimetaphan 2.5 mg before induction.
   d. A bolus of hydralazine 6.25–12.5 mg i.v. before induction.
   e. Fentanyl and droperidol have been used, in addition to conventional antihypertensive therapy (Lawes et al 1987). During preoxygenation, droperidol 5 mg and fentanyl 100 µg were given. After 5 minutes a further 100 µg of fentanyl was added. If the SAP was >170 mmHg, or the MAP >130 mmHg, trimetaphan 2.5 mg was also given. Induction of anaesthesia was only started when these pressure limits were not exceeded. It is essential to have an experienced person available to resuscitate the baby. However, this technique was claimed not to have produced significant respiratory depression in unasphyxiated neonates (Lawes et al 1987). Other regimens have included fentanyl 2.5 µg/kg and alfentanil 10 µg/kg, both of which were found to

Section 1

Eclampsia and
Severe
Pre-Eclampsia
(Pregnancy-Induced
Hypertension)

attenuate, but not abolish, the hypertensive response to intubation (Rout & Rocke 1990).

   f. Nitroglycerin modifies the hypertensive response to intubation in severe PIH (Hood et al 1985). During preoxygenation, an infusion of nitroglycerin 200 µg/ml was given until the BP was reduced by 20%. The MAP was then maintained at this level during Caesarean section. However, since nitroglycerin is a cerebral vasodilator and increases intracranial pressure, it should not be used in eclampsia, or when there is a possibility of cerebral oedema.

   g. The use of nitroprusside (Baker 1990).

   h. Alfentanil 10 µg/kg has been shown to modify the hypertensive response to intubation in the non-hypertensive pregnant patient (Dann et al 1987). It was found to be equally as good as magnesium sulphate 40 mg/kg in controlling the cardiovascular response to intubation in patients with moderate to severe PIH (Allen et al 1991). Both were superior to lignocaine 1.5 mg/kg.

7. Management of HELLP syndrome (see HELLP syndrome).

Management of eclampsia

1. Convulsions should be controlled with diazepam 5–20 mg, the airway secured and oxygenation maintained. Tracheal intubation, blood gas estimation and IPPV may be required.

2. Care should be taken to ensure that the diagnosis of eclampsia is correct. If a convulsion is not associated with hypertension and either oedema or proteinuria, or if the history and signs are atypical, then other causes must be eliminated such as cerebral haemorrhage, phaeochromocytoma or hyponatraemia. A CT scan should be performed if an intracranial aneurysm is suspected.

3. Control of hypertension (see above).

4. The only ultimate control of the eclampsia is by termination of the pregnancy, by either rapid vaginal delivery or Caesarean section.

5. If an eclamptic patient remains unconscious 4–6 hours postpartum, neurosurgical advice should be sought. A CT scan will distinguish cerebral oedema from intracranial haemorrhage. It has been suggested that the combination of diffuse white matter oedema and basal cisternal effacement is an indication for intracranial pressure monitoring (Richards et al 1986). A high intracranial pressure (N = 10–15 mmHg) may require specific treatment.

Post-delivery care

Eclampsia may still occur in the postpartum period. In the severe case, intensive monitoring and treatment should continue for 24–72 hours.

BIBLIOGRAPHY
Allen R W, James M F M, Uys P C 1991 Attenuation of the pressor response to

tracheal intubation in hypertensive proteinuric pregnant patients by lignocaine, alfentanil and magnesium sulphate. British Journal of Anaesthesia 66: 216–223

Baker A B 1990 Management of severe pregnancy-induced hypertension, or gestosis, with sodium nitroprusside. Anaesthesia and Intensive Care 18: 361–365

Barker P, Callander C C 1991 Coagulation screening before epidural analgesia in pre-eclampsia. Anaesthesia 46: 64–67

Brimacombe T 1992 Acute pharyngolaryngeal oedema and pre-eclamptic toxaemia. Anaesthesia and Intensive Care 20: 97–98

Connell H, Dalgleish J G, Downing J W 1987 General anaesthesia in mothers with severe preeclampsia/eclampsia. British Journal of Anaesthesia 59: 1375–1380

Crosby E T 1991 Obstetrical anaesthesia for patients with the syndrome of haemolysis, elevated liver enzymes and low platelets. Canadian Journal of Anaesthesia 38: 227–233

Cunningham F G, Lindheimer M D 1992 Hypertension in pregnancy. New England Journal of Medicine 326: 927–932

Dann W L, Hutchinson A, Cartwright D P 1987 Maternal and neonatal responses to alfentanil administered before induction of general anaesthesia for Caesarean section. British Journal of Anaesthesia 59: 1392–1396

Donegan M F, Bedford R F 1980 Intravenously administered lidocaine prevents intracranial hypertension during endotracheal suction. Anesthesiology 52: 516–518

Duffy B L 1988 HELLP syndrome and the anaesthetist. Anaesthesia 43: 223–225

Easterling T R, Benedetti T J, Schmucker B C et al 1990 Maternal hemodynamics in normal and preeclamptic pregnancies: a longitudinal study. Obstetrics and Gynecology 76: 1061–1069

Fox E J, Sklar G S, Hill C H et al 1977 Complications related to the pressor response to endotracheal intubation. Anesthesiology 47: 524–525

Giannotta S L, Daniels J, Golde S H et al 1986 Ruptured intracranial aneurysms during pregnancy. Journal of Reproductive Medicine 31: 139–147

Harper M A, Murnaghan G A, Kennedy L et al 1989 Phaeochromocytoma in pregnancy. Five cases and a review of the literature. British Journal of Obstetrics and Gynaecology 96: 594–606

Hood D D, Dewan D M, James F M et al 1985 The use of nitroglycerin in preventing the hypertensive response to tracheal intubation in severe preeclampsia. Anesthesia and Analgesia 63: 329–332

Lawes E G, Downing J W, Duncan P W et al 1987 Fentanyl/droperidol supplementation of rapid sequence induction controls dangerous blood pressure increases in the presence of severe pregnancy induced and pregnancy aggravated hypertension. British Journal of Anaesthesia 59: 1381–1391

Mabie W C, Ratts T E, Sibai B M 1989 The central hemodynamics of severe preeclampsia. Amercian Journal of Obstetrics and Gynecology 161: 1443–1448

Morison D H 1987 Anaesthesia and pre-eclampsia. Canadian Journal of Anaesthesia 34: 415–421

Patterson K W, O'Toole D P 1991 HELLP syndrome: a case report with guidelines for management. British Journal of Anaesthesia 66: 513–515

Ramanathan J, Sibai B M, Vu T et al 1989 Correlation between bleeding times and platelet counts in women with preeclampsia undergoing Cesarean section. Anesthesiology 71: 188–191

Redman C W G 1988 Eclampsia still kills. British Medical Journal 296: 1209–1210

Richards A M, Moodley J, Graham D I et al 1986 Active management of the unconscious eclamptic patient. British Journal of Obstetrics and Gynaecology 93: 554–562

Rocke D A, Scoones G P 1992 Rapidly progressive laryngeal oedema associated with pregnancy-aggravated hypertension. Anaesthesia 47: 141–143

Rout C C, Rocke D A 1990 Effects of alfentanil and fentanyl on induction of anaesthesia in patients with severe pregnancy-induced hypertension. British Journal of Anaesthesia 65: 468–474

Seager S J, MacDonald R 1980 Laryngeal oedema and preeclampsia. Anaesthesia 35: 360–362

Schindler M, Gatt S, Isert P et al 1990 Thrombocytopenia and platelet functional defects in preeclampsia: implications for regional anaesthesia. Anaesthesia and Intensive Care 18: 169–174

Wright J P 1983 Anesthetic considerations in eclampsia-preeclampsia. Anesthesia and Analgesia 63: 590–601

EHLERS-DANLOS SYNDROME

A group of conditions, of varying inheritance, in which there is a defect in collagen. Eleven different subtypes have been identified each showing a wide spectrum of effects, from mild to severe (Duvic & Pinnell 1986). There have been recent advances in the understanding of the genetic and molecular abnormalities of the variants (Pope 1991). Detailed descriptions are beyond the scope of this book; for further information, Pope et al 1988, Pope 1991 and Anstey et al 1991, may be consulted. The general clinical picture is one of multiple skin, connective tissue and musculoskeletal abnormalities. Cardiac defects have also been described. Anaesthesia may be required for joint dislocations, vascular or visceral rupture and surgery may be complicated by abnormal haemorrhage. Pregnancy in type IV disease is associated with a mortality of about 25%.

Preoperative abnormalities

1. The whole group is characterized by a hyperextensible and sometimes fragile, soft skin, hypermobile joints, and a tendency to bruise and bleed without definite coagulation abnormalities. Paper-tissue scars may occur over the knees, shins, forehead and chin.
2. The ecchymotic form (type IV), which involves abnormalities in type III collagen synthesis, is the most severe, although in this form the loose-jointedness and skin hyperextensibility are uncommon. Type III is the predominant collagen of blood vessels, uterus, fetal skin and the gastrointestinal tract. Complications include aneurysmal dilatation, rupture of blood vessels, and visceral rupture. Aortic dissection, similar to that in Marfan's syndrome, may occur. Type III collagen also forms 10–15% of the collagen in adult skin. Pregnancy carries a 25% mortality, and the complications of surgery can be disastrous.
3. Mitral valve prolapse, RBBB, and left anterior hemi-block have been described in association with some forms of Ehlers–Danlos (Cabeen & Kovik 1977).

Anaesthetic problems

1. The ecchymotic form (type IV) may present with uncontrollable haemorrhage, aneurysm formation and arterial or venous rupture.
2. Spontaneous perforation of a viscus, particularly the colon, may be the first event leading to the diagnosis (Sparkman 1984). Surgery may be followed by wound dehiscence, infection and recurrent perforation.
3. In types IV and VI, the use of arterial and central venous lines for monitoring, or intravascular radiological procedures, can be

accompanied by severe bleeding. Perforation of the superior vena cava has been reported during digital angiography (Driscoll et al 1984).

4. A variety of haemostatic disorders were reported in a study of 51 patients (Anstey et al 1991). Although the majority gave a history of bruising or a bleeding tendency, only 17.6% had significant abnormalities. These included platelet storage pool defects and Factors XI and XIII deficiencies. The remainder had either mild abnormalities of doubtful significance or no abnormality at all. Thus, the bleeding and bruising that occurs must be related to structural abnormalities in the skin and blood vessels.

5. Spinal or extradural anaesthesia may be complicated by an extradural haematoma. However, the use of combined spinal and extradural anaesthesia for Caesarean section has been reported in a patient with type IV disease who refused general anaesthesia (Brighouse & Guard 1992).

6. Milder forms may have postoperative wound dehiscence.

7. Venous access can be technically difficult because of the hyperextensible skin. Displacement of the cannula from a vein and venous extravasation may remain undetected.

8. If conduction defects such as RBBB and left anterior hemi-block are present, progression to complete heart block under anaesthesia could occur.

9. There is an increased risk of pneumothorax in type IV disease.

10. Mandibular hypoplasia (type VI), periodontal disease (type VIII) and recurrent mandibular joint dislocation may complicate airway management (Sacks et al 1990). In one patient, the occurrence of repeated jaw dislocations with facial ecchymosis led to the diagnosis of EDS.

11. A variety of complications may occur during pregnancy. In type I disease (30–50% cases), these were mainly associated with tissue laxity and included vaginal lacerations, abdominal hernias, ante- and postpartum haemorrhage, joint subluxations and bruising. None of these problems was associated with death. In type IV disease, however, pregnancy is associated with high mortality (Peaceman & Cruikshank 1987) and death may occur at any time. Spontaneous pulmonary artery rupture caused exsanguination during the seventh month of pregnancy (Pearl & Spicer 1981). Intrapartum deaths have resulted from aortic, uterine and vena cava rupture (Rudd et al 1983). Death occurred secondary to a postpartum haemorrhage in a patient with normal coagulation tests (Dolan et al 1980). Widespread bleeding from exceptionally fragile vessels and a ruptured splenic artery aneurysm were found at exploratory laparotomy. Postpartum deaths have resulted from spontaneous rupture of the aorta on day 1 (Rudd et al 1983), day 5 (Snyder et al 1983) and at an unspecified

time (Barabas 1972) and renal rupture on day 6 (Peaceman & Cruikshank 1987).

12. Local anaesthesia, either by intradermal infiltration or topical application (EMLA), was found not to be as effective in EDS type III as compared with controls (Arendt-Nielsen et al 1990). The reduced depth and duration of anaesthesia probably results from the looseness of the connective tissue.

Management

1. If the condition is suspected and time permits, genetic advice should be obtained to assess the type and severity.
2. Blood should be cross-matched and coagulation defects excluded.
3. Intramuscular injections must not be given in type IV and regional anaesthesia is relatively contraindicated. However, a combined spinal and extradural technique was used for Caesarean section in a patient with type IV who refused general anaesthesia (Brighouse & Guard 1992).
4. Good peripheral venous access or a cutdown should be established. The use of central venous monitoring via a large cannula, at a site where bleeding cannot be controlled by pressure, should be avoided in types IV and VI. If essential, a small needle should be used, and a peripheral site selected.
5. Particular care should be taken to avoid trauma or jaw dislocation when tracheal or nasogastric tubes are inserted.
6. During artificial ventilation, low airway pressures should be used to reduce the risk of a pneumothorax.
7. If conduction defects are present, the temporary insertion of a pacemaker should be considered.
8. Antibiotic prophylaxis is required if there is mitral valve prolapse.
9. It has been suggested that patients with type IV disease should be counselled against pregnancy, and those who become pregnant should be recommended to have termination (Peaceman & Cruikshank 1987). If this is declined, close observation for signs of vascular or bowel rupture should be maintained during labour and the early peripartum period.

BIBLIOGRAPHY

Anstey A, Mayne K, Winter M et al 1991 Platelet and coagulation studies in Ehlers–Danlos syndrome. British Journal of Dermatology 125: 155–161

Arendt-Nielsen L, Kaalund S, Bjerring P et al 1990 Insufficient effect of local analgesics in Ehlers–Danlos type III patients (connective tissue disorder). Acta Anaesthesiologica Scandinavica 34: 358–361

Barabas A P 1972 Vascular complications in the Ehlers–Danlos syndrome, with special reference to the 'arterial type' or Sack's syndrome. Journal of Cardiovascular Surgery (Torino) 13: 160–167

Brighouse D, Guard B 1992 Anaesthesia for Caesarean section in a patient with Ehlers–Danlos syndrome type IV. British Journal of Anaesthesia 69: 517–520

Cabeen W R, Kovick R B 1977 Mitral valve prolapse and conduction defects in

Ehlers–Danlos syndrome. Archives of Internal Medicine 137: 1227–1231

Dolan P, Sisko F, Riley E 1980 Anesthetic considerations for Ehlers–Danlos syndrome. Anesthesiology 52: 266–269

Driscoll S H M, Gomes A S, Machleder H I 1984 Perforation of the superior vena cava: a complication of digital angiography in Ehlers–Danlos syndrome. American Journal of Roentgenology 142: 1021–1022

Duvic M, Pinnell S P 1986 Ehlers–Danlos syndrome. In: Thiers B H, Dobson R L (eds) Pathogenesis of skin disease. Churchill Livingstone, Edinburgh

Peaceman A M, Cruikshank D P 1987 Ehlers–Danlos syndrome and pregnancy: association of type IV disease with maternal death. Obstetrics and Gynecology 69: 428–431

Pearl W, Spicer M 1981 Ehlers–Danlos syndrome. Southern Medical Journal 74: 80–81

Pope F M, Narcisi P, Nicholls A C et al 1988 Clinical presentation of Ehler's–Danlos syndrome. Archives of Disease in Childhood 63: 1016–1025

Pope F M 1991 Ehler's–Danlos syndrome. Bailliere's Clinical Rheumatology 5(2): 321–349

Rudd N L, Holbrook K A, Nimrod C et al 1983 Pregnancy complications in type IV Ehlers–Danlos syndrome. Lancet i: 50–53

Sacks H, Zelig D, Schabes G 1990 Recurrent temporomandibular joint subluxation and facial ecchymosis leading to diagnosis of Ehlers–Danlos syndrome. Journal of Oral and Maxillofacial Surgery 48: 641–647

Snyder R R, Gilstrap L C, Hauth J C 1983 Ehlers–Danlos syndrome and pregnancy. Obstetrics and Gynecology 61: 649–651

Sparkman R S 1984 Ehlers–Danlos syndrome type IV: dramatic, deceptive, and deadly. American Journal of Surgery 147: 703–704

Suzuki T, Tsuchiyama Y, Kauraguchi Y et al 1989 Anaesthesia for a patient with Ehlers Danlos syndrome and factor XIII deficiency. Masui 38: 1518–1521 (English abstr)

Wesley J R, Mahour G H, Woolley M M 1980 Multiple surgical problems in two patients with Ehlers Danlos syndrome. Surgery 87: 319–324

EISENMENGER'S SYNDROME

A rare syndrome of pulmonary hypertension associated with a reversed or bidirectional cardiac shunt, occurring through a large communication between the left and right heart. The defect may be interventricular, interatrial or aortopulmonary. The development of Eisenmenger's syndrome from the initial left-to-right shunt is usually a gradual process. Contributory factors to the pulmonary hypertension are hypoxia, high pulmonary blood flow and high left atrial pressure. Irreversible structural changes take place in the small vessels, causing pulmonary vascular obstruction and a reduction in the size of the capillary bed. The pulmonary artery pressure is the same as, or sometimes exceeds, the systemic arterial pressure. The incidence of this syndrome has decreased as a result of the more vigorous approach to diagnosis and treatment of congenital heart disease in childhood.

Preoperative abnormalities

1. Presenting symptoms include dyspnoea, tiredness, episodes of cyanosis, syncope or chest pain. Haemoptysis may occur.
2. The direction of the shunt, and hence the presence or absence of cyanosis, depends on a number of factors. These include hypoxia,

the pulmonary and systemic blood pressure differences, and the intravascular volume. It can also be affected by certain drugs.
3. CXR shows right ventricular hypertrophy, and ECG indicates varying degrees of right ventricular hypertrophy and strain.
4. Complications include thrombosis secondary to polycythaemia, air embolus and bacterial endocarditis. Cerebral abscess may follow clot embolism.

Anaesthetic problems

1. Reductions in systemic arterial pressure by myocardial depression or loss of sympathetic tone are potentially dangerous. Reversal of the shunt may occur, and sudden death has been reported. Hypovolaemia and dehydration are poorly tolerated.
2. Sinus tachycardia results from exercise or emotion, and episodes of SVT are common after the age of 30 years. The onset of atrial fibrillation is associated with a sudden deterioration in the condition of the patient.
3. The relative merits of general and regional anaesthesia are arguable. General anaesthesia tends to be favoured, since the reduction in systemic vascular resistance produced by regional blockade increases the shunt. However, successful use of extradural anaesthesia for bilateral inguinal herniorrhaphy (Selsby & Sugden 1989), and Caesarean section (Spinnato et al 1981) has been reported.
4. Pregnancy carries considerable risks and is contraindicated. Maternal mortality rates of 30% have been reported (Devitt et al 1982) whilst Caesarean section may increase the mortality to over 60%. Even termination of pregnancy may be hazardous. The diagnosis may be missed at a booking clinic. An increased haemoglobin level in early pregnancy was the only abnormality in one patient who developed unexplained cyanosis during Caesarean section for antepartum haemorrhage (Gilman 1991). Postoperative death followed cardiorespiratory failure and coagulopathy. Postmortem studies showed a persistent ductus arteriosus and pulmonary hypertension. The insertion of pulmonary artery catheters for monitoring has led to systemic and pulmonary emboli, pulmonary artery rupture and arrhythmias (Robinson 1983). Postpartum death is not uncommon. One patient died during removal of a pulmonary artery catheter on the fourth day after Caesarean section (Devitt et al 1982); another died on the sixth day (Hytens Alexander 1986). It has been argued that the risks of pulmonary artery catheters in Eisenmenger's syndrome outweigh the benefits (Robinson 1983), and that it is not always possible to obtain wedge pressures (Schwalbe et al 1990).
5. Patients are at risk from paradoxical air or clot embolism and infective endocarditis.

Management

1. Maintenance of an adequate circulating blood volume is essential. Myocardial depressants and peripheral vasodilators should be used with caution. Bradycardia must be prevented. If regional anaesthesia is used, the block should be instituted cautiously and hypovolaemia avoided. High-dose spinal morphine for the first stage of labour and pudendal block for the second stage have been used in a woman with a PDA (Pollack et al 1990). In this patient simultaneous monitoring of oxygen saturations in the right arm (predominantly preductal) and leg gave information about the right-to-left shunt.
2. It is unclear as to whether oxygen can cause pulmonary vasodilatation. Although the pulmonary vascular resistance was believed to be fixed in pulmonary hypertension, a high oxygen concentration has been shown to reduce it during Caesarean section (Spinnato et al 1981).
3. Alpha adrenergic vasopressors such as methoxamine or phenylephrine have been recommended for treatment of hypotension on induction of anaesthesia (Foster & Jones 1984). Prophylactic treatment with metararminol has been proposed (Lumley et al 1977) but, in common with other vasopressors, it also produces pulmonary vasoconstriction. Bradycardia and an intensification of cyanosis have been observed.
4. IPPV should be used with low inflation pressures.
5. Air must be completely eliminated from all intravenous lines and the extradural space located with loss of resistance to saline, not air.
6. Appropriate antibiotics are given to prevent bacterial endocarditis.
7. Low-dose heparin may reduce the risk of emboli.
8. Patients are usually advised against pregnancy. If anaesthesia is required either for termination of pregnancy or operative delivery, intensive cardiac care is indicated. Successful extradural anaesthesia has been reported for Caesarean section (Spinnato et al 1981).

BIBLIOGRAPHY

Devitt J H, Noble W H, Byrick R J 1982 A Swan–Ganz catheter related complication in a patient with Eisenmenger's syndrome. Anesthesiology 57: 335–337
Foster J M G, Jones R M 1984 The anaesthetic management of the Eisenmenger syndrome. Annals of the Royal College of Surgeons of England 66: 353–355
Gilman D H 1991 Caesarean section in undiagnosed Eisenmenger's syndrome. Report of a fatal outcome. Anaesthesia 46: 371–373
Hytens L, Alexander J P 1986 Maternal and neonatal death associated with Eisenmenger's syndrome. Acta Anaesthesiologica Belgica 37: 45–51
Lumley J, Whitwam J G, Morgan M 1977 General anesthesia in the presence of Eisenmenger's syndrome. Anesthesia and Analgesia 56: 543–547
Pollack K L, Chestnut D H, Wenstrom K D 1990 Anesthetic management of a parturient with Eisenmenger's syndrome. Anesthesia and Analgesia 70: 212–215
Robinson S 1983 Pulmonary artery catheters in Eisenmenger's syndrome: many risks, few benefits. Anesthesiology 58: 588–589
Selsby D S, Sugden J C 1989 Epidural anaesthesia for bilateral inguinal herniorrhaphy in Eisenmenger's syndrome. Anaesthesia 44: 130–132
Schwalbe S S, Deshmukh S M, Marx G F 1990 Use of pulmonary artery

Section 1

Endocarditis,
Bacterial
(Antibacterial
Prophylaxis for
Surgery)

catheterization in parturient with Eisenmenger's syndrome. Anesthesia and
Analgesia 71: 442–443
Spinnato J A, Kraynack B J, Cooper M W 1981 Eisenmenger's syndrome in pregnancy:
epidural anesthesia for elective Cesarean section. New England Journal of Medicine
304: 1215–1217

ENDOCARDITIS, BACTERIAL
(ANTIBACTERIAL PROPHYLAXIS FOR SURGERY)

A serious infection of the endocardium, most frequently affecting the
heart valves, caused by circulating micro-organisms. The uniformly fatal
disease of the pre-antibiotic era has been reduced to one with a
mortality of about 30% (Morris 1985). However its incidence has not
declined, and there has been a noticeable change in the pattern of the
disease.

Guidelines on the antibacterial prophylaxis for infective endocarditis
are regularly revised by the British Society for Antimicrobial Therapy
(Working Party 1982, Working Party 1990, Simmons et al 1992 and the
current British National Formulary). Although a number of papers have
cast doubt on the benefit and cost effectiveness of prophylaxis (Van der
Meer et al 1992) and debate continues world-wide, at present, the UK
recommendations are generally acceptable (Simmons et al 1992).

In 1981/2 a joint study between the Royal College of Physicians and
the British Cardiac Society of 544 cases of infective endocarditis has
formed the basis of a series of papers on various aspects of the disease
(Bayliss et al 1983a,b, 1984). There is an increased risk for patients with
pre-existing cardiac lesions when operations or venous procedures are
undertaken. This has implications for the anaesthetist. The patients
affected tend to be older than in the past, and with the decline in
rheumatic heart disease, the aortic valve is now more often affected than
the mitral. A proportion of patients had normal hearts, or previously
undiagnosed abnormalities. *Streptococcus* is still the predominant
organism. In some cases, the portal of entry was obvious: 19% were
probably dental in origin, 16% were from the gut, genitourinary,
respiratory tract or skin, and 5% were from procedures involving access
to the bloodstream. In 60% of cases, however, the source was unknown.
Whilst 13.7% of cases of endocarditis had had a dental procedure within
the preceding 3 months, over half of these cases had pre-existing cardiac
abnormalities, for which antibiotic prophylaxis had not been prescribed.

Any child with congenital heart disease is at risk, and endocarditis
may present with fever, anaemia and leucocytosis. If the condition
occurs in a child who has undergone open heart surgery, it carries a
high mortality (Karl et al 1987). More recently, the question has been
raised of antibiotic cover for dentistry in patients undergoing hip
replacement (Cawson 1992).

1. Factors predisposing to the development of endocarditis

Section 1

Endocarditis,
Bacterial
(Antibacterial
Prophylaxis for
Surgery)

a. High-risk patients:
  i. Prosthetic heart valves.
  ii. A previous attack of endocarditis.
b. Standard-risk patients:
  i. Congenital heart disease, especially VSD and PDA, rarely ASD.
  ii. Rheumatic heart disease.
  iii. Other cardiac abnormalities, such as mitral valve prolapse and degenerative aortic valve disease.
  iv. Previous rheumatic fever.
  v. An increased incidence in intravenous drug users, alcoholism, diabetes, renal failure, malignant disease and immunosuppression.
2. Bacteria involved in endocarditis
  Most commonly involved are *Streptococcus viridans*, *Streptococcus faecalis*, *Staphylococcus aureus* and Gram-negative organisms. In the 544 episodes studied in 1981/2, 63% were due to streptococci, 19% to staphylococci and 14% to bowel organisms (Bayliss et al 1983b). Infection with a staphyloccus carried the highest mortality (30%).
3. Types of surgery for which prophylaxis is recommended
  a. Necessary in both standard- and high-risk groups:
    i. Dental treatment including extractions, scaling, and surgery involving gingival tissues (Cawson 1983, 1992).
    ii. Genitourinary procedures, involving instrumentation (but not with clindamycin).
    iii. Upper respiratory tract procedures.
  b. Not necessary in the standard-risk but necessary in the high-risk groups:
    i. Obstetric and gynaecological procedures.
    ii. Gastrointestinal procedures.
    iii. Barium enema.
4. Recommended antibiotic prophylaxis
  a. Dental treatment without general anaesthesia
    i. Standard risk, not penicillin allergic:
       Adult: amoxycillin oral, 3g 1 hour pre. op.
       Child (5–10 years): half adult dose.
       Child (<5 years):   quarter adult dose.
    ii. Standard risk, penicillin allergic:
       Adult: clindamycin oral, 600 mg 60 minutes pre. op.
       Child (5–10 years): half adult dose.
       Child (<5 years):   quarter adult dose.
    iii. High risk:
       Adult: amoxycillin i.m. 1 g or i.v., and gentamicin i.m. 120 mg or i.v at induction and amoxycillin oral, 500 g 6 hours later.

Section 1

Endocarditis,
Bacterial
(Antibacterial
Prophylaxis for
Surgery)

Child (5–10 years): half adult dose.
Child (<5 years): quarter adult dose.

b. Dental treatment and upper respiratory tract surgery under genenral anaesthesia

i. Standard risk, not penicillin allergic:

Adult: amoxycillin i.v. 1 g before induction and 500 mg oral 6 hours later.

Or oral amoxycillin 3 g + oral probenecid 1 g 4 hours before procedure.

Child (<10 years): half adult dose.

ii. Standard risk, penicillin allergic:

Adult: vancomycin i.v. 1 g infusion over 100 min and gentamicin i.v 120 mg before induction.

Or teicoplanin i.v. 400 mg followed by gentamicin i.v. 120 mg before induction.

Or clindamycin i.v. 300 mg over 10 min and then oral or clindamycin i.v. 150 mg 6 hours later.

iii. High risk or those having been given penicillin in the preceding month:

Adult: as outlined in ii above.

Child: in ii or iii, children <14 years require teicoplanin i.v 6 mg/kg and gentamicin i.v 2 mg/kg or clindamycin half adult dose (5–10 years) or quarter adult dose (<5 years).

c. Genitourinary procedures

i. Standard risk, not penicillin allergic:

Adult: amoxycillin i.v. 1 g or i.m. and gentamicin i.v. or i.m. 120 mg at induction, amoxycillin 500 mg 6 hours later

Child (<10 years): amoxycillin half adult dose and gentamicin 2 mg/kg

ii. Standard risk, penicillin allergic and high risk:

Adult: vancomycin infusion, 1 g over 100 minutes, followed by gentamicin i.v. 120 mg before induction.

Child (<10 years): vancomycin 20 mg/kg and gentamicin 2 mg/kg by i.v. infusion

BIBLIOGRAPHY

Bayliss R, Clarke C, Oakley C M et al 1983a The teeth and infective endocarditis. British Heart Journal 50: 506–512

Bayliss R, Clarke C, Oakley C M et al 1983b The microbiology and pathogenesis of infective endocarditis. British Heart Journal 50: 513–519

Bayliss R, Clarke C, Oakley C M et al 1984 The bowel, the genitourinary tract, and

infective endocarditis. British Heart Journal 51: 339–345
Cawson R A 1983 The antibiotic prophylaxis of infective endocarditis. British Dental Journal 154: 183–184
Cawson R A 1992 Antibiotic prophylaxis for dental treatment. For hearts but not for prosthetic joints. British Medical Journal 304: 933–934
Editorial 1992 Chemoprophylaxis for infective endocarditis: faith, hope, and charity challenged. Lancet 339: 525–526
Karl T, Wensley D, Stark J et al 1987 Infective endocarditis in children with congenital heart disease: comparison of selected features in patients with surgical correction or palliation and those without. British Heart Journal 58: 57–65
Morris G K 1985 Infective endocarditis: a preventable disease? British Medical Journal 290: 1532–1533
Simmons N A, Ball A P, Cawson R A et al 1992 Antibiotic prophylaxis and infective endocarditis. Lancet 339: 1292–1293
Van der Meer J T, Van Wijk W, Thompson J et al 1992 Efficacy of antibiotic prophylaxis for prevention of native-valve endocarditis. Lancet 339: 135–139
Working Party of the British Society for Antimicrobial Chemotherapy 1982 The antibiotic prophylaxis of infective endocarditis. Lancet ii: 1323–1326
Working Party of the British Society for Antimicrobial Chemotherapy 1990 Antibiotic prophylaxis of infective endocardis. Lancet 335: 88–89

EPIDERMOLYSIS BULLOSA
(RECESSIVE DYSTROPHIC)

Epidermolysis bullosa refers to a spectrum of genetic diseases in which the primary feature is the formation of bullae in the skin or mucous membranes, either spontaneously or in response to mechanical injury (Bauer 1986). The individual types can be distinguished by genetic, clinical and pathological features. Recessive dystrophic epidermolysis bullosa, which presents at birth or in infancy, is one of the severe forms. Anaesthesia may be required for plastic surgery for syndactyly, oesophageal dilatation, skin grafting and excision of squamous cell carcinoma.

Preoperative abnormalities

1. Frictional or other trauma results in the formation of bullae in the dermis and mucous membranes. When healing takes place, scarring occurs. There appears to be a decreased number, or an absence, of anchoring fibrils in the dermis, together with an increase in collagenase activity in the blistered skin.
2. The scarring may result in flexion contractures of the limbs, fusion of digits, contraction of the mouth and fixation of the tongue.
3. Oesophageal strictures mainly involve the cervical oesophagus, and symptoms of dysphagia start in the first decade even before pathological changes are obvious (Ergun et al 1992). Anal blistering and constipation are common.
4. Protein loss from the skin results in growth failure, anaemia, hypoproteinaemia and malnutrition. Teeth are malformed and nails are shed. Dehydration and sepsis are additional problems.
5. Drug treatment may include corticosteroids, phenytoin and vitamin E.

6. There is an increased incidence of squamous cell carcinoma, amyloidosis and porphyria.

Anaesthetic problems

1. The face mask may cause bullae on the chin, nose and cheek. Conjunctival abrasions have been reported.
2. Tracheal intubation may produce bullae in the mouth which can bleed and rupture (Pratilas & Biezunski 1975). Surprisingly, there are no reports of laryngeal or tracheal bullae forming as a result of intubation. This may be because the epithelium of the larynx and trachea is of the ciliated columnar type, which appears more resilient than the squamous. In a 3-month-old child, a spontaneous bulla sited above the vocal cords resulted in stridor (Fisher & Ray 1989). There have been two reports of laryngeal stenosis, but neither patient had ever had tracheal intubation.
3. Oral airways have produced massive bullae in the mouth.
4. Microstomia from oropharyngeal scarring can cause intubation problems.
5. Venous access may be a problems because of scarring of the skin.
6. Bullae may occur at the sites of a BP cuff, ECG electrodes or adhesive tape. Shearing forces are mechanically the most damaging to the skin.
7. There is an increased risk of regurgitation and pulmonary aspiration secondary to oesophageal stricture.
8. One patient, who was rapidly turned on his side because he regurgitated, had an area of skin sheared from his shoulder (Griffin & Mayou 1993).

Management

1. Care should be taken to avoid shearing stresses to the skin whilst the patient is under anaesthesia. If feasible, the patient should be allowed to position himself on the operating table.
2. The decision whether to use a mask or intubation technique is governed by factors such as the estimated duration of the operation and the pressure required to maintain the mask in position. A review of 131 intubated cases provided no evidence that careful intubation caused laryngeal problems (James & Wark 1982). More commonly, bullae in the mouth have arisen from trauma from an oral airway, the laryngoscope or by the surgeon. Bullae have also occurred on the face due to pressure from the mask. If tracheal intubation is to be undertaken, a well-lubricated, smaller than normal size of tube, should be used. Controlled ventilation and neuromuscular blockade is advisable under these circumstances, to reduce frictional damage from the patient coughing and straining against the tube (Tomlinson 1983).

3. In the presence of an oesophageal stricture, precautions should be taken against pulmonary aspiration.
4. All instruments should be well lubricated. Petroleum jelly gauze is placed around the mask and where the anaesthetist's fingers support the chin.
5. The patient's eyes must be protected.
6. Difficulties in finding peripheral veins may mean central venous access is required.
7. Modifications to monitoring attachments, in an attempt to reduce skin damage, have been suggested (Kelly et al 1987). Moist gauze was placed underneath the BP cuff, ECG pads had their adhesive trimmed and the gel electrodes were placed under the patient's back. Adhesive tape causes shearing stresses and should be avoided if possible. When invasive monitoring is necessary, adhesive attachments can be dispensed with. Central venous and arterial lines were sutured into place in a patient having a resection of oesophageal stricture (Milne & Rosales 1980).
8. Ketamine has been used to avoid both mask anaesthesia and tracheal intubation.
9. Surgery for pseudosyndactyly has been performed under brachial plexus anaesthesia (Kelly et al 1987, Hagen & Langenberg 1988) and in combination with ketamine supplements (Kaplan & Strauch 1987).
10. Regional anaesthesia may be appropriate on occasions. Lumbar and caudal extradural and spinal anaesthesia have been described (Spielman & Mann 1984, Broster et al 1987, Yee et al 1989). The extradural catheters were not secured.

BIBLIOGRAPHY
Bauer E A 1986 Epidermolysis bullosa. In: Thiers B H, Dobson R L (eds) Pathogenesis of skin diseases. Churchill Livingstone, Edinburgh
Broster T, Placek R, Eggers G W N 1987 Epidermolysis bullosa: anesthetic management for Cesarean section. Anesthesia and Analgesia 66: 341–343
Ergun G A, Lin A N, Dannenberg A J et al 1992 Gastrointestinal manifestations of epidermolysis bullosa. A study of 101 patients. Medicine 71: 121–127
Fisher G C, Ray D A A 1989 Airway obstruction in epidermolysis bullosa. Anaesthesia 44: 449
Griffin R P, Mayou B J 1993 The anaesthetic management of patients with dystrophic epidermolysis bullosa. Anaesthesia (in press)
Hagen R, Langenber C 1988 Anaesthetic management in patients with epidermolysis bullosa dystrophica. Anaesthesia 43: 482–485
James I G, Wark H 1982 Airway management during anesthesia in patients with epidermolysis bullosa dystrophia. Anesthesiology 56: 323–326
Kaplan R, Strauch B 1987 Regional anesthesia in a child with epidermolysis bullosa. Anesthesiology 67: 262–264
Kelly R E, Koff H D, Rothaus K O et al 1987 Brachial plexus anesthesia in eight patients with recessive dystrophic epidermolysis bullosa. Anesthesia and Analgesia 66: 1318–1320
Milne B, Rosales J K 1980 Anaesthesia for correction of oesphageal stricture in a patient with recessive epidermolysis bullosa. Canadian Anaesthetists' Society Journal 27: 169–171

Pratilas V, Biezunski A 1975 Epidermolysis bullosa manifested and treated during anesthesia. Anesthesiology 43: 581–583

Spielman F J, Mann E S 1984 Subarachnoid and epidural anaesthesia for patients with epidermolysis bullosa. Canadian Anaesthetists' Society Journal 31: 549–551

Tomlinson A A 1983 Recessive dystrophic epidermolysis bullosa. Anaesthesia 38: 485–491

Yee L L, Gunter J B, Manley C B 1989 Caudal epidural anesthesia in an infant with epidermolysis bullosa. Anesthesiology 70: 149–151

EPIGLOTTITIS
(ACUTE)

An acute inflammation and swelling of the epiglottis, the aryepiglottic folds and the mucosa over the arytenoid cartilages, usually associated with *Haemophilus influenzae* type B. It occasionally results in total laryngeal obstruction, and death from hypoxia. Although epiglottitis has been considered to be primarily a paediatric disorder, with a peak incidence between the ages of 1 and 4 years, adults can also be affected and may be increasingly so. Each presents with slightly different clinical pictures. In children, the treatment of choice is short-term nasotracheal intubation until the swelling has subsided. In adults, nasotracheal intubation may also be required, but the clinical course may be less severe than in children so that an increasing number of clinicians are adopting a more conservative policy (Arndal & Andreassen 1988, Wolf et al 1990, Crosby & Reid 1991). However, sudden death is still reported, even in adults, and such a change in approach is not universally accepted.

Presentation

1. The illness is usually of sudden onset (6–12 hours), with high fever, marked constitutional symptoms, stridor, the development of a muffled voice and the absence of a harsh cough. The child is agitated and often leans forward, drooling saliva. Boys are more frequently affected than girls. Although the peak incidence has usually been thought to occur in the 2–4 years age group, there is an increasing number of cases in younger children (Emmerson et al 1991). In children less than 2 years old, the presentation may be atypical (Blackstock et al 1987).

2. Differentiation from laryngotracheobronchitis may sometimes be difficult. In a prospective study, drooling, agitation and the absence of spontaneous cough were associated with epiglottitis (Mauro et al 1988).

3. The child may present with increasing respiratory distress and cyanosis. Total airway obstruction can be sudden and without warning. Occasionally, cardiorespiratory arrest can occur before hospital admission.

4. There is a high leucocyte count, and *H. influenzae* type B is often subsequently grown from blood culture or swabs. A lateral X-ray of

the neck may show a swollen epiglottis. However, if epiglottitis is suspected, the patient must only be sent for X-ray accompanied by an experienced member of staff, in case sudden respiratory obstruction occurs.

5. Adults are more likely to present with sore throat and dysphagia. However, there is the same risk of sudden airway obstruction. Of 56 adult cases of epiglottitis, death occurred in four. Two of these were in hospital under observation, and both died before airway intervention had been undertaken (Mayosmith et al 1986).

Anaesthetic problems

1. Although the distinction between acute epiglottitis and acute laryngotracheobronchitis, the other more common cause of stridor, can frequently be made on clinical grounds, occasionally the diagnosis is difficult.
2. In children, examination of the mouth and throat, or even the distress caused by insertion of an intravenous infusion, may precipitate complete upper airway obstruction.
3. The induction of anaesthesia may abolish accessory respiratory muscle movement, and also cause obstruction.
4. Perioperative complications include cardiorespiratory arrest, accidental extubation, tracheal tube blockage, pulmonary oedema and pneumothorax. A report of 161 cases of epiglottitis revealed 45 complications in 34 patients and five deaths (Baines et al 1985). Complications included 18 episodes of cardiorespiratory arrest, 10 incidents involving accidental extubation, three cases of pneumothorax, and three episodes of pulmonary oedema following relief of the airway obstruction.
5. Pulmonary oedema has occurred after intubation in 2% children, usually those with severe obstruction progressing to respiratory arrest (Bonadio & Losek 1992).
6. The appearance of an ampicillin-resistant *H. influenzae* strain is being reported (Emmerson et al 1991).

Management

1. Acute epiglottitis represents a serious emergency which should be attended by an experienced anaesthetist whenever the diagnosis is suspected. In any child with stridor, a high index of suspicion must be maintained. Investigation should not be allowed to delay the treatment of life-threatening obstruction (Love et al 1984).
2. In children, no examination of the throat should be made, except under an anaesthetic given by an experienced anaesthetist, and preferably with an ENT surgeon present (Breivik & Klaastad 1978). In adults, it has been suggested that indirect laryngoscopy or fibreoptic bronchoscopic examination of the larynx may be

performed by a skilled endoscopist without the risk of precipitating complete obstruction (Love et al 1984, Phelan & Love 1984). This view is controversial, since it is still possible to precipitate complete airway obstruction. Should this approach be used, the endoscopist must be experienced and the facility for emergency tracheostomy immediately available.

3. Inhalation anaesthesia with halothane and oxygen, with or without nitrous oxide, is indicated. An airway should be secured first with an oral tube. This can be replaced at leisure with a suitably sized nasotracheal tube.

4. The tube must be firmly secured and an intravenous infusion set up to prevent dehydration. Bandaging of the hands will reduce the risks of extubation and decannulation.

5. In those with patients with severe obstruction, the possibility of pulmonary oedema occurring after intubation should not be overlooked. Management requires airway patency, oxygen, and in about 50% of patients IPPV and PEEP will be needed (Lang et al 1990).

6. One of the most difficult problems is the provision of sufficient humidification to prevent crusting of the tube. Examination under anaesthetic at 24 hours is advisable. Even if extubation is not possible at that stage, the tube should be changed. In the small child, partial blockage of the tube by secretions is almost invariably found. The mean duration of intubation in one series was 36 hours (Rothstein & Lister 1983). Direct observation of the epiglottis was found to be the only reliable way to determine the stage at which the tube was no longer necessary.

7. Anaesthetists are divided over the most appropriate method of respiratory management for the patient, once intubated Increasingly, IPPV is used for the period of tracheal intubation, to allow adequate sedation, oxygenation and humidification. However, in a study of 349 patients (Butt et al 1988), 83% received nasotracheal intubation and were allowed to breathe spontaneously through a condenser humidifier. No sedation was given but the patient was restrained. IPPV was only undertaken if the patient presented with complications. Criteria for extubation were: the resolution of fever to <37.5°C, time of intubation (12–16 hours), and general improvement in appearance. It was accepted that this scheme of management requires the invariable presence on the ITU of someone experienced in intubation. If the patient is allowed to breathe spontaneously, a sedative, but not a respiratory depressant, may be permitted. Accidental extubation and tracheal tube blockage are the most serious complications and can prove fatal if respiration is depressed. Whichever method is employed, facilities should be available for rapid reintubation.

8. About 80% of *H. influenzae* infections will be sensitive to ampicillin, although there is increasing evidence of ampicillin resistance (Emmerson et al 1991). For the remainder, chloramphenicol is the drug of choice. Antibiotics should be given empirically. It has been suggested that insistence on bacteriological specimens before antibiotics are given may be unnecessary and potentially hazardous.

9. The use of steroids is debatable. A retrospective non-controlled comparison between one area using them routinely and another only using them occasionally, showed no difference in outcome (Welch & Price 1983). However, in practice, steroids are often given. It has been suggested that those patients who fail the first attempt at extubation may benefit from a course of prednisolone 2 mg/kg per day for 24 hours before the second attempt (Freezer et al 1990).

10. Short-lived pulmonary oedema occasionally occurs after relief of the obstruction, and should be treated with oxygen or, if necessary, IPPV (Lang et al 1990).

BIBLIOGRAPHY

Arndal H, Andreassen U K 1988 Acute epiglottitis in children and adults. Nasotracheal intubation, tracheostomy or careful observation? Current status in Scandinavia. Journal of Laryngology and Otology 102: 1012–1016

Baines D B, Wark H, Overton J H 1985 Acute epiglottitis in children. Anaesthesia and Intensive Care 13: 25–28

Baxter F J, Dunn G L 1988 Acute epiglottitis in adults. Canadian Journal of Anaesthesia 35: 428–435

Blackstock D, Adderley R J, Steward D J 1987 Epiglottitis in young infants. Anesthesiology 67: 97–100

Bonadio W A, Losek J D 1992 The characteristics of children with epiglottitis who develop the complication of pulmonary edema. Archives of Otolaryngology and Head and Neck Surgery 117: 205–207

Breivik H, Klaastad O 1978 Acute epiglottitis in children. British Journal of Anaesthesia 50: 505–510

Butt W, Shann F, Walker C et al 1988 Acute epiglottitis: a different approach to management. Critical Care Medicine 16: 43–47

Crosby E, Reid D 1991 Acute epiglottitis in the adult: is intubation mandatory? Canadian Journal of Anaesthesia 38: 914–918

Emmerson S G, Richman B, Spahn T 1991 Changing patterns of epiglottitis in children. Otolaryngology and Head and Neck Surgery 104: 287–292

Freezer N, Butt W, Phelan P 1990 Steroids in croup: do they increase the incidence of successful extubation. Anaesthesia and Intensive Care 18: 224–228

Lang S A, Duncan P G, Shephard D A et al 1990 Pulmonary oedema associated with airway obstruction. Canadian Journal of Anaesthesia 37: 210–218

Love J B, Phelan D M, Runciman W B et al 1984 Acute epiglottitis in adults. Anaesthesia and Intensive Care 12: 264–269

Mauro R D, Poole S R, Lockhart C H 1988 Differentiation of epiglottitis from laryngotracheitis in the child with stridor. American Journal of Diseases in Children 142: 679–682

Mayosmith M J, Hirsch P J, Wodzinski S F et al 1986 Acute epiglottitis in adults. New England Journal of Medicine 314: 1133–1139

Murrage K J, Janzen V D, Ruby R R 1988 Epiglottitis: adult and pediatric comparisons. Journal of Otolaryngology 17: 194–198

Phelan D M, Love J B 1984 Adult epiglottis. Is there a role for the fiberoptic bronchoscope? Chest 86: 783–784

Rothstein P, Lister G 1983 Epiglottitis – duration of intubation and fever. Anesthesia and Analgesia 62: 785–787

Welch D B, Price D G 1983 Acute epiglottitis and severe croup. Experience in two
English regions. Anaesthesia 38: 754–759
Wolf M, Strauss B, Kronenberg J, et al 1990 Conservative management of adult
epiglottitis. Laryngoscope 100: 183–185

EPILEPSY

Epilepsy is a clinical diagnosis, based on the occurrence of at least two
seizures. A seizure is an abnormal paroxysmal discharge from a group of
neurones, resulting in a clinical manifestation or a sensory perception. It
may occur with or without loss of consciousness. The incidence of
epilepsy is 0.5–1%. It may be a symptom of an underlying pathology, in
which case there is a focal cerebral lesion. Alternatively it may be
idiopathic. In the latter there is a constitutional and sometimes
hereditary disposition to seizures, and a focal lesion is not necessarily
demonstrated. However, with the increasing use of magnetic resonance
imaging, focal lesions may be found even in apparent idiopathic
epilepsy.

Determination of the type of epilepsy is usually made on the pattern
of the fit, the age of onset, the timing and EEG changes. The
international classification of seizure types is complex and will not be
considered further. However, seizures can be broadly divided into
'partial' (which include the former terms, Jacksonian, temporal lobe and
psychomotor epilepsy) and 'generalized' (previously described as grand
mal or major convulsions). Partial seizures begin locally in the cortex
and have an aura reflective of the origin of the discharge. This type of
seizure can be further divided into simple, complex and those which
become secondarily generalized. Generalized seizures are characterized
by a sudden loss of consciousness without an aura, and bilateral
manifestations. Further subdivisions include tonic-clonic, absence and
myoclonic seizures.

Status epilepticus is a recurrence of convulsions, without intervening
periods when consciousness is recovered. At the start of status
epilepticus there is a characteristic EEG sequence of events and changes
in levels of neurotransmitters. Neuronal necrosis may occur secondary to
the accumulation of neurotransmitters. The associated mortality is about
10% and if seizures last for longer than 2 hours there may be
permanent neurological sequelae (O'Brien 1991). Those who have
recurrent episodes of status epilepticus are more prone to develop new
lesions or are more likely to die in any event.

Preoperative abnormalities

1. The interictal EEG usually shows abnormal features, but if the
   epilepsy is mild, the EEG can be normal between fits. If the
   neuronal discharge originates from a medial temporal focus, a
   specialized lead may be required to record an abnormality.

2. The nature of the lesions can now often be determined using MRI.
3. Side effects with anticonvulsants. Most cause enzyme induction and can interfere with the metabolism of other drugs. Patients receiving long-term therapy with phenytoin, phenobarbitone or primidone may develop folate deficiency and megaloblastic anaemia. Sodium valproate may interfere with haemostasis, and excessive bleeding during surgery has been reported (Tetzlaff 1991). Thrombocytopenia is the commonest defect. Its incidence is dose-related and is more common in children than in adults. Platelet dysfunction, prolonged bleeding time and hypofibrinogenaemia have been reported. Phenytoin has a narrow therapeutic range and certain drugs (including sulphonamides, cimetidine and halothane) have been known to precipitate acute phenytoin toxicity which may involve ataxia, nystagmus and respiratory depression.

Anaesthetic problems

1. Poor drug control, or non-compliance by the patient, increases the likelihood of perioperative seizures. A seizure is a highly undesirable event, since it is accompanied by marked systemic changes such as hypertension, tachycardia, respiratory and metabolic acidosis, hypoxia, and hyperthermia. Traumatic injury may occur. At a cellular level, focal increases in metabolism may cause local hypoxia or ischaemia. Rarely, recurrent postoperative fits have been reported; status epilepticus carries significant morbidity and occasionally death occurs.
2. Many anaesthetic drugs have both pro- and anticonvulsant activity. Confusion also exists in the terminology surrounding perioperative excitatory events. It is often difficult to distinguish between seizures resulting from cortical activity, and rigidity and myoclonus.
   a. Methohexitone possesses excitatory activity and is used to provoke focal discharges in epileptics undergoing surgery for focal epilepsy. Several isolated reports of fits have occurred, and in one study of 48 epileptics in whom anticonvulsants had been withheld, five had fits in association with either the induction or cessation of methohexitone (Male & Allen 1977)
   b. Etomidate may produce marked myoclonic movements on induction of anaesthesia. They are reputed not to be associated with epileptiform discharge on EEG. However, in some epileptics, increased epileptiform discharges on EEG have been seen (Opitz et al 1983, Ebrahim et al 1986). Generalized seizures have been reported with etomidate, often when given with fentanyl (Kreiger & Korner 1987). As with methohexitone, etomidate has been used to activate epileptic foci. Both generalized and focal seizures have occurred after etomidate infusions (Grant & Hutchinson 1983), and in rats, myoclonic movements have been accompanied by increases in brain glucose utilization. There is powerful

activation of beta activity on EEG, and recording from scalp electrodes may be obscured. Several authors have suggested that it should be avoided in epilepsy. However, it has been successfully used as an anticonvulsant.

c. Propofol has been associated with a number of central nervous system effects, more than 30 of which have been recorded. These have included convulsions, opisthotonus, myoclonus and prolonged unconsciousness. Prior to October 1989, 101 similar events had been reported to the Committee on Safety of Medicine (Shearer 1990). Nearly one-third of 37 patients who had seizures were epileptics (Committee on Safety of Medicines 1989). In some cases, repeated fits occurred, and in one patient, these continued for 7 days (Bredahl 1990). However, there has been little evidence of cortical epileptiform discharge on EEG. A study of EEGs recorded during propofol-induced dystonic choreiform movements showed that they were coincident with delta waves on EEG. No epileptiform EEG changes were seen and it was suggested that the movements were of subcortical rather than cortical origin (Borgeat et al 1991). In addition, decreased duration of fits during ECT has been documented (Simpson 1988) and propofol has been used for the treatment of status epilepticus.

d. During enflurane anaesthesia, EEG studies have shown that an increase in depth of anaesthesia is accompanied by the appearance of high-voltage spikes and spike waves with burst suppression. A reduction in $Paco_2$ increases the occurrence of these (Neigh et al 1971). Enflurane has been used to activate epileptic foci during surgery for epilepsy. Convulsions have occurred from minutes to several hours, and in one case, several days (Grant 1986), after enflurane anaesthesia. On another occasion, status epilepticus occurred (Nicoll 1986). However, in all cases, enflurane was not the sole agent used and, in most patients, no seizures had occurred previously. Cerebral glucose utilization studies in rats suggested activation of intercortical and corticothalamic pathways (Nakakimura et al 1988). However, in one study when enflurane was given to epileptics, EEG recordings could not demonstrate provocation of epileptic foci (Opitz et al 1977). Inhibition of seizure activity during enflurane anaesthesia has also been reported (Opitz et al 1983).

e. Rigidity and epileptiform or myoclonic movements have been noted after high-dose opioids. Simultaneous cortical EEG recordings have shown no abnormal activity in man, although animal studies have shown accompanying seizure activity on the EEG and activation of subcortical brain metabolism. High-dose pentazocine, used for cardiac surgery, has been associated with seizures. Grand mal convulsions have occurred during induction with fentanyl, but not necessarily at high dosage. In those in which EEG recording was available, no cortical seizure activity was seen. During a study of alfentanil-induced rigidity in 10 patients, the EEG showed no evidence of seizure activity, and a neurochemical mechanism has been suggested (Benthuysen et al 1986). A subsequent study of 127 patients with high-dose opioids produced similar conclusions (Ty Smith et al 1989). Pethidine has been associated with seizures, particularly when used for a long period or in patients with renal failure. Norpethidine, one of the metabolites, was probably responsible.

f. Ketamine, given to both epileptics and non-epileptics, did not show cortical or clinical seizure activity on EEG studies (Corssen et al 1974, Celisia et al 1975). However, ketamine is known to be excitatory to the thalamus and limbic system, in which it produces a seizure pattern which does not extend to the cerebral cortex (Ferrer-Allado et al 1973). Thus cortical electrodes do not reflect seizure activity. Increases in cerebral blood flow and oxygen consumption have been shown, and activation of experimentally induced corticoreticular epilepsy in cats has been reported. However, ketamine also possesses anticonvulsant properties and has been used to treat status epilepticus.

3. Patients on long-term anticonvulsant therapy may have altered responses to anaesthetic drugs. The recovery from atracurium in epileptics on long-term phenytoin, valproic acid and carbamazepine is two to three times shorter than those of non-epileptics (Tempelhoff et al 1990). There can be a similar resistance to metocurine, pancuronium and vecuronium (Bulkey et al 1987) and an increased requirement for fentanyl during craniotomy (Tempelhoff et al 1990a).

4. Anaesthetists may be involved in the management of seizures in the emergency department, but these patients are not necessarily epileptics. Seizures have been reported in association with drug abuse. In one study of emergency hospital admissions, 32 were associated with cocaine, 11 with amphetamine, seven with heroin and four with phencyclidine (Alldredge et al 1989). In 11 patients a combination of drugs was used. The seizures were usually short-lived and there were no neurological sequelae.

Management

1. Evaluation of haemostasis in patients on long-term sodium valproate.
2. Continuation of anticonvulsant medication.
3. The choice of anaesthetic agents must be left to the individual. It might be prudent to avoid those drugs which are particularly implicated in the production of clinical excitatory events or EEG excitation. However, should the use of any of these drugs be

particularly indicated, provided that adequate anticonvulsant therapy is given in the perioperative period, the risk of precipitating seizures must be slight.

4. Treatment of status epilepticus. Prompt control is important.
   a. Remove false teeth, establish an airway and give oxygen.
   b. Benzodiazepines
      i. Diazemuls 0.15–0.25 mg/kg, or 10–20 mg i.v.
      ii. Midazolam can be given either i.m. (acts in 5 minutes) or i.v. (acts in <100 s). It has been shown to be effective in status epilepticus refractory to treatment (Kumar & Bleck 1992). There is rapid entry into the brain and a swift onset of action due to its highly lipophilic nature. However, it has a short duration of action and the elimination half-life is 0.84–5.4 hours. A loading dose of 0.1–0.3 mg/kg followed by an infusion rate of 0.05–0.4 mg/kg per hour was recommended. However, when a long-term infusion is required, EEG monitoring is advisable, since there is great individual variation in requirements. It is possible to arrest clinical seizures, yet leave the patient in nonconvulsive status epilepticus.
   c. Phenytoin may be indicated, particularly for myoclonic convulsions. Give an initial loading dose of 10–15 mg/kg (250 mg/ml slowly i.v. at not more than 50 mg/min or via an infusion pump, or mixed with 0.9% saline 250 ml provided it is used immediately). For refractory convulsions, high-dose phenytoin (up to 30 mg/kg) can be used. This requires ECG monitoring on an ITU because of its effect on cardiac conduction.
   d. Take blood for anticonvulsant drugs levels, alcohol and sugar (5 ml in a fluoride tube) and serum electrolytes, calcium and blood count. Save one sample to screen for other drugs if necessary.
   e. If the patient is hypoglycaemic give 50% glucose 25 ml. Thiamine 100 mg is given if alcohol is thought likely to have been the precipitating factor.
   f. If fits cannot be controlled, the patient must be transferred to an ITU for more specialist treatment. In refractory seizures a number of other drugs have been used. These include propofol, ketamine and isoflurane (Kofke et al 1989).

BIBLIOGRAPHY

Alldredge B K, Lowenstein D H, Simon R P 1989 Seizures associated with recreational drug abuse. Neurology 39: 1037–1039

Benthuysen J L, Ty Smith N, Sanford T J et al 1986 Physiology of alfentanil-induced rigidity. Anesthesioloy 64: 440–446

Borgeat A, Dessibourg C, Popovic V et al 1991 Propofol and spontaneous movements: an EEG study. Anesthesiology 74: 24–27

Bredahl C 1990 Krampeanfald og opitotonus efter propofol anaestesi. (Seizures and opisthotonos after propofol anesthesia A possible connection). Ugeskr Laeger 152: 748–749

Bulkey R, Ebrahim Z, Roth S et al 1987 Resistance to vecuronium in patients receiving carbamazepine. Anesthesiology 67: A345

Celisia C, Chen R, Bamforth B 1975 Effects of ketamine in epilepsy. Neurology 25: 169

Committee on Safety of Medicines 1989 Current problems. No 26. Consumer's Association, London

Christys A R, Moss E, Powell D 1989 Retrospective study of early postoperative convulsions after intracranial surgery with isoflurane and enflurane anaesthesia. British Journal of Anaesthesia 62: 624–627

Corssen G, Little S, Tavakoli M 1974 Ketamine and epilepsy. Anesthesia and Analgesia 53: 319

Ebrahim Z Y, DeBoer G E, Luders H et al 1986 Effect of etomidate on the electroencephalogram of patients with epilepsy. Anesthesia and Analgesia 65: 1004–1006

Ferrer-Allado T, Brechner V L, Dymond A et al 1973 Ketamine-induced electroconvulsive phenomena in the human limbic and thalamic region. Anesthesiology 38: 333–334

Grant I S, Hutchinson G 1983 Epileptiform seizures during prolonged etomidate sedation. Lancet ii: 511–512

Grant I S 1986 Delayed convulsions following enflurane anaesthesia. Anaesthesia 41: 1024–1025

Kofke W A, Young R S K, Davis P et al 1989 Isoflurane for refractory status epilepticus: a clinical series. Anesthesiology 71: 653–659

Kreiger W, Koerner M 1987 Generalized grand mal seizure after recovery from uncomplicated fentanyl-etomidate anesthesia. Anesthesia and Analgesia 66: 284–285

Kumar A, Bleck T P 1992 Intravenous midazolam for the treatment of status epilepticus. Critical Care Medicine 20: 483–488

Male C G, Allen E M 1977 Methohexitone-induced convulsions in epileptics. Anaesthesia and Intensive Care 5: 226–230

Modica P A, Tempelhoff R, White P F 1990 Pro- and anticonvulsant effects of anesthetics (Part I). Anesthesia and Analgesia 70: 303–315

Modica P A, Tempelhoff R, White P F 1990 Pro- and anticonvulsant effects of anesthetics (Part II). Anesthesia and Analgesia 70: 433–444

Nakakimura K, Sakabe T, Funatsu Nm Maekawa T et al 1988 Metabolic activation of intercortical and corticothalamic pathways during enflurane anesthesia in rats. Anesthesiology 68: 777–782

Neigh J L, Garman J K, Harp J R 1971 The electroencephalographic pattern during anesthesia with ethrane; effects of depth of anesthesia, $Paco_2$, and nitrous oxide. Anesthesiology 35: 482–487

Nicoll J M V 1986 Status epilepticus following enflurane anaesthesia. Anaesthesia 41: 927–930

O'Brien M D 1991 Management of status epilepticus in adults. British Medical Journal 301: 918

Opitz A, Brecht S, Stenzel E 1977 Enfluran-Anestheseien bei epilptikem (Enflurane anaesthesia for epileptic patients.) Anesthetist 26: 329–332

Opitz A, Marschall M, Degen R et al 1983 General anaesthesia in patients with epilepsy and status epileticus. Advances in Neurology 34: 531–535

Paech M J, Storey J M 1990 Propofol and seizures. Anaesthesia and Intensive Care 18: 585

Shearer E S 1990 Convulsions and propofol. Anaesthesia 45: 255–256

Simpson K H, Halsall P J, Carr C M E, et al 1988 Propofol reduces seizure duration in patients having anaesthesia for electroconvulsive therapy. British Journal of Anaesthesia 61: 343–344

Tempelhoff R, Modica P A, Jellish W S et al 1990a Resistance to atracurium-induced neuromuscular blockade in patients with intractable seizure disorders treated with anticonvulsants. Anesthesia and Analgesia 71: 665–669

Tempelhoff R, Modica P A, Spitznagel E L 1990b Anticonvulsant therapy increases fentanyl requirements during anaesthesia for craniotomy. Canadian Journal of Anaesthesia 37: 327–332

Tetzlaff J E 1991 Intraoperative defect of haemostasis in a child receiving valproic acid. Canadian Journal of Anaesthesia 38: 222–224

Section 1

Epilepsy

Ty Smith N, Benthuysen J L Bickford R G et al 1989 Seizures during opioid induction – are they opioid-induced rigidiy? Anesthesiology 71: 852–862

FALLOT'S TETRALOGY

A congenital cardiac abnormality. The primary defects are pulmonary infundibular stenosis and a VSD. The VSD is sufficiently large for the pressure in both ventricles to be equal to that of the aorta. The tetralogy is completed by two secondary features – a variable degree of over-riding of the aorta, and right ventricular hypertrophy. Dynamic right ventricular outflow obstruction may occur (infundibular spasm), which is increased by sympathetic stimulation. The fraction of the right-to-left shunt depends primarily upon the relative resistances between the pulmonary (or right venticular) and systemic outflows.

Preoperative abnormalities

1. Dyspnoea may occur on exertion and is hypoxia-related. Cyanosis and finger clubbing are variable, depending on the degree of pulmonary stenosis and the size of the shunt. Polycythaemia is common. There is a pulmonary stenotic murmur, but no murmur from the VSD because of the size of the defect. Squatting is thought to reduce the fraction of the shunt by kinking the large arteries and so increasing the systemic vascular resistance. This is commonly seen in children.
2. ECG shows right atrial and right ventricular hypertrophy, right axis deviation and right bundle branch block.
3. CXR shows right ventricular hypertrophy and oligaemic lungs. In the 2.6–6% of cases which also have an absent pulmonary valve, aneurysmal dilatation of the pulmonary arteries may cause bronchial compression.
4. Initial surgery may have been undertaken to anastomose a systemic to a pulmonary artery, to improve the pulmonary blood flow and reduce cyanosis.
5. There is an increased risk of bacterial endocarditis, emboli, cerebral abscess, syncope and cyanotic attacks.

Anaesthetic problems

1. The right-to-left shunt, and hence the cyanosis, is increased by a decrease in systemic vascular resistance produced by peripheral vasodilatation. This may be caused by factors such as hypovolaemia, drugs or pyrexia.
2. Cyanosis is also made worse by an increase in pulmonary vascular resistance, or spasm of the right ventricular infundibulum. Right ventricular outflow obstruction is produced by increases in

catecholamine output, or the administration of drugs with positive inotropic effects. Anxiety, pain, hypercarbia, hypoxia and acidosis are all precipitating factors. These cyanotic attacks or 'tet' spells, which can occur when awake or under anaesthesia, may initiate a cycle of increasing hypoxia which can result in cerebral damage or death. Direct intraoperative observations of shunt direction and flow have been made with Doppler colour flow imaging using epicardial leads (Greeley et al 1989). These, in an infant and child prior to surgery, have confirmed that intracardiac right-to-left shunting is responsible for the sudden onset of cyanosis and that this is corrected as soon as the shunt is reversed by treatment. Four patients with severe life-threatening hypoxaemic spells, refractory to other treatment, responded to phenylephrine (5 μg/kg plus an infusion 0.4-2 μg/kg per min).

3. Dehydration in the presence of polycythaemia and raised plasma viscosity increases the incidence of cerebral thrombosis. Polycythaemia may be associated with coagulation defects.

4. In those patients with an absent pulmonary valve, there has been positional airway compromise secondary to bronchial compression of dilated pulmonary arteries (Hosking & Beynen 1989)

Management

1. Antibiotic cover as prophylaxis against bacterial endocarditis when appropriate.

2. A good premedication to prevent excitement and anxiety.

3. Measures aimed at reducing the right-to-left shunt. Specific treatment of cyanotic attacks include;
   a. 100% oxygen to decrease PVR.
   b. Pressor agents such as phenylephrine to increase systemic vascular resistance (Shaddy et al 1989), or fluids to correct hypovolaemia.
   c. Propranolol to decrease outflow tract obstruction. Used i.v. it was successful for an attack occurring during cardiac catheterization under local anaesthesia (Kam 1978).
   d. Deepening of light anaesthesia to reduce tachycardias associated with catecholamine output (Greeley et al 1989).
   e. Compression of the abdominal aorta. In four infants the aorta was compressed against the lumbar vertebrae sufficiently firmly to stop the femoral artery pulsations. This dramatically and immediately improved the arterial oxygen saturation (Baele et al 1991).

4. Techniques should avoid hypoxia and hypercarbia, and minimize vasodilatation and sudden increases in cardiac output. Ketamine or fentanyl with or without N_2O has been used (Shaddy et al 1989).

5. Hydration is maintained in the perioperative period and, if there is severe polycythaemia, venesection may be necessary.

6. Metabolic acidosis should be prevented or treated.

BIBLIOGRAPHY
Baele P L, Rennotte M-T E, Veyckemans F A 1991 External compression of the
    abdominal aorta reversing tetralogy of Fallot cyanotic crisis. Anesthesiology 75:
    146–149
Greeley W J, Stanley T E, Ungerleider R M et al 1989 Intraoperative hypoxemic spells
    in Tetralogy of Fallot. An echocardiographic analysis of diagnosis and treatment.
    Anesthesia and Analgesia 68: 815–89
Hosking M P, Beynen F 1989 Anesthetic management of tetralogy of Fallot with
    absent pulmonary valve. Anesthesiolog 70: 863–865
Kam C A 1978 Infundibular spasm in Fallot's tetralogy. Anaesthesia and Intensive
    Care 6: 138–140
Shaddy R E, Viney J, Judd V E et al 1989 Continuous intravenous phenylephrine
    infusion for treatment of hypoxemic spells in tetralogy of Fallot. Journal of
    Pediatrics 114: 468–470

FAMILIAL DYSAUTONOMIA
(RILEY–DAY SYNDROME)

A rare autosomal recessive neurological disease associated with
gastrointestinal dysfunction, presenting from birth and usually occurring
in Jewish children. Although most of the nervous system is involved, the
autonomic and peripheral neuronal elements are of particular concern to
the anaesthetist. A decrease in sympathetic, parasympathetic and sensory
neurones, a decrease in synthesis of noradrenaline (but with a normal
adrenal medulla) and a sensitivity to exogenous catecholamines, have
been shown. Emotional lability is common but the IQ is normal. Patients
may present for fundoplication, gastrostomy or orthopaedic procedures.

Preoperative abnormalities

1. There is a decreased sensitivity to pain and temperature, muscle
   hypotonia, incoordination and reduced tendon reflexes. Kyphosis,
   scoliosis or a combination of both are common, presumably due to
   inadequate muscle tone and impaired muscle proprioception.
2. Features include autonomic dysfunction with postural hypotension
   and lability of blood pressure, increased vagal reflexes, swallowing
   difficulties with excess salivation, gastric reflux, reduced
   gastrointestinal mobility, absent sweating and impaired temperature
   control.
3. Dysautonomic and emotional crises may be precipitated by stress and
   can be associated with elevated plasma noradrenaline and dopamine
   levels. During these there may be nausea, vomiting, hypertension,
   tachycardia, sweating and the appearance of erythematous skin
   lesions.
4. Crowded teeth, malocclusion and a smooth tongue are characteristic.
5. Respiratory symptoms are common. In a study of 65 patients
   undergoing fundoplication and gastrostomy, 55% had severe lung
   disease with increased markings or atelectasis before operation
   (Axelrod et al 1991). Only nine had clear CXRs.

Anaesthetic problems

1. Emotion and fear may precipitate a dysautonomic crisis.
2. Disorders of swallowing constitute major problem. Gastro-oesophageal reflux occurs in 95% of patients and disturbances of oropharyngeal function result in misdirected swallows with aspiration (Axelrod et al 1991). The development of lung disease secondary to recurrent pulmonary aspiration is a common feature.
3. Dysphagia for fluids results in chronic dehydration.
4. Respiratory responses to hypercarbia and hypoxia are impaired.
5. Autonomic nervous system dysfunction, apparently secondary to reduced endogenous catecholamine release, means that the patient is unable to respond to hypovolaemia and to drugs causing myocardial depression (Meridy & Creighton 1971, Foster 1983). Several cases in which either cardiac arrest or severe hypotension occurred during general anaesthesia have been reported (Kritchman et al 1959, Axelrod et al 1988).
6. Successful control of intraoperative hypotension has been obtained with both adrenaline and dopamine infusions (Stenqvist & Sigurdsson 1982). However, exaggerated responses to noradrenaline have occurred and therefore any catecholamines should be administered with caution.
7. The use of atropine is controversial. Reports exist of sensitivity to anticholinergic agents and, conversely, of pronounced reactions to vagal stimulation. Both its cautious use and its avoidance have been proposed.
8. Profound vomiting may occur in the perioperative period.
9. Temperature variations can take place.
10. Major problems have occurred in the postoperative period (Meridy & Creighton 1971, Axelrod et al 1988, 1991, Albanese & Bobechko 1987). Complications have included fever, pulmonary atelectasis or infection, aspiration, cardiovascular instability and vomiting crises. An analysis of 127 procedures in 81 patients was reported (Axelrod et al 1988). A high incidence of postoperative atelectasis after gastric surgery prompted a policy of elective artificial ventilation.

Management

1. Fundoplication with gastrostomy has been shown to improve nutrition and decrease respiratory problems (Axelrod et al 1991). The patients require careful perioperative management. Intravenous fluid therapy should be started before surgery to prevent dehydration, and anxiety treated. Diazepam is effective in controlling dysautonomic crises. Cimetidine reduces gastric secretions. Premedication with both drugs has been suggested (Axelrod et al 1988) but opiates and anticholinergics should be avoided.

2. To reduce the cardiovascular changes associated with the use of volatile agents, a moderate-dose fentanyl technique was used for major surgery in six patients (Beilin et al 1985).
3. Monitoring of arterial pressure and temperature should preferably be started before induction of anaesthesia. Vascular access is facilitated by the relative sensory deficit.
4. The uneventful use of both depolarizing and non-depolarizing neuromuscular blockers has been reported. However, the presence of hypotonia reduces their requirements, and residual neuromuscular blockade may necessitate IPPV in the postoperative period.
5. Blood and fluid loss must be replaced promptly.
6. A dopamine or an adrenaline infusion may be needed if problems occur with intraoperative hypotension. Catecholamines must be given with care, since sensitivity to their effects has been reported. Close monitoring is required, so that the blood pressure is increased, but an unacceptable tachycardia prevented.
7. IPPV is required, even for short cases, because of the impaired response to hypoxia and hypercarbia.
8. The use of local or regional techniques should be considered. Caesarean section for fetal growth retardation under local anaesthetic has been described (Leiberman et al 1991).
9. Postoperative analgesia is required for abdominal surgery. It has been suggested that in these cases, IPPV should be continued postoperatively until analgesics are no longer required (Axelrod et al 1988).
10. Vomiting crises should be treated vith gastric decompression, diazepam and cimetidine.

BIBLIOGRAPHY

Albanese S A, Bobechko W P 1987 Spine deformity in familial dysautonomia (Riley Day syndrome). Journal of Pediatric Orthopedics 7: 179–183
Axelrod F B, Donenfeld R F, Danziger F et al 1988 Anesthesia in familial dysautonomia. Anesthesiology 68: 631–635
Axelrod F B, Gouge T H, Ginsburg H B et al 1991 Fundoplication and gastrostomy in familial dysautonomia. Journal of Pediatrics 118: 388–394
Beilin B, Maayan C H, Vatashsky E et al 1985 Fentanyl anesthesia in familial dysautonomia. Anesthesia and Analgesia 64: 72–76
Foster J M G 1983 Anaesthesia for a patient with familial dysautonomia. Anaesthesia 38: 391
Kritchman M M, Schwartz H, Papper E M 1959 Experiences with general anesthesia in patients with familial dysautonomia. Journal of the American Medical Association 170: 529–533
Leiberman J R, Cohen A, Wiznitzer A et al 1991 Cesarean section by local anesthesia in patients with familial dysautonomia. American Journal of Obstetrics and Gynecology 165: 110–111
Meridy H W, Creighton R E 1971 General anaesthesia in eight patients with familial dysautonomia. Canadian Anaesthetists' Society Journal 18: 563–570

Stenqvist O, Sigurdsson J 1982 The anaesthetic management of a patient with familial dysautonomia. Anaesthesia 37: 929–932

FAMILIAL PERIODIC PARALYSES

1. Hypokalaemic periodic paralysis.
2. Hyperkalaemic periodic paralysis and paramyotonia.

There are two principal types, hypokalaemic and hyperkalaemic, both of which are autosomal dominant. In both conditions, affected individuals develop muscle weakness in association with changes in the serum potassium levels. It has been observed for some time that there is a close relationship between the clinical and electrophysiological features of hyperkalaemic periodic paralysis and paramyotonia. Some families show features of both conditions and they may in fact be allelic disorders. There appears to be genetic linkage between both hyperkalaemic periodic paralysis and paramyotonia and the gene encoding the skeletal muscle sodium channel on chromosome 17. In view of this, both conditions will be considered together.

HYPOKALAEMIC PERIODIC PARALYSIS (HypoPP)

A rare disease which usually starts in teenagers. Episodes of flaccid paralysis are precipitated by stress, cold, trauma, surgery, infections and high-carbohydrate meals. Attacks may last from several hours to 2 days. Certain muscle groups are likely to be involved more than others. It is associated with hypokalaemia but the exact mechanism for its periodic nature and its skeletal and cardiac effects is not known. Increased potassium excretion from the body is not involved. There does however seem to be an increased uptake of potassium by the cells. The cell membrane potential has been found to be reduced during attacks, making the muscle inexcitable. Insulin and glucose, steroids, thyroxine and beta stimulation can all increase cellular potassium uptake and intensify an existing hypokalaemia

Preoperative abnormalities

1. Attacks of paralysis are most likely to involve the arms, legs, trunk and neck, but usually in an asymmetric manner. Proximal muscles are mainly affected. Death may occasionally occur during an attack, secondary to respiratory failure or aspiration. Fortunately, however, the diaphragm and cranial muscles are not usually involved. The patients are more sensitive than normal to a reduction in serum potassium, such that muscle weakness may start at a level of 3 mmol/l and may become profound when <2.5 mmol/l (Ellis 1980).
2. Patients are usually taking oral potassium. Symptoms may be improved by acetazolamide. This probably acts by producing a

metabolic acidosis, thus reducing potassium uptake by the cells. Spironolactone can be used prophylactically.

3. Hypokalaemia, which can be as low as 1.6 mmol/l, may be accompanied by ECG changes such as T-wave flattening, U waves, arrhythmias, and bradycardias.
4. During an attack, the EMG shows action potential lengthening, progressing into electrical silence.
5. Thyrotoxic periodic paralysis may produce a similar picture (Fozard 1983, Robson 1985).

Anaesthetic problems

1. Attacks of paralysis can be precipitated by administration of glucose and insulin, sodium bicarbonate, diuretics, a heavy carbohydrate meal, undue stress, hypothermia, or a salt load.
2. Although patients with spontaneous attacks rarely require respiratory support, this is not always so in the postoperative period. Most case reports have shown uneventful intraoperative courses with a wide range of anaesthetic techniques employed. However, the incidence of postoperative paralysis, often developing some hours later, is about 25%. Most of these episodes have been associated with hypokalaemia (Siler & Discavage 1975, Rollman et al 1985, Lema et al 1991).
3. Occasionally the patient may be undiagnosed before surgery or he may fail to inform the medical staff. A young man developed weakness in his arms and legs in the recovery room following eye surgery (Melnick et al 1983). A family history was subsequently elicited and a serum potassium level of 3.1 mmol/l was treated with potassium infusion. The weakness had improved by the following day.
4. Hypokalaemia during surgery may be accompanied by ECG changes which are out of proportion to the measured serum potassium level.
5. The effect of muscle relaxants may be difficult to distinguish from the paralysis itself. One family had a total of 21 anaesthetics. The three patients who received neuromuscular blockers were the only ones who developed postoperative paralyses (Horton 1977).

Management

1. Stress and anxiety should be reduced by using adequate premedication. Treatment with beta adrenoceptor blockers has been reported, but only during anaesthesia.
2. Core temperature should be monitored and the theatre warmed. Precautions should be taken against heat loss during prolonged surgery.
3. ECG should be closely observed throughout the operation for the changes of hypokalaemia.

Section 1

**Familial Periodic
Paralyses**
Hypokalaemic Periodic
Paralysis (HypoPP)
Hyperkalaemic
Periodic Paralysis and
Paramyotonia (HyperPP)

4. Glucose infusions should be minimized and large sodium loads, pariticularly bicarbonate, avoided. Serum potassium levels must be monitored and hypokalaemia treated.
5. Muscle relaxants may not be required. If they are necessary, small increments can be given and the effects assessed with a nerve stimulator. The problems of distinguishing the effects of the drugs from those of the disease itself may be reduced by stimulating the facial nerve which supplies only rarely affected muscles. However, even this may be unreliable. Atracurium has been used without complication in a patient with periodic paralysis and a cardiomyopathy (Rooney et al 1988).
6. The patient's ventilation, and his serum potassium level, should be closely monitored postoperatively in an intensive care unit.

BIBLIOGRAPHY
Ellis F R 1980 Inherited muscle disease. British Journal of Anaesthesia 52: 153–164
Fozard J R 1983 Anaesthesia and familial hypokalaemic periodic paralysis. Anaesthesia 38: 293–294
Horton B 1977 Anesthetic experiences in a family with hypokalemic periodic paralysis Anesthesiology 47: 308–310
Lema G, Urzua J, Moran S et al 1991 Successful anesthetic management of a patient with hypokalemic familial periodic paralysis undergoing cardiac surgery. Anesthesiology 74: 373–375
Melnick B, Chang J-L, Larson C E et al 1983 Hypokalemic familial periodic paralysis. Anesthesiology 58: 263–265
Robson N J 1985 Emergency surgery complicated by thyrotoxicosis and thyrotoxic periodic paralysis. Anaesthesia 40: 27–31
Rollman J E, Dickson C M 1985 Anesthetic management of a patient with hypokalemic periodic paralysis for coronary bypass surgery. Anesthesiology 63: 526–527
Rooney R, Shanahan E, Sun T et al 1988 Atracurium and hypokalemic familial paralysis. Anesthesia and Analgesia 67: 782–783
Siler J N, Discavage W J 1975 Anesthetic management of hypokalemic periodic paralysis. Anesthesiology 43: 489–490

HYPERKALAEMIC PERIODIC PARALYSIS AND PARAMYOTONIA (HyperPP)

A similar, but separate, inherited disease of which three clinical variants are recognized: HyperPP with myotonia, HyperPP without myotonia and HyperPP with paramyotonia, which is cold-induced and worse on exercise. The serum potassium levels may increase by 20% during an attack, and paralysis may occur with levels no greater than 4 mmol/l. Changes in membrane potential and release of potassium from muscle have both been demonstrated. Administration of potassium can precipitate an attack although the serum potassium may remain normal. Changes in serum potassium alone cannot account for the problem. An abnormality of sodium channel function causing spontaneous depolarization has been proposed and genetic studies suggest that mutations in the gene encoding the skeletal rnuscle sodium channel are responsible.

Section 1

Familial Periodic Paralyses
Hypokalaemic Periodic Paralysis (HypoPP)
Hyperkalaemic Periodic Paralysis and Paramyotonia (HyperPP)

In a study of muscle taken from patients with periodic paralyses, several were found to have equivocal results from the contracture tests for malignant hyperthermia (Lehmann-Hom & Iaizzo 1990). No suggestion was made that these patients were susceptible to MH but, rather, that the tests lacked specificity. The significance of this is not known.

Preoperative abnormalities

1. Attacks of paralysis usually last for less than 2 hours. They are shorter than in the hypokalaemic form, and may be precipitated by hunger, cold and exercise. Mild paralysis may occur with a serum potassium >4 mmol/l and may become severe when >7 mmol/l (Ellis 1980).
2. The distribution of paralysis is similar, but the facial and tongue muscles may be involved. Percussion myotonia may be marked in an attack which can be precipitated by giving an oral potassium load and reversed with i.v. calcium gluconate.
3. EMG shows increased spontaneous activity and myotonic discharges. In paramyotonia these changes are augmented by cold.
4. ECG may show peaking of the T-waves, even prior to the episode of paralysis.
5. The serum CK level may be increased and muscle biopsy often shows nonspecific myopathic changes.
6. Symptomatic treatment includes diuretics, and antiarrhythmic drugs such as procainamide (which affects sodium influx during depolarization) and mexilitene.

Anaesthetic problems

1. Anaesthesia may precipitate paralysis, which can continue for some hours into the postoperative period (Egan & Klein 1959, Streib 1989). Although the avoidance of non-depolarizing neuromuscular blockers has been suggested, there have been several cases in which they have been used without problems (Aarons et al 1989, Ashwood et al 1992).
2. Jaw rigidity following suxamethonium, with subsequent global weakness, has been reported in two patients with HyperPP with paramyotonia (Ashwood et al 1992). However, there is no evidence of an association between malignant hyperthermia and HyperPP (Lehmann-Hom & Iaizzo 1990).
3. In paramyotonia, cold may trigger myotonia and weakness. However, successful hypothermic cardiopulmonary bypass for cardiac surgery, and subsequent rewarming, has been described (Reece et al 1983).
4. Extradural anaesthesia in a patient with paramyotonia and lupus anticoagulant has been described (Howell & Douglas 1992).

Management

1. Dextrose should be infused during the period of fasting before anaesthesia to supply carbohydrate.
2. Thiazide diuretics used prophylactically before operation will deplete body potassium. Hyperkalaemia occurring during surgery will respond to calcium gluconate or dextrose and insulin, which act by moving potassium back into the cells.
3. Warmed, sodium-containing, potassium-free, intravenous fluids should be used.
4. As with the hypokalaemic form, monitoring of serum potassium, ECG and neuromuscular function, is essential.
5. Core temperature should be monitored and attention should be paid to the maintenance of normothermia. The use of a heat and moisture exchanger, heat retaining fabrics, and a warming blanket is indicated.
6. Suxamethonium should be avoided, but non-depolarizing blockers may be used provided monitoring takes place.
7. The possible need for postoperative IPPV should be anticipated.

BIBLIOGRAPHY
Aarons J J, Moon R E, Camporesi E M, 1989 General anesthesia and hyperkalemic periodic paralysis. Anesthesiology 71: 303–304
Ashwood E M, Russell W J, Burrow D D 1992 Hyperkalaemic periodic paralysis and anaesthesia. Anaesthesia 47: 579–584
Ellis F R 1980 Inherited muscle disease. British Journal of Anaesthesia 52: 153–164
Egan T J, Klein R 1959 Hyperkalemic periodic paralysis. Pediatrics 24: 761–773
Howell P R, Douglas M J 1992 Lupus anticoagulant, paramyotonia congenita and pregnancy Canadian Journal of Anaesthesia 39: 992–996
Lehmann-Horn F, Iaizzo P A 1990 Are myotonias and periodic paralyses associated with susceptibility to malignant hyperthermia. British Journal of Anaesthesia 65: 692–697
Reece I J, Kennedy J A, Simpson J A, et al; 1983 Hypothermic cardiopulmonary bypass in paramyotonia congenita: a case report. Thorax 38: 476–477
Ricker K, Camacho L M, Grafe P et al 1989 Adynamia episodica hereditaria. What causes the weakness? Muscle and Nerve 12: 883–891
Streib E W 1989 Hypokalemic periodic paralysis in two patients with paramyotonia congenita and known hyperkalemic/exercise-induced weakness. Muscle and Nerve 12: 936–937

FAT EMBOLISM SYNDROME

Fat embolism refers to the presence of fat globules in the lung and peripheral circulation after trauma, most commonly involving fracture of the long bones (Levy 1990). The fat embolism syndrome (FES) occurs when fat emboli produce serious clinical manifestations. Main clinical features involve the lungs, the brain, and the skin. Emboli to the pulmonary capillaries are of particular clinical significance. Local endothelial damage and small vessel obstruction occur, probably due to a combination of interactions between marrow fat, free fatty acids and platelets (Gossling & Donohue 1979). The resulting increase in capillary permeability produces ventilation perfusion abnormalities and hypoxaemia. Whilst fat emboli probably occur in the pulmonary vessels in the majority of cases of long bone fracture, only a small proportion develop the classical syndrome. FES has also been reported during or after joint replacement (Green 1992) and bone marrow transplantation. In experimental animals, products of arachidonic acid metabolism, such as prostaglandins and thromboxane, are released during cemented arthroplasty and may be responsible for the haemodynamic and respiratory changes (Byrick et al 1991).

A prospective study of long bone or pelvic fractures suggested that fat embolism occurs in at least 11% of these patients and may carry a mortality of 10% (Fabian et al 1990). Pulmonary shunting is an early feature, followed by mental changes, confusion and lethargy. The authors selected a P(A–a) for O_2 of >100 mmHg as indicative of a pulmonary shunt, and this usually occurred within 24–48 hours. Laboratory tests show that changes associated with coagulopathy (decreasing Hct, thrombocytopenia and hypofibrinogenaemia) begin at the same time, or soon after, the shunt. The petechial rash appears relatively late.

Presenting problems

1. Signs and symptoms may occur immediately following injury but are often delayed for up to 48 hours.
2. Alveolar-arterial differences in oxygen (>100 mmHg) occur early, although other causes of lung injury must be excluded. An interstitial pneumonitis may present with tachycardia, dyspnoea, pyrexia, cyanosis, and frothy sputum. CXR may show bilateral pulmonary infiltrates. Florid pulmonary oedema has been reported (Hagley 1983). Respiratory failure may ensue. ECG may suggest right ventricular strain.
3. Neurological signs include an altered conscious level with confusion and restlessness, which are usually signs of cerebral hypoxia. Coma may follow (Jacobson et al 1986), occasionally without pulmonary signs. Neurological complications are frequently a cause of long-term morbidity.
4. A petechial rash, particularly over the non-dependent parts (skin folds of the upper half of the body, the conjunctivae and mucous membranes of the mouth) appears in 50–60% of cases, usually within the first 36 hours. This often occurs later than the pulmonary changes. The rash is diagnostic of the syndrome. The retina may show exudates and haemorrhages, and sometimes fat droplets can be seen in the retinal vessels.
5. A decrease in haemoglobin, hypoxaemia, acidosis and thrombocytopenia can all occur. Three fatal cases were reported in

which disseminated intravascular coagulation was a prominent feature (Hagley 1983).

6. In severe cases the mortality may range from 10–45%. Pulmonary involvement is the predominant cause of death.

Diagnosis

1. Initially, diagnosis is made on clinical grounds by the occurrence of some or all of the features appearing within 48 hours of a long bone fracture. The femoral shaft or neck, the pelvis and the tibia, are the bones most commonly involved. Rarely, fatal fat embolism has been reported during total hip replacement (Green 1992) and at closed manipulation of the hip (Van Miert et al 1991).
2. Increases in the alveolar-arterial oxygen pressure difference exceeding 100 mmHg, in the absence of other causes of lung damage. This may be accompanied by early changes suggestive of a coagulopathy.
3. Examination of the sputum and urine may show fat globules. If the patient is sufficiently cooperative during ophthalmic examination, fat may also be seen in the retinal vessels, together with exudates and haemorrhages.
4. The use of bronchoalveolar lavage has been recommended.
5. Pulmonary microvascular cytology has been used to analyze samples of capillary blood in a case of fat embolism (Castella et al 1992).
6. In a study of 42 patients following severe musculoskeletal injuries, levels of serum un-ionized calcium were significantly lower in the eight who developed the fat embolism syndrome than in those who did not (Henderson et al 1992).

Management

1. The patients who should be monitored closely and given supportive treatment in the acute phase are those with early unexplained pulmonary shunt in the absence of pulmonary injury. Respiratory management is of prime importance, since death is most commonly secondary to respiratory complications. Continual assessment of the clinical situation, including blood gases, is essential. Hypoxaemia should be initially treated with oxygen and, if necessary, with CPAP or IPPV and PEEP.
2. Early stabilization of fractures.
3. Several drugs have been suggested as specific treatment for fat embolism, but there is little objective evidence to support their use. The information on the use of corticosteroids is conflicting. Experimental evidence suggests that steroids do not influence the cardiovascular and respiratory changes (Byrick et al 1991). However, a series of 64 high-risk patients with isolated long bone injuries, but with no other injuries which might predispose to ARDS, were

studied (Schonfeld et al 1983). Methylprednisolone 7.5 mg/kg, 6-hourly for 12 doses, was given to 21 patients. None developed the fat embolism syndrome, whereas in the placebo group 9 out of the 41 did. Six cases were severe and three were mild. In another study of 55 adults with long bone fractures, in which methylprednisolone 30 mg/kg was given on admission and as a single further dose at 4 hours, a significant reduction in incidence of the FES as defined by oxygen saturations was found in the trial group (Lindeque et al 1987).

4. Cardiovascular support may be required. Crystalloid transfusion should be minimized and volume should be maintained using colloid.

BIBLIOGRAPHY

Byrick R J, Mullen J B, Wong P Y et al 1991 Prostanoid production and pulmonary hypertension after fat embolism are not modified by methylprednisolone. Canadian Journal of Anaesthesia 38: 660–667

Castella X, Valles J, Cabezuela M A et al 1992 Fat embolism syndrome and pulmonary microvascular cytology. Chest 101: 1710–1712

Chastre F, Fagon J-Y, Soler P et al 1990 Bronchoalveolar lavage for rapid diagnosis of fat embolism syndrome in trauma patients. Annals of Internal Medicine 113: 583–588.

Fabian T C, Hoots A V, Stanford D S et al 1990 Fat embolism syndrome: prospective evaluation in fractures. Critical Care Medicine 18: 42–46

Gossling H R, Donohue T A 1979 The fat embolism syndrome. Journal of the American Medical Association 241: 2740–2742

Gossling H R, Pellegrini V D 1982 Fat embolism syndrome. Clinical Orthopaedics and Related Research 165: 68–82

Green C P 1992 Fatal intra-operative fat embolism. Anaesthesia 47: 168

Hagley S R 1983 Fulminant fat embolism. Anaesthesia and Intensive Care 11: 162–166

Henderson S A, Graham H K, Mollan R A 1992 Serum and other calcium fractions in patients after severe musculoskeletal trauma. Clinical Orthopaedics and Related Research 275: 306–311

Jacobson D M, Terrence C F, Reinmuth O M 1986 The neurologic manifestations of fat embolism. Neurology 36: 847–851

Levy D 1990 The fat embolism syndrome. Clinical Orthopaedics and Related Research 261: 281–286

Lindeque B G P, Schoeman H S, Dommisse G F et al 1987 Fat embolism and the fat embolism syndrome A double-blind therapeutic study. Journal of Bone and Joint Surgery 69-B: 128–131

Schonfeld S A, Ploysongsang Y, DiLisio R et al 1983 Fat embolism prophylaxis with corticosteroids. A prospective study in high-risk patients. Annals of Internal Medicine 99: 438–443

Van Besouw J-P, Hinds C J 1989 Fat embolism syndrome. British Journal of Hospital Medicine 42: 304–311

Van Miert M, Thornington R E, Van Velzen D 1991 Cardiac arrest after massive acute fat embolism. British Medical Journal 303: 396–397

FIBRODYSPLASIA (MYOSITIS) OSSIFICANS PROGRESSIVA

A disorder of connective tissue in which there is progressive heterotopic bone formation involving axial muscles, joints, tendon and ligaments.

These changes are superimposed on a variety of congenital skeletal abnormalities which particularly affect the spine and jaw. A picture similar to that seen in ankylosing spondylitis develops, and the phrase 'stone man' has been used to describe these patients. Death commonly occurs in the third or fourth decade secondary to pneumonia. Surgery is usually required for skeletal problems, including trismus. About 600 cases have been reported in the literature and, since pregnancy is rare, new cases usually arise from fresh mutations.

Preoperative abnormalities

1. The condition usually presents with a swelling in the neck at 3 or 4 years of age. Further localized swellings form in the muscles of the neck and back over the succeeding weeks. They eventually become ossified and may ulcerate, discharging a chalky material.
2. Neck movement becomes limited, and sometimes cervical fusion occurs (Connor & Smith 1982).
3. There are characteristic abnormalities of the skeleton of the feet; a short big toe with single phalanx, sometimes with valgus deformity. Less commonly the hands may have an incurving fifth digit and short first metacarpal.
4. Trismus and jaw problems develop as a result of bony bridges forming between the mandible and the zygoma.
5. Eventually the patient develops a rigid spine and kyphoscoliosis, with ankylosis of the costovertebral and temporomandibular joints. The resulting clinical picture is similar to that seen in ankylosing spondylitis.
6. Ectopic bone formation may be precipitated by trauma.
7. Restrictive lung disease. In a study of 21 patients, the chest expansion was 1–3 cm (mean 1.4 cm), FEV_1 27–64% (mean 45%) and mean FVC 40% of normal (Connor et al 1981). By the age of 15 years there is severe limitation of chest expansion but chronic respiratory failure and cor pulmonale are not evident, probably because diaphragmatic function is adequate for the restricted mobility permitted by the disease. However, patients are prone to recurrent chest infections and death from pneumonia is common.
8. CT scan in the early stages shows that soft tissue swelling occurs before ectopic ossification. The ossification becomes evident on tomography before it can be seen on plain X-ray (Reinig et al 1986).
9. Some patients show ECG changes of RBBB or T-wave inversion in the inferior leads but there is no evidence of cardiac failure.
10. Treatment consists of calcitonin, steroids, disodium etidronate and warfarin.

Anaesthetic problems

1. Difficult intubation

   a. Limited mouth opening as a result of bony bridges between the coronoid process of mandible and the zygoma. Trismus cannot be overcome by neuromuscular blockers.
   b. Restricted neck movement secondary to soft tissue ossification in the neck, narrowing of AP diameter (hypoplasia) of vertebral bodies and fusion of posterior elements. There has been one report of atlantoaxial subluxation.

2. The presence of restrictive lung disease means that patients are prone to chest infection and pneumonia.
3. Areas of local trauma frequently form a focus for ectopic calcification. This may occur at the site of biopsies, tracheostomy and i.m or i.v. injections. Nineteen out of 20 operations for ectopic calcification in 10 patients resulted in recurrence at the site of surgery (Connor & Evans 1982).
4. Problems of positioning patients with joint contractures.
5. Pregnancy has been reported (Thornton et al 1987), but is rare. The patient had cervical and temporomandibular ankylosis, joint contractures and an inability to abduct her hips. Caesarean section was carried out under local anaesthesia with lignocaine.

Management

1. Assessment of respiratory function, treatment for, or prophylaxis against lung infection.
2. Airway assessment and management. Awake fibreoptic intubation may be required if there is trismus or neck fixation (Newton et al 1990). Otherwise, neuromuscular blockers should not be given until it can be ascertained that tracheal intubation is possible (Stark et al 1990). Tracheostomy should only be undertaken after careful consideration because of the risk of ectopic calcification. Ketamine infusions have been used for short procedures in order to avoid intubation in patients with trismus and partial fixation of the cervical vertebrae (Shipton et al 1985, Lininger et al 1989).
3. Careful positioning and padding of joints involved in contractures.

BIBLIOGRAPHY
Connor J M, Evans C C, Evans D A P 1981 Cardiopulmonary function in fibrodysplasia ossificans progressiva. Thorax 36: 419–423
Connor J M, Evans D A P 1982 Fibrodysplasia ossificans progressiva: the clinical features and natural history of 34 patients. Journal of Bone and Joint Surgery 64B: 76–83
Connor J M, Smith R 1982 The cervical spine in fibrodysplasia ossificans progressiva. British Journal of Radiology 55: 492–496
Lininger T E, Brown E M, Brown M 1989 General anesthesia and fibrodysplasia ossificans progressiva. Anesthesia and Analgesia 68: 175–176
Newton M C, Allen P W, Ryan D C 1990 Fibrodysplasia ossificans progressiva. British Journal of Anaesthesia 64: 246–250
Reinig J W, Hill S C, Fang M et al 1986 Fibrodysplasia ossificans progressiva: CT appearance. Radiology 159: 153–157
Shipton E A, Retief L W, Theron H DuT et al 1985 Anaesthesia in myositis ossificans

progressiva. A case report and clinical review. South African Medical Journal 67: 26–28

Stark W H, Krechel S W, Eggers G W N 1990 Anesthesia in 'stone man': myositis ossificans progressiva. Journal of Clinical Anesthesia 2: 332–335

Thornton Y S, Bimnbaum S J, Lebowitz N 1987 A viable pregnancy in a patient wih myositis ossificans progressiva. American Journal of Obstetrics and Gynecology 156: 577–578

FREEMAN-SHELDON SYNDROME

A congenital myopathy, usually of autosomal dominant inheritance with facial and orthopaedic deformities, otherwise known as craniocarpotarsal dysplasia. Anaesthesia may be required for inguinal hernia, orchidopexy, feeding gastrostomy, muscle biopsy or release of contractures around the mouth.

Preoperative abnorrnalities

1. A myopathy, with the development of contractures around the mouth producing the characteristic 'whistling face' appearance. Contraction of the mouth muscles contributes to microstomia and the formation of a small 'mound' on the chin. There may be hypertelorism, a small nose, a high-arched palate and an abnormal mandible with micrognathia.
2. Kyphoscoliosis may develop wlth progressive myopathy.
3. Thoracic cage deformity and myopathy of respiratory muscles may combine to produce a restrictive lung disease.
4. Contractures may also affect the limbs.
5. Diagnosis is made on EMG and muscle biopsy.

Anaesthetic problems

1. Difficult intubation may be secondary to micrognathia, microstomia and a short neck. Awake intubation was achieved with difficulty in an 11-week-old baby and after inhalational anaesthesia in two children (Laishley & Roy 1986). Successful intubation was finally achieved using a stylet in a 7-month-old (Duggar et al 1989), who was subsequently given caudal anaesthesia for surgery for club foot.
2. Muscle rigidity occurred following halothane anaesthesia in two patients (Jones & Delacourt 1992). In the first patient this did not respond to pancuronium, but relaxation occurred within 5 minutes of giving dantrolene 2 mg/kg. No hyperthermia, hyperkalaemia or cardiac arrhythmias occurred, but the following day the serum CK was 9215 iu/l. In the second, masseter muscle spasm occurred after suxamethonium and the maximum serum CK recorded was 1193 iu/l. The operation was allowed to continue, but halothane was withdrawn.

3. Difficulty in obtaining venous access secondary to hand and foot deformities has been reported. Limbs may be encased in plaster.
4. Patients are prone to develop pneumonia.

Management

1. Although the apparently uneventful use of suxamethonium has been reported (Laishley & Roy 1986), it would seem prudent to avoid it in a myopathy, particularly in view of the evidence of muscle breakdown.
2. Observe for evidence of muscle rigidity, rhabdomyolysis or hypermetabolism.
3. Assessment of intubation difficulties and appropriate management.

BIBLIOGRAPHY
Duggar R G, DeMars P D, Bolton V E 1989 Whistling face syndrome: general anesthsia and early postoperative caudal analgesia. Anesthesiology 70: 545–547
Jones R, Delacourt J L 1992 Muscle rigidity following halothane anesthesia in two patients with Freeman-Sheldon syndrome. Anesthesiology 77: 599–600
Laishley R S, Roy W L 1986 Freeman-Sheldon syndrome: report of three cases and the anaesthetic implications. Canadian Anaesthetists' Society Journal 33: 388–393

FRIEDREICH'S ATAXIA

A hereditary ataxia in which degeneration of the pyramidal and spinocerebellar tracts, and atrophy of the dorsal root ganglia, result in ataxia and combined upper and lower motor neurone lesions. Asymptomatic ECG abnormalities occur in many patients. Disorders of cardiac muscle affect about 30% of individuals and are of two types; a hypertrophic form and a dystrophic form. The condition usually presents between the ages of 5 and 15 years, with a mean of 9 years. A metabolic defect has been suggested as a cause. The disease is steadily progressive, and sudden death may occur.

Preoperative abnormalities

1. Usually presents with gait ataxia. Later the upper limbs become clumsy, with intention tremor. The cerebellar lesion causes nystagmus and dysarthria. The dorsal root lesion is associated with sensory impairment and depressed reflexes. The corticospinal tract degeneration causes progressive weakness and extensor plantar reflexes. Pes cavus is often present.
2. Cardiac abnormalities are frequent although these may simply consist of asymptomatic ECG or echocardiographic changes. In a study of 75 consecutive patients, 95% had one or more abnormalities (Child et al 1986). These consisted of ST-T wave abnormalities (79%), right axis deviation (40%), a short PR interval

(24%), an abnormal R wave in V1 (20%), abnormal inferolateral Q waves (14%) and left ventricular hypertrophy (11%) However, up to 50% of patients have clinical cardiac disease. Hypertrophic cardiomyopathy occurred in 20%, less frequently than previously thought, whilst 7% had a nonhypertrophic cardiomyopathy in which there was global hypofunction of the left ventricle. Symptoms include palpitations and chest pain. Heart failure may supervene and sudden death can occur.

3. The degree of disability progressively increases, with the development of scoliosis and need for a wheelchair being closely associated. Scoliosis occurs in 80% of patients and surgery may be required for its correction (Bird & Strunin 1984, Bell et al 1986). Chest infections are common.

4. Diabetes has been found in 18% of patients and a diabetic glucose tolerance curve in 40%.

5. The EMG is usually normal, but motor nerve conduction velocities are decreased.

Anaesthetic problems

1. Although sensitivity to non-depolarizing relaxants has been reported, this is not always so. Suggestions of a myasthenic-like response were not confirmed when a nerve stimulator was used (Bell et al 1986). However, since different muscles are affected to a variable degree, the response may depend both on the progression of the disease and the muscle group being monitored.

2. If cardiac disease is present, there is a risk of arrhythmias and heart failure. A patient having scoliosis surgery developed heart failure on the 34th postoperative day, possibly due to pulmonary emboli in addition to longstanding cardiomyopathy (Bell et al 1986). This subsequently proved fatal.

3. As the degree of scoliosis increases, or if diaphragmatic weakness develops, cardiopulmonary failure becomes a significant problem (see also Scoliosis). Chest infections readily occur.

Management

1. Assessment of respiratory reserve, and vigorous treatment of chest infections with physiotherapy and antibiotics.

2. Assessment, monitoring and treatment of cardiac lesions as appropriate.

3. Neuromuscular monitoring should be instituted, preferably before induction of anaesthesia. The monitoring of more than one muscle group may be necessary.

4. Spinal anaesthesia has been used for Caesarean section (Kubal et al 1991) and extradural anaesthesia for laparoscopic tubal ligation (Alon & Waespe 1988). However, in view of the incidence of

cardiomyopathy, caution has been advised if regional anaesthesia is considered. If a cardiomyopathy is present, full cardiac assessment is recommended (Finley & Campbell 1992).

5. Extradural narcotics were given for postoperative pain relief in a 13-year-old girl who required colorectal surgery (Campbell & Finley 1989).

BIBLIOGRAPHY

Alon E, Waespe W 1988 Epidural anaesthesie bei einer patientin mit Friedreichscher ataxie. Regional Anaesthesia 11: 58–60
Bell C F, Kelly J M, Jones R S 1986 Anaesthesia for Friedreich's ataxia. Anaesthesia 41: 296–301
Bird T M, Strunin L 1984 Hypotensive anesthesia for a patient wlth Friedreich's ataxia. Anesthesioloy 60: 377–380
Campbell A M, Finley G A 1989 Anaesthesia for a patient with Friedreich's ataxia and cardiomyopathy. Canadian Journal of Anaesthesia 36: 89–93
Child J S, Perloff J K, Bach P M et al 1986 Cardiac involvement in Friedreich's ataxia. A study of 75 patients. Journal of the American College of Cardiology 7: 1370–1378
Finley G A, Campbell A M 1992 Spinal anesthesia and Friedreich's ataxia Anesthesia and Analgesia 74: 311–312
Kubal K, Pasricha S K, Bhargava M 1991 Spinal anaesthesia in a patient with Friedreich's ataxia. Anesthesia and Analgesia 72: 257–8

GIANT AXONAL NEUROPATHY

An autosomal recessive neurological disorder of cytoplasmic intermediate filaments in which there are swollen axons with accumulation of neurofilaments (Berg et al 1972). A mild sensory neuropathy is accompanied by severe CNS involvement, mental retardation, seizures, cerebellar dysfunction and pyramidal signs. Occasionally the central nervous system abnormalities predominate (Lampl et al 1992). The condition develops in early childhood, with death occurring in adolescence, frequently secondary to muscle weakness and respiratory infection.

Preoperative abnormalities

1. Tightly kinked hair is characteristic.
2. There is profound limb weakness and wasting usually accompanied by kyphoscoliosis.
3. Diffuse demyelination is evident on CT scan and MRI.
4. EMG shows decreased sensory nerve conduction.
5. Diagnosis is confirmed by sural nerve biopsy.

Anaesthetic problems

1. Respiratory problems may occur secondary to muscle weakness.
2. Profound weakness following diazepam was reported in one patient (Mitchell & Moskovits 1991).

Management

1. Preoperative assessment of respiratory reserve.
2. Intraoperative assessment of neuromuscular function.
3. Care with respiratory depressant drugs.

BIBLIOGRAPHY
Berg B O, Rosenberg, S H, Asbury A K 1972 Giant axonal neuropathy. Pediatrics 49: 894–899
Lampl Y, Eshel Y, Ben-David E et al 1992 Giant axonal neuopathy with predominant central nervous system manifestations. Developmental Medicine and Childhood Neurology 34: 164–169
Maia M, Pires M M, Guimar E S 1988 Giant axonal disease: report three cases and review of the literature. Neuropediatrics 19: 10–15
Mitchell A, Moskovits P E 1991 Anaesthesia for a patient with axonal neuropathy. Anaesthesia 46: 469–470

GILBERT'S DISEASE
(IDIOPATHIC UNCONJUGATED HYPERBILIRUBINAEMIA)

An autosomal dominant, benign condition, in which there is a mildly elevated unconjugated bilirubin, without either structural liver disease or haemolytic anaemia. It possibly results from an impaired uptake and conjugation of bilirubin, secondary to a deficiency of glucuronyl transferase.

Preoperative abnormalities

1. Serum unconjugated bilirubin is increased, but usually to a level <50 μmol/l, and clinical jaundice is barely detectable. However, fluctuating mild jaundice may occur, particularly in the presence of stress, infection, starvation or surgery.
2. Other liver function tests are normal, and there is no haemolytic anaemia.

Anaesthetic problems

1. The condition itself is of no significance. However, the appearance of jaundice postoperatively may suggest more serious problems, and therefore the confirmation of Gilbert's syndrome as the cause is useful (Taylor 1984).
2. Starvation may elevate the bilirubin level.
3. The metabolism of morphine (Nishimura et al 1973) and papaveretum (Danks & Jackson 1991) may be delayed. Two patients were reported in whom papaveretum 10 mg caused profound sedation and respiratory depression.

Management

1. If Gilbert's disease is suspected, the administration of nicotinic acid 50 mg i.v. will double or treble the plasma unconjugated bilirubin within 3 hours. In normal patients, or in those with other liver disease, the increase will be less marked.
2. Morphine should be used with caution.
3. Early morning surgery and a dextrose infusion will reduce the increase in bilirubin produced by starvation.

BIBLIOGRAPHY
Danks J L, Jackson A F P 1991 Sensitivty to papaveretum in Gilbert's dsease. Anaesthesia 46: 998–999
Nishimura T G, Jackson S H, Cohen S N 1973 Prolongation of morphine anaesthesia in a patient with Gilbert's disease. Canadian Anaesthetists' Society Journal 20: 709–712
Taylor S 1984 Gilbert's syndrome as a cause of postoperative jaundice. Anaesthesia 39: 1222–1224

GLOMUS JUGULARE TUMOUR

A rare, slow-growing, benign vascular tumour of the glomus bodies, usually arising from the dome of the jugular bulb. It is one of the paraganglionic tumours, related to the branchial arches. The symptoms, which vary, will depend in part on local extension or invasion of structures by the tumour. The mode of presentation includes a swelling in the neck, middle ear disease, or symptoms indicative of involvement of the cerebellum, brain stem or skull base. Although normally non functional, it occasionally produces catecholamines. It must be distinguished from glomus tumours, which arise from the tympanic plexus. Surgical removal is either through the auditory canal or via a mastoid approach. If there is extensive spread, postoperative complications can be significant and radiotherapy may be a safer option (Larner et al 1992).

Preoperative abnormalities

1. Pulsatile tinnitus, hearing loss and facial paralysis can occur when the middle ear is involved.
2. Clinical signs of IX, X, XI and XII cranial nerve lesions denote extension of the tumour into the base of the skull.
3. Intracranial extension may give V and VI nerve lesions.
4. Invasion of the jugular vein or internal carotid may occur.
5. Occasionally, functioning tumours can produce catecholamines.
6. Ten per cent of patients will have another paraganglionic tumour.
7. The tumours can be visualized using carotid angiography or digital vascular imaging. Vascularity and collateral circulation need to be assessed.

8. Treatment may be by surgery, radiation or embolization.

Anaesthetic problems

1. Excision may require extensive surgery involving more than one surgical discipline. Combined or two-stage procedures may be necessary.
2. Blood loss may be heavy (Ghani et al 1983). The blood supply usually comes from the external carotid artery, but extensive tumours may also be supplied by collateral circulation from the internal carotid.
3. Occasionally, the tumour may actually involve the internal carotid artery itself or invade the jugular vein to give tumour emboli.
4. Surgery has been reported as lasting for up to 17 hours, therefore heat loss can be a problem.
5. The problems of any neurosurgical procedure, including that of air embolism.
6. Ligation of the internal carotid artery may be necessary (Braude et al 1986).

Management

1. A two-stage operation may be planned if the tumour is particularly extensive and involves two different surgical fields (Mather & Webster 1986).
2. Hypotensive anaesthesia may be required to reduce blood loss.
3. Prior radiological embolization of the tumour, to reduce haemorrhage, may be required.
4. If carotid artery ligation is contemplated, adequacy of the collateral circulation must be assessed.
5. Hypothermia and cerebral protection may be required in tumours involving the carotid artery. A technique has been described in which moderate hypothermia, normocarbia, normotension and thiopentone infusion provided successful cerebral protection for resection of an extensive tumour which involved the internal carotid (Braude et al 1986).

BIBLIOGRAPHY

Braude B M, Hockman R, McIntosh W A et al 1986 Management of a glomus jugulare tumour with internal carotid artery involvement. Anaesthesia 41: 861–865

Ghani G A, Sung Y-F, Per-Lee J H 1983 Glomus jugulare tumours – origin, pathology and anesthetic considerations. Anesthesia and Analgesia 62: 686–691

Larner J M, Hahn S S, Spaulding C A et al 1992 Glomus jugulare tumors. Long-term control by radiation therapy. Cancer 69: 1813–1817

Mather S P, Webster N R 1986 Tumours of the glomus jugulare. Anaesthesia 41: 856–860

GLUCAGONOMA

A rare glucagon-secreting tumour of the alpha cells of the pancreatic islets, the majority of which have metastasized at the time of presentation. One of the group of tumours classified as APUDomas. Glucagon causes glycogenolysis, release of insulin and catecholamines, protein breakdown, lipolysis and ketogenesis. In addition, it is known to have positive inotropic and chronotropic effects, which are not prevented by beta adrenoceptor blockers. There have been only four cases reported in the anaesthetic literature.

Preoperative abnormalities

1. The patient, more frequently a woman, may present with a bullous skin condition known as necrolytic migratory erythema (Price et al 1989).
2. There may be weight loss, anaemia and diarrhoea.
3. Glucose tolerance tests may show mild or frank diabetes.
4. Basal plasma glucagon levels are increased.
5. Plasma pancreatic polypeptide levels are often increased.
6. Somatostatin analogues may provide palliation.

Anaesthetic problems

1. There is an increased incidence of venous thrombosis.
2. Wide fluctuations in plasma glucagon levels have been reported to occur during handling of the tumour (Nicoll & Catling 1985). The levels recorded were, however, less than those needed to produce pharmacological effects, and no cardiovascular changes were seen.
3. Fluctuations of blood sugar also occurred in three cases reported by Boskovski et al (1991), but the levels were not clinically significant.
4. Other endocrinopathies may coexist, including insulinoma and phaeochromocytoma (see APUDomas).

Management

1. Evidence of secretion of other neuroendocrine hormones should be sought.
2. Careful monitoring of intraoperative cardiovascular function and blood glucose levels.
3. Octreotide may be an effective treatment for the glucagonoma syndrome (Wynick & Bloom 1991).

BIBLIOGRAPHY

Boskovski N A, Chapin J W, Becker G L et al 1991 Anesthesia for glucagonoma resection. Journal of Clinical Anesthesia 3: 48–52

Friesen S R 1982 Tumors of the endocrine pancreas. New England Journal of Medicine 306: 580–590

Nicoll J M V, Catling S J 1985 Anaesthetic management of glucagonoma. Anaesthesia
40: 152–157
Price M L, Darley C R, Kirkham N 1989 The glucagonoma syndrome. Journal of the
Royal Society of Medicne 82: 553–554
Wynick D, Bloom S R 1991 Clinical Review 23. The use of long-acting somatostatin
analog octreotide in the treatment of gut neuroendocrine tumours. Journal of
Clinical Endocrinology and Metabolism 73: 1–3

GLUCOSE-6-PHOSPHATE DEHYDROGENASE DEFICIENCY

A sex-linked hereditary abnormality in which the activity or stability of
the enzyme glucose-6-phosphate dehydrogenase (G6PD) is markedly
diminished. It is most commonly found among blacks and people of
Mediterranean origin but also in North European and South East Asian
populations. G6PD is an essential enzyme for glucose metabolism in the
pentose phosphate pathway within the RBC. This pathway is ultimately
involved in the production of reduced glutathione, and the reduction of
methaemoglobin within the RBC. When G6PD activity is impaired, the
accumulation of methaemoglobin and a deficiency of reduced
glutathione alter cell integrity. Globin precipitates (Heinz bodies) are
produced and the RBCs become more prone to haemolysis. Several
variants of the A and B G6PD subtypes have been described, resulting
in different clinical severity.

Management is directed towards avoiding oxidant stimulants which
initiate haemolysis (Martin & Casella 1991).

Preoperative abnormalities

1. With rare exceptions, the only clinical manifestation of G6PD
   deficiency is haemolytic anaemia. Usually the anaemia is episodic
   and is associated with stress, most notably drug administration,
   infection, the newborn period and, in certain individuals, exposure
   to fava beans (favism). Drugs known to cause haemolysis in G6PD-
   deficient subjects include the antimalarials, primaquine and
   chloroquine, the sulphonamides, tolbutamide, nitrofurantoin, the
   sulphones, methylene blue, nalidixic acid, high-dose aspirin, vitamin
   C, vitamin K, phenacetin and nitrates. Chloramphenicol, quinidine
   and quinine affect those with the Mediterranean form of the
   condition only. Two to five days after ingestion of one of these
   drugs, there may be abdominal pain and jaundice associated with a
   decrease in haemoglobin level. Heinz bodies appear in the blood
   during this period.
2. Chronic non-spherocytic haemolytic anaemia, with jaundice, and
   splenomegaly may be seen occasionally. The anaemia is not usually
   severe, but in some instances the need for frequent transfusions has
   been reported.
3. There is an increased incidence of cataracts and vitreous
   haemorrhage.

Anaesthetic problems

1. Drug-induced haemolysis can occur after administration of any of the above drugs. However, haemolysis has occurred intraoperatively in the absence of these (Sazama et al 1980) and the possibility that it was initiated by a stress reaction, or red cell damage during cardiopulmonary bypass, was considered.

2. Infants are more susceptible to oxidative stress than are adults (Martin & Casella 1991).

3. The appearance of postoperative jaundice may cause confusion as to its origin (Shapley & Wilson 1973).

4. G6PD-deficient individuals may be sensitive to toxic doses of prilocaine and sodium nitroprusside, not as a result of methaemoglobinaemia, as sometimes stated, but because of the concurrent production of oxidizing chemicals which can produce haemolysis (Smith & Snowdon 1987). If clinically significant toxic methaemoglobinaemia occurs in a G6PD-deficient patient, methylene blue is ineffective in treatment and may itself cause haemolysis (Rosen et al 1971, Smith & Snowdon 1987).

5. Malignant hyperthermia was thought to have occurred in a patient with G6PD deficiency (Younker et al 1984). However, there was no mention of confirmation of the diagnosis of MH with contracture testing.

Management

1. Elective surgery should not be undertaken during a haemolytic episode.

2. Agents known to produce haemolysis should be avoided. Particular care should be taken not to exceed the maximum safe doses of sodium nitroprusside or prilocaine (Smith & Snowdon 1987, Martin & Casella 1991).

3. A folic acid supplement may be required.

BIBLIOGRAPHY

Martin L D, Casella E S 1991 Anesthesia and glucose-6-phosphate dehydrogenase deficiency in a child with congenital heart disease. Journal of Cardiothoracic and Vascular Anesthesia 5: 596–599

Rosen P J, Johnson C, McGehee W G et al 1971 Failure of methylene blue treatment in toxic methemoglobinemia. Association with glucose-6-phosphate dehydrogenase deficiency: Annals of Internal Medicine 75: 83–86

Sazama K, Klein H G, Davey R J et al 1980 Intraoperative hemolysis: the initial manifestation of glucose-6-phosphate dehydrogenase deficiency. Archives of Internal Medicine 140: 845–846

Shapley J M, Wilson J R 1973 Post-anaesthetic jaundice due to glucose-6-phosphate dehydrogenase deficiency. Canadian Anaesthetists' Society Journal 20: 390–392

Smith C L, Snowdon S L 1987 Anaesthesia and glucose-6-phosphate dehydrogenase deficiency. Anaesthesia 42: 281–288

Younker D, DeVore M, Hartlage P 1984 Malignant hyperthermia and glucose-6-phosphate dehydrogenase deficiency Anesthesiology 60: 601–603

GLYCOGEN STORAGE DISEASES

A group of genetic diseases in which there are defects in enzymes concerned with either the breakdown or the branching of glycogen.

The Cori classification is:

I = von Gierke's	V = McArdle's
II = Pompe's	VI = Hers'
III = Cori's, Forbes	VII = Thompson
IV = Andersen's	VIII = Tarin

Type	Enzyme deficiency	Affected organs
I	glucose-6-phosphatase	liver and kidneys
II	alpha-1,4 glucosidase	skeletal and cardiac muscle
III	amylo-1,6 glucosidase	liver, skeletal and cardiac muscle and blood cells
IV	amylo-1,4 to 1,6-transglucosidase	liver, skeletal and cardiac muscle and blood cells
V	muscle phosphorylase	muscle
VI	liver phosphorylase	liver and white blood cells
VII	phosphoglucomutase	muscle
VIII	muscle fructokinase	muscle and red blood cells

The commoner of the diseases are dealt with under the individual names; see von Gierke's, Pompe's, McArdle's and Hers' diseases.

BIBLIOGRAPHY
Casson H 1975 Anaesthesia for portacaval bypass in patients with metabolic disease. British Journal of Anaesthesia 47: 969–975
Cox J M 1968 Anesthesia and glycogen-storage disease. Anesthesiology 29: 1221–1225
Edelstein G, Hirshman C A 1980 Hyperthermia and ketoacidosis during anesthesia in a child with glycogen storage disease. Anesthesiology 52: 90–92
Ellis F R 1980 Inherited muscle disease. British Journal of Anaesthesia 52: 153–164

GOLDENHAR'S SYNDROME

An inherited condition, alternatively known as oculoauriculovertebral dysplasia. Two criteria are required for the diagnosis; an eye abnormality associated with any two of the following three – ear, mandibular or vertebral anomalies (Feingold & Baum 1978). Anaesthesia is needed for ocular surgery.

Preoperative abnormalities

1. Ocular abnormalities include coloboma of the eyelid, epibulbar dermoid, subconjunctival lipoma and defects of the extraocular muscles.
2. Micrognathia, maxillary hypoplasia, cleft or high arched palate.
3. Orthopaedic abnormalities include: vertebral anomalies (40%), club foot, congenital dislocation of the hip, Sprengel's deformity and radial limb defects.

4. A range of cardiac defects (35%) have been reported – Fallot's tetralogy, ventricular septal defect, transposition of the great vessels and total anomalous pulmonary venous drainage.
5. Mental retardation is usual.
6. There may be abnormalities of the immune system.

Anaesthetic problems

1. Difficulties in tracheal intubation have been reported (Stehling 1978, Cooper & Murray-Wilson 1987, Mohandas & Selvarajah 1988, Madan et al 1990). In the latter series only one patient out of 17 had problems. These difficulties may be secondary to either facial or vertebral abnormalities.
2. Problems of associated congenital heart disease.

Management

1. Careful clinical assessment of upper airway problems. A child with a history of respiratory distress underwent respiratory inductance plethysmography and pulse oximetry before surgery, to assess the patency of the upper airway during sleep. Since there was no evidence of severe obstruction, inhalation induction was undertaken (Aoe et al 1990).
2. Intubation problems may be resolved by tracheostomy (Stehling 1978), retrograde intubation (Cooper & Murray-Wilson 1987) or fibreoptic intubation using a guide wire.
3. Management of associated abnormalities, such as in a neonate with transposition of the great vessels and hydrocephalus (Scholtes et al 1987).

BIBLIOGRAPHY

Aoe T, Kohchi T, Mizuguchi T 1990 Respiratory inductance plethysmography and pulse oximetry in the assessment of upper airway patency in a child with Goldenhar's syndrome. Canadian Journal of Anaesthesia 37: 369–371

Cooper C M S, Murray-Wilson A 1987 Retrograde intubation. Management of a 4.8-kg, 5-month infant. Anaesthesia 42: 1197–1200

Feingold M, Baum J 1978 Goldenhar's syndrome American Journal of Diseases of Children 132: 136–138

Madan R, Trikha A, Ventataraman R K et al 1990 Goldenhar's syndrome: an analysis of anaesthetic management. A retrospective study of seventeen cases. Anaesthesia 45: 49–52

Mohandas K, Selvarajah S 1988 Failed intubation in a case of oculoauriculovertebral dysplasia (Goldenhar's syndrome). Medical Journal of Malaysia 43: 255–258

Scholtes J L, Veyckemans F, Obbergh L V et al 1987 Neonatal anaesthetic management of a patient with Goldenhar's syndrome with hydrocephalus. Anaesthesia and Intensive Care 15: 338–340

Stehling L 1978 Goldenhar's syndrome and airway management. American Journal of Diseases of Children 132: 818

GOODPASTURE'S SYNDROME

A general term applied to a combination of glomerulonephritis and pulmonary haemorrhage, which may be caused by a variety of disease processes (Holdsworth et al 1985). Frequently, but not invariably, it is rapidly progressive. It is typically associated with antibodies to glomerular basement membrane (anti-GBM), detectable in plasma by radioimmunoassay and by immunofluorescence techniques on muscle biopsy. These cross-react with alveolar basement membrane, although those individuals with lung haemorrhage are usually smokers, and those with isolated anti-GBM nephritis are non-smokers. Systemic vasculitides such as PAN and Wegener's granulomatosis may also cause lung haemorrhage and renal failure.

Preoperative abnormalities

1. Usually presents with cough, dyspnoea, haemoptysis which may be massive, and anaemia.
2. The pulmonary lesions proceed to interstitial fibrosis and haemosiderin deposits. Lung function tests show a restrictive type of abnormality.
3. Glomerulonephritis, which usually follows or coincides with pulmonary lesions, may produce proteinuria, haematuria and casts. The end-result is renal failure.
4. Treatment may be with corticosteroids for pulmonary haemorrhage, cytotoxic drugs to stop renal damage and plasmapheresis to remove antibodies.

Anaesthetic problems

1. Poor respiratory function with hypoxaemia and respiratory alkalosis.
2. Pulmonary haemorrhage that may, on occasions, be life-threatening (Klasa et al 1988).
3. Impaired renal function and sometimes renal failure.
4. Hypochromic anaemia and a high ESR.
5. Patients may be on immunosuppressives or steroids, or undergoing plasma exchange, with the aim of reducing the antibody titre.

Management

1. Preoperative assessment of lung function and, in particular, arterial blood gases. Elective pulmonary surgery should not be undertaken during periods of active haemorrhage.
2. Assessment of renal function and appropriate management.
3. A successful pregnancy has been managed (Yankowitz et al 1992) and required regular assessment of pulmonary and renal function. The use of steroids was associated with hyperglycaemia requiring control with insulin. Plasmapheresis was necessary.

BIBLIOGRAPHY
Holdsworth S, Boyce N, Thomson N M et al 1985 The clinical spectrum of acute glomerulonephritis and lung haemorrhage (Goodpasture's syndrome). Quarterly

Journal of Medicine 55: 75–86
Klasa R J, Abboud R T, Ballon H S et al 1988 Goodpasture's syndrome: recurrence
    after a five-year remission. American Journal of Medicine 84: 751–755
Yankowitz J, Kuller J A, Thomas R L 1992 Pregnancy complicated by Goodpasture
    syndrome. Obstetrics and Gynecology 79: 806–808

GUILLAIN–BARRÉ SYNDROME

A collective name given to a group of acute ascending polyneuropathies
in which motor involvement predominates. Some may have an
immunological basis, and antecedent infection, surgery and
immunizations have all been implicated in their development. Progress
is variable with advancement for 1–3 weeks, a plateau phase of several
weeks followed by slow improvement (Ropper 1992). There is a mortality
of 5–20%, whilst in 3% of patients the disease becomes chronic or
relapsing. Deaths occur from sepsis, ARDS, pulmonary emboli
and unexplained cardiac arrest. The anaesthetist may be involved in
treatment of respiratory insufficiency, or for surgery.

Preoperative abnormalities

1. Muscle weakness usually starts in the legs and progresses upwards,
   at a variable rate. Cranial nerve involvement, usually of the bulbar
   and facial nerves, may occur in up to 50% of cases, although
   involvement of other nerves has been described. One patient arrived
   in hospital in coma, with absent brainstem reflexes (Coad & Byrne
   1990) and the diagnosis was only made after CSF protein levels of
   2 g/l were found. In some cases there is respiratory insufficiency and
   an inability to clear secretions. IPPV is required in respiratory failure
   in 10–23% cases. Loss of tendon reflexes may occur.
2. Mild paraesthesias in the toes and fingertips may precede the muscle
   weakness.
3. Muscle pain or aching is common (50–76%). Two distinct types are
   reported; deep muscular pain with tenderness, and burning or
   hyperaesthesia in the extremities.
4. Autonomic dysfunction may produce cardiovascular instability and
   an impairment of normal compensatory vasoconstrictor responses
   (Lichtenfeld 1971). Changes of position can be accompanied by
   marked decreases in blood pressure. Attacks of sweating,
   tachycardia and hypertension may occur. Brady- and
   tachyarrhythmias may necessitate pacemaker insertion. Sudden
   deaths have occurred, probably secondary to arrhythmias. It has
   been suggested that the lack of respiratory variation in heart rate,
   which is characteristic of autonomic dysfunction, occurs more often
   in the group of patients with respiratory muscle weakness, who
   require IPPV (Oakley 1984). In those patients with autonomic

complications the mortality rate may be as high as 13%, although in specialist units a rate of only 1.3% has been quoted (Winer 1992).

5. The CSF protein content is raised, with no increase in cell count.

Anaesthetic problems

1. If the intercostal muscles are affected, respiration and sputum clearance may be compromised. Bulbar weakness may result in pulmonary aspiration and segmental collapse. One patient had such severe involvement of the cranial nerves that an initial, mistaken diagnosis of brain stem death was made (Coad & Byrne 1990). Subsequently, full recovery took place.
2. Autonomic dysfunction can produce postural variations in blood pressure and marked hypotension on induction of anaesthesia. Cardiovascular collapse has occurred immediately after the administration of a spinal anaesthetic (Perel et al 1977). This was thought to be caused by a combination of hypotension secondary to sympathetic blockade, and a 30°C head-up tilt.
3. Pain may be a troublesome feature and is difficult to treat.
4. Administration of suxamethonium may be associated with transient severe hyperkalaemia. In one patient, asystole after suxamethonium was subsequently followed by rhabdomyolytic renal failure (Hawker et al 1985).
5. Hyponatraemia may occasionally occur, as a result of inappropriate ADH secretion.
6. Guillain-Barré syndrome (GBS) may occasionally occur during prenancy so that decisions are required about the method of analgesia, anaesthesia and delivery (McGrady 1987). Cardiac arrest after suxamethonium was reported in a pregnant patient who had recovered from GBS (Feldman 1990).

Management

1. In the presence of decreasing respiratory function, IPPV may be required. Vital capacity should be measured 4-hourly during the phase of deterioration. The use of accessory muscles of respiration, and the reduction of vital capacity to 1 litre (or 15 ml/kg), presages respiratory failure (Ferner et al 1987). Facial weakness is an ominous sign. The institution of IPPV may be accompanied by hypotension. Tracheostomy is required when prolonged ventilation is anticipated.
2. In patients who require IPPV, continuous cardiac monitoring is required. It has been suggested that regularity of the heart rate, measured by minimal R–R interval variation on deep breathing, may indicate autonomic failure and the possibility of sudden death as a result of arrhythmias (Oakley 1984) (see Autonomic failure). Pacemaker insertion may have to be considered. When tachycardia compromises cardiac output, beta adrenoceptor blockade may be considered. Esmolol has been used for this purpose (Calleja 1990).

3. Extradural opiates have been given for the treatment of intractable pain (Connelly et al 1990).
4. General care includes:
   a. Physiotherapy for the chest, with passive movements for the limbs.
   b. Nasogastric feeding. Constipation should be anticipated, with the use of stool softeners or enemas.
   c. Psychological management. The patient may be very frightened, and constant reassurance is needed. Depression is a frequent problem in the later stages.
5. Reports of the efficacy of plasma exchange show variable results. On balance, plasmapheresis appears to be safe and has been shown to accelerate recovery and shorten the time for IPPV, particularly if it is instituted early (Hughes 1985).
6. Steroids are now not recommended.
7. There are isolated reports of the use of intravenous high-dose immunoglobulins (Rajah 1992) and preliminary trials suggest that it is at least as effective as plasma exchange (Winer 1992, van der Meche & Schmitz 1992).
8. If general anaesthesia is required, suxamethonium should be avoided, even after recovery from GBS.
9. Extradural anaesthesia has been used both for Caesarean section and for pain relief (McGrady 1987, Connelly et al 1990).

BIBLIOGRAPHY
Calleja M A 1990 Autonomic dysfunction and Guillain–Barré syndrome. The use of esmolol in its management. Anaesthesia 45: 736–737
Coad N R, Byrne A J 1990 Guillain–Barré syndrome mimicking brainstem death. Anaesthesia 45: 456–457
Connelly M, Shagrin J, Warfield C 1990 Epidural opioids for the management of pain in a patient with the Guillain–Barré syndrome. Anesthesiology 72: 381–383
Feldman J M 1990 Cardiac arrest after succinylcholine administration in a pregnant patient recovered from Guillain–Barré syndrome. Anesthesiology 72: 942–944
Ferner R, Barnett M, Hughes R A C 1987 Management of Guillain–Barré syndrome. British Journal of Hospital Medicine 38: 525–530
Hawker F, Pearson I Y, Soni N et al 1985 Rhabdomyolytic renal failure and suxamethonium. Anaesthesia and Intensive Care 13: 208–209
Hughes R A C 1985 Plasma exchange for Guillain–Barré syndrome British Medical Journal 291: 615–616
Lichtenfeld P 1971 Autonomic dysfunction in the Guillain–Barré syndrome. American Journal of Medicine 50: 772–780
McGrady E M 1987 Management of labour and delivery in a patient with Guillain–Barré syndrome. Anaesthesia 42: 899–900
Oakley C M 1984 The heart in the Guillain–Barré syndrome. British Medical Journal 288:94
Perel A, Reches A, Davidson J T 1977 Anaesthesia in the Guillain–Barré syndrome. Anaesthesia 32: 257–260
Rajah A 1992 The use of high-dose intravenous immunoglobulins in Guillain–Barré syndrome. Anaesthesia 47: 220–222
Ropper A H 1992 The Guillain–Barré syndrome. New England Journal of Medicine 326: 1130–1136
Van der Meche F G A, Schmitz P I M and the Dutch Guillain–Barré Study Group 1992 A randomized trial comparing intravenous immune globulin and plasma

exchange in Guillain–Barré syndrome. New England Journal of Medicine 326: 1123–1129

Winer J 1992 Guillain–Barré syndrome revisited. British Medical Journal 304: 65–66

HAEMOGLOBINOPATHIES
(see also THALASSAEMIA)

Normal haemoglobin (HbA) consists of a colourless protein, globin, which is made up from two alpha and two beta polypeptide chains, and four haem radicals. The haem radical is a porphyrin structure, at the centre of which is a hexavalent iron atom. Four of the valencies are occupied by the nitrogen atoms of pyrrole rings, and the fifth by one of the globin polypeptide chains. The last one is therefore free, for haemoglobin to transport oxygen in a reversible combination.

The haemoglobinopathies rest from inherited structural alterations in one of the globin chains. The thalassaemias, on the other hand, result from inherited defects in the rate of synthesis of one or more of the globin chains.

Types of haemogtobinopathies

1. Sickle cell disease and allied disorders.
2. Haemoglobinopathies producing cyanosis.
3. Haemoglobinopathies associated with unstable haemoglobin.
4. Haemoglobinopathies producing polycythaemia.

Types of normal haemoglobin

HbA Normal adult haemoglobin. Has two alpha and two beta chains. Ninety-eight per cent of adult molecule is in this form.

HbF Fetal haemoglobin. Has two alpha and two gamma chains. Is gradually replaced during the first 6 months of life, but varying amounts may persist in the haemoglobinopathies and modify the disease severity.

HbA2 Forms 2.5% of adult haemoglobin. Has two alpha and two delta chains.

SICKLE CELL DISEASE

A genetic abnormality of haemoglobin synthesis involving the substitution of valine for glutamic acid at the sixth amino acid position in the beta chain of the globin molecule. It occurs most frequently in blacks of African origin and in some Mediterranean races. Resistance to malaria occurs.

Sickle cell disease A general term encompassing all abnormal combinations in which HbS forms a part, e.g. HbSS, HbSC, HbThal.

Sickle cell anaemia   Refers to HbSS only.
Sickle cell trait   Refers to HbAS.
The homozygous form (HbSS, sickle cell anaemia) affects 0.25% of the UK black population, while the heterozygous form (HbAS, sickle cell trait) affects up to 10%. In HbAS, the red blood cells contain 20–45% HbS, whereas in HbSS the content is 85–95% HbS.

The solubility of deoxygenated HbS is much lower than that of HbA and it has a tendency to gel. A decreased oxygen tension within the red cells is associated with stacking of the haemoglobin molecules into long crystals. The cell membrane is deformed by these molecular changes, and the red cell takes on a sickle shape. Dehydration promotes this tendency, and sickling increases the blood viscosity. Once initiated the process can be self perpetuating. Obstruction of blood vessels to organs may occur, and results in tissue infarction. Oxygenation can reverse the sickling process in the initial stages, but when repeated episodes have taken place, cell membrane changes tend to make it irreversible.

Haemolytic anaemia and jaundice occur as a result of premature destruction of these abnormal RBCs. The mean red cell life will depend on the percentage of abnormal haemoglobin within an individual cell. Cells with a majority of abnormal haemoglobin can have their life reduced from 120 days to less than 20.

In sickle cell anaemia, variable increases in fetal haemoglobin of up to 20% can occur. The levels may be genetically determined. High levels of HbF are advantageous, as its mixture with HbS will increase the solubility of the reduced haemoglobin and thus decrease the severity of the disease. Levels of HbF of 10% protect against stroke and avascular necrosis, whilst those above 20% reduce painful crises and pulmonary complications (Davies & Wonke 1991).

Preoperative abnormalities

1. Sickle cell screening (Sickledex) is a rapid diagnostic test which detects the presence of HbS, but does not distinguish HbSS from HbAS or HbSC. For elective procedures the genotype should be determined by haemoglobin electrophoresis.
2. Patients with HbSS have a severe haemolytic anaemia, whereas those with HbAS usually have a normal haemoglobin. The clinical severity of HbSC varies. Some individuals with HbSC are virtually asymptomatic, but half of them will develop symptoms during childhood and most others become symptomatic in adolescent or adult life.
3. Sickle cell disease is associated with small vessel occlusion and episodes of infarction in affected organs. These may involve bone, bone marrow, liver, spleen, brain and lung. The episodes cause pain, pyrexia and tachycardia. Reduced oxygen tension and acidosis cause sickling of red cells. The increased viscosity encourages stasis

and sludging, which in turn produces occlusion, ischaemia and infarction. Further hypoxia and acidosis perpetuate the cycle.

4. Renal problems may occur in both HbAS and HbSS. Papillary necrosis and haematuria can develop as a result of sickling in the juxtamedullary glomeruli. The concentrating capacity of the kidney is reduced and at least 2 litres of fluid per day is required to excrete the normal osmolar load.
5. In HbSS, varying crises can occur.
   a. The vaso-occlusive problems have been described.
   b. Sequestration crises occur particularly in infants and young children, and result from massive sudden pooling of red cells, especially in the spleen. It is the main cause of infant death in the first year of life.
   c. An aplastic crisis is due to sudden marrow depression, and is generally associated with infection, especially viral.
   d. Haemolytic crises sometimes occur in association with glucose-6-phosphate dehydrogenase deficiency following drug therapy.
6. Infants less than 6 months old have high percentages of HbF, and therefore may not require transfusion.
7. Chest syndrome is a term used for recurrect episodes of chest pain, fever and the presence of pulmonary infiltrates on CXR. The aetiology is unclear, but multiple microinfarctions may contribute. An alternative theory is that rib infarction causes pleuritis and splinting of the ribs leading to atelectasis (Rucknagel et al 1991).
8. Sickle cell lung disease, which comprises both perfusion and diffusion defects, results in progressive changes in blood gases and lung function. This complication contributes to the mortality in young people from pulmonary failure and cor pulmonale (Powars et al 1988). Recurrent episodes of intravascular sickling and acute chest syndrome appear to be two of the risk factors for the development of lung disease.
9. There is an increased incidence of morbidity and mortality associated with *Streptococcus pneumoniae* in the first 3 years of life. Penicillin prophylaxis started before 4 months reduced the incidence of pneumococcal infection.
10. Cardiovascular adaptations to sickle cell anaemia occur, even in the steady state. These consist of an increased cardiac output (70–100% higher for given Hb level) and a reduced systemic vascular resistance. Doppler ultrasound techniques showed that these changes are further accentuated in a sickle cell crisis, possibly as a result of shunting (Singer et al 1989).

Anaesthetic problems

1. Sickling of red blood cells may be precipitated by hypoxia, acidosis, cold and hyperosmolality. Organ infarction, ischaemia and further

hypoxia may result. The postoperative period is often the most hazardous time. Increased sickling of red blood cells occurs, with progressive decreases in the saturation of haemoglobin with oxygen.

In HbSS:
a. 100% saturation – Some sickling occurs.
b. 65% saturation – 75% of cells are sickled.
c. 50% saturation – all cells are sickled.
d. The critical Pao_2 for irreversible sickling is 5.5 kPa.

In HbAS:
a. If 40% HbS, sickling starts at 40% saturation.
b. The critical Pao_2 for irreversible sickling is 2.7 kPa.

2. Sickle cell trait does carry a small risk. Sudden deaths during exercise, and splenic infarcts at altitude have been reported in the US forces literature. There appears to be an association between sickle cell trait and cerebral infarction that is more than coincidental (Radhakrishnan et al 1990). Despite statements to the contrary, anaesthesia for those with the sickle cell trait has not been entirely free from complications.

Adequate oxygenation cannot always be guaranteed during anaesthesia and recovery. Superior sagittal sinus thrombosis occurred in a child following eye surgery (Dalal et al 1974).

Failure to detect airway obstruction and cyanosis in the recovery room resulted in hypoxic fits, cerebral infarction and subsequent death in a patient with HbAS (personal communication). In another case, cardiac arrest and subsequent maternal death occurred during Caesarean section (Anaesthetic Advisory Committee to the Chief Coroner of Ontario 1987). It was postulated that aortocaval compression had occurred, and its relief at delivery allowed the sudden return of hypoxic, acidotic and sickled blood to the heart.

3. Patients with sickle cell states who are shocked, hypoxic and acidotic are difficult to resuscitate.

4. The reduced concentrating capacity of the kidney, which tends to be progressive, means that the patient cannot compensate for dehydration. Renal manifestations of the disease may result in end-stage renal disease requiring chronic haemodialysis or renal transplantation (Gyasi et al 1990).

5. Some cases of von Willebrand's disease have been reported in association with HbSS and HbAS in patients presenting with haematuria.

6. Children less than 3 years old are at risk from sepsis, usually pneumococcal, and from acute splenic sequestration.

7. Problems of pain relief, either postoperatively, or following sickle cell crisis.

8. Cholelithiasis is common and reported incidences vary from 4–55%, depending on the method of diagnosis. laparoscopic techniques are

becoming common (Ware et al 1992). Nine patients had RBC transfusions to reduce HbS levels and increase the Hb to 10 g/dl. In one patient conversion to open cholecystectomy was required because of intraoperative hypoxaemia and high pulmonary airway pressures (Cunningham & Schlanger 1992). The patient was only admitted on the morning of surgery and no formal assessment of lung disease had been made.

9. Problems of adenotonsillectomy (Derkay et al 1991).
10. Postoperative deaths from pulmonary embolism and acute chest syndrome have been reported (Gray et al 1991).

Section 1

Haemoglobinopathies
Sickle Cell Disease

Management

1. Diagnosis
   Sickle cell screening should be done in at-risk populations before anaesthesia, even when the Hb is normal. A normal haemoglobin can also occur in patients with HbSC, and yet severe sickling take place.
2. Manoeuvres to prevent sickling of red blood cells.
   a. Hypoxia in both the arterial and venous sides of the circulation must be avoided. Monitoring of both arterial and central venous Po_2 may be useful. Transcutaneous Po_2 measurement has been suggested, but does not always reflect arterial, or regional Po_2 (Dhamee et al 1982).
   b. Acidosis must not occur. A mild respiratory alkalosis can be maintained by IPPV. Alkalinization with sodium bicarbonate has been suggested, although significant degrees of alkalosis may impair oxygen release (see e.).
   c. Body temperature is maintained. Hypothermia increases sickling and blood viscosity, which result in stasis.
   d. Local circulatory stasis is prevented. Increased oxygen extraction, possibly producing dangerously low venous Po_2 levels despite a normal Po_2, is avoided. Vasopressors should be avoided. Although it has been recommended that tourniquets should not be used, two studies suggest that they are safe provided oxygenation and acid-base status are normal (Stein & Urbaniak 1980, Adu-Gyamfi et al 1993). During labour, precautions against aortocaval compression are essential. Extradural anaesthesia was reported to have improved a sickle cell crisis involving the extremities, in a patient in active labour (Finer et al 1988).
   e. Dehydration, which increases sickling, has to be avoided. The decreased concentrating capacity of the kidney accentuates the problem. To prevent dehydration, in the immediate preoperative period, 10 ml/kg per h of Hartmann's solution, with 44–50 mmol sodium bicarbonate added to each litre, has sometimes been recommended. This also maintains a mild alkalosis, but not all authorities agree that this is either necessary or effective.

f. Elective surgery should not take place in the presence of infection, as a crisis may be precipitated.
3. Measures to reduce the amount of HbS.
These are controversial. The complexity of each technique has tended to vary inversely with the number of patients reported. Since the highest incidence of the disease occurs in countries where facilities may be limited, this is perhaps not surprising. Series of 505 (Oduro & Searle 1972) and 284 (Homi et al 1979) general anaesthetics given to patients with various haemoglobinopathies, have been published. Six patients died in each group. All deaths occurred in the postoperative period, and in only two was there any suggestion that the anaesthetic management might have contributed. One patient, who had an elective procedure in spite of a preoperative pyrexia, died of pneumonia. The second, a man with a head injury, received sedation during a carotid angiogram. It should not be overlooked that in one of the series (Homi et al 1979) only 21% of the 202 patients with HbSS received a preoperative blood transfusion.
In contrast, transfusion as a means of reducing the relative amounts of HbS before, or during, surgery has been encouraged. It has been suggested that for, major surgery, the aim should be a reduction of HbS to 30%, in the presence of a haematocrit of 36% (Esseltine et al 1988).
Each technique has its indications, advantages and disadvantages:
a. Preoperative transfusion only if the haemoglobin is below a certain level (Homi et al 1979).
b. Preoperative transfusion of 15–20 ml/kg packed red cells, 1–2 days before elective, or immediately before emergency surgery (Janik & Seeler 1980).
c. Serial transfusions during a 10–15 day preoperative period.
d. Exchange transfusion either pre- or intraoperatively (Riethmuller et al 1982, Talacki & Ballas 1990). Partial exchange transfusion has also been used during pregnancy (Nagey et al 1981).
If operative transfusion is required, fresh blood, which has high 2,3-diphosphoglycerate levels, is preferable.
4. Management of vaso-occlusive crisis.
a. General measures of rest, warmth, rehydration and simple analgesics.
b. Treat infection promptly.
c. Pain relief. Patient-controlled analgesia with morphine was compared with i.v. morphine for sickle cell crisis and found to be equally safe and effective (Gonzalez et al 1991).
d. Chemotherapeutic agents such as hydroxyurea (Davies 1991).
5. Although the use of a cell-saver has been proposed (Romanoff et al 1988), this has been questioned because of the 50% incidence of sickling that was observed when the processed blood was examined

under the microscope (Brajtbord et al 1989). This was attributed to the cell-saver washing process.

6. Hydroxyurea administration increases the production of fetal haemoglobin (Rodgers et al 1990, Goldberg et al 1990), but trials are needed to show whether or not there is clinical benefit. No effect was seen from the use of erythropoietin (Goldberg et al 1990).

7. In a few centres, bone marrow transplantation is being performed (Davies 1991).

BIBLIOGRAPHY

Adu-Gyamfi Y, Sankarankutty M, Marwa S 1993 Use Of a tourniquet in patients with sickle-cell disease. Canadian Journal of Anaesthesia 40: 24–27

Anaesthesia Advisory Committee to the Chief Coroner of Ontario 1987 Intraoperative death during Caesarean section in a patient with sickle cell trait. Canadian Journal of Anaesthesia 34: 67–70

Brajtbord D, Johnson D, Ramsay M et al 1989 Use of the cell saver in patients with sickle cell trait. Anesthesiology 70: 878

Cunningham A J, Schlanger M 1992 Intraoperative hypoxemia complicating laparoscopic cholecystectomy in a patient with sickle hemoglobinopathy. Anesthesia and Analgesia 75: 838–843

Dalal F Y, Schmidt G B, Bennett E J et al 1974 Sickle-cell trait. A report of postoperative neurological complication. British Journal of Anaesthesia 46: 387–388

Davies S C 1991 The vaso-occlusive crisis of sickle cell disease. Time for coordinated trials of new treatment. British Medical Journal 302: 1551–1552

Davies S C, Wonke B 1991 The management of haemoglobinopathies Bailliere's Clinical Haematology 4.2: 361–389

Derkay C S, Bray G, Milmoe G J et al 1991 Adenotonsillectomy in children with sickle cell disease. Southern Medical Journal 84: 205–208

Dhamee M S, Whitesell R C, Munshi C 1982 Towards safer anaesthesia in sickle cell states. Anaesthesia 37: 94–95

Esseltine D W, Baxter M R N, Bevan J C 1988 Sickle cell states and the anaesthetist. Canadian Journal of Anaesthesia 35: 385–403

Finer P, Blair J, Rowe P 1988 Epidural analgesia in the management of labour pain and sickle cell crisis. Anesthesiology 68: 799–800

Francina A, Chassard D, Baklouti F et al 1989 Open-heart surgery in a patient with a high oxygen affinity haemoglobin variant. Anaesthesia 44: 31–33

Goldberg M A, Brugnara C, Dover G J et al 1990 Treatment of sickle cell anemia with hydroxyurea and erythropoietin. New England Journal of Medicine 323: 366–372

Gray A, Anionwu E N, Davies S C et al 1991 Patterns of mortality in sickle cell disease in the United Kingdom. Journal of Clinical Pathology 44: 459–463

Gonzalez E R, Bahal N, Hansen L A et al 1991 Intermittent injection vs patient-controlled analgesia for sickle cell crisis pain. Comparison in patients in the emergency department. Archives of Internal Medicine 151: 1373–1378

Gyasi H K, Zurroug A W, Matthew M et al 1990 Anaesthesia for renal transplantation in sickle cell disease. Canadian Journal of Anaesthesia 37: 778–785

Homi J, Reynolds J, Skinner A et al 1979 General anaesthesia in sickle cell disease. British Medical Journal 1: 1599–1601

Janik J, Seeler R A 1980 Perioperative management of children with sickle cell haemoglobinopathy. Journal of Pediatric Surgery 15: 117–120

Nagey D A, Garcia J, Welt S I 1981 Isovolumetric partial exchange transfusion in the management of sickle cell disease during pregnancy. American Journal of Obstetrics and Gynecology 141: 403–407

Oduro K A, Searle J F 1972 Anaesthesia in sickle cell states: a plea for simplicity. British Medical Journal 4: 596–598

Pollack C V Jr, Jorden R C, Kolb J C 1991 Usefulness of empiric chest radiography and urinalysis testing in adults with acute sickle cell pain crisis. Annals of Emergency Medicine 20: 1210–1214

Powars D P Weidman J A, Odom-Maryon T et al 1988 Sickle cell chronic lung
    disease: prior morbidity and the risk of pulmonary failure. Medicine 67: 66–75
Radhakrishnam K, Thacker A K, Maloo J C et al 1990 Sickle cell trait and stroke in
    the young adult. Postgraduate Medical Journal 66: 1078–1080
Riethmuller R, Grundy E M, Radley-Smith R 1982 Open heart surgery in a patient
    with homozygous sickle cell disease. Anaesthesia 37: 324–327
Rodgers G P 1991 Recent approaches to the treatment of sickle cell anemia. Journal of
    the American Medical Association 265: 2097–3101
Rodgers G P, Dover G J, Noguchi C T et al 1990 Haematologic responses of patients
    with sickle cell disease to treatment with hydroxyurea. New England Journal of
    Medicine 322: 1037–1045
Romanoff M E, Woodward D G, Bullard W G 1988 Autologous blood transfusion in
    patients with sickle cell trait. Anesthesiology 68: 820–821
Rucknagel D L, Kalinyak K A, Gelfand M J 1991 Rib infarcts and acute chest
    syndrome in sickle cell diseases. Lancet 337: 831–833
Singer M, Boghossian S, Bevan D H et al 1989 Hemodynamic changes during sickle
    cell crisis. American Journal of Cardiology 64: 1211–1213
Stein R E, Urbaniak J 1980 Use of the tourniquet during surgery in patients with
    sickle cell haemoglobinopathies. Clinical Orthopaedics and Related Research 151:
    231– 233
Talacki C A, Ballas S K 1990 Modified method of exchange transfusion in sickle cell
    disease. Journal of Clinical Apheresis 5: 183–187
Ware R E, Kinney T R, Casey J R et al 1992 Laparoscopic cholecystectomy in young
    patients with sickle hemoglobinopathies. Journal of Pediatrics 120: 58–61

HAEMOLYTIC URAEMIC SYNDROME

A syndrome of thrombocytopenia, haemolytic anaemia, renal vascular
injury and renal failure. It occurs most commonly in infants and young
children. In adults it tends to be associated with viral toxins,
immunosuppressive drugs, oral contraceptives or occur postpartum.
There is widespread vascular endothelial damage with deposition of
fibrin, and intravascular haemolysis. All organs are affected, although
the kidney is primarily involved. The prognosis in children is reasonably
good, whereas in adults the renal failure is usually irreversible.

Preoperative abnormalities

1. In young children, the presenting problem is usually gastroenteritis
   with bloody diarrhoea.
2. Progression occurs to haemolytic anaemia and renal failure. The
   exact mechanism and sequence of events is not known. However,
   the primary lesion appears to be one of renal vascular endothelial
   injury, possibly due to lipid peroxidation (Neild 1987). Factor VIII is
   released from the endothelium, and platelet aggregation, with
   subsequent thrombosis and necrosis, occurs. A deficiency of
   prostacyclin has also been demonstrated. The oxidant injury may
   also damage the red cells, which then become more susceptible to
   destruction. A consumptive coagulopathy is well recognized.
3. In adults, there may be a relevant drug history. Mitomycin C,
   5-fluorouracil and oral contraceptives have all been implicated.
   The syndrome can occur postpartum, and occasionally there may
   be a family history.

4. Hepatosplenomegaly may be present.
5. There is widespread organ involvement and the condition merges imperceptibly with thrombotic, thrombocytopenic purpura. Cardiac, neurological, and hepatic problems have been described.

Anaesthetic problems

1. Anaesthesia may be required for the creation of arteriovenous shunts for renal dialysis (Johnson & Rosales 1987).
2. Haematological problems include anaemia, thrombocytopenia and, occasionally, coagulation abnormalities.
3. Cardiovascular complications include hypertension, pericardial effusion, and heart failure.
4. Neurological complications include fits, unconsciousness, and hemiplegia.
5. Hepatic dysfunction may occur.

Management

1. Most of the patients are children, therefore peritoneal dialysis is the treatment of choice. If fluid overload and hyperkalaemia are already present, haemodialyis may be needed before the administration of a general anaesthetic.
2. Fresh frozen plasma may be of benefit.
3. Control of hypertension and fluid and electrolyte balance may be needed.
4. During anaesthesia, a technique using IPPV, isoflurane and atracurium, with neuromuscular monitoring, has been suggested (Johnson & Rosales 1987). Postoperative IPPV may be required.
5. Steroids are not indicated. Heparin is sometimes used.

BIBLIOGRAPHY
Johnson G D, Rosales J K 1987 The haemolytic uraemic syndrome and anaesthesia. Canadian Journal of Anaesthesia 34: 196–199
Neild G 1987 The haemolytic uraemic syndrome: A review. Quarterly Journal of Medicine 63: 367–376

HAEMOPHILIA A
(AND HAEMOPHILIA B)

Haemophilia A is a sex-linked recessive inherited coagulation disorder, associated with reduced levels of Factor VIII. Males are affected, whilst females are the carriers. Occasional instances of female deficiency have been described where the mother is a carrier and the father has haemophilia A. Haemophilia A is clinically indistinguishable from haemophilia B (Christmas disease), which is a rarer condition associated with a deficiency of Factor IX. Haemophilia A will be dealt with in detail, but the principles of the anaesthetic management of haemophilia B are similar.

Preoperative abnormalities

1. The clinical severity is related to Factor VIII levels as measured by clotting assay. The factor level can be expressed as iu/ml, or as a percentage of normal. The normal range is 50–200 iu/ml, or 50–200%

Factor level (%)	Clinical severity	Type of bleeding
<1	severe	frequent spontaneous bleeding
2–5	moderate	variable – some spontaneous bleeding; severe bleeding after trauma
6–15	mild	bleeding on trauma
>15	very mild	bleeding only after severe trauma

2. Spontaneous bleeding affects mainly joints and muscles. Inadequately treated, recurrent joint bleeds can lead to ankylosis and permanent joint deformities.
3. Coagulation tests detect the abnormality in intrinsic pathway with prolongation of partial thromboplastin generation. Whole blood clotting time is usually normal except in the most severe cases. Bleeding time is normal. Definitive diagnosis by Factor VIII:C assay.
4. Treatment is by replacement of deficient Factor VIII.
5. Complications of treatment include production of Factor VIII antibodies (6–10%), Factor VIII inhibitors in 3.6–25% patients (Ehrenforth et al 1992), allergic reactions, and transmission of viruses, especially hepatitis C (Tedder et al 1991), hepatitis B and HIV.

Anaesthetic problems

1. High risk of transmitting hepatitis B or C.
2. Need to avoid i.m. injections and regional anaesthesia. Special care is required during laryngoscopy and tracheal intubation.
3. Problems of venous access.
4. Although Factor VIII levels in female carriers are usually 50%, there may be a wide range of Factor VIII:C activity. An 11-month-old girl who required adenoidectomy had a level of 22% and needed perioperative treatment (Harrison et al 1991).

Management

1. Advice of a haematologist, and knowledge of an individual patient's history is essential.
2. Sources of Factor VIII concentrate:
   a. Cryoprecipitate. Average Factor VIII content is about 2 iu/ml. It is only suitable for treatment in children or mild haemophiliacs.

b. Human freeze-dried Factor VIII. Both NHS and commercial preparations are available. All preparations are now heat treated to eliminate HIV infections.

c. Animal freeze-dried Factor VIII. Commercially produced bovine and porcine with high potency of animal Factor VIII. The material is highly antigenic and is indicated for patients with high-titre Factor VIII antibodies.

$$\text{Dose in units of Factor VIII} = \frac{\% \text{ rise needed} \times \text{patients weight in kg}}{1.5-2}$$

3. Prior to major surgery, patients should be tested to exclude Factor VIII antibodies, and assess the response to Factor VIII infusion.

4. During surgery, the infusion therapy should be controlled by specific factor assay. The amount and duration of treatment depends on the response to Factor VIII infusion, and its half-life (between 7–22 hours, with an average of 12 hours). It also depends on the nature of the operation and the time taken for the wound to heal.

   In severe haemophilia A it is usual to give an immediate preoperative dose of 50 iu/kg of Factor VIII, and on the evening of operation a second dose of 25 iu/kg. The pre- and postinfusion Factor VIII level should be measured for the first dose. On the second day, 25 iu/kg is given twice daily and continued for 7–10 days. A safe objective is to keep the postinfusion Factor VIII near 100% and the preinfusion level near 50% for the first postoperative week. Daily assays are thus needed for the first week, then less frequently. After 7–10 days, it is usually safe to reduce the frequency of doses from twice to once daily. If Factor VIII level is found to be particularly low in individual patients, then more frequent administration of Factor VIII is needed.

5. In mild haemophiliacs undergoing minor surgery or dental extraction, i.v. infusion of desmopressin in a dose of 0.3 µg/kg in 50 ml saline 0.9% will give a short-term increase in Factor VIII. Water retention may occur. Stimulation of the fibrinolytic system necessitates the simultaneous use of tranexamic acid.

6. Dental surgery may be carried out if covered by a single dose of Factor VIII, 25–30 iu/kg. Tranexamic acid 10 mg/kg i.v. is given initially, then 15 mg/kg t.d.s. orally is continued for 10 days. Postoperatively, infection predisposes to bleeding, so prophylactic antibiotics are needed.

7. The presence of Factor VIII antibody is a contraindication to surgery, except where life saving. Under such circumstances large doses may have to be given (Rizza 1984).

8. In three large retrospective studies of surgery in haemophilia and related disorders, individual problem cases were discussed. (Sampson et al 1979, Kasper et al 1985, Kitchens 1986). The safety of elective surgery performed in large centres was emphasized. However, the incidence of postoperative bleeding varied from 5%

(Sampson et al 1979) to 23% (Kasper et al 1985). A range of Factor VIII levels were achieved, but the minimum level required to prevent postoperative bleeding is still to be determined. Average trough levels of about 30% in the first 5 days have been recorded and have led to the suggestion that the previously recommended levels were not necessary (Sampson et al 1979). On the contrary, there are cases in which postoperative bleeding occurred despite adequate levels of Factor VIII (Kasper et al 1985). Increasing Factor VIII doses three-fold, from 600 to 2000 iu/kg per operation, to raise the trough levels from 37% to 70%, did not reduce the incidence of postoperative bleeding. It was concluded that Factor VIII levels could not be the only determinant of bleeding in haemophilia.

9. Analgesia must be carefully managed. In the above series, persistence of bleeding was sometimes related to the inadvertent use of aspirin-containing compounds or NSAIDs. Mild pain should be treated with paracetamol, pentazocine, dihydrocodeine or buprenorphine. Opiate analgesics should be used with caution to prevent addiction.

HAEMOPHILIA B (CHRISTMAS DISEASE)
(SEE ALSO HAEMOPHILIA A)

A sex-linked recessive inherited coagulation disorder associated with reduced levels of factor IX.

Preoperative abnormalities

1. For clinical features and severity see Haemophilia A.
2. Coagulation tests detect the abnormality in intrinsic pathway and the definitive diagnosis is made on Factor IX assay.

Anaesthetic problems
See Haemophilia A.

Management

1. The principles of treatment for major surgery and dental extraction are the same as in Haemophilia A. However, desmopressin is not effective in Factor IX deficiency.
2. Treatment is by replacement with Factor IX concentrates (both NHS and commercial)
   The recovery of Factor IX is less than in Factor VIII, so the dose required is greater:

   $$\text{Dose in units of Factor IX} = \frac{\%\text{ rise needed} \times \text{patients weight in kg}}{0.9}$$

BIBLIOGRAPHY
Ehrenforth S, Kreuz W, Scharrer I et al 1992 Incidence of development of factor
    VIII and factor IX inhibitors in haemophiliacs. Lancet 339: 594–598
Harrison H C, Lammi A 1991 Adenoidectomy in a girl with haemophilia. Journal of
    Otology and Laryngology 105: 957–958
Kasper C K, Boylen A L, Ewing N P et al 1985, Hematologic management of
    hemophilia A for surgery. Journal of the American Medical Association 253: 1279–
    1283.
Kitchens C S 1986 Surgery in hemophilia and related disorders. Medicine 65: 34–45
Rizza C R 1984 Haemophilia A and B. Prescribers' Journal 24: 77–78.
Sampson J F, Hamstra R, Aldrete J A 1979 Management of hemophiliac patients
    undergoing surgical procedures. Anesthesia and Analgesia 58: 133–135.
Tedder R S, Briggs M, Ring C et al 1991 Hepatitis C antibody profile and viraemia
    prevalence in adults with severe haemophilia. British Journal of Haematology 79:
    512–515

HALLERVORDEN-SPATZ DISEASE

A rare autosomal recessive disease of the basal ganglia, most probably
involving iron and lipid metabolism. The clinical syndrome is one of
onset in childhood, progressive dementia, choreoathetosis, dystonia and
spasticity. Hallervorden-Spatz disease is technically a postmortem
diagnosis. Only after death can the histological features of iron
deposition in the substantia nigra and pallidal nuclei, with gliosis,
demyelination and axonal swelling, be confirmed.

Preoperative abnormalities

1. Clinical features are those of dyskinesia, spasticity, torticollis,
   increasing scoliosis and severe mental retardation. Pigmentary
   degeneration of the retina has been described.
2. The spontaneous appearance of an NMS-like syndrome has been
   reported; hyperthermia, rigidity, impaired conscious level and
   autonomic imbalance (Hayashi et al 1993).
3. Occasionally, late-onset disease may occur. One patient presented
   with Parkinsonian features in a family in which all children died
   before the age of 25 (Jankovic et al 1985).
4. Sea-blue histiocytes are seen on bone marrow examination.

Anaesthetic problems

1. Oropharyngeal rigidity has been reported (Roy et al 1983).
2. Swallowing disorders are common and patients tend to choke on
   food and secretions.
3. Noxious stimuli may intensify the dystonia.
4. It has been suggested that these patients may present spontaneously
   with clinical features similar to those of neuroleptic malignant
   syndrome, but in the absence of precipitating neuroleptic drugs
   (Hayashi et al 1993).

Management

1. Increasing depth of anaesthesia caused relaxation of rigidity, torticollis and some scoliosis (Roy et al 1983). The dystonia returned on emergence.
2. Suxamethonium should be avoided.
3. The use of dantrolene for hyperthermia and muscle rigidity has been described (Hayashi et al 1993).

BIBLIOGRAPHY

Jankovic J, Kirkpatrick J B, Blomquist K A et al 1985 late-onset Hallervorden-Spatz disease presenting as familial parkinsonism. Neurology 35: 227–234
Hayashi K, Chihara E, Sawa T et al 1993 Clinical features of neuroleptic syndrome in basal ganglia disease. Spontaneous presentation in a patient with Halleruorden-Spatz syndrome in the absence of neuroleptic drugs. Anaesthesia 48: 499–502
Roy R C, McClain S, Wise A et al 1983 Anesthestic management of a patient with Hallervorden-Spatz disease. Anesthesiology 58: 382–384
Williams D J, Ironside J W 1989 Liver and pituitary abnormalities in Hallervorden-Spatz disease. Journal of Neurology, Neurosurgery and Psychiatry 52: 1410–1414

HEART BLOCK
(see also SICK SINUS SYNDROME)

A patient may present for surgery either with a permanent pacemaker implanted, or with a bradyarrhythmia which may require the insertion of a temporary transvenous pacemaker for the perioperative period. Increasing numbers of pacemakers are being implanted, and in some cases increasingly complex electronic devices are being used.

Preoperative abnormalities

1. Heart block may be congenital or acquired, and the latter either acute or chronic.
    Congenital heart block may occur alone, or in association with other cardiac abnormalities. As an isolated phenomenon it is relatively benign, since the block to conduction is at the level of the AV node. The ventricular pacemaker is proximal to the bifurcation of the bundle of His, so the QRS complexes are narrow, and the ventricular conduction system intact. The rate is relatively high and can vary from 40 to 80 per minute, and may increase with exercise. However, sudden death may occasionally occur.
    In chronic acquired heart block the defect is more distal in the conducting system. The AV junction or bundle branches are usually involved, the QRS complexes are wide, the heart rate is lower and not increased by exercise. The prognosis is generally worse, but ultimately depends on the underlying cause.
2. Heart block can be divided into three types:
    a. First-degree AV block: P–R interval prolonged beyond 0.21 s.

b. Second-degree AV block:
  i. Type I. Progressive P–R lengthening until a complete failure of conduction and a beat is dropped (Wenkebach phenomenon).
  ii. Type II. Intermittent failure of AV conduction without preceding prolongation of P–R interval. This type is of more serious significance than type I, and often progresses to third degree AV block.
c. Third-degree AV block: Complete dissociation of the atria and ventricles due to failure of atrial impulses to be transmitted.
3. Patients may present with syncopal (Stokes-Adams) attacks, fatigue, angina or heart failure.

Anaesthetic problems

1. Patients with second-degree heart block, particularly type II, may progress to complete heart block under anaesthesia, since most volatile agents prolong cardiac conduction.
2. Those with complete heart block may be unable to compensate for a fall in cardiac output by increasing their ventricular rate. Organ blood flow, significantly that to the myocardium and brain, may be dramatically reduced. When increases in stroke volume can no longer compensate for slow heart rates, cardiac failure occurs.
3. When patients with heart block are anaesthetized, there is no method of monitoring the adequacy of cerebral blood flow and hence there is the risk of cerebral damage.
4. The problems of the underlying cause. The commonest cause of third-degree AV block in the elderly is idiopathic fibrosis. However, other causes include coronary artery disease, cardiomyopathy, drugs and cardiac surgery.
5. The use of surgical diathermy in the presence of pacemakers may produce complications:
  a. With an older type of pacemaker, ventricular fibrillation has been reported rarely (Titel & El-Etr 1968).
  b. Inhibition of demand pacemaker function (Wajszczuk et al 1969) or interference with AV sequential pacemaker (Dressner & Lebowitz 1988).
  c. 'Phantom' reprogramming of a programmable pacemaker (Domino & Smith 1983).
  d. Idiosyncratic responses in multiprogrammable pacemakers. In one case, interference with the quartz crystal clock was interpreted as impending battery failure and the pacemaker went into a slow back-up mode aimed at preserving battery life (Shapiro et al 1985).
  e. Asystole occurred as a result of the diathermy indirectly causing battery drainage and pacemaker failure (Mangar et al 1991).

6. In order to prevent pacemaker inhibition during diathermy, the placing of a strong magnet over the pulse generator has, in the past, been recommended (Simon 1977). This is said to change a demand pacemaker (VVI) to an asynchronous one (VOO). With modern pacemakers this should not be done because it may allow the electromagnetic waves of the diathermy to reprogramme and change the firing rate of the pacemaker.

7. Pacemaker failure can occur during anaesthesia. Generator failure has occurred on induction of anaesthesia after administration of suxamethonium (Finfer 1991). Myopotentials were thought to have inhibited pacemaker function. Generator failure may also occur if the stimulator threshold increases above the maximum output of the generator. This has been attributed to endocardial burns following defibrillation (Finfer 1991) and the use of unipolar diathermy during TURP (Kellow 1993).

8. Pacemaker failure occurred after a magnetic instrument mat was placed on the chest of a patient before surgery started (Purday & Towey 1992). In this particular pacemaker, the application of a magnet activated the test sequence for determining the stimulation threshold for capture. This chain of events was confirmed subsequently in the cardiology clinic, using the magnetic mat.

9. Special problems may occur with rate-responsive pacemakers (Andersen & Madsen 1990). Changes during surgery and anaesthesia can act as a stimulus to a rate increase and result in unphysiological pacing rates. For example, respiration-sensing pacemakers may respond to manual hyperventilation by producing a tachycardia. This was initially interpreted as a sign of light anaesthesia and later on as hypovolaemia, in a patient undergoing a TURP. The pulse rate only returned to normal when the anaesthetist stopped manual ventilation in order to set up a blood transfusion (Madsen & Andersen 1989). A movement-sensing pacemaker may respond to vigorous surgical stimulation. Intraoperative somatosensory evoked potentials acted as a stimulus causing pacemaker-mediated tachycardia (Merritt et al 1988).

10. Pacemaker failure may occur during surgery. This may be due to loose connections, battery failure, displacement of a lead or a change in pacemaker threshold.

11. Ventricular demand pacemakers do not allow sequential AV contraction, therefore left ventricular systolic performance may be decreased when pacing takes over (Ducey et al 1991). Reprogramming of the pacemaker or therapeutic suppression may be required.

12. Halothane increases the pacing threshold and should be avoided.

13. Potential problems for patients undergoing extracorporeal shock wave lithotripsy (ESWL) (Celentano et al 1992). One episode of bradycardia which responded to isoprenaline was reported, but in

general cardiac pacemakers do not seem to be damaged. In a survey of 98 units undertaking ESWL, complications were minor and in only one patient was the pacemaker spontaneously deprogrammed by lithotripsy (Drach et al 1990).

14. Patients with pacemakers should not undergo magnetic resonance imaging. The magnet may cause pacemaker failure, reprogramming or microshock.

Management

1. The indications for insertion of a transvenous pacemaker before surgery are sometimes debatable, but may include:
   a. Sinoatrial node dysfunction producing a brady/tachyarrhythmia syndrome.
   b. Second- or third-degree AV block
   c. LBBB and first-degree heart block.
   d. Bifascicular block. RBBB in combination with posterior fascicular block often progresses to third-degree heart block. It has therefore been suggested that bifascicular block is an indication for a temporary pacemaker. However, some authors believe this to be unnecessary (Rooney et al 1976). No complications occurred during extradural anaesthesia in patients with RBBB and left anterior fascicular block who were asymptomatic (Coriat et al 1981).

   It has also been suggested that a temporary pacemaker is unnecessary in congenital complete heart block, especially in children, since the rate is usually relatively high and the prognosis good. However, should problems occur, temporary transvenous cardiac pacing takes time to initiate. In a prospective survey of 153 insertions, the median time was found to be 20 minutes (Donovan & Lee 1984).

2. If a permanent pacemaker is already in place, information on its mode of function should be sought (Horgan 1984). All patients with pacemakers are regularly reviewed in a pacemaker clinic. Its markings, date of insertion and battery life should be checked.
   a. Pacemaker markings:
   I Chamber paced:
   V = ventricle, A = atrium, D = dual (A & V).
   II Chamber sensed:
   V = ventricle, A = atrium, D = dual (A & V), O = none.
   III Mode of response:
   T = triggered, I = inhibited, D = dual (T or I), O = none.
   IV Programmable functions:
   P = programmable (rate and/or output), M = multiprogrammable, C = communicating, O = none, R = rate-response.

V Special anti-tathyarrhythmic functions:

  B = bursts of impulses, N = normal rate competition, S = scanning response, E = externally activated.

b. Pacemaker type and function.

The most common type of pacemaker in use is VVI. The chamber paced is the ventricle, as is the chamber sensed, and the pacemaker is inhibited by spontaneous ventricular activity.

A programmable pacemaker is one in which certain parameters such as rate, sensitivity, output and refractory period, can be changed non-invasively. This is accomplished by the use of a programmer, which sends electromagnetic coded signals to the pacemaker. Some of the multiprogrammable ones have extremely complex functions to treat difficult arrthythmias and to anticipate problems such as battery failure.

Although VVI will be the most frequently encountered, other types of pacemaker may be needed on occasions, to cope with individual requirements or pacing problems (Shaw & Whistance 1986, Andersen & Madsen 1990). Some of these are associated with particular individual problems during anaesthesia. If a complex rate-responsive pacemaker is encountered, Andersen & Madsen's article should be consulted.

  i. Maintenance of atrial transport. Atrial demand pacemakers (AAI) are useful in sick sinus syndrome, when atrioventricular conduction is intact. It is haemodynamically advantageous if atrial synchrony is maintained, since an atrial contribution to ventricular filling may improve the cardiac output by up to 30%, as compared with that produced by VVI pacemakers. This may be important for patients with ventricular pacing, who are experiencing symptoms suggestive of the pacemaker syndrome. Dizziness or syncope may result from hypotension due to loss of atrioventricular synchrony, or to retrograde ventriculoatrial conduction.

  ii. Rate responsiveness to exercise. Dual-chamber pacemakers (e.g. DDD), can stimulate both chambers in sequence, and if atrial activity is normal they allow a 'physiological' response to exercise. When there is sinus disease, other variables will have to be used to assess body activity. A new generation of rate-responsive pacemakers has been developed which are responsive to various physiological variables such as respiration, temperature, Q-T interval, myocardial contractility, oxygen saturation and blood pH changes.

  iii. Antitachycardia pacemakers. These have been designed to detect tachycardias, then terminate them by breaking the re-entrant circuit.

c. Pacemaker threshold

If possible, a cardiologist should be asked to check the pacing threshold, which is the minimum voltage necessary for the pacing stimulus to capture the ventricles consistently. Pacemaker function depends on both electrical and non-electrical factors. The threshold for capture is dependent upon cellular factors such as acid-base balance, hypoxia, potassium and drugs. If the threshold increases, there may be intermittent failure of pacing. If the threshold decreases there is a risk of inducing ventricular fibrillation.

d. Detection of pacemaker dysfunction

The occurrence of syncope may suggest pacemaker dysfunction. A 10% decrease in heart rate in a fixed rate pacemaker may indicate impending battery failure. An irregular heart rate in a VVI pacemaker means that R waves are not being sensed.

3. The use of diathermy.

Advice is still usually given that this should only be used if really necessary. Although many of the modern pacemakers are said to be safe with diathermy, problems have been encountered (Mangar et al 1991, Kellow 1993). As pacemakers have become more complex, with programmes both to detect and eliminate external electrical interference, and to provide back-up for programme or battery failure, so idiosyncratic complications may arise. Two cases of apparent pacemaker malfunction have been reported, which were a direct result of the complex back-up functions of the pacemaker (Shapiro et al 1985).

If diathermy is needed:

a. Place the indifferent electrode of the diathermy on the same side as the operating site and as far away from the pacemaker as possible;

b. Limit its frequency and duration of use, and keep the diathermy current as low as possible.

c. Use a bipolar rather than a unipolar diathermy.

d. Check the patient's pulse for inhibition of pacemaker function.

e. With a programmable pacemaker, it might be helpful to have the programmer itself available in theatre, so that the programming could be checked at the end of the operation. However, in many cases this is not feasible.

4. Pacemaker failure (Donovan & Lee 1984)

Whenever a pacemaker is in place, atropine, adrenaline and isoprenaline should be available, for use in the event of pacemaker failure.

If failure to pace occurs with a temporary pacemaker:

a. Try reversing the polarity.

b. Try increasing the output to maximum.

c. Change to VOO (asynchronous) mode.

d. Check that the connections are intact.

e. Change the whole unit, or the batteries.

f. If using a bipolar lead, try each as unipolar.

g. Turn the patient into the left lateral position to improve electrode contact.

h. Change the pacing lead.

5. If pacing with a ventricular demand pacemaker results in decreased cardiac output, pacemaker suppression may be required. A peripheral nerve stimulator on the ipsilateral shoulder was used to provide a stimulus which suppressed the pacemaker and allowed a patient's normal sinus rhythm to return the blood pressure and cardiac output to normal (Ducey et al 1991).

6. Monitoring of pulse and blood pressure
   Blood pressure should be carefully monitored. If the ECG is susceptible to diathermy influence, then other methods of pulse observation, such as palpation or an oesophageal stethoscope, should be used to detect pacemaker inhibition. Direct arterial monitoring is advisable in major cases.

7. In patients requiring extracorporeal shock wave lithotripsy, the presence of a cardiologist and equipment for emergency transvenous pacing has been recommended (Drach et al 1990, Celentano et al 1992).

8. Should defibrillation be required, the paddles should be positioned as far away from the generator as possible, preferably in an anterior/posterior position. Loss of capture may occur subsequently secondary to an endocardial burn and an increase in stimulus output may be required.

BIBLIOGRAPHY

Andersen C, Madsen G M 1990 Rate-responsive pacemaker and anaesthesia. A consideration of possible implications. Anaesthesia 45: 472–476

Bloomfield P, Bowler G M R 1989 Anaesthetic management of a patient with a permanent pacemaker. Anaesthesia 44: 42–46

Celentano W J, Jahr J S. Nossaman B D 1992 Extracorporeal shockwave lithotripsy in a patient with a pacemaker. Anesthesia and Analgesia 74: 770–772

Coriat P, Harari A, Ducardonet A et al 1981 Risk of advanced heart block during extradural anaesthesia in patients with right bundle branch block and left anterior hemiblock. British Journal of Anaesthesia 53: 545–548

Domino K B, Smith T C 1983 Electrocautery-induced reprogramming of a pacemaker using a precordial magnet. Anesthesia and Analgesia 62: 609–612

Donovan K D, Lee K Y 1984 Indications for and complications of temporary transvenous cardiac pacing. Anaesthesia and Intensive Care 13: 63–70

Drach G W, Weber C, Donovan J M 1990 Treatment of pacemaker patients with extracorporeal shock wave lithotripsy: experience from 2 continents. Journal of Urology 143: 895–896

Dressner D L, Lebowitz p W 1988 Atrioventricular sequential pacemaker inhibition by transurethral electrosurgery. Anesthesiology 68: 599–601

Ducey J P, Fincher C W Baysinger C L 1991 Therapeutic suppression of a permanent ventricular pacemaker using a peripheral nerve stimulator. Anesthesiology 75: 533–536

Finfer S R 1991 Pacemaker failure on induction of anaesthesia. British Journal of Anaesthesia 66: 509–512

Horgan J H 1984 Cardiac pacing. British Medical Journal 288: 1942–1944

Kellow N H 1993. Pacemaker failure during transurethral resection of the prostate. Anaesthesia 48: 136–138.

Madsen G M, Andersen C 1989 Pacemaker-induced tachycardia during general anaesthesia: a case report. British Journal of Anaesthesia 63: 360–361.

Mangar D, Atlas G M, Kane P B 1991 Electrocautery-induced pacemaker malfunction. Canadian Journal of Anaesthesia 38: 616–618.

Merritt W T, Brinker J A, Beattie C 1988 Pacemaker mediated bradycardia induced by intraoperative somatosensory evoked potential stimuli. Anesthesiology 69: 766–768.

Purday J P, Towey R M 1992 Apparent pacemaker failure caused by activation of ventricular threshold test by a magnetic instrument mat during general anaesthesia. British Journal of Anaesthesia 69: 645–646.

Rooney S-M, Goldiner P L, Muss E 1976 Relationship of right bundle branch block and marked left axis deviation to complete heart block during general anaesthesia. Anesthesiology 44: 64–66.

Shapiro W A, Roizen M F, Singleton M A et al 1985 Intraoperative pacemaker complications. Anesthesiology 63: 319–322.

Shaw D B, Whistance A W T 1986 Clever pacemakers. Hospital Update: 843–852.

Simon A B 1977 Perioperative management of the pacemaker patient. Anesthesiology 46: 127–131.

Titel J H, El-Etr A A 1968 Fibrillation resulting from pacemaker electrodes and electrocautery during surgery. Anesthesiology 29: 845–846.

Wajszczuk W J, Mowry F M, Dugan N L 1969 Deactivation of a demand pacemaker by transurethral electrocautery. New England Journal of Medicine 280: 34–35.

HELLP SYNDROME
(see also ECLAMPSIA)

A rare complication of pregnancy-induced hypertension (PIH), it is characterized by Haemolysis, Elevated Liver enzyme activity and Low Platelet count. Reported to occur in 5–10% patients with PIH, it carries a maternal mortality of 2–24% and a perinatal mortality of 8–40%. A high proportion of the patients will require operative delivery; in a series of 33 patients presenting over 5 years, 94% required Caesarean section (Crosby 1991). In another study of 112 cases, there were two maternal deaths, two patients had ruptured liver haematomas and nine had renal failure (Sibai et al 1986).

Preoperative abnormalities

1. The presence of PIH or eclampsia, although this is not always severe.
2. Clinical signs include epigastric pain and tenderness, hypertension, proteinuria, nausea and vomiting. Upper abdominal pain and nausea or vomiting are the commonest presenting complaints (Crosby 1991).
3. Thrombocytopenia is present.
4. Jaundice and disordered liver function. Rarely, liver rupture has been reported (Sibai et al 1986).
5. Hypovolaemia and decreasing urine output.
6. Other complications have included adult respiratory distress syndrome, acute renal failure and abruptio placenta.

7. Abnormalities of coagulation (other than thrombocytopenia) are not commonly observed and some authors have concluded that DIC is not a complication. However, it occurred in 3 out of 33 in one series (Crosby 1991). In addition, close observation suggests that some coagulation activation does take place. One study compared coagulation in 15 consecutive patients with HELLP syndrome with 12 who had pregnancy-induced hypertension alone. Sensitive and specific coagulation assays showed that patients with the HELLP syndrome had a compensated DIC. These abnormalities persisted over several days indicating that there was a continuing, but mild trigger to the coagulation system (de Boer et al 1991). It has been suggested that fibrin deposition may occur and may be responsible for the liver, kidney and placental dysfunction in these patients.

Anaesthetic problems

1. Care of the ill parturient with PIH (See Eclampsia).
2. Possible bleeding problems secondary to thrombocytopenia. Frequently, extradural catheters are in place before the syndrome is recognized, and persistent bleeding into the extradural space has been reported (Sibai et al 1986).
3. Problems of expediting delivery.
4. Management of other complications such as renal failure and ARDS.
5. Thirty one per cent of patients present postpartum.
6. The differential diagnosis is from haemolytic uraemic syndrome and thrombotic thrombocytopenic purpura.

Management

1. Investigations include Hb, white cell count, platelet count, partial thromboplastin time, fibrinogen concentration, FDP, liver function tests, and urea and electrolyte concentrations.
2. Ill patients may need to be transferred to an ITU where close monitoring of CVP and urinary output can take place. Hypovolaemia should be treated and a urine output of 0.5 ml/kg per hour maintained.
3. FFP and platelets are required to increase the platelet count to more than 50 000/mm^3. Patterson & O'Toole (1991) described the management of Caesarean section for twins in a patient with a platelet count of 22 000/mm^3, haemolytic anaemia and abnormal liver function tests. CVP and urinary output were monitored. Fresh frozen plasma and 6 units of platelets increased the platelet count to 50 000/mm^3 and a hydralazine infusion controlled the arterial blood pressure.
4. Control of hypertension and, if general anaesthesia is required, treatment to attenuate the hypertensive response to tracheal intubation (see Eclampsia and PIH).

5. The baby should be delivered expeditiously, preferably vaginally, if the gestation is beyond 34 weeks. However, Caesarean section is usually required, and unless an extradural catheter is already sited, general anaesthesia is necessary.
6. Should an extradural catheter be in place when thrombocytopenia develops (Duffy 1988), a neurological assessment must be carried out before each top up. Otherwise, extradural anaesthesia should not be undertaken.
7. Monitor on the ITU for at least 48 hours.

BIBLIOGRAPHY

Aarnoudse J G, Houthoff W J, Weits J et al 1986 A syndrome of liver damage and intravascular coagulation in the last trimester of normotensive pregnancy. A clinical and histopathological study. British Journal of Obstetrics and Gynaecology 93: 145–155.

Barton J R, Sibai B M 1991 Care of the pregnancy complicated by HELLP syndrome. Obstetric and Gynecology Clinics of North America 18: 165–179.

Crosby E T 1991 Obstetrical anaesthesia for patients with the syndrome of haemolysis, elevated liver enzymes and low platelets. Canadian Journal of Anaesthesia 38: 227–233.

de Boer K, Buller H R, Ten Cate J W et al 1991 Coagulation studies in the syndrome of haemolysis, elevated Liver enzymes and low platelets. British Journal of Obstetrics and Gynaecoloy 98: 42–47

Duffy B L. 1988 HELLP syndrome and the anaesthetist. Anaesthesia 43: 223–225

Patterson K W, O'Toole D P 1991 HELLP syndrome: a case report with guidelines for management. British Journal of Anaesthesia 66: 513–515

Sibai B M, Taslimi M M, El-Nazer A et al 1986 Maternal-perinatal outcome associated with the syndrome of hemolysis, elevated liver enzymes, and low platelets in severe preeclampsia-eclampsia. American Journal of Obstetrics and Gynecology 155: 501–509

Weinstein L 1982 Syndrome of hemolysis, elevated liver enzymes and low platelet count: a severe consequence of hypertension of pregnancy. American Journal of Obstetrics and Gynecoloy 142: 159–167

HEPATITIS (VIRAL)

A number of different viruses cause individual types of hepatitis:

1. Hepatitis A virus (HAV).
2. Hepatitis B virus (HBV).
3. Hepatitis C (previously known as non-A non-B hepatitis virus).
4. Epstein-Barr virus (EBV: in infectious mononucleosis).
5. Cytomegalovirus.
6. Herpes simplex virus.

HEPATITIS A

Usually occurs in children and has an incubation period of between 15 and 40 days. Spread is primarily gastrointestinal. Serological diagnosis depends on finding antibody in the IgM plasma fraction in the acute stage, and subsequently in the IgG fraction, which indicates immunity.

Gamma globulin is of prophylactic value. HAV accounts for only about 20% of adult hepatitis.

HEPATITIS B

Is of particular interest to the anaesthetist and is considered in some detail.

Epidemiology

Hepatitis B has a long incubation period, of 2–6 months, and was initially thought to be spread only by the parenteral route. Until the 1960s, HAV and HBV infections were clinically indistinguishable, other than by inference from a history of blood transfusion, the incubation period, or by epidemiological studies.

Studies on institutionalized mentally retarded children not only confirmed the differences in incubation period between the two diseases, but unexpectedly showed that both viruses could be transmitted either orally or parenterally. HBV could therefore be transmitted by close physical contact, and actual skin penetration was not essential. Differentiation between the two diseases by inference, from a history of parenteral transmission, was therefore no longer reliable.

Australia antigen

An antibody was discovered in a haemophiliac which reacted with the serum of an Australian aborigine. This new antigen was therefore named the Australia antigen. It was later found to be associated only with serum hepatitis. Subsequent widespread testing for the Australia antigen revealed that particular populations had a higher incidence of the antigen than others. Amongst these were leukaemics, haemophiliacs, institutionalized patients, drug abusers, patients with chronic renal failure on dialysis, those of Central African origin and paid blood donors in the USA.

Australia antigen and renal dialysis units

Patients with renal failure proved to be a particular problem. They often had a mild form of hepatitis and readily became asymptomatic carriers. The widespread contact with blood and dialysis patients on haemodialysis units facilitated HBV transmission so that in the late 1960s many dialysis units had epidemics of hepatitis. Screening of all blood donors, barrier techniques, and the provision of separate facilities for infected patients, has resulted in HBV no longer being epidemic in British renal units after 1973. However, this is not so with all units abroad, so any relaxation of strict screening of patients may still have serious effects.

Serological markers (Tedder 1980)

The Australia antigen is now known as hepatitis B surface antigen (HBsAg) and denotes current HBV infection. Antibody (antiHBs) means past infection and present immunity. If HBV is treated with detergent, the core structure with its antigen HBcAg is released. AntiHBc is normally present in excess and therefore free HBcAg is never detected in serum. The presence of AntiHBc indicates past or present infection and levels may be very high in carriers. A further antigen (HBeAg), is detectable in the early stages of infection and in some carriers.

HEPATITIS C

This is the commonest type of hepatitis associated with blood transfusion, and routine testing of blood donors for antibodies to components of the hepatitis C virus began in the UK in 1991 (Fagan 1991). Hepatitis C accounts for about half of the non-A, non-B hepatitis post transfusion. There is evidence for sexual transmission (Tedder et al 1991).

Anaesthetic problems of hepatitis B virus

1. There is a small risk of infection from a patient with HBV. Transmission can occur by accidental inoculation, by splashing infected material into the eye or, occasionally, by ingestion of virus-containing material.
2. If infection occurs and the anaesthetist is not immune, acute hepatitis may manifest itself after 2–6 months. Occasionally it is fatal. The majority of patients will be normal afterwards and the antigen usually disappears from the serum within 4 weeks. A few patients may develop chronic liver disease.
3. After infection, some apparently healthy people become carriers of the antigen and therefore are potentially dangerous to other people.
4. HBV is resistant to destruction by physical methods.

Management

1. Selective patient screening
   Patients admitted to hospital who fall into one of the increased risk categories should be screened. These may include drug addicts, haemophiliacs, homosexuals, renal patients, those with tattoos, and patients who have had recent jaundice. Elective surgery should be delayed in patients with acute hepatitis until they are no longer infectious.
2. A carrier state is confirmed when at least two specimens over a period of a few months have similar HBeAg levels. Carriers are divided into 'simple', who are of low infectivity, and 'super' carriers who are highly infectious. These can be distinguished serologically (Tedder 1980).

3. The DHS has now advised that certain hospital staff, including those working in operating theatres, should be vaccinated against HBV. Guidelines on hepatitis B and AIDS have been issued by the Association of Anaesthetists (1988).
4. The wearing of gloves should be a routine for all procedures in which contact with blood or other secretions is anticipated. At present this practice is low, even amongst anaesthetists (O'Donnell & Asbury 1992a, b).
5. If accidental inoculation of a member of staff occurs from a HBsAg patient, screening of that member should be immediately performed. If there is evidence of immunity, nothing more need be done. If not, passive immunization with HB immunoglobulin should be carried out within 24–48 hours and again at 1 month. Active immunization can be given at the same time. The genetically engineered vaccines (e.g. Engerix B) have replaced those from human sources.
6. Operating theatre management of HBsAg-positive patients.
   a. The patient should be last on the theatre list.
   b. Minimise the number of staff in theatre.
   c. Staff should wear gown, gloves, masks and visors.
   d. Attempt to use only disposable linen and instruments.
   e. Meticulous attention must be paid to prevention of needle-stick injuries. Accidents should be reported.
   f. Surfaces will require decontamination with sodium hypochlorite.
   g. Metal should be treated with glutaraldehyde.

7. Blood samples and pathological specimens.
   a. Specimens should be taken by qualified staff.
   b. Do not squirt blood or sheath needles.
   c. Specimens and needle disposal box should be labelled 'hepatitis risk'. Check that the specimen tube is intact.
   d. Keep tests to a minimum and, if suspected, screen first.
   e. Seal the tube inside a plastic bag, do not use staples; attach forms to the outside.
   f. Simply wash blood off unbroken skin and clean surfaces with sodium hypochlorite.
   g. If skin is pierced, clean, allow to bleed, then seal.
   h. Consider giving hepatitis immunoglobulin.
   i. The patient should be followed up.

BIBLIOGRAPHY

Association of Anaesthetists 1988 AIDS and hepatitis B. Guidelines for Anaesthetists. Association of Anaesthetists, London

Browne R A, Chernesky H B 1984 Viral hepatitis and the anaesthetist. Canadian Anaesthetists' Society Journal 31: 279–286

du Moulin G C, Hedley-Whyte J 1983 Hospital-associated viral infection and the anesthesiologist. Anesthesiology 59: 51–65

Fagan E A 1991 Testing for hepatitis C virus. Panels of antigens and antibodies are most practical. British Medical Journal 303: 535–536

O'Donnell N G, Asbury A J 1992a The occupational hazard of human immunodeficiency virus and hepatitis. I Perceived risks and preventive measures adopted by anaesthetists: a postal survey. Anaesthesia 47: 923–928
O'Donnell N G, Asbury A J 1992b The occupational hazard of human immunodeficiency virus and hepatitis B virus. II. Anaesthesia 47: 929–935
Oxman M N 1984 Hepatitis-B vaccination of high-risk hospital personnel. Anesthesiology 60: 60: 1–3
Tedder R S 1980 Hepatitis B in hospitals. British Journal of Hospital Medicine 23: 266–279
Tedder R S, Gilson R J C, Briggs M et al 1991 Hepatitis C virus: evidence for sexual transmission. British Medical Journal 302: 1299–1302

HEPATORENAL SYNDROME

A loosely applied term, often used whenever hepatic and renal problems coexist. It initially referred to the renal failure which occasionally follows surgery for obstructive jaundice, particularly if the serum bilirubin is >145 µmol/l. Some hepatologists feel that it should only be used for unexplained renal failure complicating hepatic cirrhosis (Hishon 1981). The prevention of renal failure after surgery in jaundiced patients is considered here, although the bibliography covers wider aspects.

Presenting problems

1. Jaundice is produced by obstruction of the biliary tree, usually by stones, tumour or stricture. Conjugated bilirubin fails to reach the gut. Alkaline phosphatase levels frequently exceed 210 iu/l.
2. Hepatocellular damage inevitably occurs if the obstruction has been present for any length of time. Serum transaminase levels may be moderately increased.
3. Pruritus and bradycardia may accompany severe jaundice.
4. An absence of bile salts from the gut impairs the absorption of vitamin K and causes a prolonged prothrombin time.

Management

1. Preoperative prophylactic measures will reduce the incidence of postoperative renal failure in jaundiced patients. Initially, the problem was thought to be due to anoxia and the toxic effects of bilirubin. The protective function of i.v. mannitol has been demonstrated (Dawson 1965, Baum et al 1969). Adequate preoperative hydration is required. This is followed by mannitol 10%, 0.5–1 g/kg to promote a urine output of at least 50 ml/h. It may not be universally successful in preventing renal problems.
2. The renal problems have been linked with endotoxaemia. Portal endotoxaemia has been demonstrated, at operation, in patients with obstructive jaundice (Bailey 1976). Those who additionally had a peripheral endotoxaemia developed a significant decrease in

creatinine clearance. It has also been suggested that the absence of bile salts allows endotoxin to be absorbed from the gut. Oral administration of sodium taurocholate, 1 g t.d.s for 48 hours, has been shown to be protective (Evans et al 1982). n patients with serum bilirubin levels above 145 μmol/l, it was recommended that a combination of mannitol with fluids, antibiotics and bile salts be used.

BIBLIOGRAPHY

Bailey M E 1976 Endotoxins, bile salts and renal function in obstructive jaundice. British Journal of Surgery 63: 774–778

Baum M, Stirling G A, Dawson J L 1969 Further study into obstructive jaundice and ischaemic renal damage. British Medical Journal 2: 229–231

Dawson J L 1965 Postoperative renal function in obstructive jaundice: effect of a mannitol diuresis. British Medical Journal 1: 82–86

Evans H J R, Torrealba V, Hudd C et al 1982 The effect of preoperative bile salt administration on postoperative renal function in patients with obstructive jaundice. British Journal of Surgery 69: 706–708

Hishon S 1981 The hepatorenal syndrome. Hospital Update 7: 1027–1035

HEREDITARY ANGIONEUROTIC OEDEMA
(See also C1 ESTERASE INHIBITOR DEFICIENCY)

A symptom complex of intermittent painless, non-itching, swelling of subcutaneous tissue, respiratory mucosa and intestinal walls. Acute attacks are commonly precipitated by trauma or stress, and can last from a few hours up to 4 days. Often presenting in adolescence, it is an autosomal dominant condition in which there is a deficiency or abnormality of the inhibitor of the activated first component of complement (C1 inhibitor). Complement, whose major function is to eliminate antigen, is present in serum and a number of other body fluids, and is a mediator of immunological tissue damage (Powell 1984). The complement system is a cascade resembling the clotting sequence, in which a series of normally inactive proteins sequentially activate each other. The complement cascade is initially activated by either the classical or the alternate pathway. It is normally kept under control by inhibitors or, when activated, by the spontaneous decay of the active component. The kinin-generating and fibrinolytic systems are also involved and the oedema appears to be due to generation of a peptide which causes increased capillary permeability. The hereditary form is responsible for only a small proportion of cases of angio-oedema.

Preoperative abnormalities

1. Attacks of angioneurotic oedema can be precipitated by trauma or stress, or there may be no obvious cause. There may be serious consequences if the oedema involves the airway or leads to intestinal obstruction. The oedema does not respond to treatment with steroids, antihistamines or adrenaline.

2. A family history of the disease is usually elicited. In the past, the development of acute laryngeal oedema has carried a high mortality.
3. Plasma C1 inhibitor levels are below normal. During attacks there is a low C4 and often a low C2. Levels remain normal in 15% of cases, but a functional abnormality exists (Powell 1984).
Measurement of serum C4 titre is a good screening test during symptomatic periods. If the levels are normal, the condition is excluded. If levels are low, then assay of C1 inhibitor is warranted (Sim & Grant 1990).
4. Some patients with disabling symptoms may be on long-term therapy with stanozolol or danazol.

Anaesthetic problems

1. Patients may present spontaneously with acute upper airway obstruction from laryngeal oedema. Emergency tracheostomy may be needed (Hamilton et al 1977).
2. Surgery involving tooth extraction or tracheal intubation carries a risk of initiating an attack. Fatal laryngeal oedema has been reported after dental extraction (Wall et al 1989).
3. Attacks of abdominal pain may result from intestinal oedema. Unless the diagnosis is made, patients may be submitted to unnecessary surgery (Beck et al 1973).
4. Although it has been suggested that pregnancy provides a protective effect against attacks, complications may still arise (Stiller et al 1984), and abdominal pain may become a diagnostic problem (Chappatte & de Swiet 1988). A maternal death from hypovolaemia has also been reported. This was secondary to widespread oedema in a patient with absent serum C1 esterase inhibitor (Postnikoff & Pritzker 1979). The terminal episode started with perineal oedema in association with episiotomy infection, 48 hours after delivery, and the immediate cause of death was pericardial effusion, pulmonary, and laryngeal oedema.

Management

1. Attacks of glottic oedema can be treated with FFP, which contains C1 inhibitor. A single transfusion will maintain the level for between 1 and 4 days. Clinical improvement has been seen within 40 minutes. There is a theoretical risk that an attack may be exacerbated, due to the C2 and C4 content of FFP.
2. In patients presenting with acute abdominal pain, the diagnosis of intestinal oedema may be confirmed by a barium meal and follow-through examination. Administration of FFP has been shown to relieve symptoms within 2–3 hours (Beck et al 1973).
3. If elective or emergency surgery is required, prophylaxis can be achieved with FFP. Preferably, 2 units of FFP should be given 24 hours in advance. C1 inhibitor levels are increased for up to 4 days.

4. For prophylaxis, either danazol (a progestogen) 200 mg t.d.s, or stanozolol (an anabolic steroid) 2.5–10 mg daily, can also be given. Danazol increases the plasma levels of C1 esterase inhibitor and C4 (Gelfand et al 1976), probably by influencing hepatic synthesis of the inhibitor. It starts to act within 24 hours, and is at a maximum at 1–2 weeks. If possible, 10 days' treatment should be given before surgery.

5. The use of local or regional anaesthesia has been proposed.

6. Facilities for tracheostomy should be available in life-threatening conditions.

7. Extradural analgesia has been used for vaginal delivery (Wingtin & Hardy 1989).

8. For severe cases, purified C1 esterase inhibitor can be obtained from Immuno Limited (Rye Lane, Dunton Green, Sevenoaks, Kent TN14 5HB, UK). It may also be useful in patients in whom danazol fails to increase the C1 esterase inhibitor concentrations, in those who are at risk of upper airway oedema, and for children and pregnant women, in whom danazol is contraindicated (Laxenaire et al 1990).

BIBLIOGRAPHY

Beck P, Wills D, Davies G T et al 1973 A family study of hereditary angioneurotic oedema. Quarterly Journal of Medicine 42: 317–339.
Chappatte O, de Swiet M 1988 Hereditary angioneurotic oedema and pregnancy. Case reports and review of the literature. British Journal of Obstetrics and Gynaecology 95: 938–942
Gelfand J A, Sherins R J, Alling D W et al 1976 Treatment of hereditary angioedema with danazol. New England Journal of Medicine 295: 1444–1448
Hamilton A G, Bosley A R J, Bowen D J 1977 Laryngeal oedema due to hereditary angioedema. Anaesthesia 32: 265–267
Hopkinson R B, Sutcliffe A J 1979 Hereditary angioneurotic oedema. Anaesthesia 34: 183–186
Laxenaire M-C, Audibert G, Janot C 1990 Use of purified C1 esterase inhibitor in patients with hereditary angioedema. Anesthesiology 72: 956–957
Poppers P J 1987 Anaesthetic implications of hereditary angioneurotic oedema. Canadian Journal of Anaesthesia 34: 76–78
Postnikoff I M, Pritzker K P H 1979 Hereditary angioneurotic edema: an unusual case of maternal mortality. Journal of Forensic Sciences 24: 473–478
Powell R J 1984 Serum complement levels. British Journal of Hospital Medicine 32: 104–110
Rodgers G K, Galos R S, Johnson J T 1991 Hereditary angioedema: case report and review of management. Otolaryngology, Head and Neck Surgery. 104: 394–398
Sim T C, Grant J A 1990 Hereditary angioedema: its diagnostic and management perspectives. American Journal of Medicine 88: 656–664
Stiller R J, Kaplan B M, Andreoli J W Jr 1984 Hereditary angioedema and pregnancy. Obstetrics and Gynecology 64: 133–135
Wall R T, Frank M, Hahn M 1989 A review of 25 patients with hereditary angioedema requiring surgery. Anesthesiology 71: 309–311
Wingtin L N, Hardy F 1989 Epidural block during labour in hereditary angioneurotic oedema. Canadian Journal of Anaesthesia 36: 366

HEREDITARY SPHEROCYTOSIS

A familial haemolytic anaemia of autosomal dominant inheritance in which premature destruction of intrinsically abnormal erythrocytes occurs in the spleen. Variation in abnormalites of the membrane may influence the clinical severity and the stage at which haemolysis first presents (Eber et al 1990).

Preoperative abnormalities

1. Small spherocytic red blood cells are present in the peripheral blood. The surface to volume ratio is altered and the normal discoid shape is lost. Cells have an increased osmotic fragility, their survival time is reduced and there is marrow hyperplasia.
2. Splenomegaly, mild haemolytic anaemia and acholuric jaundice.
3. A raised reticulocyte count by up to 20%.
4. An increased incidence of gallstones and leg ulcers.
5. RBC survival times are improved by splenectomy.

Anaesthetic problems

1. Splenectomy is needed in the majority of patients.
2. Cholecystectomy may be required.

Management

Prophylactic pneumococcal vaccine may be required if splenectomy is undertaken.

BIBLIOGRAPHY

Eber S W, Ambrust R, Schroter W 1990 Variable clinical severity of hereditary spherocytosis: relation to erythrocytic spectrum, concentration, osmotic fragility and autohemolysis. Journal of Pediatrics 117: 409–416

HERS' DISEASE
(CORI TYPE VL GLYCOGEN STORAGE DISEASE)

One of the glycogen storage diseases in which there is liver phosphorylase or phosphorylase b kinase deficiency (Hers et al 1989). It is similar to type I, von Gierke's disease, but is less severe.

Preoperative abnormalities

1. Hepatomegaly occurs from increased glycogen stores in the liver.
2. There is a tendency to hypoglycaemia and a variable response to glucagon and adrenaline (Cox 1968).
3. Children may present with failure to thrive.
4. Tends to be less severe than type I disease. In a series of patients having portacaval shunt surgery for metabolic diseases, the single type Vl case was the only one not to require parenteral nutrition (Casson 1975).

Anaesthetic problems
Hypoglycaemia and acidosis can occur after starvation.

Management
A dextrose infusion, to prevent an acidosis at the beginning of surgery, should be given during the period of preoperative starvation.

BIBLIOGRAPHY
Casson H 1975 Anaesthesia for portacaval bypass in patients with metabolic diseases. British Journal of Anaesthesia 47: 969–975
Cox J M 1968 Anesthesia and glycogen storage disease. Anesthesioloy 29: 1221–1225
Hers H-G, van Hoof F, de Barsy T 1989 glycogen storage diseases. In: Scriver CR et al (eds) The metabolic basis of inherited disease. McGraw-Hill, New York

HOMOCYSTEINURIA

One of the aminoacidurias, this autosomal recessive metabolic disease results from a deficiency of cystathionine beta-synthase, which catalyzes the reaction of homocysteine and serine to produce cystathionine (Watts 1987). Large amounts of homocysteine and methionine are found in the blood and the urine. Excess homocysteine causes a loss of endothelial cells from the intima of blood vessels, exposing collagen and allowing platelet thrombi to form on the surface. There is platelet consumption, and a reduction in platelet count. The decrease in cysteine, which is an important constituent of the cross linkages in collagen, produces a weakened collagen. There is fragmentation of elastic tissue of large arteries (Carson et al 1965).

Homocysteinaemia has been found to be an independent risk factor in young individuals with vascular disease (Clarke et al 1991). After diagnostic criteria had been determined (peak serum homocysteine levels following methionine loading), 123 patients with vascular disease presenting before the age of 55 were compared with 27 normal, matched individuals. Hyperhomocysteinaemia was found in 42% with cerebrovascular disease, 28% with peripheral vascular disease and 30% with coronary artery disease, but not in the normal subjects. In 18 of the 23 patients with hyperhomocysteinaemia, cystathionine beta-synthase deficiency was confirmed.

Preoperative abnormalities

1. Abnormalities include lens dislocation, ligamentous laxity, elongated extremities similar to Marfan's syndrome, but without the hyperextensiblity of joints, kyphoscoliosis, and brittle, light coloured hair. If the condition is not diagnosed and treated early, mental retardation occurs.
2. Homocysteine, which is not normally present in the urine, occurs in large amounts, as does methionine.

3. The irritant effect on the vascular endothelium causes platelet aggregation and subsequent thromboembolism. Major thromboembolic episodes occurred in 5 out of a series of 10 patients (Carson et al 1965).

4. Treatment consists of a diet which is low in methionine but contains cysteine supplements. Pyridoxine, dipyramidole and acetyl salicylic acid may be used to decrease platelet adhesion. Vitamin B12 and folic acid are also given.

Anaesthetic problem

1. Thomboembolism, which can be fatal, may occur in association with surgery. Problems are not confined to the homozygous individual. Cerebral infarction, which occurred 11 days after Caesarean section was the presenting feature in a heterozygote (Minkhorst et al 1991).

2. Patients may have increased insulin levels resulting in hypoglycaemia.

3. Regional anaesthesia has certain theoretical disadvantages. Penetration of a large extradural blood vessel might initiate thrombosis, as may the accompanying venous stasis of the lower limbs.

4. Anaesthesia for the surgery of lens dislocation is most frequently reported (Frost 1980, Grover et al 1979, Parris & Quimby 1982).

5. There are increased risks in pregnancy, and maternal deaths have been reported secondary to thromboses (Minkhorst et al 1991, Constantine & Green 1987). There is a high incidence of fetal loss and unsuccessful pregnancies (Burke et al 1992).

Management

1. Dehydration must be avoided, and a good cardiac output and peripheral perfusion maintained.

2. Blood viscosity and platelet adhesiveness can be reduced by dextran, and the prior administration of pyridoxine.

3. Dextrose infusion will prevent hypoglycaemia.

4. Early mobilization and low-dose heparin therapy decreases the chance of postoperative thromboembolism.

BIBLIOGRAPHY

Burke G, Robinson K, Refsum H et al 1992 Intrauterine growth retardation, perinatal death, and maternal homocysteine levels. New England Journal of Medicine 326: 69–70

Carson N A J, Dent C E, Field C M B et al 1965 Homocystinuria. Journal of Pediatrics 66: 565–583

Clarke R, Daly L, Robinson K et al 1991 Hyperhomocysteinemia: an independent risk factor for vascular disease. New England Journal of Medicine 324: 1149–1155

Constantine G, Green A 1987 Untreated homocystinuria: a maternal death in a woman with four pregnancies. British Journal of Obstetrics and Gynaecology 94: 803–806

Frost P M 1980 Anaesthesia ad homocystinuria. Anaesthesia 35: 918–919
Grover V K, Malhotra S K, Kaushik 5 1979 Anaesthesia and homocystinuria.
    Anaesthesia 34: 913–914
Minkhorst A G, van Dongen P W, Boers G H et al 1991 Cerebral infarction after
    caesarean section due to heterozygosity for homocystinuria; a case report. European
    Journal of Obstetrics, Gynecology and Reproductive Biology 40: 241–243
Parris W C V, Quimby C W 1982 Anesthetic considerations for the patient with
    homocysteinuria. Anesthesia and Analgesia 61: 708–710
Watts R W E 1987 Inborn errors of metabolism. In: Weatherall D J, Ledingham J G G,
    Warrel D A (eds) Oxford Textbook of Medicine. Oxford Scientific Publications,
    Oxford

HUNTER'S SYNDROME
(see HURLER'S SYNDROME and MUCOPOLYSACCHARIDOSES)

HUNTINGTON'S CHOREA

A degenerative neurological disorder inherited as an autosomal
dominant. Progressive degradation and death of neurones is
accompanied by an alteration in the levels of many neurotransmitters
(Martin & Gusella 1986). The onset occurs between 30 and 45 years
and death frequently follows within 10–15 years of the first symptoms.

Preoperative abnormalities

1. Clinical features are progressive and include choreiforrn movements,
   ataxia, dysarthria and dementia. Sleep and anaesthesia usually
   abolish the chorea, which may not return until several hours
   following the anaesthetic
2. The chorea may be preceded by several years of gradually increasing
   personality changes and mental deterioration.
3. Patients with the clinical disease may be taking a variety of drugs to
   improve the chorea, including the butyrophenones, phenothiazines
   and tetrabenazine.

Anaesthetic problems

1. Despite the use of a variety of agents, four of the 16 cases reported
   in the anaesthetic literature, were accompanied by prolonged apnoea
   or recovery (Davies 1966, Gualandi & Bonfanti 1968, Blanloeil et al
   1982). Barbiturate (Davies 1966) and suxamethonium (Gualandi &
   Bonfanti 1968) sensitivities have been suggested as the likely causes.
   Plasma cholinesterase measurement was not mentioned. Subsequent
   papers have, however, reported successful anaesthetics in which one
   or both of these agents were given (Farina & Rauscher 1977,
   Browne & Cross 1981, Costarino & Gross 1985), whilst others used

alternative agents (Lamont 1979, Johnson & Heggie 1985, Rodrigo 1987, Kaufman & Erb 1990). Assessment of the possible causative factors for either prolonged apnoea or delayed recovery from anaesthesia, must take account of:

a. A higher than expected incidence of atypical plasma cholinesterase (the fluoride resistant gene E_1f) has been confirmed in patients with Huntington's chorea (Whittaker 1980).

b. These patients are often receiving a variety of powerful psychotropic drugs including phenothiazines and butyrophenones, and tetrabenazine, a drug which depletes stores of cerebral biogenic amines. Any of these drugs may interact with anaesthetic agents.

c. In advanced cases, there are gross atrophic changes in the cerebral cortex and basal ganglia.

d. Patients are frequently wasted and of poor nutritional status.

2. Dysphagia and abnormalities of pharyngeal and laryngeal function may predispose to aspiration in the perioperative period. Videofluoroscopic studies identified coughing on foods, choking on liquid and episodes of aspiration (Kagel & Leopold 1992).

Management

1. Blood should be taken for plasma cholinesterase levels and dibucaine and fluoride numbers, even if it is not intended to use suxamethonium. Their documentation may be of subsequent value. Should suxamethonium be required in the absence of the results, or if non-depolarizing agents are used, neuromuscular monitoring is essential.

2. The dosages of all anaesthetic agents should be kept to a minimum, bearing in mind the pathology of the disease itself, preoperative medication, and the general nutrition of the patient.

3. Case reports of individual patients have encouraged the use of midazolam for induction (Rodrigo 1987), a propofol bolus for induction and an infusion for maintenance (Kaufman & Erb 1990).

BIBLIOGRAPHY

Blanloeil Y, Bigot A, Dixneuf B 1982 Anaesthesia in Huntington's chorea Anaesthesia 37: 695–696

Browne M G, Cross R 1981 Huntington's chorea. British Journal of Anaesthesia 53: 1367

Costarino A, Gross J B 1985 Patients with Huntington's chorea may respond normally to succinylcholine. Anesthesiology 63: 570

Davies D D 1966 Abnormal response to anaesthesia in a case of Huntington's chorea. British Journal of Anaesthesia 38: 490–491

Farina J, Rauscher L A 1977 Anaesthesia and Huntington's chorea. British Journal of Anaesthesia 49: 1167–1168

Gualandi W, Bonfanti G 1968 Un caso di apnea prolungata in corea di Huntington. Acta Anaesthesiologica (Padova) 19: 235–238

Johnson M K, Heggie N M 1985 Huntington's chorea: a role for the newer anaesthetic
    agents. British Journal of Anaesthesia 57: 235–236
Kagel M C, Leopold N A 1992 Dysphagia in Huntington's disease: a 16-year
    retrospective. Dysphagia 7: 106–114
Kaufman M A, Erb T 1990 Propofol for patients with Huntington's chorea.
    Anaesthesia 45: 889–890
Lamont A S M 1979 Brief report: Anaesthesia and Huntington's chorea. Anaesthesia
    and Intensive Care 7: 189–190
Martin J B, Gusella J F 1986 Huntington's disease. Pathogenesis and management.
    New England Journal of Medicine 315: 1267–1276
Rodrigo M R C 1987 Huntington's chorea: midazolam, a suitable induction agent?
    British Journal of Anaesthesia 59: 388–389
Whittaker M 1980 Plasma cholinesterase variants and the anaesthesia. Anaesthesia
    35: 174–197

HURLER'S, HURLER-SCHEIE, SCHEIE'S AND HUNTER'S SYNDROMES
(see also MUCOPOLYSACCHARIDOSES)

The mucopolysaccharidoses (MPS) are a group of inherited connective tissue syndromes which result from deficiencies of specific enzymes responsible for the degradation of mucopolysaccharides (glycoaminoglycans). Mucopolysaccharides are constituents of normal connective tissue and are composed of repeating disaccharide units connected to protein. They are normally broken down in the cell lysosomes to monosaccharides and amino acids. In the absence of certain enzymes, intermediate products of degradation accumulate. Cell size increases and cell function is impaired. The effects depend upon the enzyme defect and the specific organs involved.

Hurler's, Hurler-Scheie and Scheie's syndromes are all type I MPS. Hunter's, type II, is similar to Hurler's, but less severe and with no mental retardation. All four are considered together here because they produce similar anaesthetic problems, and are the most difficult of the MPS types with which the anaesthetist might have to deal.

Patients often present with otolaryngological problems, including serous otitis media, sensorineural deafness and upper airway obstruction. In a study of 45 children, every patient had at least one head and neck complication (Bredenkamp et al 1992). Anaesthesia is most likely to be required for repeated ENT procedures, the repair of inguinal or umbilical herniae, and, more recently, amnion transplant (King et al 1984) and bone marrow transplantation.

Preoperative abnormalities

Hurler's syndrome (type IH: gargoylism)

1. Craniofacial. Hypertelorism, frontal bossing, depressed nasal bridge, coarse features, irregular and broadly spaced teeth, gum hypertrophy, macroglossia and corneal opacities.
2. Respiratory. Mouth breathing, airway obstruction, profuse secretions, pectus excavatum, frequent respiratory infections and sleep apnoea.

3. Cardiac. Coronary artery disease resulting from intimal deposition of mucopolysaccharides, valvular lesions, pulmonary hypertension and cardiac failure.
4. Skeletal. Dwarfing, short neck, kyphoscoliosis and claw hand. Atlantoaxial instability has been described.
5. Mental status. Subnormal.
6. Other organs. Hepatosplenomegaly, umbilical and inguinal herniae.
7. Deficient enzyme. L-iduronidase
8. Prognosis. Death within the first decade.

Scheie's (type IS)

1. Craniofacial. Corneal clouding, prognathism and macroglossia.
2. Respiratory. Airway involvement, but less severe.
3. Cardiac. Aortic regurgitation.
4. Skeletal. Normal stature, short neck, deformity of hands and feet.
5. Mental status. Normal.
6. Other organs. Glaucoma, herniae and carpal tunnel syndrome.
7. Deficient enzyme. L-iduronidase.

Hurler–Scheie (type IH/S)
(Intermediate between Hurler and Scheie)

Hunter's (type II)
X-linked recessive, similar to Hurler's but less severe. There is evidence of two distinct groups, mild and severe. This distinction is based on the presence or absence of progressive mental retardation (Young & Harper 1982).

1. Craniofacial. Coarse facies, deafness and papilloedema.
2. Respiratory. Upper airway involvement from soft tissue deposition, excessive secretions.
3. Cardiac. Coronary intimal thickening, valvular disease and heart failure. Heart disease is the commonest cause of death.
4. Skeletal. Dwarfism, claw hands and stiff joints.
5. Mental status. Normal in the mild form, progressive retardation in the severe.
6. Other organs. Hepatosplenomegaly. The majority of patients have either umbilical or inguinal herniae.
7. Deficient enzyme. Iduronate sulphatase

Anaesthetic problems

1. Airway maintenance and induction difficulties. Reviews of patients with MPS have noted that more than 50% had airway-related problems (Baines & Keneally 1983, Kempthorne & Brown 1983, King et al 1984, Herrick & Rhine 1988). The majority were either

Hurler or Hunter MPS. Difficulties in airway maintenance appear to stem in part from obstruction by soft tissue deposits in the mouth, the tongue and the pharyngeal tissues, and in part from excess, and frequently purulent, tracheobronchial secretions.

2. Tracheal intubation difficulties were again reported in more than 50% of cases. The above problems are compounded by the large head and hypertelorism. Complete failure to intubate occurred in three patients, another had a hypoxic cardiac arrest (Kempthorne & Brown 1983) but was resuscitated, and one died (Young & Harper 1982). It has been noted that the larynx is often smaller than anticipated. In one series, tracheostomy was required in four patients, either for sleep apnoea or for failed intubation on induction of anaesthesia (Ruckstein et al 1990). Failure to intubate a patient before surgery for aortic and mitral valve replacement prompted the institution of cardiopulmonary bypass whilst undertaking mask ventilation of the lungs (Nicolson et al 1992). Multiple attempts to intubate the patient subsequently culminated in the use of a retrograde tracheal technique.

3. Venous access may be a problem (King et al 1984).

4. Atlanto-occipital instability may occur on occasions, and a spastic quadriplegia has been reported in Hurler's (Brill et al 1978).

5. Fatal postoperative respiratory obstruction has been reported secondary to glottic oedema in an abnormal larynx (Hopkins et al 1973). Emergency tracheostomy proved difficult because of hard, thickened cartilage.

6. Sleep apnoea secondary to upper airway obstruction, with oxygen desaturation and hypercarbia during sleep, has been reported (Ruckstein et al 1990). This may result in cardiac failure and growth retardation (Stevens 1988). In a study of 21 patients, 50% had a clinical history of sleep apnoea and 90% had evidence of it on polysonography (Semenza & Pyeritz 1988).

7. Tracheostomy may be required.

8. Pulmonary oedema has occurred secondary to relief of airway obstruction in a patient undergoing fibreoptic intubation (Wilder & Belani 1990).

Management

1. Asssessment of the airway and possible intubation difflculties is essential. Examination of previous anaesthetic notes may indicate problems. Occasionally, a CT scan of the airway may be helpful. Parents should be warned that tracheostomy may be required.

2. Cardiological evaluation is required.

3. Cervical spine should be screened to detect atlantoaxial instability.

4. A drying agent is essential, and sedatives best avoided in these patients.

5. It has been claimed that inhalation inductions are difficult, and intravenous agents are dangerous (Herrick & Rhine 1988). Awake fibreoptic intubation should be considered, but even this is not free of risk (Wilder & Belani 1990) and should only be carried out by those experienced in the technique. Neuromuscular blockers should not be used until the airway is ensured.

6. A nasal airway has been thought to be more effective than an oral one (Brown 1984) and can be left in place until the patient is awake. Lateral X-rays in two patients have shown that an oral airway pushes the epiglottis down and backwards to occlude the laryngeal inlet, whereas a nasal airway keeps it forward. Preoperative tracheostomy has been reported in patients with known failed intubation (Baines & Keneally 1983). Secretions may still block the tube. The domiciliary use of a nasopharyngeal tube has been described in a patient with cardiac failure and episodes of profound nocturnal hypoxaemia (Stevens 1988).

7. Local anaesthetic techniques should be considered. Spinal anaesthesia has been employed in a patient with a previous failed intubation (Sjogren & Pedersen 1986). Combined continuous spinal analgesia and general anaesthesia were used for upper abdominal surgery in a patient with Hurler-Scheie syndrome (Sethna & Berde 1991).

8. Tracheostomy may be required, either for failed tracheal intubation or to treat obstructive sleep apnoea.

BIBLIOGRAPHY

Baines D, Keneally J 1983 Anaesthetic implications of the mucopolysaccharidoses. Anaesthesia and Intensive Care 11: 198–202

Bredenkamp J K, Smith M E, Dudley J P et al 1992 Otolaryngologic manifestations of the mucopolysaccharidoses. Annals of Otology, Rhinology and Laryngology 101: 472–478

Brill C B, Rose J S, Godmilow L et al 1978 Spastic quadriparesis due to C1-C2 subluxation in Hurler syndrome. Journal of Pediatrics 92: 441–443

Brown T C K 1984 The airway in mucopolysaccharidoses. Anaesthesia and Intensive Care 12: 178

Herrick I A, Rhine E J 1988 The mucopolysaccharidoses and anaesthesia: a report of clinical experience. Canadian Journal of Anaesthesia 35: 67–73

Hopkins R, Watson J A, Jones J H, et al 1973 Two cases of Hunter's syndrome. The anaesthetic and operative difficulties in oral surgery. British Journal of Oral Surgery 10: 286–299

Kempthorne P M, Brown T C K 1983 Anaesthesia and the mucopolysaccharidoses. Anaesthesia and Intensive Care 11: 203–207

King D H, Jones R M, Barnett M B 1984 Anaesthetic considerations in the mucopolysaccharidoses. Anaesthesia 39: 126–131

Nicolson S C, Black A E, Kraras C M 1992 Management of a difficult airway in a patient with Hurler-Scheie syndrome during cardiac surgery. Anesthesia and Analgesia 75: 830–832

Ruckstein M J, Macdonald R E, Clarke J T R et al 1990 The management of otolaryngological problems in the mucopolysaccharidoses: a retrospective review. The Journal of Otolaryngology 20: 177–183

Semenza G L, Pyeritz R E 1988 Respiratory complications of mucopolysaccharide storage disorders. Medicine 67: 209–219

Sethna N F, Berde C B 1991 Continuous subarachnoid analgesia in two adolescents with severe scoliosis and impaired pulmonary function. Regional Anesthesia 16: 333–336

Sjogren P, Pedersen T 1986 Anaesthetic problems in Hurler-Scheie syndrome. Report of 2 cases. Acta Anaesthesiologica Scardanavica 30: 484–486

Stevens I M 1988 Domiciliary use of nasopharyneal intubation for obstructive sleep apnoea in a child with mucopolysaccharidosis. Anaesthesia and Intensive Care 16: 493–494

Wilder R T, Belani K G 1990 Fiberoptic intubation complicated by pulmonary edema in a 12-year-old child wth Hurler syndrome. Anesthesiology 72: 205–207

Young I D, Harper P S 1982 Mild form of Hunter's syndrome: clinical delineation based on 31 cases. Archives of Diseases in Childhood 57: 828–836

HYDATID DISEASE

Hydatid cysts are the larval stage of the tapeworm, *Echinococcus granulosus*. Dogs are the main hosts. Man and sheep are intermediate hosts. Hydatid disease is not uncommon among the mid-Wales farming communities and up to 26% of farm dogs in this area have *E. granulosus* (Morris 1981). If the ova are ingested by man, embryos are released when the chitinous coat is digested. These enter the liver by the portal vein. They may be destroyed or they may develop into a cyst. In man, the cysts are found in the liver (65%), lung (25%), muscles (5%), bone (3%) and brain (1%).

Each cyst is two layered and contains straw coloured fluid in which there are free scolices, brood capsules containing scolices, and daughter cysts. Around the cyst is an area of compressed host tissue and fibrosis known as the pericyst. In 5–10% of cases the cyst will die, and calcification may occur (Lewis et al 1975).

Preoperative abnormalities

1. Hepatic cysts occur most frequently in the right lobe. Bacterial infection may result in a liver abscess. Rupture into a bile duct, or bile duct obstruction may occur and produce biliary colic. There may be jaundice. The number and location of the cysts can be shown on CT scan or ultrasound.

2. Pulmonary cysts can present with haemoptysis, dyspnoea, cough or chest pain. CXR may show a variety of appearances including an oval opacity, evidence of bronchial fistula formation, or rupture of the cyst with the development of a fluid level.

3. Eosinophilia occurs in about 30% cases. The Casoni skin test is still used for screening. Immunoelectrophoresis is the most specific test. Complement fixation test is positive in up to 80% cases. Haemagglutination test detects a specific antibody.

Anaesthetic problems

1. Pulmonary hydatid cysts can cause bronchial obstruction and occasionally they may rupture into the airway. If this happens,

flooding of the lungs occurs, with widespread dissemination of the scolices.

2. Hydatid fluid is highly antigenic, and rupture of a cyst has occasionally produced sudden death from an anaphylactic reaction (Jakubowski & Barnard 1971).
3. Cerebral cysts can produce raised intracranial pressure.
4. Scolicidal agents are potentially toxic and their use in combination with surgery may increase the complication rate.

Management

1. Surgical removal is indicated, except in older patients with small cysts (Behrns & van Heerden 1991). Meticulous care must be taken to avoid rupture and spread of the fertile scolices.
2. Relatively new drugs, such as mebendazole and albendazole, are being tested as scolicidal agents. However, there is no evidence that they are effective in the treatment of pulmonary hydatid (Aggarawal & Wali 1991).
3. Pulmonary cysts. Protective formalin-soaked packs are placed around the wound, an incision is made through the pericyst and the cyst is carefully extruded by the anaesthetist, using gentle hand ventilation (Saidi 1977).
4. Because of the risk of an anaphylactic reaction, adrenaline, metaraminol, isoprenaline and steroids must be immediately available (Lewis et al 1975).

BIBLIOGRAPHY
Aggarawal P, Wali J P 1991 Albendazole in the treatment of pulmonary echinococcosis. Thorax 46: 599–560
Behrns K E, van Heerden J A 1991 Surgical management of hepatic hydatid disease. Mayo Clinic Proceedings 66: 1193–1197
Jakubowski M S, Barnard D E 1971 Anaphylactic shock during operation for hydatid disease. Anesthesiology 34: 197–199
Lewis J W, Koss N, Kerstein M D 1975 A review of echinococcal disease. Annals of Surgery 181: 390–396
Morris D L 1981 The management of hydatid disease. British Journal of Hospital Medicine 25: 586–595
Saidi F 1977 A new approach to the surgical treatment of hydatid cyst. Annals of the Royal College of Surgeons 59: 115–118

HYPERCALCAEMIA

When artefactual causes of an increased serum calcium level have been excluded, the commonest causes of hypercalcaemia are malignancy and hyperparathyroidism. Sarcoidosis, thyrotoxicosis and vitamin D toxicity are uncommon. Other causes are extremely rare. Occasionally, a patient with hypercalcaemia may present for anaesthesia. Severe hypercalcaemia (>3.2 mmol/l) may be dangerous and, in consultation with a physician, urgent lowering of the level may be required.

Preoperative abnormalities

1. Any malignancy with destructive bone metastases can produce hypercalcaemia, by increased bone resorption and reduced urinary excretion of calcium. Hypercalcaemia occurs in about 10% of cancer patients. The commonest causes are breast carcinoma, myeloma, bronchial, and renal carcinoma. If the serum albumin is low, adjustment for this should be made:

   Adjusted calcium = Measured calcium + 0.02 × (mean normal albumin – measured albumin)

   where Ca is in mmol/l and albumin in g/l.
2. Hypercalcaemia and an increased parathyroid hormone level (PTH) is diagnostic of hyperparathyroidism, but treatment may be required before the result is available.
3. Carcinoma of the lung or a renal cell carcinoma may rarely release a parathormone-like substance, leading to hypercalcaemia.
4. Symptoms of hypercalcaemia may be vague. They include general muscle weakness, apathy, gastrointestinal complaints such as nausea, vomiting, constipation and pancreatitis, weight loss, thirst, polyuria, polydipsia and mental disturbances, progressing to unconsciousness. Renal stones may form. Symptoms do not usually occur until the serum calcium is >3.2 mmol/l. ECG may show an abnormally short Q-T interval.

Anaesthetic problems

1. A hypercalcaemic patient may be severely dehydrated.
2. Hypercalcaemia may precipitate serious arrhythmias. Fatal intraoperative cardiac arrest occurred in a young man with a serum calcium level of 5.6 mmol/l, despite attempts to reduce the levels (Murphy 1992).
3. Digitalis toxicity is exacerbated by a high serum calcium level.
4. If rapid sequence induction is undertaken in the presence of hypercalcaemia, 1.4 times the normal dose of suxamethonium will be required (Roland et al 1991).

Management

1. Replacement of extracellular fluid by rehydration is the first and most important manoeuvre. A diuresis causes excretion of calcium in the urine. An infusion of 1 litre of sodium chloride 0.9% 3–4 hourly for 24 hours should reduce the serum calcium by 0.5 mmol/l. Loop diuretics can be added, but not until adequate fluid repletion is achieved. Thiazide diuretics should not be used because they increase tubular reabsorption of calcium. Fluid balance and serum potassium levels require careful monitoring.

2. Corticosteroids can be used, although there is some question about their efficiency. Calcitonin (100–400 iu s.c. 8-hourly) reduces mobilization of calcium from bone and will also produce an early, but transient effect (48–72 hours) on calcium levels.

3. The use of diphosphonates (e.g. etidronate), which may reduce osteoclastic bone resorption, is being investigated (Stevenson 1985).

4. Mithramycin, a cytotoxic antibiotic, has hypocalcaemic properties, but its action is delayed and myelosuppression, hepatic and renal toxicity are a problem (Brada & Horwich 1986).

BIBLIOGRAPHY
Brada M, Horwich A 1986 Oncological emergencies. Hospital Update 12: 799–812
Drugs ard Therapeutics Bulletin 1990 Treating cancer-associated hypercalcaemia. Drugs and Therapeutics Bulletin 28: 85–87
Murphy J P 1992 Fatal hypercalcaemic crisis. British Journal of Hospital Medicine 18: 677–678
Roland E, Villers S, Lequeau F et al 1991 Succinylcholine dose-response in hyperparathyroidism. Aresthesioloy 75: A808
Stevenson J C 1985 Malignant hypercalcaemia. British Medical Journal 291: 421–422
Tisell L-E, Hedback G, Jansson S et al 1991 Management of hyperparathyroid patients with grave hypercalcemia. World Journal of Surgery 15: 730–737

HYPERTENSION
(ACUTE EMERGENCY)

Patients receiving antihypertensive medication frequently present for surgery, and the need for continuity of therapy in the perioperative period is well recognized. Recent articles have reviewed the current management of hypertension, and discussed the benefits and limitations of long-term therapy (Smith & Littler 1987, Heagerty 1988).

The management of patients presenting with untreated hypertension depends upon the level of the diastolic blood pressure and the surgical circumstances. For elective surgery, provided that the diastolic pressure does not exceed 110 mmHg, there is no evidence of increased cardiac complications (Goldman & Caldera 1979). Patients with persistent diastolic levels above this should be referred to a physician for leisurely treatment.

Urgent surgery may be required in patients with diastolic blood pressures of 110–120 mmHg. A number of drugs given before or during anaesthesia have been reported to attenuate, although not necessarily abolish, untoward haemodynamic and arrhythmic responses to noxious stimuli such as laryngoscopy and tracheal intubation. These include a benzodiazepine premedication, beta adrenoceptor blockers, moderate-to-high doses of fentanyl or alfentanil, droperidol, verapamil and lignocaine. These have been administered either individually, or in varying combinations (Donegan & Bedford 1980, Prys-Roberts 1984, Dann et al 1987, Lawes et al 1987, Yaku et al 1992).

The occurrence of severe untreated hypertension (a diastolic pressure >130 mmHg) in the perioperative period is known to be associated with an increased morbidity and mortality. Potential complications include cerebral haemorrhage, hypertensive encephalopathy, left ventricular failure, renal failure and vascular damage to the eyes.

A number of agents exist for the treatment of acute hypertension (Editorial 1991). The choice depends on the cause, the accompanying pathology, monitoring facilities and familiarity with the use of the drug. Therapy should be extremely cautious, since restoration of normal blood pressure has been associated with myocardial infarction, stroke, and blindness. This is particularly true in the elderly. There are probably few occasions on which the blood pressure needs to be reduced more quickly than over a number of hours, and probably days.

Acute treatment of severe hypertension may be required:
   a. If there is a need for urgent surgery.
   b. If uncontrolled hypertension arises in the perioperative period.
   c. For specific clinical problems such as phaeochromocytoma, PIH, acute aortic dissection and left ventricular failure.

Drugs used in the more urgent treatment of hypertension

Nifedipine
A calcium channel blocker which relaxes smooth muscle. Produces tachycardia, headache, flushing and sweating.
   a. Route: sublingual or oral.
   b. Dose: 10 mg.
   c. Onset: 5–10 min (sublingual), 20 min (oral).
   d. Max effect: 30 min (sublingual), 40 min (oral).
   e. Duration: 3 hours (sublingual), 8–12 hours (oral).

Captopril
An angiotensin-converting-enzyme inhibitor, which inhibits the conversion of angiotensin I to angiotensin II. Also used in heart failure as an adjunct to diuretics and digoxin, but first-dose hypotension may occur when patients in heart failure are receiving loop diuretics. Found to be as effective and safe in hypertensive emergencies as sublingual nifedipine (Angeli et al 1991).
   a. Route: oral, sublingual.
   b. Dose: 12.5–25 mg.
   c. Onset: sublingual 20–30 min.
   d. Duration: mean 4 hours.

Hydralazine
A direct dilator of arterioles. Produces tachycardia and an increase in cardiac output. Should therefore be avoided in myocardial ischaemia or LVF.
   a. Route: i.v., i.m. or by infusion
   b. Dose: 5–20 mg, given slowly over 20 min. Can repeat after 30 min.
   c. Onset: 3–6 min.
   d. Duration: 3–6 hours (i.v.), 4–8 hours (i.m.)

Diazoxide
A direct dilator of arterioles. Causes sodium and water retention.
Tachycardia and increased cardiac oxygen consumption means that it is
contraindicated in myocardial ischaemia and LVF.
  a. Route: i.v.
  b. Dose: 30–300 mg i.v. incremental doses in a supine patient. Can
     be repeated up to three times in 24 hours
  c. Onset: 3–5 min.
  d. Max effect: 20–40 min.
  e. Duration: 4–12 hours.

Minoxidil
A potent orally active vasodilator. Direct dilator of arterioles, with little
effect on capacitance vessels. A reflex tachycardia and fluid retention
means that beta blockers and diuretics must be given in addition. For
severe hypertension when other drugs have failed.
  a. Route: oral
  b. Dose: 2.5 mg b.d., increasing by 5–10 mg each 3 days up to
     maximum of 25 mg b.d.
  c. Onset: 20 min.
  d. Max effect: 2–3 hours.
  e. Duration: half-life 3 hours but effects may persist beyond 24
     hours.

Labetalol
A combined alpha and beta adrenergic blocker. The beta effects are three
to seven times more powerful than the alpha effects. It is not very
effective if the patient is already taking antihypertensives. Potentially
dangerous in phaeochromocytoma.
  a. Route: i.v., i.m. or infusion.
  b. Dose: 10–50 mg i.v., infusion 2 mg/min to a maximum of 200 mg.
  c. Onset: i.v. 5–20 min.
  d. Duration: 3–4 hours.

Sodium nitroprusside
Direct-acting vasodilator. Increases coronary artery blood flow and
decreases pulmonary artery pressure. Unstable in solution in the light
therefore requires covering with aluminium foil. Must be discarded if
blue. Direct arterial monitoring is required.
  For acute use, the maximum safe dose is 1.5 mg/kg. If used long
term, cyanide and thiocyanate levels must be monitored. With toxic
levels there is severe metabolic acidosis and progressive hypotension. If
accidental overdose occurs, sodium thiosulphate (25 ml 50% solution
over 10 min) or dicobalt edetate (300 mg over 10 min then 50 ml 50%
glucose) is given.

   a. Route: by infusion only.
   b. Dose: 50 mg in 500 ml gives 100 μ/ml; titrate by effect, starting at 0.5 μg/kg per min.
   c. Onset: 1–5 min.
   d. Duration: 2–5 min.

Trimetaphan

A ganglion blocking agent and direct peripheral vasodilator. Causes tachycardia, tachyphylaxis and pupillary dilatation. Maximum dose 1 g.
   a. Route: by infusion only.
   b. Dose: 500 mg in 500 ml, start at 3–4 mg/min.
   c. Onset: 1–5 min.
   d. Duration: 5–10 min.

Phentolamine

An alpha adrenoceptor blocker and direct vasodilator. Used specifically for hypertensive crises associated with phaeochromocytoma or adrenaline overdose.
   a. Route: i.v. or infusion.
   b. Dose: 2.5–5 mg each 5 min (i.v.), 5–60 mg over 10–30 min at a rate of 0.1–2 mg/min (infusion).
   c. Onset: 2–5 min (i.v.).
   d. Duration: 10–15 min.

Clonidine

A centrally acting alpha stimulant which reduces sympathetic outflow from the brain stem vasomotor centre. May produce a decrease in cerebral blood flow. Use with caution in cerebrovascular disease.
   a. Route: i.m. or i.v.
   b. Dose: 300 μg i.m., 150–300 i.v. over 5–10 min, to a maximum of 750 μg in 24 hours.
   c. Onset: 5 min (i.m.), immediate (i.v.).
   d. Duration: 5–6 hours (i.m.), 3–4 hours (i.v.).

BIBLIOGRAPHY

Angeli P, Chieza M, Caregaro L et al 1991 Comparison of sublingual captopril and nifedipine in immediate treatment of hypertensive emergencies. Archives of Internal Medicine 151: 678–682

Dann W L, Hutchinson A, Cartwright D P 1987 Maternal and neonatal responses to alfentanil administered before induction of general anaesthesia for Caesarean section. British Journal of Anaesthesia 59: 1392–1396

Donegan M E, Bedford R F 1980 Intravenously administered lidocaine prevents intracranial hypertension during endotracheal suction. Anesthesiology 52: 516–518

Editorial 1991 Hypertensive emergencies. Lancet 338: 220–221.

Goldman L, Caldera D L 1979 Risks of general anesthesia and elective operation in the hypertensive patient. Anesthesiology 50: 285–292

Heagerty A M 1988 Recent advances in therapy for hypertension. British Journal of Anaesthesia 61: 360–364

Lawes E G, Downing J W, Duncan P W et al 1987 Fentanyl/droperidol supplementation of rapid sequence induction controls dangerous blood pressure increases in the presence of severe pregnancy-induced (PIH) and pregnancy aggravated (PAH) hypertension. British Journal of Anaesthesia 59: 1381–1391

Prys-Roberts C 1984 Anaesthesia and hypertension. British Journal of Anaesthesia 56: 711–724
Smith S A, Littler W A 1987 Drugs used in the treatment of hypertension. In: Kaufman L (ed) Anaesthesia Review 4. Churchill Livingstone, Edenburgh
Yaku H, Mikawa K, Maekawa N et al 1992 Effect of verapamil on the cardiovascular response to tracheal intubation. British Journal of Anaesthesia 68: 85–89
Walters B N J 1984 Urgent treatment of acute hypertension. British Journal of Hospital Medicine 10 49–52

HYPONATRAEMIA

Occurs in about 10% of the hospital population (Flear et al 1981). Serum sodium levels <120 mmol/l, which are considered to be dangerous, are found in only 0.2% of patients. Chronic levels lower than this may be tolerated surprisingly well. However in the acute situation, levels between 120 and 125 mmol/l have sometimes produced convulsions.

Hyponatraemia is usually secondary to water overload, and may occur preoperatively as a result of some underlying illness or therapy, or postoperatively secondary to enthusiastic overhydration with non-salt-containing fluids. After operation most patients have been shown to have increased plasma levels of ADH. In addition, a number of drugs possess antidiuretic properties. The administration of large amounts of simple dextrose solutions can therefore cause fluid retention and hyponatraemia.

If possible, the primary cause should be determined. Therapeutic measures, if required, differ considerably, and depend on the aetiology. In many cases an underlying illness may simply require treatment, while water intake should be restricted whenever appropriate.

Rapid intravenous correction of hyponatraemia in the presence of postoperative water intoxication has been associated with death and cerebral damage. Rapid changes in brain hydration due to osmotic gradients may be responsible (Arieff 1986, Swales 1987, Sterns 1992). It is illogical to treat an excess of water with more water and salt.

Causes

1. Dilutional hyponatraemia
   a. Excess water intake. Water retention can occur due to the perioperative infusion of large volumes of non-salt-containing glucose solutions. Oxytocin and opiates, both of which have antidiuretic properties, given during labour or prostaglandin termination of pregnancy can compound the problem (Feeney 1982). In patients treated with beta adrenergic stimulants to suppress premature labour, retention of water is thought to be one of the contributing factors towards the rare development of pulmonary oedema (Hawker 1984). Surgery is normally

associated with increased serum ADH levels. The use of certain drugs, such as vasopressin, DDAVP and steroids, will tend to exacerbate the situation. The features of the TURP syndrome (see Section 2) are in part due to hyponatraemia, secondary to absorption of glycine from the prostatic venous sinuses during prostatectomy.

b. Decreased water clearance. May be secondary to appropriate, or inappropriate secretion of ADH. The syndrome of inappropriate ADH (SIADH) is said to occur with a variety of conditions. It may be associated with a tumour, most frequently bronchial carcinoma, thoracic disease, IPPV, the Guillain-Barré syndrome, rabies, tetanus and a variety of cerebral problems such as injury, meningitis or primary tumours. It also occurs in those who are brain dead. However, it has also been suggested that the hyponatraemia associated with CNS lesions is iatrogenic, occurring secondary to excessive administration of fluids (Bouzarth & Shenkin 1982).

2. Loss of body solutes

   a. Loss of sodium. Causes include diuretics, gastrointestinal losses, renal disease, adrenal insufficiency, withdrawal of steroid therapy, salt depletion and severe hypothyroidism.

   Further causes of solute loss have been suggested (Flear et al 1981), but there is controversy about their significance.

   b. Loss of intracellular anions and potassium. If solute is lost, cells become hypo-osmolar. To prevent cell shrinkage, the plasma osmolality falls and hyponatraemia is produced.

   c. Membrane defects result in leakage of cellular contents. This may occur in sick cell syndrome, associated for example, with heart failure.

   d. In cachexia, the catabolic state results in impaired production of intracellular anions.

   Doubt has been cast on the concept of sick cell syndrome (Leaf 1974, Bichet & Schrier 1982), since the leakage of intracellular solute into the extracellular fluid should be capable of being demonstrated by a positive osmolal gap (measured – calculated osmolality) and a normal serum osmolality. Some studies have failed to confirm this.

3. Increase in solute in plasma

   Results in a redistribution of water to maintain osmotic balance. Can occur in:

   a. An infusion of mannitol.

   b. Sudden hyperglycaemia.

   c. The sick cell syndrome (see above).

   It is suggested that serious illness may cause cell membrane defects which result in loss of intracellular solutes into the extracellular fluid, which in turn pulls out intracellular water. Hyponatraemia occurs, but if this theory is correct, the plasma osmolality should remain normal, and an osmolal gap should be shown.

4. Excess of large paraprotein or lipid molecules
   May decrease the fractional water content of plasma and give a falsely low sodium level (pseudohyponatraemia).
5. Reduction of plasma proteins
   At physiological pH these contribute to the anions. A reduction may result in a compensatory fall in sodium.

Problems

1. Cerebral complications. A decreased conscious level and fits may occur. The level at which this appears is variable, often depending on the rapidity with which the hyponatraemia had developed. Fits can occur in acute hyponatraemia when plasma sodium levels are <123 mmol/l, but patients with chronic hyponatraemia appear to tolerate levels which are much lower than this.
2. Pulmonary oedema may occur.
3. Complications during correction. Although severe hyponatramia in itself may be dangerous, it has been suggested that its rapid correction may be even more so (Arieff 1986, Sterns et al 1986, Sterns 1992). This view has, however, challenged (Narins 1986). In the proponents' series (Arieff 1986, Sterns et al 1986), retrospective studies of 15 and 6 patients respectively, seemed to indicate that rapid correction of hyponatraemia with i.v. saline was associated with sudden deterioration, brain damage, and death. This deterioration, which usually took place after correction of the serum levels, has been termed 'osmotic demyelination syndrome' (Sterns et al 1986), and the pathological changes found in the brain described as central pontine myelinolysis. Although the subject is controversial, there is increasing evidence in favour of the view that the hyponatraemia is less damaging than its rapid correction (Brunner et al 1990, Sterns et al 1989, Laureno & Karp 1988). In one of the studies, data over a 15-year period had been collected on 15 previously healthy women who developed severe hyponatraemia after elective surgery (Arieff 1986). The average preoperative serum sodium level of 138 mmol/l decreased to 108 mmol/l about 48 hours after surgery. Fits and respiratory arrest occurred in all patients and in each case seemed to be associated with rapid correction of the hyponatraemia; 27% died, 13% had limb paralyses and 60% remained in a persistent vegetative state. The presenting picture was one of SIADH, and a number of the patients had received drugs with antidiuretic properties. Significantly, the original hypotonic state was entirely iatrogenic. All patients had been given large volumes of only dextrose-containing fluids and were in an average net positive fluid balance of 7.5 litres. After the diagnosis of hyponatraemia had been made, sodium chloride in a variety of

concentrations was given. Some patients recovered consciousness as the serum sodium level increased, only to lapse into coma subsequently.

Diagnosis

A number of investigations may be required for the evaluation of hyponatraemia, although in many cases not all are necessary.

a. Plasma electrolytes, urea, creatinine and glucose.
b. Plasma osmolality.
c. Urine osmolality and urinary sodium, 24 hours if possible.
d. Serum proteins.
e. Plasma cortisol.
f. Serum lipids.
g. Body weight changes.

1. Dilutional hyponatraemia
   May be diagnosed on history alone. During prostaglandin termination or in labour, the administration of more than 3.5 litres of dextrose 5% with oxytocin has been associated with water intoxication and fits (Feeney 1982). Postoperative hyponatraemia may be a combination of dilution with 5% dextrose and an elevated ADH level. Hyponatraemia, low plasma osmolality, a urine osmolality of about 3–4 times that of the plasma, and a high urinary sodium is highly suggestive of SIADH. Causes of SIADH should be sought.

2. Loss of body solutes
   When there is sodium depletion, the urinary sodium excretion may be <20 mmol/24 h, or a single sample concentration may be <10 mmol/l. In renal disease or heart failure these measurements may not be reliable. Hypokalaemia and alkalosis may indicate total body potassium depletion.

3. Increase in solute in plasma
   Iso-osmotic redistribution of water takes place when there is a sudden increase in a solute. This may occur in hyperglycaemia, and possibly in the sick cell syndrome. When the integrity of the cell membrane is impaired, some leakage of organic solutes is allowed into the extracellular fluid. The movement of solute is accompanied by water. If this happens, hyponatraemia should be accompanied by a normal plasma osmolality and an osmolal gap.

4. Pseudohyponatraemia
   Hyponatraemia in the presence of a normal plasma osmolality may also indicate a paraproteinaemia or high serum triglyceride levels. If these are removed during estimation, the sodium concentration will be found to be normal.

5. Decrease in serum cations or increase in anions
   Hypoproteinaemia or paraproteinaemia may alter the electrochemical balance resulting in a compensatory reduction in serum sodium.

Management

1. Dilutional hyponatraemia
   Prevention is important, since many of the causes are iatrogenic.
   a. Excess water intake. Large quantities of dextrose 5% should not
   be administered perioperatively when antidiuretic factors may be
   operating. If oxytocin is required, sodium chloride 0.9% may be
   used as an alternative vehicle. Should an electrolyte solution be
   contraindicated, a syringe pump may be used, or the total
   volume of dextrose 5% limited to 2 litres in 24 hours.
   Water restriction should be used as the primary management.
   Should intravenous correction be required, caution is advisable.
   In severe symptomatic hyponatraemia, a correction rate of as little
   as 6–8 mmol/l per day has been proposed, despite the fact that
   it may take several days to achieve a level of between 120 and
   130 mmol/l (Stems 1992). Diuretic therapy has also been
   recommended.
   b. Inappropriate ADH secretion. Water is restricted and potassium
   given. If unsuccessful, demeclocycline 0.9-1.2 g/day is given in
   divided doses reducing to a daily maintenance dose of 600-900
   mg/day. The renal excretion of water is enhanced by blocking
   the renal tubular effect of ADH.
2. Loss of body solutes
   a. Loss of sodium. Treatment of the underlying illness is usually
   sufficient. Intravenous saline 0.9% may be required. Hypertonic
   solutions should be avoided because of the risk of producing
   sudden osmotic gradients.
   b. Diuretics must be discontinued if hypokalaemia is suspected.
3. Increase in solutes in plasma
   Treatment of diabetes, if present. If a diagnosis of sick cell
   syndrome is confirmed, the underlying disease should be treated.
   Occasionally the use of glucose, insulin and potassium may assist
   the cell membrane to return to normal. Initially 100 ml 50%
   dextrose, 20 units soluble insulin and potassium chloride should be
   used. Subsequent dosage will depend on blood glucose and
   potassium.
4. Pseudohyponatraemia
   There is an osmolar gap, vhich is the difference between the
   calculated and measured plasma osmolalities. Osmolality is a
   measure of the total solute content of body fluids (or the number of
   particles in a given weight of solvent). Since most of the measured
   osmolality in healthy patients comes from urea, glucose, sodium and
   its anions, attempts have been made to find the best formula for the
   calculated osmolality, in order to detect an unmeasured osmolar
   component, such as alcohol, glycine, trichloroethane,
   hyperproteinaemia or hyperlipidaemia (Worthley et al 1987).

Comparing varying types of patients and five different formulae, the most appropriate was:

$$\text{Calculated osmolality} = 2 \times Na + urea + glucose.$$

BIBLIOGRAPHY

Arieff A 1 1986 Hyponatremia, convulsions, respiratory arrest and permanent brain damage after elective surgery in healthy women. New England Journal of Medicine 314: 1529–1535

Bichet D, Schrier R W 1982 Evidence against concept of hyponatraemia and 'sick cells'. Lancet 1: 742

Bouzarth W F, Shenkin H A 1982 Is 'cerebral hyponatraemia' iatrogenic? Lancet 1: 1061–1062

Brunner J E, Redmond J M, Haggar A M et al 1990 Central pontine myelinolysis and pontine lesions after rapid correction of hyponatraemia: a prospective magnetic imaging study. Annals of Neurology 27: 61–66

Feeney J G 1982 Water intoxication and oxytocin. British Medical Journal 285: 243

Flear C T G, Gill G V, Burn J 1981 Hyponatraemia: mechanisms and management. Lancet 2: 26–31

Hawker F 1984 Pulmonary oedema associated with beta 2 sympathomimetic treatment of premature labour. Anaesthesia and Intensive Care 12: 143–151

Laureno R, Karp B I 1988 Pontine and extrapontine myelinolysis following rapid correction of hyponatraemia. Lancet i: 1439–1441

Leaf A 1974 Hyponatraemia. Lancet 1: 1119–1120

Narins R G 1986 Therapy of hyponatremia. New England Journal of Medicine 314: 1573–1575

Sterns R H, Riggs J E, Schochet S S Jr 1986 Osmotic demyelination syndrome following correction of hyponatremia. New England Journal of Medicine 314: 1535–1542

Sterns R H, Thomas D J, Herndon R M 1989 Brain dehydration and neurologic deterioration after rapid correction of hyponatraemia. Kidney International 35: 69–75

Sterns R H 1992 Severe hyponatraemia: the case for conservative management. Critical Care Medicine 20: 534–539

Swales J D 1987 Dangers in treating hyponatraemia. British Medical Journal 294: 261–262

Swales J D 1991 The management of hyponatraemia. British Journal of Anaesthesia 67: 146–153

Worthley L I G, Guerin , Pain R W 1987 For calculating osmolality – the simplest formula is the best. Anaesthesia and Intensive Care 15: 199–202

HYPOTHYROIDISM

Hypothyroidism may be primary, or secondary to pituitary or hypothalamic disease. Autoimmune thyroiditis is the commonest primary cause, whilst the sequelae of surgical or radioiodine treatment of thyroid disease are also common. Deficiency of circulating thyroid hormone results in retardation of all body functions.

The condition may be subclinical, mild or severe. It akects all systems of the body and the presentations are protean. Mild disease may be unnoticed preoperatively, but can be responsible for delayed recovery from anaesthesia.

After successful treatment, both TSH and T4 levels should be normal. Replacement therapy must be cautious so as not to precipitate myocardial ischaemia or heart failure. In severe, untreated hypothyroidism, elective surgery must be postponed. If emergency surgery has to be undertaken, the mortality is high. However, in the case of patients with severe angina who require coronary artery surgery, the surgery may have to take precedence. The management of cardiac bypass surgery in patients with hypothyroidism, has been described (Finlayson & Kaplan 1982). Thyroxine was not given until after myocardial revascularization. Reduced doses of diazepam and opiates were used for anaesthesia. Digoxin and steroids were also given during operation.

Preoperative abnormalities

1. Delay in the relaxation phase of reflexes, dry skin, a husky voice, loss of the outer part of the eyebrows and weight gain. In severe disease there is lethargy, bradycardia, hypothermia and respiratory depression. Deposition of a mucinous substance causes thickening of the subcutaneous tissues producing a non-pitting oedema. Myxoedematous infiltration of the vocal cords and tongue can occur. Cardiovascular complications include ischaemic heart disease, bradycardia, pericardial effusion and cardiac failure. Neurological complications may involve carpal tunnel syndrome, polyneuritis, myopathy and cerebellar syndrome. About 72% of patients have paraesthesia or a sensory neuropathy (Beghi et al 1989). Psychiatric disturbances may be marked.
2. A raised TSH, and decreased T4 and sometimes T3. It should be remembered that depression of T4 alone often occurs in ill patients who are not hypothyroid. Acute hypothyroidism has been been described in a severely ill surgical patient (Mogensen & Hjortso 1988).
3. Anaemia, which may be microcytic or macrocytic, hyponatraemia, lactic and respiratory acidosis, inappropriate ADH secretion with severe hyponatraemia, and hypoglycaemia are features of myxoedema coma.
4. The ECG is of low voltage with flattened or inverted T waves, and CXR may show mild cardiac enlargement.
5. Associated diseases include diabetes mellitus, pernicious anaemia and Addison's disease.

Anaesthetic problems

1. Severe hypotension, and even cardiac arrest, has been reported after induction of anaesthesia (Abbott 1967, Levelle et al 1985).
2. There is extreme sensitivity to anaesthetic agents, narcotics and analgesics (Kim & Hackman 1977).
3. Anaesthesia, or intercurrent illness such as pneumonia, may precipitate hypothyroid coma (Sherry & Hutchinson 1984, Gilbert

et al 1992). This carries a mortality of 50%, even when there is optimal treatment.

4. Hypothermia readily occurs under anaesthesia (Abbott 1967).
5. A completely absent response to peripheral nerve stimulation has been reported (Miller et al 1989). Subsequent investigation showed a sensorimotor polyneuropathy. After treatment the response to nerve stimulation became normal.
6. Respiratory responses are impaired and there may be obstructive sleep apnoea. Muscle weakness may predispose to respiratory failure.

An obese patient with undiagnosed myxoedema had severe hypotension on induction, and postoperative respiratory failure. It was difficult to wean her off the ventilator. On the sixth day, when it was noticed that the oxygen consumption index was extremely low, the diagnosis of myxoedema was made and confirrned biochemically (Levelle et al 1985).

7. Rapid treatment of hypothyroidism may precipitate myocardial infarction or failure.
8. Adrenocortical insufficiency may also be present.
9. Large goitres may cause tracheal narrowing.
10. In the presence of a low BMR, IPPV readily results in hypocapnoea which decreases cerebral blood flow. Since cerebral oxygen consumption is not reduced, a relative reduction in cerebral oxygenation may result.
11. Impaired haemostasis has been recorded secondary to Factor VII deficiency (Ford & Carter 1990).

Management

1. In severe hypothyroidism, elective surgery should be cancelled whilst treatment is instituted. Patients with angina requiring coronary artery bypass surgery may be an exception to this rule (Finlayson & Kaplan 1982, Drucker & Burrow 1985). With milder forms of the disease, the case for cancellation is less clear. In a study of 59 patients with mild or moderate hypothyroidism (with matched controls), no evidence was found to justify deferring surgery until the hypothyroidism had been corrected (Weinberg et al 1983).
2. Adequate treatment of hypothyroidism, using 100–200 μg 1-thyroxine daily, takes time to achieve. Particular caution is required in the elderly, or in those with cardiac disease. In these patients, the dose should be reduced to 25 μg per day, increasing only at 3- to 4-weekly intervals. With overt hypothyroidism, it may take 6 months to restore metabolism to normal. A normal T4 and TSH signal adequate treatment. The half-life of 1-thyroxine is 1–2 weeks.

3. Severe hypothyroidism requiring urgent surgery, and myxoedema coma are probably the only indications for intravenous thyroid replacement.

   a. A single dose of lyothyronine sodium 50 μg slowly then 25 μg 8-hourly. ECG control should be used.

   b. Hydrocortisone 100 mg 6-hourly and intravenous fluids, including dextrose, may also be required.

4. If urgent surgery is needed in severe disease, careful cardiovascular monitoring is essential. There is minimal reserve. Dehydration and fluid overload are both poorly tolerated. Inotropic agents may produce severe arrhythmias and myocardial ischaemia.

5. Controlled ventilation with CO_2 monitoring to avoid hypocapnoea. Postoperative IPPV may be needed.

6. Core temperature should be monitored. A warming blanket, high theatre temperature and an infusion warmer will reduce hypothermia.

7. All drugs should be administered with caution.

BIBLIOGRAPHY

Abbott T R 1967 Anaesthesia in untreated myxoedema: report of two cases. British Journal of Anaesthesia 39: 510–514

Beghi E, Delodovici M L, Bogliun G et al 1989 Hypothyroidism and polyneuropathy. Journal of Neurology, Neurosurgery and Psychiatry 52: 1420–1423

Drucker D J, Burrow G N 1985 Cardiovascular surgery in the hypothyroid patient. Archives of Internal Medicine 145: 1585–1587

Finlayson D C, Kaplan J A 1982 Myxoedema and open heart surgery: anaesthesia and intensive care unit experience. Canadian Anaesthetists' Society Journal 29: 543–549

Ford H C, Carter J M 1990 Haemostasis in hypothyroidism. Postgraduate Medical Journal 66: 280–284

Gilbert R E, Thomas G W, Hope R N 1992 Coma and thyroid dysfunction. Anaesthesia and Intensive Care 20: 86–87

Gorman C A 1988 Thyroid function testing: a new era. Mayo Clinic Proceedings 63: 1026

Kim J M, Hackman L 1977 Anaesthesia for untreated hypothyroidism: report of 3 cases. Anesthesia and Analgesia 56: 299–302

Levelle J P, Jopling M W, Sklar G S 1985 Perioperative hypothyroidism: An unusual postanesthetic diagnosis. Anesthesiology 63: 195–197

Miller L R, Benumof J L, Alexander L et al 1989 Completely absent response to peripheral nerve stimulation in an acutely hypothyroid patient. Anesthesiology 71: 779–781

Mogensen T, Hjortso N-C 1988 Acute hypothyroidism in a severely ill surgical patient. Canadian Journal of Anaesthesia 35: 74–75

Murkin J M 1982 Anesthesia and hypothyroidism. Anesthesia and Analgesia 61: 371–383

Sherry K M, Hutchinson I L 1984 Postoperative myxoedema. A report of coma and upper airway obstruction. Anaesthesia 39: 1112–1114

Simons R J, Simon J M, Demers L M et al 1990 Thyroid dysfunction in elderly hospitalized patients. Effect of age and severity of illness. Archives of Internal Medicine 150: 1249–1253

Smallridge R C 1992 Metabolic and anatomic thyroid emergencies: a review. Critical Care Medicine 20: 276–291

Weinberg A D, Brennan M D, Gormon C A et al 1983 Outcome of anaesthesia and surgery in hypothyroid patients. Archives of Internal Medicine 143: 893–897

INFECTIOUS MONONUCLEOSIS

A common viral infection, caused by the Epstein–Barr virus, which produces a variety of clinical patterns and spectrum of severity. Two rare complications of the disease may occasionally involve the anaesthetist:

1. Acute upper airway obstruction.
2. Guillian–Barré syndrome and bulbar paralysis.

Preoperative abnormalities

1. The three main types are:
   a. Anginose: pharyngitis and adenitis.
   b. Glandular: predominantly lymphadenopathy and mild fever.
   c. Febrile: a prolonged generalized illness with fever.
2. Diagnosis may be confirmed by the Monospot test and specific serology, as well as the presence of a lymphocytosis, with atypical lymphocytes on blood film.
3. Rare complications include thrombocytopenia (Cyran et al 1991) and acute splenic rupture.

Anaesthetic problems

1. There have been several reports of upper airway obstruction from lymphoid hyperplasia of Waldeyer's ring and oedema of the faucial arch, epiglottis and aryepiglottic fold (Wolfe & Rowe 1980), and lingual tonsils (Har-El & Josephson 1990). Cardiac arrest has been reported during tracheostomy (Lee 1969). Apnoea and hypoxia on inhalation induction (Konarzewski et al 1991) and fatalities have occurred (Carrington & Hall 1986).
2. In one near-fatal case, a cervical and parapharyngeal abscess resulted in gross oedema of the epiglottic, subglottic, and postcricoid regions (Westmore 1990).
3. Emergency tonsillectomy does not necessarily immediately improve stridor. Stridor and episodes of sleep apnoea persisted in one patient for 48 hours after surgery (Konarzewski et al 1991).
4. Liver function may be impaired.
5. Infectious mononucleosis is occasionally complicated by the Guillain–Barré syndrome or bulbar palsies (Maddern et al 1991). Deaths have been associated with respiratory failure, aspiration and pneumonia.
6. Acute mucosal bleeding may occur, sometimes associated with thrombocytopenia (Johnsen et al 1984).

Management

1. Although upper airway obstruction may be a feature in patients requiring hospital admission, it is generally mild and responds to conservative treatment. The use of a soft nasopharyngeal airway has been suggested, and in 25 cases of airway obstruction thus treated, only one patient required tracheostomy (Synderman & Stool 1982). However, occasionally severe airway obstruction develops. It is therefore recommended that patients with even slight respiratory embarrassment be observed in a place with ENT and anaesthetic facilities (Johnsen et al 1984).

2. Some surgeons consider 'hot' tonsillectomy to be the treatment of choice. If an anaesthetic is required for adenotonsillectomy, facilities for immediate tracheostomy must be available. A case of stridor was described in which an attempted awake visualization of the pharynx under local anaesthetic precipitated tonsillar bleeding. Immediate tracheostomy was performed under local anaesthesia, followed by a general anaesthetic for tonsillectomy (Catling et al 1984). Cardiac arrest has also been reported during tracheostomy under local anaesthesia (Lee 1969).

3. Bulbar paralysis may be another indication for tracheostomy (Wolfe & Rowe 1980).

4. Successful treatment of thrombocytopenia using gamma globulin has been described (Cyran et al 1991).

BIBLIOGRAPHY

Carrington P, Hall J I 1986 Fatal airway obstruction in infectious mononucleosis. British Medical Journal 292: 195

Catling S J, Asbury A J, Latif M 1984 Airway obstruction in infectious mononucleosis. Anaesthesia 39: 699–702

Cyran E M, Rowe J M, Bloom R E 1991 Intravenous gammaglobulin treatment for immune thrombocytopenia associated with infectious mononucleosis. American Journal of Hematology 38: 124–129

Har-El G, Josephson J S 1990 Infectious mononucleosis complicated by lingual tonsillitis. Journal of Laryngology and Otology 104: 651–653

Johnsen T, Katholm M, Stangerup S-E 1984 Otolaryngological complications in infectious mononucleosis. Journal of Laryngology and Otology 98: 999–1001

Konarzewski W, Walker P, Donovan A 1991 Upper airway obstruction by enlarged tonsils. Anaesthesia 46: 595–596

Lee M D 1969 Respiratory obstruction in glandular fever. Journal of Laryngology and Otolaryngology 83: 617–622

Maddern B R, Werkhaven J, Wessel H B et al 1991 Infectious mononucleosis with airway obstruction and multiple cranial nerve paresis. Otolaryngology and Head and Neck Surgery 104: 529–532

Synderman N L, Stool S E 1982 Management of airway obstruction in children with infectious mononucleosis. Otolaryngology and Head and Neck Surgery 90: 168–170

Westmore G A 1990 Cervical abscess: a life-threatening complication of infectious mononucleosis. Journal of Laryngology and Otology 104: 358–359

Wolfe J A, Rowe L D 1980 Upper airway obstruction in infectious mononucleosis. Annals of Otology, Rhinology and Laryngology 89: 430–433

INSULINOMA

A rare, insulin-secreting pancreatic islet cell tumour, which may be benign or malignant. Malignancy occurs in about 10% of cases. In the majority, the tumour is solitary and resection is curative. A small number of insulinomas are associated with MEN I, in which case they are usually multiple.

Preoperative abnormalities

1. The symptoms of episodic hypoglycaemia may be suggestive of central nervous system disease, hysteria, epilepsy, sympathetic overactivity, behavioural problems or intoxication. Patients may complain of sweating, hunger, palpitations, or exhibit various focal neurological deficits coinciding with cerebral hypoglycaemia. Symptoms are either spontaneous, or induced by an overnight fast or controlled insulin infusion. They frequently occur before breakfast or during vigorous exercise. In a study of 25 patients, the median time of severe symptoms of cerebral hypoglycaemia was 2 years, and one-third of patients had had hypoglycaemic seizures (Doherty et al 1991). Hypoglycaemia may occur in pregnancy or postpartum. One patient was found to be comatose on the second morning after delivery (Garner & Tsang 1989).

2. Elevated fasting plasma insulin, and C-peptide levels in the presence of hypoglycaemia confirm the diagnosis. Fasts must be closely supervised.

3. Medical control of insulin secretion may be achieved by diazoxide, a somatostatin analogue or streptozotocin.

4. A small percentage of insulinomas form part of a multiple endocrine neoplasia syndrome (MEN I).

5. Diagnosis may require ultrasound or CT scan, MRI, angiography or selective portal venous sampling.

Anaesthetic problems

1. Hypoglycaemia under anaesthesia. Permanent neurological damage may result, but the approach to management of the blood sugar during surgery remains controversial. To prevent hypoglycaemia, the administration of dextrose 25% via a central venous infusion, whilst checking the plasma glucose at regular, but unspecified intervals, has been suggested (Chari 1977). A contrary view is that surgery should only take place in hospitals equipped with an artificial pancreas (Roizen 1981). This device performs on-line glucose

estimations and automatically administers glucose/insulin i.v. as necessary (Pulver et al 1980). Others have withheld glucose except when the blood glucose decreased below 3 mmol/l (Lamont & Jones 1978). This was based on the premise that a rebound hyperglycaemia after insulinoma resection indicated complete removal of the tumour. Thus, if glucose were to be given, the sign would be masked. The reliability of this sign has, however, been questioned.

Records of 38 operations for insulinoma in which glucose had not been given, were studied (Muir et al 1983), to establish:
a. whether intermittent, as opposed to continuous, sampling of glucose protected the patient from hypoglycaemia.
b. whether the maintenance of moderate hypoglycaemia to subsequently establish complete removal was safe.
c. whether rebound hyperglycaemia was consistent and indicative of complete surgical removal.
   It was concluded that:
d. provided the glucose level was above 3.3 mmol/l, intermittent sampling, at 15-minute intervals was safe.
e. the deliberate witholding of intraoperative glucose was potentially dangerous.
f. although rebound hyperglycaemia often occurred it was of no predictive value during the operation.
2. Hyperglycaemia may occur for the first few postoperative days as a result of persistent high levels of hormones with hyperglycaemic effects.
3. A possible interaction between diazoxide and thiopentone has been suggested (Burch & McCleskey 1981). Two patients on diazoxide infusions developed hypotension on induction of anaesthesia. Diazoxide inhibits insulin release, has peripheral vasodilator effects, and is strongly protein bound. Mechanisms associated with competition for binding sites between the two drugs were postulated.
4. Intraoperative tumour localization may be difficult.

Management

1. Since hyperglycaemic rebound is not predictive of complete removal of the insulinoma during operation, moderate hypoglycaemia would appear to be both unnecessary, and potentially dangerous (Muir et al 1983). Maintenance of a plasma glucose level between 5.5 and 8.5 mmol/l, with estimations at 15-minute intervals, is recommended.
2. Care must be taken to avoid either hyper- or hypoglycaemia. In patients treated with diazoxide, rapid infusion of dextrose 5% was

found to produce high glucose levels (Burch & McCleskey 1981). It was suggested that the rate be limited to 2 ml/kg per h.

3. Serial intraoperative measurements of serum insulin levels have been used for retrospective corroboration of the success of surgery (Krentz et al 1990). Intraoperative ultrasound may improve tumour localization (Rothmund et al 1990).

4. Close cardiovascular monitoring during induction of anaesthesia is essential, especially in patients having diazoxide infusions, when hypotension may be a problem.

5. Sevoflurane anaesthesia, which is claimed to suppress insulin secretion, has been used (Matsumoto & Saki 1992).

BIBLIOGRAPHY

Burch P C, McLeskey C H 1981 Anesthesia for patients with insulinoma treatment with oral diazoxide. Anesthesiology 55: 472–475

Chari P, Pandit S K, Kataria R N et al 1977 Anaesthetic management of insulinoma. Anaesthesia 32: 261–264

Doherty G M, Doppman J L, Shawker T N et al 1991 Results of a prospective strategy to diagnose, localize, and resect insulinomas. Surgery 110: 989–996

Garner P R, Tsang R 1989 Insulinoma complicating pregnancy presenting with hypoglycaemic coma after delivery: a case report and review of the literature. Obstetrics and Gynecology 73: 847–849

Krentz A J, Hale P J, Baddeley R M et al 1990 Intra-operative blood glucose and serum insulin concentrations in the surgical management of insulinoma. Postgraduate Medical Journal 66: 24–27

Lamont A S M, Jones D 1978 Anaesthetic management of insulinoma. Anaesthesia and Intensive Care 6: 261

Matsumoto M, Sakai H 1992 Sevoflurane anesthesia for a patient with insulinoma (English Abstr) Masui 41: 446–449

Muir J J, Endres S M, Offord K et al 1983 Glucose management in patients undergoing operation for insulinoma removal. Anesthesiology 59: 371–375

Pulver J J, Cullen B F, Miller D R et al 1980 Use of the artificial beta cell during anesthesia for surgical removal of insulinoma. Anesthesia and Analgesia 59: 950–952

Roizen M F 1987 Preoperative evaluation of patients with diseases that require special preoperative evaluation and intraoperative management. In: Miller R D (ed) Anesthesia. Churchill Livingstone, Edinburgh

Rothmund M, Angelini L, Brunt L M et al 1990 Surgery for benign insulinoma: an international review. World Journal of Surgery 14: 393–398

JEHOVAH'S WITNESSES
(see Section 3)

JUVENILE HYALINE FIBROMATOSIS

A rare inherited condition which includes skin lesions, gingival hypertrophy, painful flexion contractures of joints and destruction of bone. Anaesthesia may be required for Nissen's fundoplication, orthopaedic or skin surgery.

Preoperative abnormalities

1. Painful flexion contractures of all large joints and the radiological appearance of osteopenia and cortical defects, particularly in the humerus and femur (O'Neill & Kasser 1989).
2. Oral lesions, in particular gingival hyperplasia, and sometimes anal mucosal hypertrophy.
3. Skin lesions presenting as firm brown nodules of the face, nose, palate, ears, and neck.
4. Growth retardation secondary to vomiting and feeding difficulties. Recurrent infections which may be fatal (Bedford et al 1991).
5. Kidney, lung, and gastrointestinal tract may be involved.

Anaesthetic problems

1. Difficulties in intubation can result from gingival hypertrophy and contractures involving the cervical spine and temporomandibular joints. Tissue hyperplasia may involve the larynx.
2. Flexion contractures of joints, which are not lessened under anaesthesia, and may interfere with positioning and patient monitoring.
3. Gastro-oesophageal reflux may occur.

Management

1. Assessment of organ involvement.
2. Estimation of intubation difficulties. Awake fibreoptic intubation was performed in a 13-month-old child using a bronchoscopically placed stylet as a guide (Vaughn et al 1990).

BIBLIOGRAPHY
Aldred M J, Crawford P J 1987 Juvenile hyaline fibromatosis. Oral Surgery, Oral Medicine and Oral Pathology 63: 71–77
Bedford C D, Sills J A, Sommelet-Olive D et al 1991 Juvenile hyaline fibromatosis: a report of two severe cases. Journal of Pediatrics 119: 404–410
O'Neil D B, Kasser J R 1989 Juvenile hyaline fibromatosis. A case report and review of musculoskeletal manifestations. Journal of Bone and Joint Surgery A 71: 941–944
Vaughn G C, Kaplan R F, Tieche S 1990 Juvenile hyaline fibromatosis: anesthetic management. Anesthesiology 72: 201–203

KEARNS-SAYRE SYNDROME

A rare multisystem disorder, one of a group of structural mitochondrial defects known as mitochondrial myopathies, in which external ophthalmoplegia is associated with neural, retinal, and cardiac abnormalities (Tulinius et al 1991).

Preoperative abnormalities

1. Progressive ophthalmoplegia develops in early adulthood, before the age of 20 years.
2. Retinal pigmentation occurs.
3. There may be proximal limb muscle weakness, and sometimes bulbar involvement and cerebellar ataxia.
4. Heart block. The incidence of cardiac conduction defects increases with age, and syncope or sudden death may occur in the fourth decade.
5. Endocrinopathies may occur. Renal tubular acidosis and tetany have been reported (Eviatar et al 1990).

Anaesthetic problems

1. Conduction defects, including bundle branch block and complete heart block, have been described (Kenny & Wetherbee 1990).
2. In the presence of muscle weakness, an abnormal response to muscle relaxants might be anticipated. However, neuromuscular studies using both suxamethonium and pancuronium have been performed in a patient. There was a normal response to both of these drugs, and no hyperkalaemia occurred after suxamethonium (D'Ambra et al 1979).

Management

1. Conduction defects may necessitate preoperative transvenouspacemaker insertion.
2. Neuromuscular monitoring ts advisable.

BIBLIOGRAPHY

D'Ambra M N, Dedrick D, Savarese J J 1979. Kearns-Sayre syndrome and pancuronium-succinylcholine-induced neuromuscular blockade. Anesthesiology 51: 343–345.
Eviatar L, Shanske S, Gauthier B et al 1990 Kearns-Sayre syndrome presenting as renal tubular acidosis. Neurology 40: 1761–1763
Kenny D, Wetherbee J 1990 Kearns-Sayre syndrome in the elderly: mitochondrial myopathy with advanced heart block. American Heart Journal 120: 440–443
Tulinius M H, Holme E, Kristiansson B et al 1991 Mitochondrial encephalomyopathies in childhood. II Clinical manifestations and syndromes. Journal of Pediatrics 119: 251–259

KLIPPEL–FEIL SYNDROME

An inherited autosomal dominant condition in which skeletal abnormalities, particularly in the cervical spine, may be associated with genitourinary and cardiac anomalies.

Preoperative abnormalities

1. A short webbed neck, with restricted movement and undescended, winged scapulae. Several cervical vertebrae may be fused or reduced in number. The base of the skull may be flattened (platybasia) and the thoracic vertebrae occasionally involved. Kyphoscoliosis and spinal cord anomalies may occur. The syndrome has been classified according to the pattern of vertebral fusion:

   Type I   Block fusion of all cervical and some upper thoracic vertebrae.
   Type II   Fusion of one or two parts. Often C2/3 and C5/6.
   Type III   Types I and II combined with lower thoracic or lumbar involvement.

2. Significant genitourinary abnormalities were found in 64% of patients in one series (Moore et al 1975). Problems included renal agenesis, ectopia and malrotation, and penile hypospadias.
3. An incidence of congenital heart disease of 4–14% has been reported. Lesions include patent ductus arteriosus, coarctation of the aorta, and mitral valve prolapse.
4. Maxillofacial abnormalities may occur.
5. Deafness occurs in about one-third of patients.

Anaesthetic problems

1. A short neck and fused cervical vertebrae may contribute to difficulties in tracheal intubation.
2. If cervical instability is present, there is a risk of spinal cord injury. Quadriplegia has been reported after minor trauma (Elster 1984). In one patient, paraesthesia and weakness occurred on neck extension (Hall et al 1990). Magnetic resonance imaging of the spinal canal undertaken in 20 children showed stenoses of 9 mm or less in 25% of patients (Ritterbusch et al 1991) and subluxation of 5 mm or greater in 25%. Several children had spinal cord abnormalities in addition.
3. Sleep apnoea has been reported.
4. The trachea may be short (15 or fewer rings compared with the normal 17). This increases the risk of accidental bronchial intubation (Wells et al 1989).
5. Kyphoscoliosis may reduce respiratory reserve.

Management

1. X-rays of the cervical spine will indicate the types of cervical anomaly, and flexion and extension views, the presence of any instability. If, on questioning, any symptoms suggestive of spinal cord compression are elicited, the use of MRI should be considered to evaluate the abnormalities (Rutterbusch et al 1991).

2. Potential intubation difficulties must be assessed. Awake intubation may be appropriate and has been described for cholecystectomy (Daum & Jones 1988) and for Caesarean section in a patient with Klippel-Feil syndrome, congenital hydrocephalus and pregnancy-induced hypertension (Burns et al 1988). An inhalation induction was described in a neonate with coincidental Klippel–Feil and a craniocervical encephalocoele (Naguib et al 1986).
3. If cardiac defects are diagnosed, prophylactic antibiotic therapy will be necessary.

BIBLIOGRAPHY

Burns A M, Dorje P, Lawes E G, et al 1988 Anaesthetic management of Caesarean section for a mother with pre-eclampsia, the Klippel–Feil syndrome and congenital hydrocephalus. British Journal of Anaesthesia 61: 350–354

Daum R E O, Jones D J 1988 Fibreoptic intubation in Klippel–Feil syndrome. Anaesthesia 43: 18–21

Elster A D 1984 Quadriplegia after minor trauma in the Klippel–Feil syndrome. Journal of Bone and Joint Surgery 66A: 1473–1474

Hall J E, Simmons E D, Danylchuk K et al 1990 Instability of the cervical spine and neurological involvement in Klippel–Feil syndrome. A case report. Journal of Bone and Joint Surgery 72A: 460–462

Moore W B, Matthews T J, Rabinowitz R 1975 Genitourinary anomalies associated with Klippel–Feil syndrome. Journal of Bone and Joint Surgery 57A: 355–357

Naguib M, Farag H, Ibrahim A E W 1986 Anaesthetic considerations Klippel–Feil syndrome. Canadian Anaesthetists' Society Journal 33: 66–70

Ritterbusch J F, McGinty L D, Spar J et al 1991 Magnetic resonance imaging for stenosis and subluxation in Klippel–Feil syndrome. Spine 16: S539–541

Wells A L, Wells T R, Landing B H et al 1989 Short trachea, a hazard in tracheal intubation of neonates and infants: syndromal association. Anesthesiology 71: 367–373

LARYNGEAL PAPILLOMATOSIS

Benign warty tumours of the larynx which occur in children and are caused by one or more of the human papillomaviruses, mostly type 11, but sometimes type 6. They arise most commonly on the true vocal cords with extension onto the ventricles. Frequently recurrent, they may also be present in other parts of the respiratory tract.

Preoperative abnormalities

1. Usually presents in early childhood with hoarseness, cough, respiratory distress, or stridor secondary to upper airway obstruction. Of 90 patients whose symptoms presented between birth and age 11 years, nearly half occurred before the age of 2, 90% had a voice change, 44% airway obstruction and 39% stridor (Cohen et al 1980).
2. Chronic airway obstruction may lead to pulmonary hypertension, right ventricular hypertrophy, cor pulmonale and polycythaemia (Hawkins & Udall 1979).

3. Regression may occur at puberty.
4. Tracheal involvement is more frequent than was previously thought (Weiss & Kashima 1983), although current techniques in management are reducing the incidence of tracheal spread (Crockett et al 1987b).

Anaesthetic problems

1. Upper respiratory tract obstruction, usually in young infants, although a fatal case of laryngeal papillomatosis in pregnancy secondary to laryngeal obstruction has been described (Helmrich et al 1992).
2. Numerous anaesthetics may be required. In one series, 66% of the patients had multiple diffuse disease and each required an average of 15.9 anaesthetics (Cohen et al 1980).
3. Tracheostomy and tracheal intubation may seed papillomas and cause distal spread of the disease. In the past, tracheal intubation seemed to predispose to this. The combination of laser treatment with Venturi and jet ventilation techniques may minimize viral spread (Crockett et al 1987b).
4. Tracheobronchial papillomatosis may occur in 2–26% of cases of laryngeal papillomatosis. A case was reported in which an absence of ventilation of the right lung was noticed during resection of laryngeal papillomata in a 10-year-old child. At bronchoscopy, a large papilloma was found to be occluding the right main bronchus. Tracheostomy had been performed in this child at an earlier stage (Callander 1986).
5. Laser treatment is not complication free. In a study of 890 resections in 66 patients, although the immediate complication rate was low, delayed tissue damage occurred in 36% children and 17% adults (Crockett et al 1987a). The more severe the disease, the greater the likelihood of late complications.
6. Airway fires have occurred during laser treatment. Ignition of the surgeon's glove resulted in entrainment of burning vapours into the airway by the Venturi (Wegryznowicz et al 1992), and burns were sustained by both patient and surgeon.
7. There is a small risk of virus spread to the staff. A laser surgeon who had previously treated anogenital condylomas developed laryngeal papillomatosis. Both of these tumours harbour papillomaviruses of the same viral types, therefore it was speculated that the laser plume had carried virus particles (Hallmo & Naess 1991). However, analysis of the smoke plume from laser-treated laryngeal papilloma studies did not reveal the presence of human papillomavirus, unless direct suction contact had been made with the lesion (Abramson et al 1990).

Management

1. Interferon has been claimed to eliminate papilloma in 40% children and reduce their growth rate in 30% (Crockett et al 1987a). However, lesions that are unresponsive to interferon treatment may regularly require endoscopy and resection or laser excision.

2. For management of anaesthesia for laser surgery of airway lesions, see Section 3.

3. A rigid bronchoscope should be available in case of sudden obstruction of the airway by a papilloma.

4. Tracheostomy should be avoided unless life saving. In one series, a low incidence of tracheobronchial papillomata (3.3%) was thought to be due to the low incidence of tracheostomy (4%) in that particular hospital when compared with that (10%) in the cases referred from elsewhere (Cohen et al 1980).

5. If avoidance of tracheal intubation reduces the chance of spread, a technique using inhalation anaesthesia and local anaesthetic spray, apnoea (Hawkins & Joseph 1990), or insufflation of halothane and oxygen (or air in the case of laser surgery), can be commended. In a series, less than one-third of the 1047 anaesthetics were given through a tracheal tube or a tracheostomy (Cohen et al 1980). Although it has been suggested that a Venturi technique should be avoided (Weiss & Kashima 1983), jet ventilation with laser surgery now seems to be the treatment of choice (Crockett et al 1987a, b). However, care should be taken to avoid airway fires (see Section 3, Anaesthesia for laser surgery of the airway).

6. Precautions against the spread of the virus to staff include the use of eye protection and gloves. Since the aspirate is potentially infective, disposable suction canisters and tubing should be used.

7. Postoperative humidification of oxygen is recommended.

8. Preoperative corticosteroids have been claimed to reduce postoperative oedema but their use is arguable. Laser techniques are increasingly being used for laryngeal lesions and seem to be associated with less immediate postoperative complications.

9. If severe obstructive symptoms are present, the airway must be secured before general anaesthesia is given.

10. Airway manipulation in small children is often complicated by coughing, excess secretions and laryngeal spasm. An infusion of procaine (2% solution in 5% dextrose) 1 mg/kg per min i.v., was found to produce much smoother operating conditions when compared with identically anaesthetized matched controls. Recovery was more rapid and there were no signs of toxicity (Lawson et al 1979).

BIBLIOGRAPHY

Abramson A L, DiLorenzo T P, Steinberg B M 1990 Is papillomavirus detectable in the plume of laser-treated laryngeal papilloma? Archives of Otolaryngology and Head and Neck Surgery 116: 604–607

Callander C C 1986 Tracheobronchial papillomatosis: Anaesthetic implications. Anaesthesia and Intensive Care 14: 201–202

Cohen S R, Geller K A, Seltzer S et al 1980 Papilloma of the larynx and tracheobronchial tree in children. Annals of Otolaryngology 89: 497–503

Crockett D M, Scamman F L, McCabe B F et al 1987a Venturi jet ventilator for microlaryngoscopy: technique, complications, pitfalls. Laryngoscope 97: 1326–1330

Crokett D M, McCabe B F, Shive C J 1987b Complications of laser surgery for recurrent respiratory papillomatosis. Annals of Otology Rhinology and Laryngology 96: 639–644

Hallmo P, Naess O 1991 Laryngeal papillomatosis with human papillomavirus DNA contracted by a laser surgeon. European Archives of Otolaryngology 248: 425–427

Hawkins D B, Udall J N 1979 Juvenile laryngeal papillomas with cardiomegaly and polycythemia. Pediatrics 63: 156–157

Hawkins D B, Joseph M M 1990 Avoiding wrapped endotracheal tubes in laser laryngeal surgery: experiences with apneic anesthesia and metal Laser Flex endotracheal tubes. Laryngoscope 100: 1283–1287

Helmrich G, Stubbs T M, Stoerker J 1992 Fatal maternal laryngeal papillomatosis in pregnancy: a case report. American Journal of Obstetrics and Gynecology 166: 524–525

Lawson N W, Rogers D, Seifen A et al 1979 Intravenous procaine as a supplement to general anesthesia for carbon dioxide laser resection of laryngeal papillomas in children. Anesthesia and Analgesia 58: 492–496

Wegrzynowicz E S, Jensen N F, Pearson K S et al 1992 Airway fire during jet ventilation for laser excision of vocal cord papillomata. Anesthesiology 76: 468–469

Weiss M D, Kashima H K 1983 Tracheal involvement in laryngeal papillomatosis. Laryngoscope 93: 45–48

LESCH–NYHAN SYNDROME

An X-linked recessive disorder of purine metabolism in which there is an absence of hypoxanthine guanine phosphoribosyl transferase (HGPRT) activity. There is primary purine overproduction with hyperuricaemia, gout, and choreoathetoid spasticity.

Preoperative abnormalities

1. Mental retardation, choreoathetoid movements, spasticity and bizarre episodes of self mutilation.
2. Hyperuricaemia results in a nephropathy and urinary tract calcification. Death frequently results from renal failure in the third decade.
3. Arthritis and gouty tophi occur.
4. A B-lymphocyte immune deficiency may result in an increased susceptibility to infection.
5. Urinary uric acid levels are always increased and serum urate usually so.

Anaesthetic problems

1. Self mutilation may result in scarring of the mouth region.
2. Patients are susceptible to aspiration pneumonitis.

3. Abnormal adrenergic responses and decreased monoamine oxidase activity have been reported (Larson & Wilkins 1985).

Management

1. Teeth extraction may be required to reduce the trauma from self mutilation.
2. Suxamethonium should probably not be used (Larson & Wilkins 1985).

BIBLIOGRAPHY
Larson L O, Wilkins R G 1985 Anesthesia and the Lesch-Nyan Syndrome. Anesthesiology 63: 197–199

LUDWIG'S ANGINA

Cellulitis of the floor of the mouth which can be produced by any infection. Gram-positive cocci (usually streptococci) are most common, but sometimes gram-negative rods or anaerobes are responsible. In 50% of cases more than one organism is isolated (Moreland et al 1988). It is most frequently precipitated by dental infection involving the second and third lower molars, but trauma can be contributory.

Before antibiotics or in the untreated patient, fatalities have occurred (Iwu 1990). In the post-antibiotic era the mean age of patients is 29 years. They are usually previously fit, but most have dental disease. The condition may also occur in immunocompromized or diabetic patients.

Preoperative abnormalities

1. Bilateral submandibular swelling proceeding to brawny swelling of the neck. Although the submandibular space is primarily involved in Ludwig's angina, spread into adjacent fascial spaces may occur. A detailed account of the anatomy of spread of infection can be consulted (Lindner 1986).
2. Elevation of the tongue caused by cellulitis of floor of the mouth.
3. Dysphagia secondary to swelling, and trismus.
4. Upper airway obstruction.
5. Other complications include bacteraemia, aspiration, empyema, mediastinitis, internal jugular vein thrombosis and pericarditis.
6. Fever, leucocytosis and increased ESR.

Anaesthetic problems

1. Trismus, not necessarily relieved by muscle relaxants, may make oral intubation difficult or impossible.
2. Upper airway obstruction, resulting in hypoxia.

3. Intravenous induction of anaesthesia may be hazardous because it can result in apnoea and an inability to maintain ventilation on a mask (Loughnan & Allen 1985).
4. After fibreoptic intubation with a polyvinylchloride nasotracheal tube, difficulties were experienced in withdrawing the bronchoscope (Chung & Liban 1991). When the bronchoscope was successfully removed, obstruction again occurred and was found to be the result of compression of the tube by severe supraglottic swelling.

Management

1. Aggressive early treatment with antibiotics reduces airway problems and the need for surgical intervention.
2. Airway maintenance in the compromised airway. Signs of airway obstruction, dyspnoea or dysphagia may indicate the need for tracheostomy. In these cases, sedative premedication should be avoided.
3. Surgical drainage with or without tooth extraction.
4. Anaesthesia for surgery in which there is trismus, but no airway obstruction
   a. Awake fibreoptic intubation but with facilities for emergency tracheostomy available.
   b. Inhalation induction and laryngoscopy. If the trismus relaxes and the vocal cords can be seen, a neuromuscular blocker can be given.
   c. Tracheostomy.
5. If there is significant stridor, a tracheostomy under local anaesthesia may be considered.

BIBLIOGRAPHY
Chung R A, Liban J B 1991 Ludwig's angina and tracheal tube obstruction. Anaesthesia 46: 228–229
Iwu C O 1990 Ludwig's angina: report of seven cases and review of current concepts of management. British Journal of Oral and Maxillofacial Surgery 28: 189–193
Lindner H H 1986 The anatomy of the fasciae of the face and neck with particular reference to the spread and treatment of intraoral infections (Ludwig's) that have progressed into adjacent fascial spaces. Annals of Surgery 204: 705–714
Loughnan T E, Allen D E 1985 Ludwig's angina. The anaesthetic management of nine cases. Anaesthesia 40: 295–297
Moreland L W, Corey J, McKenzie R 1988 Ludwig's angina. Report of a case and review of the literature. Archives of Internal Medicine 148: 461–466
Patterson H C, Kelly J H, Stome M 1982 Ludwig's angina: an update. Laryngoscope 92: 370–377
Schwartz H C, Bauer R A, Davis N J et al 1974 Ludwig's angina: use of fiberoptic laryngscopy to avoid tracheostomy. Journal of Oral Surgery 32: 608–611

LYSERGIC ACID DIETHYLAMIDE (LSD) ABUSE

LSD is a psychedelic drug, which can either be synthesized, or obtained naturally from the seeds of *Rivea corymbosa* (morning glory), or ergot fungus on rye. Its effect is almost entirely on the CNS and it rapidly produces tolerance. Intoxicated patients are liable to injure themselves and be unaware of it. Respiratory depression has been reported.

Preoperative abnormalities

1. The onset of CNS effects occurs 40 minutes after an oral dose. Hallucinations may last for 2 hours and the biological half-life is 3 hours (Caldwell 1981).
   Effects (Caldwell 1981):

0.5–1 µg/kg	Euphoria and a degree of visual, auditory or tactile disturbances.
1 µg/kg	Increases sensory distortion.
2 µg/kg	Alarming hallucinations.
0.2 mg/kg	Possible lethal threshold.

2. Central autonomic stimulation occurs, probably mediated via the hypothalamus. Parasympathetic and sympathetic effects include tremors, tachycardia, hypertension, fever, piloerection, mydriasis, lacrimation, and hyper-reflexia.
3. LSD has analgesic properties.
4. Tolerance to both autonomic and psychic effects is produced rapidly, but dependence does not occur.
5. LSD produces EEG changes.

Anaesthetic problems

1. Injury may be sustained without the patient being aware of it.
2. Hypertension, tachycardia and fever occur with toxic doses.
3. Interaction with belladonna alkaloids may occur.
4. Some inhibition of cholinesterase activity has been reported and theoretically it may prolong the action of suxamethonium.
5. Exaggerated responses to other sympathomimetic amines may occur.
6. Increased toxicity of ester-type local anaesthetics has been suggested (McGoldrick 1980).

Management

1. Heart rate, blood pressure and temperature should be monitored continuously.
2. Persistent sympathetic effects during general anaesthesia can be treated with alpha and beta adrenoceptor blockers:

Phentolamine	1–2 mg and repeat, or infusion of 0.1-2 mg/min.
Propranolol	0.5 mg at 10-min intervals to a maximum of 5 mg.
Metoprolol	1–2 mg/min up to 5 mg. Repeat at 5-min intervals to a total of 10–15 mg.

3. If sedatives are required, a benzodiazepine or chlorpromazine is probably suitable.
4. Anticholinergics should be avoided if the patient shows signs of toxicity, as the effects of LSD may be enhanced.
5. If the effects of LSD are still present, less analgesia will be needed. Opiates should be used cautiously in case of respiratory depression (McCammon 1986).
6. The concomitant use of other sympathomimetics should be avoided.

BIBLIOGRAPHY
Caldwell T B 1990 Anesthesia for patients with behavioral and environmental disorders. In: Katz J, Benumof J, Kadis L (eds) Anesthesia and uncommon diseases. W B Saunders, Philadelphia
McCammon R L 1986 Anesthesia for the chemically dependent patient. International Anesthesia Research Society Review Course Lecutres 47–55
McGoldrick K E 1980 Anesthetic implications of drug abuse. Anesthesiology Review 7: 12–17

MALIGNANT HYPERTHERMIA

A rare pharmacogenetic condition, or possibly a spectrum of conditions, of complex inheritance. Malignant hyperthermia (MH) usually presents during general anaesthesia with a syndrome indicative of greatly accelerated muscle metabolism. Occasionally, it has been induced by severe exercise (Britt 1988, Hackl et al 1991). The exact defect is unknown. Dysfunction of the sarcoplasmic reticulum and abnormalities of intracellular ionic calcium are thought to play an important role, with the secondary and possibly synergistic effects of the sympathetic nervous system (Gronert et al 1988). The primary release of calcium is normal, but there is thought to be an enhanced calcium-induced release of calcium from the sarcoplasmic reticulum by agents known to induce MH (Fletcher 1987). Studies on erythrocytic membranes suggest that there may be a generalized membrane permeability defect. Genetic studies indicate that the MH gene is on chromosome 19, in a position close to the ryanodine receptor gene (Levitt et al 1991). At present, the in-vitro contracture tests are being compared with genetic linkage studies to see if there should be any alteration to the criteria for diagnosis (MacKenzie et al 1991).

The cardinal signs include hyperthermia, and respiratory and metabolic acidosis, with or without muscle rigidity. MH can be precipitated by a number of drugs, known as 'trigger' agents. Until recently the mortality was high but it has now been dramatically reduced from about 70% to 24% (Ellis et al 1986), although this decrease is less than had been predicted. The reduction has been achieved by:

1. An increased awareness of the condition.

2. More intensive patient monitoring for sensitive indicators, such as ET_{CO_2}, which assist early diagnosis.
3. Availability of an i.v. form of dantrolene sodium, a drug which has played an important role in the treatment of MH.

In the past, the diagnosis has been made too readily on clinical grounds alone. In retrospect, a number of cases previously thus identified in the literature may well not have been true MH. In 1984 the European MH Groups (Ellis et al 1984) agreed a protocol for the diagnosis of the condition. This was subsequently modified (European MH Group 1985). In 1989, a North American MH Group also reported (Larach 1989). It is hoped that the standardization of in-vitro tests and diagnostic classification will allow further elucidation of the precise defect. Case reports should now only be given credence when the diagnosis has been confirmed according to these criteria.

Is MH associated with other conditions?
During anaesthesia, patients with a number of other disorders have developed clinical syndromes which have certain features in common with MH, and as a result were labelled as being 'associated with an increased risk of MH'.

These assertions have, in general, proved not to be true (Brownell 1988, Ellis 1990), except in the case of central core disease (see Central core disease) and the King syndrome. However, there are certain other neuromuscular conditions which have been associated with acute rhabdomyolysis, hyperkalaemia, a high CK level, mild pyrexia and acidosis, and yet in-vitro testing usually shows the patient not to be MH-susceptible. These include muscular dystrophy, spinal muscular atrophy, the myotonias and periodic paralysis and neuroleptic malignant syndrome.

Muscular dystrophies
The muscular dystrophies are most prone to present with features in common with MH under anaesthesia, sometimes with a fatal outcome. Contracture testing for MH was negative in two children, one with Becker's muscular dystrophy and the other with DMD (Gronert et al 1992). It was considered that the MH-like features seen during anaesthesia were a result of alterations in the muscle membrane secondary to the dystrophy itself. Exposure to volatile agents and suxamethonium might increase membrane permeability and it is suggested that compensatory hypermetabolism results from attempts to re-establish membrane stability and prevent calcium flux.

Spinal muscular atrophy
A 13-year-old child developed acute rhabdomyolysis in association with dental anaesthesia using suxamethonium and halothane (Personal

observation). On the day following surgery, the serum CK level was in excess of 252 000 u/l. Investigation 4 years later was negative for MH, but electron microscopy suggested a subclinical spinal muscular atrophy. Rhabdomyolysis had presumably been precipitated by suxamethonium.

Myotonia syndromes and the periodic paralyses
More recently, Lehman-Horn and Iaizzo (1990) have subjected muscle from patients with myotonia or periodic paralyses to in vitro contracture tests for MH. Four out of 44 gave positive tests and 10 were equivocal. All the positive tests were in patients with myotonic dystrophy, and eight patients with hyperkalaemic periodic paralysis had equivocal results. The significance of this is not yet known. However, neither the patients nor their families had experienced problems with general anaesthesia.

Neuroleptic malignant syndrome
Investigation of six survivors of the neuroleptic malignant syndrome (NMS) revealed that five were negative for MH, and one result was equivocal (Krivosic-Horber et al 1987). This would suggest that NMS is a distinct entity, but sharing with MH common clinical features, and a response to dantrolene.

Sudden infant death syndrome
The suggestions of an association between sudden infant death syndrome (SIDS) and MH has been disputed (Ellis et al 1988).

Heat–stroke
Heat-stroke may produce a picture similar to that of MH (Britt 1988). Muscle biopsy and in vitro contracture tests were performed in two patients who had developed severe exercise-induced rhabdomyolysis (Hackl et al 1991). In one, the tests proved to be positive although the clinical patterns were indistinguishable. The frequency of exercise-induced symptoms (muscle pains, cramp and stiffness) is reported to be greater in those patients undergoing muscle biopsy who are MHS than those who are MHN (Hackl et al 1991).

Presentation
1. A family history of MH may be elicited. Confirmatory tests may or may not have been performed. According to standard criteria agreed by members of the European Malignant Hyperpyrexia Group (1985), the current diagnoses are:
   a. MHS: definite susceptibility to MH.
   b. MHN: non-susceptible subject from a proven MH pedigree.
   c. MHE: equivocal result; consider as MHS.

2. The clinical signs and symptoms of MH can be broadly divided into two categories. It is critical to remember this when a suspicion of MH is raised during anaesthesia.
   a. signs of metabolic stimulation.
   b. signs of abnormal muscle activity.
   However, it must be remembered that other conditions may cause one or other or both. Signs of both may occur with Duchenne (or other) muscular dystrophy, spinal muscle atrophy, myotonia congenita, McArdle's disease and carnitine palmitoyl transferase deficiency.
3. Signs of metabolic stimulation
   a. Hypercarbia. Tachypnoea occurs in a spontaneously breathing patient, whilst in the paralyzed patient, there is an apparently increased requirement for muscle relaxants. Both states are initially due to stimulation of respiration by a rising alveolar CO_2. If a capnograph is used, an increase in ET_{CO_2} may be the earliest sign of MH.
   b. Metabolic acidosis. In early reports of fulminating cases, an arterial pH of less than 7.0 was not uncommon. Severe acidosis may have been responsible for the cases in which sudden death occurred unexpectedly in the operating theatre.
   c. Arrhythmias.
   d. Hyperthermia.
   e. Hypoxaemia. In the later stages, cyanosis may result from a combination of a massive increase in oxygen consumption, and ventilation perfusion defects.
4. Signs of abnormal muscle activity
   a. Failure of the jaw to relax after suxamethonium. An increase in tone in the masseter muscle is a normal response to suxamethonium and in some patients the tension developed may be marked (Leary & Ellis 1990, Saddler et al 1990). However, masseter muscle rigidity (MMR) may also be an early sign of MH. Susceptibility to MH was found in about half of a series of 77 patients who developed masseter rigidity (Rosenberg & Fletcher 1986). It was therefore suggested that any patient who developed MMR after suxamethonium should be assumed to be MH susceptible and anaesthesia terminated. However, a 1% incidence of MMR was found in children receiving halothane and suxamethonium (Carroll 1987) and it soon became apparent that MMR was not exclusive to MH. (See also Section 2, Masseter muscle rigidity).
   b. Rigidity of certain, but not necessarily all, groups of muscles. Although a non-rigid group has been described, it is not yet known whether this is a different biochemical process, or an earlier stage of the same process. A contracture of the muscle

actually takes place and if the process is not aborted, oedema, and subsequently ischaemia, of the muscle can develop.

c. Hyperkalaemia. Potassium may be released in large quantities, particularly after the use of suxamethonium.

d. Myoglobinuria and renal failure may result.

e. A greatly elevated serum CK. This may be in excess of 100 000 iu/l.

5. Disseminated intravascular coagulation may occur in advanced cases.

6. Cerebral and pulmonary oedema can occur.

Management

1. Criteria for preoperative diagnosis. Following a strict protocol (Ellis et al 1984, European MH Group 1985. North American Malignant Hyperthermia Group 1989), a quadriceps muscle biospy, which includes the motor point, is subjected to:
   a. A static caffeine test.
   b. A static halothane test.
   c. A dynamic halothane test.
   The results should allow classification of patients into the three groups: MHS, MHN and MHE.

2. A patient who is known to be MHS, MHE, or possibly has a family history of MH, should be given a non-triggering anaesthetic.
   a. Known triggering agents include:
      i. All the inhalational agents including desflurane (Wedel et al 1991) and sevoflurane (Otsuka et al 1991).
      ii. Suxamethonium.
   b. Agents not definitely implicated but avoidance suggested (Gronert 1980):
      i Phenothiazines.
      ii. Atropine.
   Discussion continues over the safety of giving calcium, which may be needed to treat severe hyperkalaemia. Avoidance of its use has been suggested, but there is clinical and experimental evidence against it acting as a trigger agent (Murakawa et al 1988, Gronert et al 1986). Although avoidance of the use of ketamine has been suggested in the past (Gronert 1980), its use in a total of 76 MH- susceptible swine did not produce signs of MH (Derschwitz et al 1989). It was considered that, should there be a particular indication for ketamine, it could be used, provided that end-tidal CO, is monitored.
   c. Agents thought to be safe, or for use if necessary, include:
      i. Thiopentone.
      ii. Nitrous oxide.
      iii. Opiates.
      iv. Droperidol.

    v. Pancuronium, vecuronium.

    vi. Benzodiazepines.

    vii. Bupivacaine.

    viii. Propofol has now been used widely, both clinically and experimentally (Raff & Harrison 1989, Krisovic-Horber et al 1989, Allen 1991, McKenzie et al 1992) without evidence of triggering MH.

    ix. Amide local anaesthetics (Allen 1991).

3. The routine use of dantrolene preoperatively in MHS and MHE patients remains controversial. There is now no indication for the use of oral dantrolene, in view of its side effects and the uncertainty of achieving therapeutic levels (Harrison 1988). Many believe that it is sufficient to give a non-triggering anaesthetic, provided that an entirely volatile agent-free anaesthetic machine is used, the monitoring of ET_{CO_2} is available, and intravenous dantrolene is readily to hand.

    [Decontamination of a machine may be achieved by flushing it with oxygen 12 l/min for 6 minutes (McGraw & Keon 1989)]. Of 956 patients who had muscle biopsy without pretreatment with dantrolene, only four developed mild MH episodes, all of which responded to general measures (Cunliffe & Britt 1987).

    Occasionally, treatment may be considered to be appropriate before prolonged surgery, in which case, dantrolene i.v. 2.4 mg/kg should be given, but only after induction of anaesthesia.

4. If an unexpected intraoperative diagnosis of MH is made, the treatment required will depend upon the severity of the reaction at the time of diagnosis. The patient's susceptibility, the promptness of the diagnosis and hence the dose of the triggering agent received, are all important factors.

    A short exposure and rapid diagnosis may mean that the syndrome can be aborted at the initial stage of treatment. Nowadays, the increased quality of monitoring means that the fulminant case is rarely seen. However, it also means that there is an increase in the number of aborted or doubtful cases. All the early signs of MH are non-specific. It is therefore the responsibility of the anaesthetist, should the possibility of MH be raised, to gain as much information as possible at the time of the event.

5. What should be done if there are mild symptoms and signs which could be part of the MH syndrome, but which could equally well be secondary to other factors? It is recommended that attention be paid to the following features (Ellis et al 1990):

    a. Good record keeping of time sequence of clinical events

        i. MMR (duration and degree).

        ii. Presence or absence of generalized rigidity.

        iii. Arrhythmias.

        iv. Tachypnoea with signs of CO_2 production.

    v. Cyanosis.

    vi. Increase in core temperature.

  b. Laboratory tests

    i. Arterial blood gases.

    ii. Serum potassium.

    iii. Initial, 12- and 24-hour serum CK.

    iv. Evidence of myoglobinuria.

Serial serum CK levels taken under these circumstances are most important. Whilst the CK is normally of little diagnostic help in MH in the absence of a triggering event, if an anaesthetic has been given which is associated with evidence of hypermetabolism, it may be of considerable value. If the CK level is high, it is likely that the event that occurred was of significance. It may not necessarily be MH, but could be associated with one or another of a variety of conditions. These include Duchenne muscular dystrophy, spinal muscular atrophy, myotonia congenita, myotonic dystrophy, McArdle's disease or carnitine palmitoyl transferase deficiency.

6. Management of a fulminant episode of malignant hyperthermia. The fulminant MH syndrome may require the whole scheme to be executed rapidly, whereas in the mild case only the triggering agents need be stopped.

  a. Stop the use of all MH trigger agents. Terminate surgery if possible. Observe the ECG and capnograph.

  b. Delegate one person to prepare dantrolene sodium 1 mg/kg.

  c. Record core temperature, pulse rate and blood pressure every 5 min.

  d. Estimate arterial pH and blood gases. Hypercarbia should be treated with vigorous hyperventilation, acidosis with sodium bicarbonate 2–4 mmol/kg. Oxygenation must be maintained.

  e. Save one venous sample for serum CK and send one for electrolytes and serium calcium estimations.

  f. Give dantrolene sodium i.v. 1 mg/kg. Repeat at 10-min intervals if necessary, up to a maximum of 10 mg/kg.

  g. If the syndrome is severe, treat the symptoms. Cool the patient and treat hyperkalaemia if necessary.

  h. Keep the first urine sample for myoglobin estimation. Measure urine output. If obvious myoglobinuria occurs, give intravenous fluids, and mannitol or frusemide to promote urine flow.

  i. The use of steroids is controversial, but may be indicated for cerebral oedema in the severe case.

  j. Repeat the serum CK estimation at 24 hours.

  k. Treat DIC if necessary.

  l. Dantrolene may need to be repeated for up to 24 hours as further retriggering may occur. It half-life is only 5 hours.

7. With general awareness of MH and increased use of monitoring, the occurrence of a postoperative pyrexia sometimes results in the patient being informed that 'there might be a small chance that you are susceptible to malignant hyperthermia'. Whilst such caution is commendable, in the absence of other positive features of MH this statement has enormous implications for the patient, the family, and for their subsequent anaesthetists. With such a history, the odds of the patient being MHS are negligible, yet once this spectre has been raised, subsequent anaesthetists may feel obliged to treat the patient as MHS. Since, on the basis of such a vague history, in vitro testing would never be undertaken, the ghost cannot be laid to rest.

Under such circumstances, my preference is to administer an anaesthetic in which ventilation is controlled, but an inhalational agent is given. Blood is taken for serum CK levels before and after operation, and ET_{CO_2} and temperature are monitored continuously during surgery. If these prove to be normal, the patient is told that he is not susceptible, and is given a letter outlining the strategy that was undertaken.

8. The social implications for a family in whom a diagnosis of malignant hyperthermia has been made, particularly in certain cultures, may be devastating (Fletcher 1987, Ellis 1988). In addition, despite warning their surgeons in advance, they frequently face surgical delays or cancellations by anaesthetists who are unfamiliar with administration of non-triggering anaesthetics.

BIBLIOGRAPHY

Allen G 1991 Propofol and malignant hyperthermia. Anesthesia and Analgesia 73: 359

Britt B A 1988 Combined anesthetic- and stress-induced malignant hyperthermia in two offspring of malignant hyperthermia-susceptible parents. Anesthesia and Analgesia 67: 393–399

Brownell A K W 1988 Malignant hyperthermia: relationship to other diseases. British Journal of Anaesthesia 60: 303–308

Carroll J B 1987 Increased incidence of masseter spasm in children with strabismus anesthetised with halothane and succinyl choline. Anesthesiology 67: 559–561

Cunliffe M, Lerman J, Britt B A 1987 Is prophylactic dantrolene indicated for MHS patients undergoing elective surgery? Anesthesia and Analgesia 66: S35

Dershwitz M, Sreter F A, Ryan J F 1989 Ketamine does not trigger malignant hyperthermia in susceptible swine. Anesthesia and Analgesia 69: 501–503

Ellis F R 1988 The diagnosis of MH: its social implications. British Journal of Anaesthesia 60: 251–252

Ellis F R 1990 Predicting malignant hyperthermia. British Journal of Anaesthesia 64: 411–412

Ellis F R, Halsall P J 1984 Suxamethonium spasm. British Journal of Anaesthesia 56: 381–384

Ellis F R, Halsall PJ, Christian A S 1990 Clinical presentation of suspected malignant hyperthermia during anaesthesia in 402 probands. Anaesthesia 45: 838–841

Ellis F R, Heffron J J A 1985 Clinical and biochemical aspects of malignant hyperpyrexia. In: Recent advances in anaesthesia and analgesia 15. Churchill Livingstone, Edinburgh

Ellis F R, Fletcher R, Halsall P 1984 A protocol for the investigation of malignant hyperpyrexia by the European Malignant Hyperpyrexia Group. British Journal of Anaesthesia 56: 1267–1269

Ellis F R, Halsall P J, Harriman D G F 1986 The work of the Leeds Malignant
    Hyperpyrexia Unit, 1971–1984. Anaesthesia 41: 809–815
Ellis F R, Halsall P J, Harriman D G F 1988 Malignant hyperpyrexia and sudden
    infant death syndrome. British Journal of Anaesthesia 60: 28–30
European MH Group 1985 Laboratory diagnosis of malignant hyperpyrexia
    susceptibility (MHS). British Journal of Anaesthesia 57: 1038
Fletcher R 1987 4th International Hyperpyrexia Workshop. Report of a meeting.
    Anaesthesia 42: 206
Gronert G A 1980 Malignant hyperthermia. Anesthesiology 53: 395–423
Gronert G A, Ahern C P, Milde J et al 1986 Effect of CO_2, calcium, digoxin and
    potassium on cardiac and skeletal muscle in malignant hyperthermia susceptible
    swine. Anesthesiology 64: 24–28
Gronert G A, Mott J, Lee J 1988 Aetiology of malignant hyperthermia. British Journal
    of Anaesthesia 60: 253–267
Gronert G A, Fowler W Cardinet G H et al 1992 Absence of malignant hyperthermia
    contractures in Becker-Duchenne dystrophy at age 2. Muscle and Nerve 15: 52–56
Hackl W, Winkler M, Mauritz W et al 1991 Muscle biopsy for diagnosis of malignant
    hyperthermia susceptibility in two patients with severe exercise-induced myolysis.
    British Journal of Anaesthesia 66: 138–140
Harrison G G 1988 Dantrolene – dynamics and kinetics. British Journal of Anaesthesia
    60: 279–286
Krivosic-Horber R, Adnet P, Guevart E 1987 Neuroleptic malignant syndrome and
    malignant hyperthermia. British Journal of Anaesthesia 59: 1554–1556
Krivosic-Horber R, Reyfort H, Becq M C et al 1989 Effect of propofol on malignant
    hyperthermia susceptible pig model. British Journal of Anaesthesia 62: 691–693
Leary N P, Ellis F R 1990 Masseteric muscle spasm as a normal response to
    suxamethonium. British Journal of Anaesthesia 64: 488–492
Lehmann-Horn F, Iaizzo P A 1990 Are myotonias and periodic paralyses associated
    with susceptibility to malignant hyperthermia. British Journal of Anaesthesia 65:
    692–697
Levitt R C, Meyer D, Fletcher J E et al 1991 Molecular genetics and malignant
    hyperthermia. Anesthesiology 75: 1–3
McGraw T T, Keon T P 1989 Malignant hyperthermia and the clean machine.
    Canadian Journal of Anaesthesia 36: 530–532
MacKenzie A E, Allen G, Lahey D et al 1991 A comparison of the caffeine halothane
    muscle contracture test with the molecular genetic diagnosis of malignant
    hyperthermia. Anesthesiology 75: 4–8
McKenzie A J, Couchman K G, Pollock N 1992 Propofol is a 'safe' anaesthetic agent
    in malignant hyperthermia susceptible patients. Anaesthesia and Intensive Care 20:
    165–168
Murakawa M, Hatano Y, Magaribuchi T et al 1988 Should calcium administration be
    avoided in treatment of hyperkalaemia in malignant hyperthermia? Anesthesiology
    67: 604–605
North American Malignant Hyperthermia Group 1989 Standardization of the caffeine
    halothane muscle contracture test. Anesthesia and Analgesia 69: 511–519
Otsuka H, Komura Y, Mayumi T et al 1991 Malignant hyperthermia during
    sevoflurane anesthesia in a child with central core disease. Anesthesiology 75: 699–
    700
Raff M, Harrison G G 1989 The screening of propofol in MHS swine. Anesthesia and
    Analgesia 68: 750–751
Rosenberg H, Fletcher J E 1986 Masseter muscle rigidity and malignant hyperthermia
    susceptibility. Anesthesia and Analgesia 65: 161–164
Saddler J M, Bevan J C, Plumley M H et al 1990 Jaw muscle tension after
    succinylcholine in children undergoing strabismus surgery. Canadian Journal of
    Anaesthesia 37: 21–25

Wedel D J, laizzo P A, Milde J H 1991 Desflurane is a malignant of malignant hyperthermia in susceptible swine. Anesthesiology 74: 508–512

MARCUS-GUNN JAW WINKING PHENOMENON

A rare congenital abnormality in which there appears to be abnormal connections between the external pterygoid and ocular muscles. This results in ptosis, which can be partly corrected by the patient either opening the jaw or moving it to the contralateral side. A number of other abnormal reflexes may occur.

Preoperative abnormalities

1. Ptosis is present, but lid retraction is associated with jaw opening.
2. Abnormal pupillary reflexes may occur.

Anaesthetic problems

Unusual oculocardiac reflexes were reported during three separate operations on the eyelid in a young man with Marcus-Gunn syndrome (Kwik 1980). Arrhythmias, which appeared on manipulation of the eyelid and also occurred in the recovery room, included premature atrial contractions, wandering pacemaker, and bradycardia.

Management

1. It has been suggested that the use of IPPV and a retrobulbar block may decrease the incidence of arrhythmias (Kwik 1980).
2. ECG monitoring should begin in the anaesthetic room and be continued in the recovery room.

BIBLIOGRAPHY
Kwik R S H 1980 Marcus-Gunn syndrome associated with an unusual oculo-cardiac reflex. Anaesthesia 35: 46–49

MARFAN'S SYNDROME

An autosomal dominant inherited condition involving a connective tissue deficit, probably affecting the microfibrillar component of elastic fibres. Tensile strength of collagen is reduced, while its elasticity is increased. Skeletal, cardiovascular and ocular features occur. The diagnosis is made on clinical grounds and there are variable manifestations of the condition. At least two of the following four criteria should be present: a family history of the condition, the ocular, cardiovascular, or skeletal features (Pyeritz & McKusick 1979).

In the past, premature death in the third to fifth decade was common. The biochemical defect makes the aorta susceptible to dilatation and dissection, so that aortic dissection and valvular regurgitation were responsible for about 90% of these deaths. However, with the use of regular, non-invasive cardiovascular assessment and more aggressive prophylactic surgery, the prognosis has improved (Marsalese et al 1989).

Surgery may be required for the correction of the cardiac, ophthalmic, and orthopaediac features of the disease. This may include elective or emergency aortic surgery or cardiac valve replacement.

Preoperative abnormalities

1. Skeletal abnormalities include arachnodactyly, a high arched palate, increased length of tubular bones, scoliosis (40–70%), pectus excavatus and ligamentous laxity.
2. Ectopia lentis occurs in up to 80% of cases. Patients are prone to myopia and retinal detachment.
3. Cardiovascular complications are the commonest cause of death. Structural changes in the heart and great vessels may be present and can result in mitral or aortic regurgitation, dissecting aortic aneurysm, aortic root or pulmonary artery dilatation and coronary artery disease. Mitral valve prolapse and acute aortic valve prolapse can also occur. Pathological changes in the arteries include cystic degeneration of the media and replacement of elastic fibres by mucoid material. Estimation of aortic size and valvular dysfunction may require echocardiography, cardiac catheterization or MRI. In young people aged less than 20 years, the prevalence of serious cardiovascular complications is low, but aortic root diameter does increase with age and serious complications are similar to those that occur in adults (El Habbal 1992). Mitral valve prolapse and aortic root dilatation are the commonest (Hirata et al 1992). Mitral valve prolapse tends to be symptomatic but aortic root dilatation is silent, unless there is dissection or regurgitation.
4. In the pregnant patient there is a risk of aortic arch dissection in the third stage of labour.

Anaesthetic problems

1. A number of deaths have been reported in association with surgery but there has been no consistent cause of death. In a study of 13 patients, two of four who died had been assessed as having no cardiovascular involvement (Verghese 1984). Neither had, however, undergone echocardiography. In a report of general life-expectancy, cardiovascular complications accounted for 95% of deaths in those patients in whom a definite diagnosis was confirmed.
2. Hypotonia and ligamentous laxity may predispose the patient to accidental injury during anaesthesia. Joints, including the temporomandibular, are prone to dislocation.

3. Scoliosis, hypotonia, a high incidence of emphysema, lung cysts, spontaneous pneumothoraces and honeycomb lungs all increase the risk of intra- and postoperative pulmonary complications. Midtracheal obstruction and respiratory distress occurred after Harrington rod placement in a patient with scoliosis (Mesrobian & Epps 1986). This was attributed to a combination of structural weakness of cartilage and skeletal abnormalities.

4. If ascending aortic dilatation already exists, especially if it is greater than 6 cm in an adult, the risk of rupture is high and hypertensive peaks may predispose to aortic dissection (Pyeritz & McKusick 1979).

Management

1. Detailed examination of the cardiovascular system is essential and should include assessment of aortic size, and a search for evidence of aortic or mitral regurgitation, coronary artery disease and heart failure. Echocardiography has been suggested as being mandatory in all patients requiring surgery (Wells & Podolakin 1987).

2. High pulsatile pressures must be avoided to reduce the risks of aortic dissection. Beta adrenoceptor blocker therapy has decreased the risk of sudden death in animal models (Wells & Podolakin 1987). However, haemodynamic studies suggest that acute beta blockade is not necessarily beneficial (Yin et al 1989). Dynamic aortic studies in patients given i.v. propranolol 0.15 mg/kg showed that short-term beta blockers exacerbated the primary abnormality of aortic wall motion in Marfan's (which is an increase in the magnitude of the wave reflections), causing additional stress to the aortic wall. The abnormality was ameliorated by nitroprusside, a vasodilator.

3. Direct arterial monitoring may assist in the process of controlling sudden increases in blood pressure, but may carry a higher than normal risk of damage to the artery.

4. Therapeutic abortion may be indicated if pregnancy occurs. Should this not be acceptable, elective Caesarean section is recommended. Nitroglycerin was used to control the blood pressure in Caesarean section performed at 31 weeks' gestation in a patient with progressive aortic dissection (Hayashi et al 1991).

BIBLIOGRAPHY

El Habbal M H 1992 Cardiovascular manifestations of Marfan's syndrome in the young. American Heart Journal 123: 752–757

Hayashi M, Terai T, Nishikawa K et al 1991 General anesthesia for cesarean section in a patient with Marfan's syndrome associated with dissecting aortic aneurysm. (English abstr). Masui 40: 622–626

Hirata K, Triposkiadis F, Sparks E et al 1992 The Marfan syndrome: cardiovascular physical findings and diagnostic correlates. American Heart Journal 123: 743–752

Marsalese D L, Moodie D S, Vacante M et al 1989 Marfan's syndrome: natural history and long-term follow-up of cardiovascular involvement. Journal of the American College of Cardiology 14: 422–428

Mesrobian R B, Epps J L 1986 Midtracheal obstruction after Harrington rod placement in a patient with Marfan's syndrome. Anesthesia and Analgesia 65: 411–413

Pyeritz R E, McKusick V A 1979 The Marfan syndrome; diagnosis and management. New England Journal of Medicine 300: 772–777

Verghese C 1984 Anaesthesia in Marfan's syndrome. Anaesthesia 39: 917–922

Wells D G, Podolakin W 1987 Anaesthesia and Marfan's syndrome: case report. Canadian Journal of Anaesthesia 34: 311–314

Yin F C P, Brin K P, Ting C-T et al 1989 Arterial hemodynamic indexes in Marfan's syndrome. Circulation 79: 854–862

MASTOCYTOSES

A rare and complex group of diseases in which there are abnormal aggregations of mast cells within the skin, and in other organs (Austen 1992). Bone, liver, spleen and lymph nodes are most commonly affected. When the skin alone is involved, the condition is known as urticaria pigmentosa. This mostly occurs in infants and children, may be associated with mastocytomas, and is relatively benign (Coleman et al 1980).

Systemic mastocytosis occurs in about 10% of cases. The various forms of this which occur in adult life may be associated with intermittent symptoms varying from a mild disturbance, to the occasional fatal attack. These episodes are associated with mast cell disruption and the resultant release of one or more of a number of biochemical substances from granules within the cells. Histamine and heparin were thought to be the most important of these, although other enzymes such as chymases, tryptases and hydrolases may be released. Prostaglandin D2 has also been implicated as being a cause of symptoms in certain patients who failed to respond to histamine antagonists (Roberts et al 1980). Mast cells also produce cytokines (such as the interleukins) involved in adaptive immunity and tissue inflammatory response (Austen 1992). Other substances which may be released in small amounts include the leukotrienes, serotonin, and hyaluronic acid. Among the precipitating factors are trauma, surgery, extremes of temperature, toxins, alcohol, and a variety of drugs.

Preoperative abnormalities

1. Symptoms are variable, and can include episodic attacks of itching, urticaria, dermographia, headache, flushing, syncope, palpitations, abdominal pain, diarrhoea, nausea, and vomiting. The flush is bright red and lasts for about 20 minutes, in contrast to that associated with carcinoid, which is more cyanotic and lasts for less than 10 minutes. Delay in diagnosis is frequent. The mean duration of symptoms before diagnosis in a series of 26 patients was found to be 2 years (Webb et al 1982).

2. Skin lesions vary in type and colour, but small, reddish brown maculopapular lesions are common. A positive Darier's sign may be demonstrated. Light stroking of the affected skin with a blunt, but pointed, object produces dermographia (due to localized urticaria) and a flare.

3. When bones are affected, the patient may present with unexpected bone loss or compression fractures secondary to osteoporosis.

4. Hepatomegaly and splenomegaly are common.

5. Increased gastric acid secretion is associated with duodenal ulceration. In one study, all patients with gastrointestinal symptoms were found to have increased plasma histamine levels and these correlated with basal gastric acid output (Chemer et al 1988).

6. Skin biopsy shows an increased number of mast cells (>5 per high-power field). Diagnosis may also be made on bone or liver biopsy.

7. Increased blood and urinary levels of histamine, and urinary prostaglandin D2 metabolite levels, may be demonstrated.

8. Certain groups of patients may develop various haematological abnormalities, including malignancies. Anaemia, leucocytosis and thrombocytopenia were the commonest problems (Horny et al 1990), although thrombocythaemia has been reported (Le Tourneau et al 1991). Coagulation studies are occasionally abnormal.

Anaesthetic problems

1. Disruption of mast cells may produce severe cardiovascular effects. Drugs reported to have precipitated symptoms in individual patients include salicylates, opiates, polymyxin, thiopentone lignocaine, gallamine, and d-tubocurarine.

2. Surgery, endoscopy, regional and general anaesthesia can also produce life-threatening complications. In one series, complications occurred in six out of 42 cases (Parris et al 1986). Hypotension and bronchospasm were the most frequently encountered. Intraoperative cardiovascular collapse occurred during pancreatic biopsy (Desborough et al 1990). A massive increase in plasma histamine levels was associated with hypotension, flushing, and a profound decrease in systemic vascular resistance. This patient had experienced a similar, but less severe episode, during upper gastrointestinal endoscopy.

3. Although heparin may also be released, it has rarely been reported as producing clinically significant problems. However, in the patient described above, the APTT became prolonged to 150 seconds during pancreatectomy, subsequent to his episode of cardiovascular collapse.

4. If systemic mastocytosis is present and an anaphylactoid reaction occurs, the reaction is likely to be more severe than in a normal patient. It has been suggested that this particularly applies to blood transfusion reactions (Scott et al 1983).

5. Although cutaneous mastocytosis in children is usually thought to be free of anaesthetic problems (James et al 1987) profound hypotension and flushing were reported during surgery in a patient with asymptomatic urticaria pigmentosa (Hosking & Warner 1987).

Management

1. Symptoms should be controlled preoperatively by the use of H1 receptor antagonists (terfenadine, chlorpheniramine), H2 receptor antagonists (cimetidine, ranitidine or famotidine), and prostaglandin inhibitors (indomethacin or salicylates). Sodium cromoglycate, a mast cell stabilizer, improves preoperative symptoms.
2. Plasma histamine levels did not increase during a portacaval shunt in a patient who was treated with histamine antagonists and cromoglycate (Smith et al 1987). However, plasma histamine has a short half-life and is difficult to measure. Plasma tryptase may be a better indicator of mast cell activation in systemic mastocytosis, since it is released together with histamine from mast cells and is present in the blood for several hours (Schwartz et al 1987).
3. Preoperative intradermal skin testing, with drugs likely to be used during anaesthesia, is recommended (Parris et al 1986). Positive skin tests occurred in 15 out of a series of 42 patients. Drugs likely to produce reactions should be avoided. It has been suggested that, since most patients are receiving histamine antagonists at the time of surgery, greater concentrations should be used than those employed for testing after anaphylactoid reactions (Lerno et al 1990). The standard procedure of 0.01–0.02 ml of a dilute solution (10^{-4}–10^{-6}) to raise a 1–2 mm wheal is recommended for drug-related anaphylactoid reactions (Fisher 1984). Lerno et al recommend that concentrations of 10^{-2} or 10^{-3} should be used in systemic mastocytosis. A positive reaction is a wheal of at least 10-mm diameter appearing within 10 minutes and lasting at least 30 minutes.
4. Sedation with a benzodiazepine helps to reduce anxiety.
5. It is recommended that adrenaline, both as a 1 in 1000 bolus and as an infusion of 1 mg in 25 ml saline, should be available for immediate use to heat severe hypotension (Parris et al 1986). An initial dose of 5–8 µg/kg followed by an infusion of 5–10 µg/kg/min is recommended (Lerno et al 1990).
6. There have been no reports of inhalational agents causing degranulation of mast cells. Ether-linked anaesthetics, such as isoflurane, may actually inhibit degranulation.
7. Care should be taken to avoid precipitating factors such as trauma, hypothermia and hyperthermia (Parris et al 1981).
8. Dextrans are probably better avoided (Scott et al 1983).

BIBLIOGRAPHY

Austen K F 1992 Systemic mastocytosis. New England Journal of Medicine 326: 639–640

Cherner J A, Jensen R T, Dubois A et al 1988 Gastrointestinal dysfunction in systemic mastocytosis: a prospective study. Gastroenterology 95: 657–667

Coleman M A, Liberthson R R, Crone R K et al 1980 General anesthesia in a child with urticaria pigmentosa. Anesthesia and Analgesia 59: 704–706

Desborough J P, Taylor I, Hattersley A et al 1990 Massive histamine release in patient with systemic mastocytosis. British Journal of Anaesthesia 65: 833–836

Fisher M M 1984 Intradermal testing after anaphylactoid reaction to anaesthetic drugs: practical aspects of performance and interpretation. Anaesthesia and Intensive Care 12: 115–120

Horny H P, Ruck M, Wehrmann M et al 1990 Blood findings in generalized mastocytosis: evidence of frequent occurrence of myeloproliferative disorders. British Journal of Haematology 76: 186–193

Hosking M R, Warner M A 1987 Sudden intraoperative hypotension in a patient with asymptomatic urticaria pigmentosa. Anesthesia and Analgesia 66: 344–346

James P D, Krafchik B R, Johnston A E 1987 Cutaneous mastocytosis in children: anaesthetic considerations. Canadian Journal of Anaesthesia 34: 522–524

Lerno G, Slaats G, Coenen E et al 1990 Anaesthetic management of systemic mastocytosis. British Journal of Anaesthesia 65: 254–257

Le Tourneau A, Gaulard P, D'Agay M F et al 1991 Primary thrombocythaemia associated with systemic mastocytosis: a report of five cases. British Journal of Haematology 79: 84–89

Parris W C V, Sandidge R C, Petrinely G 1981 Anesthetic management of mastocytosis. Anesthesiology Review 8: 32–35

Parris W C V, Scott H W Smith B E 1986 Anesthetic management of systemic mastocytosis: experience with 42 cases. Anesthesia and Analgesia 65: S117

Roberts L J, Sweetman B J, Lewis R A et al 1980 Increased production of prostaglandin D2 in patients with systemic mastocytosis. New England Journal of Medicine 303: 1400–1404

Scott H W, Parris W C V, Sandidge P C et al 1983 Hazards in operative management of patients with systemic mastocytosis. Annals of Surgery 197: 507–514

Schwartz L B, Metcalfe D D, Miller J S et al 1987 Tryptase levels as an indicator of mast cell activation in systemic anaphylaxis and mastocytosis. New England Journal of Medicine 316: 1622–1626

Smith G B, Gusberg R J, Jordan R H et al 1987 Histamine levels and cardiovascular responses during splenectomy and splenorenal shunt formation in a patient with systemic mastocytosis. Anaesthesia 42: 861–867

Webb T A, Li C-Y, Yarn L T 1982 Systemic mast cell disease: a clinical and hematopathologic study of 26 cases. Cancer 49: 927–938

McARDLE'S SYNDROME

A type V glycogen storage disease, which appears as an autosomal recessive myopathy. Skeletal muscle is mainly involved, although reports of cardiac muscle and ECG abnormalities have appeared. It results from the single enzyme defect of muscle phosphorylase. Failure of conversion of glycogen into lactate results in increased muscle glycogen. Patients with myophosphorylase deficiency do not become acidotic during exercise and it has been suggested that hyperkalaemia may contribute significantly to the drive to breathe, especially during heavy exercise (Paterson et al 1990). Males are more commonly affected than females. There was one report of dual pathology in a patient with excess muscle fatiguability – McArdle's disease coexisted with MH (Isaacs et al 1989).

Attempts to improve exertional myalgia in McArdle's with dantrolene were unsuccessful.

Preoperative abnormalities

1. Symptoms of cramp, stiffness, muscle pains, and fatiguability on exercise may appear in childhood. Muscle contractions are relieved by rest. A family history may be elicited.
2. Occasional episodes of myoglobinuria can occur after strenuous exercise. This was associated with the development of renal failure (McMillan et al 1989) in a patient who had previously been asymptomatic.
3. Progressive atrophy of muscle may occur in the fifth decade.
4. The diagnosis can be made with neurohistochemical techniques, or by demonstrating decreased venous lactate and pyruvate concentrations with ischaemic exercise. NMR can be used to demonstrate muscle phosphorylase deficiency and EMG shows a decrease in evoked muscle response, after supramaximal stimuli.

Anaesthetic problems

1. Suxamethonium may cause myoglobinuria, with the risk of renal failure.
2. The use of a limb tourniquet may result in muscle atrophy.
3. Shivering can produce muscle damage.

Management

1. Suxamethonium should not be given. Atracurium has been used in a child (Rajah & Bell 1986) and vecuronium in an adult (Tzabar & Ross 1990), without producing myoglobinuria or serum CK elevation. The use of alcuronium during a Caesarean section has also been reported (Coleman 1984). A peripheral nerve stimulator must be used.
2. A tourniquet should only be applied if absolutely essential.
3. Core temperature should be monitored. The operating theatre must be warm. A heated mattress and blood warmer are required for long operations, to avoid shivering and heat loss. Patients are intolerant of a hypermetabolic state (Ellis 1980).
4. A usable energy source such as dextrose, fructose or lactate should be given during the procedure and continued until oral intake is resumed.
5. If myoglobinuria occurs, i.v. fluids and mannitol should be given to reduce the possibility of renal failure.

BIBLIOGRAPHY
Coleman P 1984 McArdle's disease. Problems of anaesthetic management for
    Caesarean section. Anaesthesia 39: 784–787

Ellis F R 1980 Inherited muscle disease. British Journal of Anaesthesia 52: 153–164
Isaacs H, Badenhorst M E, Du Sautoy C 1989 Myophosphorylase B deficiency and
    malignant hyperthermia. Muscle Nerve 12: 203–205
McMillan M A, Hallworth M J, Doyle D et al 1989 Acute renal failure due to
    McArdle's disease. Renal Failure 11: 23–25
Paterson et al 1990 Changes in arterial K^+ and ventilation during exercise in normal
    subjects and subjects with McArdle's syndrome. Journal of Physiology 429: 339–
    348
Rajah A, Bell C F 1986 Atracurium and McArdle's disease. Anaesthesia 41: 93
Tzabar Y, Ross D G 1990 Vecuronium and McArdle's disease. Anaesthesia 45: 697

MEDIASTINAL MASSES

The mediastinum lies between the right and left pleural cavity and is divided at the level of the sternal angle into the superior and inferior mediastinum. The latter is further divided into posterior, middle or anterior mediastinum. When a patient presents with a mediastinal mass, two features provide clues about its nature – the site, and the age of the patient.

In babies they are likely to be bronchial cysts, teratomas or secondary to oesophageal duplication. In infants and children, the commonest masses are neurogenic in origin, and are in the posterior mediastinum. In adults, middle mediastinal masses are usually carcinoma or lymphoma, although achalasia of the oesophagus has been reported (King & Strickland 1979). Anterior masses are frequently related to the thymus or thyroid. Posterior masses are often neurogenic in origin.

Patients with mediastinal masses may present for diagnostic procedures or thoracotomy. Bronchoscopy, lymph node biopsy, mediastinoscopy and staging laparotomy are the commonest operations.

Anaesthesia in a patient with a large mediastinal mass may be extremely hazardous because several important structures can be compressed. The superior vena cava, the tracheal bifurcation, the pulmonary artery and the aortic arch are all adjacent. The literature continues to report fatalities in patients with superior vena caval (SVC) obstruction, or compression of the trachea or a main bronchus (Mackie 1987).

Preoperative abnormalities

1. SVC obstruction
    Is diagnosed on clinical examination. It is four times more likely to occur with right-sided lesions than it is with those on the left, and will be more severe when the obstruction is below the azygos vein. At postmortem examination, actual venous thrombosis has been found to be present in more than one-third of cases of SVC obstruction (Lokich & Goodman 1975). Most masses which cause SVC obstruction are malignant.

    Initially there is dilatation of the veins in the neck and upper thorax. Distension is most prominent when the patient is supine, but the veins do not collapse on sitting or standing. Subsequently there is progression to oedema of the face (with periorbital and conjunctival oedema and proptosis), the arms and the breasts to give a peau d'orange appearance. In these latter cases, signs and symptoms of cerebral oedema may develop, and increasing respiratory difficulty secondary to laryngeal oedema may indicate the need for urgent radiotherapy or chemotherapy.

2. Signs of airway obstruction or invasion
A careful history and, in particular, questioning about positional respiratory difficulty, stridor, dyspnoea, and non-productive cough. Obstruction is often intermittent and worse on lying supine. Patients often prefer to sit up. Presumably the supine position is associated with a decrease in thoracic volume (Pullerits & Holzman 1989). One child with intermittent upper airway obstruction was mistakenly diagnosed as having inhaled a foreign body (Ahktar et al 1991). Children with mediastinal masses are particularly at risk.

   Lesions may progress rapidly, therefore a recent CXR is essential. A normal PA X-ray does not exclude obstruction. Anterior-posterior compression of the trachea may only be demonstrated on a penetrated lateral view. In difficult cases, a CT scan of the airway can be invaluable since the diameter of the trachea and the site of obstruction can be measured accurately (Azizkhan et al 1985, Barker et al 1991). A reduction in tracheal diameter to 50% or less is usually associated with symptoms. Sometimes it may be helpful to additionally examine dynamic airway function. This can be seen directly on fibreoptic bronchoscopy using local anaesthesia, or by constructing flow-volume loops. Reduction in maximum expiratory flows may warn of the possibility of obstruction after tracheal extubation.

3. Myocardial or pericardial involvement
Arrhythmias can occur, or the patient may have signs of a pericardial effusion. In cases of cardiac tamponade, there is respiratory distress and pulsus paradoxus. There may be cyanosis and syncope on straining (Keon 1981). Echocardiography should confirm the diagnosis.

4. Obstruction of the pulmonary artery. As a result of direct compression.

5. Spinal cord involvement. Can occur in posterior mediastinal tumours.

6. Recurrent laryngeal nerve problems. Primarily occur with left sided lesions.

7. Systemic non-metastatic effects of tumours, such as hormone secretion, neuropathies, and myasthenia gravis.

Anaesthetic problems

1. In the presence of SVC obstruction, if a venous wall is breached anywhere in the area which drains into the SVC, severe haemorrhage will occur. Drugs given via venous access in the arm will have a significantly delayed action. Cyanosis of the face and upper trunk and increased central venous pressure occurred following general anaesthesia in a patient subsequently found to have a tumour encasing and obstructing the superior vena cava (Riley et al 1992).

2. In cases of severe obstruction, cerebral and glottic oedema may occur.

3. There can be tracheal compression or invasion. Sudden respiratory obstruction can happen at any stage of the anaesthetic. It most commonly occurs after administration of a muscle relaxant and tracheal intubation (Bray & Fernandes 1982, O'Leary & Tracey 1983, Azizkhan et al 1985), but problems have also been encountered during inhalation induction (Mackie & Watson 1984, John & Narang 1988), after reversal of neuromuscular blockade and tracheal tube withdrawal (Prakash et al 1988), and in the recovery room (Bittar 1975). Deaths continue to be reported (Neuman et al 1984, Levin et al 1985, Northrip et al 1986).

   Difficulty in inflation of the lungs after intubation might be a result of external pressure, producing distortion or obstruction of the tube. However, it is more probably due to the change in lung mechanics which occurs during anaesthesia and after administration of a muscle relaxant. During spontaneous respiration there is a subatmospheric intrapleural pressure and a widening of airways on inspiration. Administration of a muscle relaxant will alter the support of the bronchial tree such that, in the presence of external pressure, collapse of the airway can occur and cause complete obstruction. Softening of the tracheal wall may contribute to this. In most of the cases described, partial relief of the obstruction coincided with the return of spontaneous respiration or recovery of consciousness.

4. Pulmonary oedema occurred after tracheal extubation in a patient following biopsy of an anterior mediastinal tumor (Price & Hecker 1987).

5. Pulmonary artery involvement will decrease pulmonary perfusion and cardiac output.

6. Myocardial or pericardial involvement results in arrhythmias, and occasionally cardiac tamponade. Fatal collapse on induction of anaesthesia has been described in two children (Keon 1981, Halpern et al 1983), both of whom were found at autopsy to have lymphomas involving the heart and infiltrating the pericardium and pulmonary artery. Cardiovascular collapse has also occurred on

induction of anaesthesia without evidence of tracheal obstruction or tamponade.

7. Spinal cord involvement occurs most commonly in children with neurogenic tumours.

Management

1. Full assessment, as already outlined, is important before embarking on general anaesthesia. Children are particularly at risk and close collaboration between the specialties is essential (Azizkhan et al 1985).

2. If there are obvious signs of SVC obstruction, then urgent radiotherapy or chemotherapy is probably indicated before surgical intervention, although this has been disputed (Yellin et al 1990). Radiotherapy reduces the size of the tumour, as well as the degree of venous obstruction, provided that actual venous thrombosis has not occurred. If thrombosis is suspected, fibrinolytic agent or anticoagulants may be used (Lokich & Goodman 1975).

3. Should there be any suggestion of tracheal obstruction, surgery ought to be performed under local anaesthetic if possible. After the passage of a double-lumen tube under local anaesthesia, a patient breathed spontaneously until the chest was opened (Younker et al 1989). If local anaesthetic techniques are not possible, an inhalational induction should be administered and no muscle relaxants given (Sibert et al 1987). In the symptomatic patient, radiotherapy must be undertaken before surgery. Five life- threatening complications were associated with intubation anaesthesia in 74 cases of untreated mediastinal or hilar Hodgkin's disease (Piro et al 1976). By contrast, no complications were seen in 24 cases with mediastinal involvement when anaesthesia took place after initial radiotherapy, or in 78 anaesthetics where there was no mediastinal disease. If severe airway obstruction occurs unexpectedly, an improvement may be obtained by moving the patient from the supine to the lateral or prone position (Prakash et al 1988, Ahktar et al 1991). Direct laryngoscopy, which straightens the trachea, may relieve the obstruction, and rigid bronchoscopy may be life-saving (John & Narang 1988). In this patient, microlaryngeal tubes were passed over bougies, down each main bronchus, past the obstruction. The tubes remained in place until the fifth day of chemotherapy. Planned extracorporeal oxygenation may be indicated under certain circumstances (Hall & Friedman 1975).

BIBLIOGRAPHY

Akhtar T M, Ridley S, Best C J 1991 Unusual presentation of acute upper airway obstruction caused by an anterior mediastinal mass. British Journal of Anaesthesia 67: 632–634

Section 1

Mediastinal Masses

Azizkhan R G, Dudgeon D L, Buck J R et al 1985 Life-threatening airway obstruction as a complication to the management of mediastinal masses in children. Journal of Pediatric Surgery 20: 816–822

Barker P, Mason R A, Thorpe M H 1991 Computerised axial tomography of the trachea. A useful investigation when a retrosternal goitre causes symptomatic tracheal compression. Anaesthesia 46: 195–198

Bittar D 1975 Respiratory obstruction associated with induction of general anesthesia in a patient with mediastinal Hodgkin's disease. Anesthesia and Analgesia 54: 399–403

Bray R J, Fernandes F J 1982 Mediastinal tumour causing airway obstruction in anaesthetised children. Anaesthesia 37: 571–575

Hall D K, Friedman M 1975 Extracorporeal oxygenation for induction of anesthesia in a patient with an intrathoracic tumor. Anesthesiology 42: 493–495

Halpern S, Chatten J, Meadows A T et al 1983 Anterior mediastinal masses: anesthesia hazards and other problems. Journal of Pediatrics 102: 407–410

John R E, Narang V P S 1988 A boy with an anterior mediastinal mass. Anaesthesia 43: 864–866

Keon T P 1981 Death on induction of anesthesia for cervical node biopsy. Anesthesiology 55: 471–472

King D M, Strickland B 1979 An unusual cause of thoracic inlet obstruction. British Journal of Radiology 52: 910–913

Levin H, Bursztein S, Heifetz M 1985 Cardiac arrest in a child with an anterior mediastinal mass. Anesthesiology 64: 1129–1130

Lokich J J, Goodman R 1975 Superior vena cava syndrome. Journal of the American Medical Association 231: 58–61

Mackie A 1987 Anesthetic management of mediastinal masses – again. Anesthesia and Analgesia 66: 696

Mackie A M, Watson C B 1984 Anaesthesia and mediastinal masses. Anaesthesia 39: 899–903

Neuman G G, Weingarten A E, Abramowitz R M et al 1984 The anesthetic management of the patient with an anterior mediastinal mass. Anesthesiology 60: 144–147

Northrip D R, Bowman K B, Tsueda K 1986 Total airway occlusion and superior vena cava syndrome in a child with an anterior mediastinal mass. Anesthesia and Analgesia 65: 1079–1082

O'Leary H T, Tracey J A 1983 Mediastinal tumours causing airway obstruction. Anaesthesia 38: 66–67

Piro A J, Weiss D R, Hellman S 1976 Mediastinal Hodgkin's disease: a possible danger for intubation anaesthesia. International Journal of Radiation, Oncology, Biology, Physics 1: 415–419

Prakash V B S, Abel M O, Hubmayr R D 1988 Mediastinal mass and tracheal obstruction during general anesthesia. Mayo Clinic Proceedings 63: 1004–1011

Price S L, Hecker B R 1987 Pulmonary oedema following obstruction in a patient with Hodgkin's disease. British Journal of Anaesthesia 59: 518–521

Pullerits J, Holzman R 1989 Anaesthesia for patients with mediastinal masses. Canadian Journal of Anaesthesia 36: 681–688

Riley R H, Harris L A, Davis W J et al 1992 Superior vena cava syndrome following general anesthesia. Anaesthesia and Intensive Care 20: 229–232

Sibert K S, Biondi J W, Hirsch N P 1987 Spontaneous respiration during thoracotorny a patient with a mediastinal mass. Anesthesia and Analgesia 66: 904–907

Yellin A, Rosen A, Reichert N et al 1990 Superior vena cava syndrome – the myth – the facts. American Review of Respiratory Disease 141: 1114–1118

Younker D, Clark R, Coveler L 1989 Fiberoptic endobronchial intubation for resection of a mediastinal mass. Anesthesiology 70: 144–146

MENDELSON'S SYNDROME
(PULMONARY ASPIRATION SYNDROME SEE SECTION 2)

MILLER'S SYNDROME

A recently described syndrome of postaxial acrofacial dysostosis.

Preoperative abnormalities

1. Craniofacial abnormalities similar to those found in Treacher Collin's syndrome, including micrognathia and cleft palate.
2. Limb and cardiac defects, including ASD, VSD and PDA, also occur.
3. The patient is usually of normal intelligence.
4. Multiple anaesthetics may be required for plastic surgery.

Anaesthetic problems

So far only a single case has been reported in the anaesthetic literature (Richards 1987). The potential anaesthetic problems were:

1. Intubation difficulties due to micrognathia.
2. Postoperative respiratory obstruction.
3. Limb shortening causing venous access problems.
4. Difficulties with positioning of the patient.

Management

The following were recommended (Richards 1987):

1. Identification of cardiac problems, if present.
2. An inhalation induction to anticipate intubation difficulties.
3. Support for the limbs is required to prevent stress on joints, nerves and blood vessels.

BIBLIOGRAPHY
Richards M 1987 Miller's syndrome. Anaesthetic management of postaxial acrofacial dysostosis. Anaesthesia 42: 871–874

MITRAL VALVE DISEASE

Two main problems confront the anaesthetist when dealing with a patient with cardiac valvular disease. The first is that of the preoperative assessment of the severity of the lesion, and the degree of myocardial dysfunction resulting from it. The second, and crucial to the conduct of anaesthesia, is an understanding of the compensatory mechanisms which may have taken place. These will depend on whether the valvular disease is acute or longstanding.

The pathophysiology and compensatory mechanisms of an acute valve lesion following endocarditis or myocardial infarction are very different from those of chronic valve disease, in which gradual compensatory cardiac hypertrophy or dilatation has taken place. In either case, the aim is to give an anaesthetic which will cause as little disturbance as possible to these compensatory mechanisms.

The serious effects of decompensation range from pulmonary oedema and hypoxia, to a severe decrease in left ventricular output resulting in myocardial ischaemia, infarction or arrhythmias. Whilst in mild disease there may be few problems, severe valvular disease requires close cardiovascular monitoring, a careful choice of anaesthetic technique, and anticipation and cautious correction of the factors causing decompensation.

MITRAL STENOSIS

Normal left ventricular filling is restricted by the decreased area across the stenosed valve. The normal area of the valve is 4 cm^2. Symptoms appear when this is reduced to about 2.5 cm^2; below 1 cm^2 symptoms are severe.

Compensation is normally achieved by increasing the pressure gradient across the mitral valve, and is dependent upon atrial contraction and the duration of diastole. Decompensation often begins with the onset of atrial fibrillation associated with a fast ventricular rate.

Preoperative abnormalities

1. The pulse may be irregular as a result of atrial fibrillation. Palpation of the precordium may reveal a palpable first sound ('tapping apex beat'). On auscultation there may be an opening snap (the closer to the second sound, the more severe the stenosis), followed by a mid-diastolic murmur, with presystolic accentuation if the patient remains in sinus rhythm. The loudness of the murmur is no guide to severity, and may be inaudible if the cardiac output is low, in neglected disease. Atrial fibrillation causes decompensation by decreasing the left ventricular filling time and by reducing cardiac output. This is manifest clinically by cool, possibly cyanosed peripheries, and a low-volume pulse. A malar flush is common.
2. Left atrial pressure (LAP) is increased, while dilatation and hypertrophy of the left atrium occurs. When LAP increases, so does pulmonary capillary pressure, and when this exceeds colloid osmotic pressure (25–30 mmHg), pulmonary oedema develops. A sudden increase in LAP may be precipitated by tachycardia due to exercise, emotion, fever, pregnancy, or by an arrhythmia. A proportion of the patients will develop irreversible pulmonary hypertension, right ventricular hypertrophy, pulmonary and tricuspid regurgitation, and occasionally right heart failure.

3. Chest X-ray shows left atrial enlargement, with a prominent left atrial appendage and double contour of the right heart border. Kerley B lines may be present. ECG may show P mitrale. Definitive diagnosis is by echocardiography which allows precise measurement of left atrial dimensions and demonstration of the abnormal movement of the thickened or calcified valve cusps. If combined with Doppler techniques, valve area can be estimated.
4. In the presence of AF, systemic thromboembolism may occur.
5. The patient is usually taking digoxin, and sometimes beta adrenoceptor blockers and anticoagulants.
6. Symptomatic history is a good guide to severity. Dyspnoea on mild exertion, with episodes of paroxysmal nocturnal dyspnoea, indicate a LAP of 15–20 mmHg. Occasionally angina occurs.

Anaesthetic problems

1. Tachycardia or fast atrial fibrillation reduces diastolic filling time and may precipitate pulmonary oedema.
2. Large decreases in systemic vascular resistance may result in severe hypotension, since there is limited capacity to increase cardiac output in compensation.
3. Volume overload may produce pulmonary oedema; conversely, hypovolaemia, accentuated by diuretics, may reduce cardiac output.
4. Myocardial depressant drugs can cause severe hypotension.
5. The Trendelenberg position may result in hypoxia and pulmonary oedema.
6. Hypoxia and acidosis can cause pulmonary vasoconstriction.
7. Nitrous oxide may be unsafe if pulmonary vascular resistance is increased (Schulte-Sasse et al 1982).
8. Bacteraemia during surgery or instrumentation carries the risk of bacterial endocarditis.

Management

1. Prophylactic antibiotics are required for any surgery which carries a risk of producing a bacteraemia. This includes dental, genitourinary and bowel operations, and childbirth (See Endocarditis, bacterial).
2. AF must be controlled before surgery.
3. Whilst digoxin is the mainstay of treatment, care should be taken to prevent tachycardia. Atropine should be avoided. A sedative premedication reduces anxiety. An adequate depth of anaesthesia and good analgesia are essential. High-dose alfentanil was used for emergency Caesarean section in a patient with severe mitral stenosis, and the baby responded to a single dose of naloxone (Batson et al 1990). Extradural opiates were used for postoperative pain.

4. Inotropic agents, particularly a dilating inotrope such as dobutamine, may be required to treat hypotension, although they can worsen pulmonary vasoconstriction.
5. Myocardial depressants should be avoided if possible.
6. Prevention of peripheral vasoconstriction due to cold, pain and hypovolaemia, is essential. A CVP will assist the assessment of volume requirement for optimum right ventricular function. In severe mitral stenosis and before corrective surgery, it may be necessary to use dilating agents such as nitroprusside or nitrates. IPPV may be life saving.
7. The degree of monitoring used depends upon the severity of the lesion and the magnitude of the surgery. In the absence of pulmonary hypertension the changes in CVP will mirror those in the left atrium. However, if it is present, the PAWP does not correlate very well with the LAP.
8. If there is right ventricular dysfunction, nitrous oxide should be avoided.
9. In obstetrics, extradural anaesthesia may be appropriate for delivery or Caesarean section. The use of PAP monitoring to demonstrate the beneficial effects of extradural anaesthesia in a patient during delivery, has been reported (Hemmings et al 1987). The technique of bedside measurement of pulmonary artery and pulmonary capillary wedge pressures has been well described (George & Banks 1983).

MITRAL REGURGITATION

Causes include rheumatic endocarditis (in which case the lesion is frequently mixed), mitral valve prolapse, papillary muscle dysfunction, or rupture of chordae tendinae. The latter conditions usually follow myocardial infarction. There is a difference in pathophysiology between chronic regurgitation and that of acute onset. In the acute event, the regurgitated volume depends upon the duration of systole the size of the orifice, and the systolic pressure gradient across the valve. Volume loading will increase the size of the orifice, but if the volume is too low the contractility will be suboptimal.

Preoperative abnormalities

1. An apical pansystolic murmur radiating to the axilla.
2. During systole a part of the stroke volume enters the aorta, whilst the rest is regurgitated into the left atrium. The ratio between the two depends upon the degree of incompetence and the impedance of each pathway.
3. There is left ventricular hypertrophy secondary to an increased work-load, and in severe chronic cases left ventricular failure may

eventually occur. In acute mitral regurgitation pulmonary oedema occurs early (McLintic et al 1992).

4. During diastole the left atrium has to eject the normal pulmonary venous flow as well as the regurgitated fraction. Left atrial dilatation therefore takes place.
5. AF usually only occurs in mixed lesions or in advanced cases.
6. Chest X-ray will show left atrial dilatation and left ventricular hypertrophy. Echocardiography provides precise information about chamber dimensions, wall thickness and movement, and will demonstrate a rheumatic or prolapsing valve.
7. In general, in a patient with rheumatic mitral regurgitation, the progression of exercise intolerance is slow, unless complications such as heart failure or bacterial endocarditis occur. If, however, the regurgitation follows myocardial infarction, there may be sudden onset of acute pulmonary oedema and death.

Anaesthetic problems

1. Even when the disease is mild, there is a greater risk of bacterial endocarditis than with any other valve lesion.
2. There is a risk of systemic embolism and the patient may be receiving anticoagulants.
3. An increase in systemic vascular resistance will increase the regurgitated volume and decrease the cardiac output.
4. Hypovolaemia will decrease the LAP and the stroke work.
5. A bradycardia can worsen the regurgitation, since distortion of the valve may be enhanced by an increased diameter of the ventricle during diastole.

Management

1. Prophylactic antibiotics will be required when appropriate.
2. Situations in which there is heat loss, untreated pain and hypovolaemia, all of which cause peripheral vasoconstriction, should be avoided.
3. Left atrial filling pressure should be maintained to increase the forward output of the left ventricle. Hypovolaemia must therefore be avoided.
4. A mild tachycardia is advantageous, to avoid excess diastolic filling of the ventricle and valve distortion.

MITRAL VALVE PROLAPSE (MVP)

The recognition of this condition has increased with the advent of echocardiography, although there is argument about its diagnosis, significance and prognosis (Oakley 1984). It has been reported to occur in up to 5% of healthy patients. However, the diagnosis is a non-specific one, and would appear to cover a wide spectrum, with considerable variations in clinical significance. A chance finding on echocardiography in thin, young patients who are asymptomatic, is probably not of importance. In older patients who are symptomatic, and have elongated or ruptured chordae tendinae or pathological valve changes, the prognosis may be less good. Each patient should be assessed in relation to the clinical symptoms and findings. Patients with previously undiagnosed MVP may occasionally present with arrhythmias during anaesthesia.

Preoperative abnormalities

1. Abnormalities vary from slight prolapse of the posterior mitral valve leaflet with no regurgitation, to gross prolapse associated with substantial regurgitation as the ventricles contract. The first is probably an anatomical variation, the second can arise from pathological changes in the chordae tendinae or valve leaflets.
2. MVP has also been found in a number of genetic conditions in which there are connective tissue defects. These include Marfan's and Ehlers-Danlos syndromes, and pseudoxanthoma elasticum.
3. The patient is frequently asymptomatic, but symptoms such as syncope, chest pain, and palpitations may feature. There is an increased incidence of bacterial endocarditis and a small risk of cerebral embolism.
4. Clinical signs may include a mid-systolic click and a late systolic murmur. If gross regurgitation occurs during systole, then left atrial dilatation and left ventricular hypertrophy may be present. Atrial and ventricular arrhythmias may occur and there are occasional reports of sudden death.

Anaesthetic problems

1. The degree of valve prolapse is increased by anything that reduces ventricular volume, thus resulting in redundancy of the mitral leaflet (Thiagarajah & Frost 1983). Conversely, prolapse is reduced by increases in ventricular volume. The following situations may accentuate valve prolapse:
   a. Increased myocardial contractility.
   b. Decreased preload resulting from hypovolaemia or sympathetic nervous system blockade.
   c. Tachycardia, which reduces the time for ventricular filling.
   d. High airways pressure produced by straining.
2. Most case reports are of unexpected atrial or ventricular arrhythmias arising in the perioperative period, and in more than half of the cases the diagnosis was made postoperatively on echocardiography (Krantz et al 1980, Thiagarajah & Frost 1983, Berry et al 1985).

Occasionally, ventricular fibrillation, profound bradycardia, or actual cardiac arrest can occur (Cheng 1990). In one patient, two episodes of asystole occurred during attempted diagnostic extradural block (Abraham & Lees 1989), although its association with mitral valve prolapse was unclear (Cheng 1990).

Management

1. The anaesthetic technique in MVP should aim to minimize the effects of factors known to worsen the prolapse.
   a. Avoid sympathetic stimulation and increases in myocardial contractility. A good premedication relieves anxiety. Atropine, and agents producing arrhythmias, are avoided. Hypoxia, hypercarbia and acidosis are prevented. Avoid light anaesthesia. If tachycardia occurs in spite of these manoeuvres, propranolol can be used.
   b. Prevent hypovolaemia. Circulating blood volume is maintained by expansion of the intravascular volume,
   c. Minimize decreases in systemic vascular resistance. Sympathetic blockade produced by regional anaesthesia may worsen the prolapse. However, sometimes there may be no choice. Extradural anaesthesia was required for Caesarean section in a patient with MVP, asthma and pneumonia (Alcantara & Marx 1987). The importance of adequately preloading the patient, and fractionating the doses of local anaesthetic, were stressed. Hypotension secondary to sympathetic blockade should be treated with a dilute phenylephrine solution, rather than with ephedrine. Induced hypotension may also worsen the prolapse and should preferably not be used (Thiagarajah & Frost 1983).
2. High airway pressures should be avoided.
3. Prophylactic antibiotics for bacterial endocarditis are required.

BIBLIOGRAPHY

Abrahams Z A, Lees DC 1989 Two cardiac arrests after needle puncture in a patient with mitral valve prolapse: Psychogenic? Anesthesia and Analgesia 69: 126–128

Alcantara L C, Marx C F 1987 Cesarean section under epidural analgesia in a parturient with mitral valve prolapse. Anesthesia and Analgesia 66: 902–903

Batson MA, Longmire 5, Csontos E 1990 Alfentanil for urgent caesarean section in a patient with severe mitral stenosis and pulmonary hypertension Canadian Journal of Anaesthesia 37: 685–688

Berry F A, Lake C L, Johns R A et al 1985 Mitral valve prolapse – another cause of intraoperative arrhythmias in the pediatric patient. Anesthesiology 62: 662–664

Cheng T O 1990 Cardiac arrest and mitral valve prolapse. Anesthesia and Analgesia 70: 229

George R J D, Banks R A 1983 Bedside measurement of Pulmonary capillary wedge pressure. British Journal of Hospital Medicine 29: 286–291

Hemmings C T, Whalley D G, O'Connor P J et al 1987 Invasive monitoring and anaesthetic management of a parturient with mitral stenosis. Canadian Journal of Anaesthesia 34: 182–185

Krantz J M, Viljoen J F, Schermer R et al 1980 Mitral valve prolapse. Anesthesia and Analgesia 59: 379–383

Leonard J C 1979 Mitral valve disease. British Journal of Hospital Medicine 22: 204–212

McLintic A J, Metcalfe M J, Ingram K S et al 1992 Acute mitral regurgitation: physiological and pharmacological considerations in the management of a critically ill patient. Anaesthesia and Intensive Care 20: 373–376

Oakley C M 1984 Mitral valve prolapse: harbinger of death or variant of normal? British Medical Journal 288: 1853–1854

Schulte-Sasse U, Hess W, Tarnow J 1982 Pulmonary vascular responses to nitrous oxide in patients with normal and high pulmonary vascular resistance. Anesthesiology 57: 9–13

Thiagarajah S, Frost E A M 1983 Anaesthetic considerations in patients with mitral valve prolapse. Anaesthesia 38: 560–566

MORQUIO'S SYNDROME
(See also MUCOPOLYSACCHARIDOSES)

One of the mucopolysaccharidoses (type IV), this autosomal recessive connective tissue disorder results from the abnormal metabolism of certain polysaccharides (Baines & Keneally 1983, Kempthorne & Browne 1983). Excessive amounts of some metabolites of these substances are laid down in the body tissues and result in a variety of defects. Skeletal, cardiac, eye, and hearing problems develop, but there is no mental retardation. Death frequently occurs before the age of 30.

Preoperative abnormalities

1. Skeletal abnormalities include dwarfism, kyphosis, genu valgum, hand deformity, joint mobility, pigeon chest, vertebral flattening with wide disc spaces, and neck instability from hypoplasia of the odontoid peg. Spinal cord compression may develop in late childhood with slow-onset paraplegia. The face is flattened, and the teeth may be widely spaced, and have defective enamel.
2. Restrictive lung disease secondary to kyphoscoliosis.
3. Cardiac infiltration can affect both the mitral and aortic valves and late-onset aortic regurgitation may occur. In an echocardiographic study of 10 patients, six had abnormalities mainly involving the aortic or mitral valves (John et al 1990). However, these lesions were haemodynamically relatively mild. Heart disease may also develop secondary to the progressive chest deformity.
4. Corneal opacities commonly develop.
5. Nerve deafness may occur.
6. Inguinal herniae are common and may require surgery.
7. Excess keratin sulphate is found in the urine.

Anaesthetic problems

1. Atlantoaxial subluxation may occur and result in spinal cord transection, particularly in relation to traumatic events (Lipson 1977). A rapid rate of progression of myelopathy has been reported, with the risk of acute quadriparesis or sudden death from

respiratory arrest. Atlantoaxial instability may not always be the cause of neurological problems. In a myelographic study of 13 patients, odontoid dysplasia and a hypoplastic dens was found in every case (Stevens et al 1991). However, the atlantoaxial stability was said to be mild, and if severe spinal cord compression was present, it was secondary to anterior extradural soft tissue thickening rather than the subluxation. Both features were described in a child who developed a hemiparesis after a fall (Ashraf et al 1991). Acute tetraplegia, and subsequent death from pneumonia, was reported in an 8-year-old girl having a myelogram under general anaesthesia (Beighton & Craig 1973). Displacement of the atlas on the axis was found to have occurred. This was attributed to excess movement of the head during the anaesthetic.

2. Respiratory function may be impaired (Hope et al 1973), and upper airway obstruction and chest deformities may contribute to postoperative respiratory problems. Respiratory failure and subsequent death from pneumonia occurred in a patient following radical cervical lymph node resection for melanoma of the scalp (Jones & Croley 1979). Infiltration of upper airway structures with glycosaminoglycans may cause upper airway obstruction in the perioperative period (Berkowitz et al 1990).

3. Intubation difficulties have been described resulting from facial deformity and redundant pharyngeal mucosa (Jones & Croley 1979).

4. Upper airway obstruction has been produced by head flexion (Pritzker et al 1980).

5. Obstructive sleep apnoea.

Management

1. A careful assessment of respiratory function is required so as to detect those patients with seriously impaired reserve. in view of the increased risk of major postoperative problems, and the reduced life expectancy, a decision to embark on non-essential major surgery should not be made lightly.

2. Cervical spine X-rays should be examined for signs of C 1/C2 instability, and pre-existing neurological defects documented. If hypoplasia of the dens or instability is suspected, some means of immobilizing the neck is required to prevent flexion damage to the spinal cord. The management of appendicectomy in a young boy, who already had paraplegia from spinal cord compression, was described (Birkinshaw 1975). The child lay prone with his head propped on his hands and a plaster cast was applied to his head, back and sides. When the plaster was dry the patient was carefully rolled into a supine position. After an inhalation induction with halothane, intubation was achieved with deep ether anaesthesia.

3. If intubation difficulties are suspected, either an inhalation induction or an awake intubation should be considered.

4. If there are cardiac lesions, prophylaxis for endocarditis is required.

BIBLIOGRAPHY
Ashraf J, Crockard H A, Ransford A O et al 1991 Transoral decompression and
    posterior stabilisation in Morquio's disease. Archives of Diseases in Childhood 66:
    1318–1321
Baines D, Keneally J 1983 Anaesthetic implications of the mucopolysaccharidoses: A
    fifteen year experience in a Children's Hospital. Anaesthesia and Intensive Care
    11: 198–202
Beighton P, Craig I 1973 Atlanto-axial subluxation in the Morquio syndrome. Journal
    of Bone and Joint Surgery 55B: 478–481
Berkowitz I D, Raja S N, Bender K S et al 1990 Dwarfs: pathology and anesthetic
    implications. Anesthesiology 73: 739–759
Birkinshaw K J 1975 Anaesthesia in a patient with an unstable neck: Morquio's
    syndrome. Anaesthesia 30: 46–49
Hope E O S, Farebrother M J B, Bainbridge D 1973 Some aspects of respiratory
    function in three siblings with Morquio–Brailsford disease. Thorax 28: 335–343
John R M, Hunter D, Swanton R H 1990 Echocardiographic abnormalities in type IV
    mucopolysaccharidoses. Archives of Diseases in Childhood 65: 746–749
Jones A E P, Croley T F 1979 Morquio syndrome and anesthesia. Anesthesiology 51:
    261–262
Kempthorne P M, Brown T C K 1983 Anaesthesia and the mucopolysaccharidoses: A
    survey of techniques and problems. Anaesthesia and Intensive Care; 11: 203–207
Lipson S J 1977 Dysplasia of the odontoid process in Morquio's syndrome causing
    quadriparesis. Journal of Bone and Joint Surgery 59A: 340–344
Pritzker M R, King R A, Kronenberg R S 1980 Upper airway obstruction during head
    flexion in Morquio's disease. American Journal of Medicine 69: 467–470
Stevens J M, Kendall B E, Crockard H A et al 1991 The odontoid process in Morquio-
    Brailsford's disease. The effects of spinal fusion. Journal of Bone and Joint Surgery
    73: 851–858

MOTOR NEURONE DISEASE
(AMYOTROPHIC LATERAL SCLEROSIS)

A progressive degenerative disease of the motor system of unknown
aetiology. It involves both upper and lower motor neurones and presents
in late middle age with muscle weakness and fasciculations. Bulbar
palsies are a common and distressing feature, and involvement of non-
motor pathways is increasingly being recognized (Tandan & Bradley
1985). The prognosis is poor, and in about 50% of cases death occurs
within 3 years of onset. In the early stages there is an increased risk of
bony injury from falls, and later in the disease anaesthetists may be
involved in ventilatory care. The importance of supportive treatment in
terminal management has been emphasized (O'Brien et al 1992).

Preoperative abnormalities

1. A combination of signs and symptoms of upper and lower motor
    neurone disease. Muscle cramps, weakness, wasting, fasciculations,
    spasticity, hyper-reflexia, and extensor plantar reflexes, may coexist
    with bulbar signs. These include impairment of speech, swallowing
    and laryngeal reflexes which cause distressing symptoms such as

dysphagia, drooling, choking, and dysarthria. The ocular muscles are spared. The disease is progressive.

2. EMG indicates muscle denervation and shows fibrillation potentials.
3. A form of the disease may occur in conjunction with a carcinoma, usually bronchial.

Anaesthetic problems

1. Administration of suxamethonium has been reported to have produced marked hyperkalaemia and cardiovascular collapse (Beach et al 1971).
2. Patients may be sensitive to the effects of non-depolarizing muscle relaxants (Rosenbaum et al 1971).
3. There is a risk of perioperative pulmonary aspiration and airway obstruction in cases in which bulbar signs are present.
4. Postoperative respiratory insufficiency may occur.
5. The ethical problems involved in the conflict between preserving life and minimizing suffering in the later stages of the disease (Newrick & Langton Newer 1984).

Management

1. In view of the report of cardiovascular collapse secondary to hyperkalaemia, the use of suxamethonium should be avoided.
2. If non-depolarizing drugs are essential, small doses are given initially and neuromuscular function monitored.
3. If bulbar muscle function is impaired, precautions should be taken to prevent perioperative pulmonary aspiration.
4. The use of extradural anaesthesia for lower abdominal surgery has been reported in three patients (Kochi et al 1989).
5. Silverstein et al (1991) stress the importance of regularly allowing patients an opportunity to discuss the possibility of ventilatory support and express their views about cardiopulmonary resuscitation.
6. In advanced cases of the disease, careful consideration should be given to the appropriateness of surgery, particularly when there is bulbar involvement. Severe problems may arise once a patient is committed to IPPV. However, in some patients, respiratory muscle weakness may present as shortness of breath early in the disease. In these patients, non-invasive respiratory support at night may produce symptomatic benefit (Howard et al 1989). The use of phrenic nerve pacing is being tried for ventilatory support (Editorial 1990).
7. Muscle pains may be a prominent and distressing feature. The response to opiates has been shown to be good and there is no evidence that the course or duration of the disease is affected (O'Brien et al 1992). Oral morphine, either as an elixir or slow-

release preparation, is the opioid of choice, accompanied by a laxative. An antiemetic may be needed in the early stages.

BIBLIOGRAPHY

Beach T P, Stone W A, Hamelberg W 1971 Circulatory collapse following succinylcholine: report of a patient with diffuse lower motor neurone disease. Anesthesia and Analgesia 50: 431–437

Editorial 1990 Phrenic nerve pacing in quadriplegia. Lancet 336: 88–90

Howard R S, Wiles C M, Loh L 1989 Respiratory complications and their management in motor neuron disease. Brain 112: 1155–1170

Kochi T, Oka T, Mizuguchi T 1989 Epidural anesthesia for patients with amyotrophic lateral sclerosis. Anesthesia and Analgesia 68: 410–412

Newrick P G, Langton-Hewer R 1984 Motor neurone disease: can we do better? British Medical Journal 289: 539–542

Norris F H 1992 Motor neurone disease. Treating the untreated. British Medical Journal 304: 459–460

O'Brien T, Kelly M, Saunders C 1992 Motor neurone disease: a hospice perspective. British Medical Journal 304: 471–473

Rosenbaum K J, Neigh J L, Strobel G E 1971 Sensitivity to non-depolarising muscle relaxants in amyotrophic lateral sclerosis. Anesthesiology 35: 638–641

Silverstein M D, Stocking C B, Antel J P 1991 Amyotrophic lateral sclerosis and life-sustaining therapy: patients' desires for information, participation in decision making, and life-sustaining therapy. Mayo Clinic Proceedings 66: 906–913

Tandan R, Bradley W G 1985 Amyotrophic lateral sclerosis. Part I. Clinical features, pathology and ethical issues in management. Annals of Neurology 18: 271–280

MOYA MOYA DISEASE

A rare abnormality of the cerebral circulation, first described in Japan, in which gradual occlusion or severe stenosis of the internal carotid arteries occurs. Cerebral angiography shows a fine hazy network of vessels (the moya-moya collaterals) around the base of the brain. Patients usually present with signs of cerebrovascular insufficiency, either in childhood or as adults.

Preoperative abnormalities

1. The patient may present with a variety of features suggestive of inadequate cerebral blood flow. These may range from transient ischaemic attacks to fixed neurological deficits.
2. Cerebral angiography demonstrates the occluded arteries and the abnormal 'net-like' collateral circulation.
3. Normal cerebral blood flow may be reduced by as much as a half.
4. In adults there is an increased incidence of intracranial aneurysms.

Anaesthetic problems

1. Hyperventilation can produce a reduction in arterial P_{CO_2} which may compromise the already poor cerebral circulation. Cases have been described in which hypocapnoea during anaesthesia was associated with a deterioration in neurological status. No deterioration occurred

in those patients in whom normocapnoea was maintained (Sumikawa & Nagai 1983, Bingham & Wilkinson 1985). Anaesthesia using pancuronium, fentanyl, and 0.5–1% isoflurane, while maintaining normocapnoea, was used in eight procedures on seven patients (Brown & Lam 1987). It has been suggested, however, that short periods of hypocapnoea may be tolerated in patients, provided a potent inhalational agent is being used as a cerebral vasodilator at the same time (Martino & Warner 1991).

2. In one series, four out of seven patients were found to have abnormal ECGs. One 27-year-old developed a ventricular tachycardia during surgery (Brown & Lam 1987).
3. Postoperatively, subjects are prone to develop fits.
4. The diagnosis may not always be known before surgery. A 5-year-old child was given spinal anaesthesia for circumcision. Two hours after surgery he developed recurrent seizures and a left hemiparesis lasting for 10 days (Yasukawa et al 1988). The occurrence of subsequent transient ischaemic attack was suggestive of a compromised cerebral circulation, and carotid angiography showed the picture of moya moya disease.

Management

1. Surgical treatment is directed towards increasing the cerebral blood flow. Various surgical manoeuvres have been tried, including anastomosis of the superficial temporal to the middle cerebral artery, encephaloduroarteriosynangiosis, and encephalo-omental synangiosis.
2. The maintenance of an $ETco_2$ between 5.5 kPa and 6 kPa has been recommended (Yamagishi et al 1991, Chadha et al 1990).
3. Normothermia should be maintained.

BIBLIOGRAPHY
Bingham R M, Wilkinson D J 1985 Anaesthetic management in Moya-moya disease. Anaesthesia 40: 1198–1202
Brown S C, Lam A 1987 Moya-moya disease. A review of clinical experience and anaesthetic management. Canadian Journal of Anaesthesia 34: 71–75
Chadha R, Singh S, Padmanabhan V 1990 Anaesthetic management in moyamoya disease. Anaesthesia and Intensive Care 18: 120–123
Jacob R, Kausalya R 1990 Moyamoya disease. Anaesthesia and Intensive Care 18: 582
Karasawa J, Tuoho H, Ohnishi H et al 1992 Long-term follow-up study after extracranial-intracranial bypass surgery for anterior circulation ischaemia in childhood moyamoya disease. Journal of Neurosurgery 77: 84–89
Martino J D, Warner C O 1991 Hypocarbia during anaesthesia in children with moyamoya disease. Canadian Journal of Anaesthesia 38: 942–943
Sumikawa K, Nagai H 1983 Moya-moya disease and anesthesia. Anesthesiology 58: 204–205
Yasukawa K, Akagawa S, Nakagawa Y et al 1988 Convulsions and temporary hemiparesis following spinal anesthesia in a child with moya moya disease. Anesthesiology 69: 1023

Yamagishi N et al 1991 Anesthetic management of revascularisation for Moyamoya disease (English abstr.) Masui 40: 1132–1137

MUCOPOLYSACCHARIDOSES (MPS)

A group of inherited connective tissue syndromes which result from enzyme deficiencies. The mucopolysaccharides, (or glycosaminoglycans) are constituents of connective tissue, and are made up of repeating disaccharide units connected to protein. They are normally broken down in the cell lysosomes to monosaccharides and amino acids. In the absence of certain enzymes, accumulation of intermediate products of the degradation process takes place. These substances increase cell size and cause impairment of function. The effects depend upon the enzyme defect, and the specific organs involved. The disease progresses with age, and life-expectancy is greatly reduced.

Surgery is required most frequently for inguinal and umbilical herniae, ENT, orthopaedic, or neurosurgical operations. In a review of 43 children, every patient was found to have at least one complication involving the head and neck, and in more than a half, ENT surgery was required (Bredenkamp et al 1992).

More recently there have been attempts to replace missing enzymes by regular implantation of tissue such as human amnion (King et al 1984), but there has been little evidence of success. Although these syndromes are rare, the more commonly encountered ones provide a considerable anaesthetic challenge, primarily because of airway problems The classification of syndromes is shown below. Some are dealt with under their individual names. Abnormalities in the least common types are included here.

TYPE I

Type IH	Hurler's syndrome (gargoylism) (see Hurler's syndrome)
Type IS	Scheie's syndrome (see Hurler's syndrome)
Type IH/S	Hurler-Scheie's (see Hurler's syndrome)

TYPE II   Hunter's syndrome (see Hurler's syndrome)

TYPE III   Sanfilippo's syndrome
Craniofacial: mild coarsening of facial features.
Skeletal: none.
Cardiac: none.
Mental: severe progressive retardation.
Other organs: none.
Anaesthetic: difficult intubation has been reported (Kempthorne & Brown 1983).

TYPE IV   Morquio's syndrome (see Morquio's syndrome)

TYPE VI   Maroteaux–Lamy syndrome
Craniofacial: coarse features and macroglossia.

Skeletal: kyphosis, flat vertebrae, genu valgum.

Cardiac: none.

Mental: normal.

Other organs: none.

Anaesthetic: four out of six patients had either a difficult airway or difficult intubation (Baines & Keneally 1983, Kempthorne & Brown 1983). Atlantoaxial instability has been reported.

TYPE VII   B-glucuronidase

TYPE VIII   ? like Morquio's and Sanfilippo's syndromes

BIBLIOGRAPHY
Baines D, Keneally J 1983 Anaesthetic implications of the mucopolysaccharidoses. Anaesthesia and Intensive Care 11: 198–202
Bredenkamp J K, Smith M E, Dudley J P et al 1992 Otolaryngologic manifestations of the mucopolysaccharidoses. Annals of Otology, Rinology and Laryngology 101: 472–478
Herrick I A, Rhine E J 1988 The mucopolysaccharidoses and anaesthesia. Canadian Journal of Anaesthesia 35: 67–73
Kempthorne P M, Brown T C K 1983 Anaesthesia and the mucopolysaccharidoses. Anaesthesia and Intensive Care 11: 203–207
King D H, Jones R M, Barnett M B 1984 Anaesthesia and the mucopolysaccharidoses. Anaesthesia 39: 126–131
Ruckenstein MJ, MacDonald R E, Clarke J T et al 1991 The management of otolaryngological problems in the mucopolysaccharidoses: a retrospective review. Journal of Otolaryngology 20: 177–183

MUSCULAR DYSTROPHY
(see also DUCHENNE MUSCULAR DYSTROPHY)

A group of inherited muscle disorders. The severe Duchenne type, which is the most common, also produces the most serious anaesthetic problems This condition is described separately. Precise diagnosis is not always possible, but the other types are less severe (Ellis 1980). In general, dystrophies other than Duchenne do not affect the muscles of respiration or swallowing, and cardiac involvement is less common. However, marked sensitivity to curare was reported with ocular muscular dystrophy (Robertson 1984), and therefore neuromuscular monitoring is mandatory in these patients. Episodes of acute hypermetabolism and rhabdomyolysis sometimes occur during anaesthesia, and several authors have suggested an association between muscle dystrophies and malignant hyperthermia. However, contracture testing in two children, one with Becker's, the other with Duchenne, were negative (Gronert et al 1992) and these authors considered that the MH-like features seen during anaesthesia were a result of alterations in the muscle membrane secondary to the dystrophy itself. Exposure to volatile agents and suxamethonium might increase membrane permeability, and compensatory hypermetabolism is suggested to result from attempts to re-establish membrane stability and prevent calcium flux.

X-linked

1. Duchenne (severe). In this condition anaesthesia has been associated with a number of serious and sometimes fatal complications (see Duchenne muscular dystrophy).
2. Becker (mild). Although this dystrophy is less severe than the Duchenne type, an anaesthetic death associated with acute rhabdomyolysis, hyperkalaemia and hypocalcaemia has been reported (Bush & Dubowitz 1991).
3. Emery-Dreifuss. Features include fixed muscle contractures with flexion of the elbow and shortening of tendo Achilles, limitation of neck flexion, progressive muscle weakness and wasting (humeroperoneal), cardiomyopathy with heart block and atrial arrhythmias (Miller et al 1985). Arrhythmias occurred in all affected men over the age of 35 years, and a proportion of female carriers had ECG abnormalities (Bialer et al 1991). Although the muscle dystrophy itself is relatively benign, sudden death may occur. Subarachnoid anaesthesia has been described in a young man for Achilles tendon lengthening (Morrison & Jago 1991).

Autosomal recessive

4. Severe.
5. Mild limb girdle: with facial involvement
                     without facial involvement.

Autosomal dominant

6. Facioscapulohumeral (Landouzy-Dejerine) onset in adolescence, first affecting the shoulders, facial weakness, winging of scapulae, proximal arm wasting. Slowly progressive. Uneventful anaesthesia using atracurium showed no increased sensitivity, but a more rapid recovery time than normal (Dressner & Ali 1989).
7. Distal.
8. Ocular.
9. Oculopharyngeal (Landrum & Eggars 1992).

BIBLIOGRAPHY
Bialer M G, McDaniel N L, Kelly T E 1991 Progression of cardiac disease in Emery-Dreifuss muscular dystrophy. Clinical Cardiology 14: 411–416
Bush A, Dubowitz V 1991 Fatal rhabdomyolysis complicating general anaesthesia in a child with Becker muscular dystrophy. Neuromuscular Disorders 1: 204–210
Dressner D L, Ali H H 1989 Anaesthetic management of a patient with facioscapulohumeral muscular dystrophy. British Journal of Anaesthesia 62: 331–334
Ellis F R 1980 Inherited muscle disease. British Journal of Anaesthesia 52: 153–164
Gronert G A, Fowler W, Cardinet G H et al 1992 Absence of malignant hyperthermia contractures in Becker–Duchenne dystrophy at age 2. Muscle and Nerve 15: 52–56

Landrum A L, Eggers G W N 1992 Oculopharyngeal dystrophy: an approach to anesthetic management. Anesthesia and Analgesia 75: 1043–1045
Miller R G, Layzer R B, Mellenthin M A et al 1985 Emery–Dreiluss muscular dystrophy with autosomal dominant transmission. Neurology 35: 1230–1233
Morrison P, Jago R H 1991 Emery–Dreifuss muscular dystrophy. Anaesthesia 46: 33–35
Robertson J A 1984 Ocular muscular dystrophy. A cause of curare sensitivity. Anaethesia 39: 251–253

MYASTHENIA GRAVIS

An autoimmune disease of the neuromuscular junction involving the postjunctional acetylcholine receptors. Specific autoantibodies have been identified and microscopic changes in the membrane demonstrated. Not only is there a reduction in the number of acetylcholine receptors at the postjunctional membrane so that the safety margin is decreased, but there also appears to be a variation in the functional ability of the antibodies to block the receptors (lDrachman 1978). It appears that there are two populations of receptors, with half-lives of 12 days and 12 hours respectively. Both types of receptor may be decreased in myasthenia gravis.

The condition is characterized by muscle weakness and fatiguability on repeated use of that muscle. Females are more commonly affected than males, in a 2:1 ratio. There is an association with thymic enlargement and thymomas, both benign and malignant.

Preoperative abnormalities

1. Symptoms are primarily those of increasing muscle weakness and neuromuscular fatigue which improve after resting. Muscles of the eye and face are affected early in the disease and result in ptosis and diplopia. Bulbar palsy may produce swallowing and speech difficulties, and neck muscles may be affected. Sometimes respiratory muscle involvement occurs early. Variable progression or remission may occur. The involvement of particular muscle groups is inconstant, but proximal muscles of the upper limbs are affected more frequently than the lower limbs.
2. Antibodies against acetylcholine receptors are found in 80–90% of patients with myasthenia gravis.
3. Diagnosis may be confirmed by demonstrating an improvement within 10–30 seconds of giving edrophonium i.v. 2–10 mg. This lasts for about 5 minutes.
4. Current treatment includes:
   a. Immunological suppression to eliminate the antibody. Azathioprine or steroids are used, and benefit 90% of cases. This has become the first line of treatment.
   b. Thymectomy, increasingly via the transcervical approach.
   c. Symptomatic relief with anticholinesterase preparations which potentiate the effects of acetylcholine. Pyridostigmine and

neostigmine are most commonly used. Concurrent use of atropine or propantheline may be required to block muscarinic effects, such as intestinal colic.

d. Plasma exchange, for short-term treatment, particularly in a crisis.

Anaesthetic problems

1. The operation
   Anaesthesia may be required for thymectomy, or for other incidental surgery. Thymectomy is performed via either a median sternotomy or a transcervical approach. The former produces the greater anaesthetic difficulties.
2. The variables
   The main problem revolves around the anaesthetist's ability to anticipate and manage three variables:
   a. The muscle weakness produced by the patient's disease.
   b. His preoperative anticholinesterase medication.
   c. The surgeon's requirement for muscle relaxation. Adequate respiratory function must be maintained in the pre- and postoperative period, and yet adequate intraoperative muscle relaxation may be needed for surgical access.
3. Neuromuscular blockers
   Myasthenics may or may not have an increased sensitivity to non-depolarizing blockers. Unexpected sensitivity or apnoea may represent the first signs of myasthenia. In one patient with an undiagnosed thymoma, total paralysis after pancuronium 1 mg was associated with a high titre of antiacetylcholine receptor antibodies, but without clinical manifestations of the disease (Enoki et al 1989). A patient with sero-negative ocular myasthenia also had marked sensitivity to only 2 mg vecuronium (Kim & Mangold 1989). Sensitivity may also occur when the patient is in remission (Lumb & Calder 1989).

   The blockade of the acetylcholine receptors by antibody resembles partial curarization, therefore the amount of a drug required to produce effective paralysis is often reduced. There is, however, wide patient variation in response. The actual amount of drug needed will depend upon factors such as the stage of the disease, the presence or absence of a remission, the actual muscles being tested and whether or not anticholinesterase medication has been given preoperatively. In addition, the responses of the peripheral and bulbar muscles may be very different, particularly when there is bulbar involvement (Baraka 1992a). Using a cumulative dose plus infusion technique, Eisenkraft et al (1989) found that the ED50 and ED95 of vecuronium in 10 myasthenics was 53% and 56%, respectively.

   Responses to suxamethonium vary widely. Resistance to

suxamethonium has been reported (Wainwright & Broderick 1987, Eisenkraft et al 1988). However the use of 1.5 mg/kg has been reported to give good intubating conditions with recovery in 10–15 minutes (Baraka & Tabboush 1991). In an EMG study of eight children, resistance to suxamethonium was usually seen (Brown et al 1990). However, if the patient is in remission, resistance may not occur (Abel et al 1991). Baraka (1992b) studied the plasma cholinesterase levels in three myasthenic patients about to undergo thymectomy, two of whom were receiving pyridostigmine therapy. He found that the levels correlated with the recovery time from suxamethonium. Both patients treated with pyridostigmine had decreased plasma cholinesterase activity, and in these patients there was prolongation of neuromuscular block with suxamethonium.

4. Volatile agents will increase muscle weakness and isoflurane has twice as potent a depressant effect on neuromuscular transmission in myasthenics as halothane (Nilsson & Muller 1990).

5. Excess anticholinesterase
   Excessive amounts of an anticholinesterase may itself cause increased muscle weakness and this can be confused with that due to the myasthenia. Experimentally, an excess of anticholinesterase has been shown to reduce the number of functioning receptors. Thus, a patient in a cholinergic crisis may require IPPV.

6. Respiratory dysfunction or prolonged apnoea
   Respiratory muscle or bulbar weakness may occur pre- or postoperatively and can predispose the patient to pulmonary aspiration, chest infection or respiratory failure.

7. Immunosuppression may lead to neutropenia and serious infection.

Management

1. Management of neuromuscular blockade
   The method of management depends on the severity of the myasthenia, the type of operation, and the anaesthetist's personal preference. In a series of 100 cases of transcervical thymectomy (Girnar et al 1976), those patients with mild myasthenia were given half their normal dose of pyridostigmine, while those with severe disease received their full dose. Anaesthesia and intubation were achieved with thiopentone, nitrous oxide, oxygen, and either halothane or ethrane. IPPV was maintained without a muscle relaxant and 92 patients were extubated successfully within 2 hours of operation. In two patients having trans-sternal thymectomy, thoracic extradural anaesthesia was given in combination with light general anaesthesia (Burgess & Wilcosky 1989). The avoidance of neuromuscular blockers and the use of postoperative extradural fentanyl allowed early extubation.

   Upper abdominal surgery requires a greater degree of muscle relaxation than can be produced by inhalation agents alone. With the advent of clinical neuromuscular monitors, good control can be achieved using only small doses of a drug. Atracurium, in five patients with moderate to severe myasthenia, was found to be 1.7–1.9 times more potent than in normal individuals (Smith et al 1989). The satisfactory use of atracurium in incremental doses has been reported (MacDonald et al 1984, Ward & Wright 1984). Whilst the final doses required to produce 90-95% blockade varied from 0.05 mg/kg to 0.33 mg/kg, it was agreed that with atracurium, a relatively rapid rate of spontaneous recovery took place when compared with other relaxants. Sensitivity to vecuronium has been shown and its degree was related to the titre of acetylcholine receptor antibodies (Nilsson & Meretoja 1990). Vecuronium 0.02–0.04 mg/kg was used in six patients for thymectomy, without problems in reversal (Hunter et al 1985). Alternatively, if a rapid sequence induction is required, suxamethonium 1.5 mg/kg will give good intubating conditions.

2. Muscle relaxant reversal and anticholinesterases
   Either reversal of muscle relaxants, or restoration of respiration in the myasthenic, may be achieved by the routine use of neostigmine and atropine. However, care must be taken not to give a dose in excess of the patient's normal requirements, otherwise a cholinergic crisis may occur (Eisencraft & Papatestas 1988). Equivalent doses are:

Neostigmine i.v.	1 mg
Neostigmine oral	30mg
Pyridostigmine i.v.	4 mg
Pyridostigmine oral	120mg

   The patient's usual anticholinesterases may have to be given i.v. until oral medication can be taken.

3. Postoperative care
   All patients require postoperative high-dependency facilities. Some patients will need postoperative IPPV. The surgical approach to the thymus is still controversial. A transcervical technique is being increasingly used, rather than the more traumatic trans-sternal route. The cervical approach is associated with a reduced requirement for prolonged postoperative IPPV.

4. Will scoring systems predict patients who will require prolonged IPPV?
   The contradictory reports of the sensitivity of such scoring systems are probably due in part to the variation in the surgical approach to the thymus. A scoring system utilizing four factors and claiming a predictive sensitivity of 100% has been devised (Leventhal et al 1980). The factors were:
   a. Length of disease greater than 6 years.
   b. Concomitant respiratory disease.
   c. Pyridostigmine requirement of >750 mg/day.

d. Vital capacity of <2.9 litres.

All the patients had trans-thoracic thymectomy.

In another paper, these predictors were utilized in 92 patients, and a sensitivity of only 37.5% was achieved (Eisencraft et al 1986). However, all of these patients had a transcervical thymectomy, which involved a much lower (8.7%) requirement for postoperative IPPV. This was a significant improvement on previously reported series of trans-sternal procedures, for which the IPPV rates varied from 33% to 50%. A further attempt to utilize the scoring system included both approaches to the thymus, and a variety of non-thymectomy operations (Grant & Jenkins 1982). In the thymectomy group, only three out seven who required IPPV were predicted. In contrast, none of the 24 non-thymectomy patients needed ventilation, despite 11 having scores of >10.

5. Tracheostomy

Occasionally, tracheostomy may be required, but only if ventilation is prolonged and excess secretions are a problem.

6. Respiratory failure in myasthenia

Respiratory failure in myasthenic patients may be secondary to either a myasthenic or a cholinergic crisis. IPPV should be instituted, anticholinesterase therapy stopped, and then only cautiously reintroduced after testing with i.v. edrophonium. An improvement suggests a myasthenic cause, and deterioration, a cholinergic crisis. Facilities should be available for the rapid institution of IPPV. The use of an atracurium infusion for prolonged IPPV and tracheobronchial toilet has been described (Pollard et al 1989).

BIBLIOGRAPHY

Abel M, Eisenkraft J B, Patel N 1991 Response to suxamethonium in a myasthenic patient during remission. Anaesthesia 46: 30–32

Baraka A, Tabboush Z 1991 Neuromuscular response to succinylcholine–vecuronium sequence in three myasthenic patients undergoing thymectomy. Anesthesia and Analgesia 72: 827–830

Baraka A 1992a Anaesthesia and myasthenia gravis. Canadian Journal of Anaesthesia 39: 476–486

Baraka A 1992b Suxamethonium block in the myasthenic patient. Correlation with plasma cholinesterase. Anaesthesia 47: 217–219

Brown T C K, Gebert R, Meretoja O A et al 1990 Myasthenia gravis in children and its anaesthetic implications. Anaesthesia and Intensive Care 18: 466–472

Burgess F W, Wilcosky B 1989 Thoracic epidural anesthesia for transsternal thymectomy in myasthenia gravis. Anesthesia and Analgesia 69: 529–531

Drachman D B 1978 Myasthenia gravis. New England Journal of Medicine 298: 186–193

Drachman D B 1987 Present and future treatment of myasthenia gravis. New England Journal of Medicine 316: 743–745

Eisenkraft J B, Papatestas A E, Kahn C H et al 1986 Predicting the need for postoperative mechanical ventilation in myasthenia gravis. Anesthesiology 65: 79–82

Eisenkraft J B, Papatestas A E 1988 Anaesthesia for trans–sternal thymectomy in myasthenia gravis. Annals of the Royal College of Surgeons of England 70; 257–258

Eisenkraft J B, Book W J, Mann S M, Papatestas A E, Hubbard M 1988 Resistance to succinylcholine in myasthenia gravis: a dose-response study. Anesthesiology 69: 760–763

Eisenkraft J B, Book W J, Papatestas A E et al 1989 Sensitivity to vecuronium in myasthenia gravis: a dose-response study. Anesthesia and Analgesia 68: S80

Enoki T, Naito Y, Hirokawa Y et al 1989 Marked sensitivity to pancuronium in a patient without clinical manifestations of myasthenia gravis. Anesthesia and Analgesia 69: 840–842

Girnar D S, Weinreich A I 1976 Anesthesia for transcervical thymectomy in myasthenia gravis. Anesthesia and Analgesia 55: 13–17

Grant R P, Jenkins L C 1982 Prediction of the need for postoperative mechanical ventilation in myasthenia gravis: thymectomy compared with other surgical procedures. Canadian Anaesthetists' Society Journal 29: 112–116

Hunter J M, Bell C F, Florence A M et al 1985 Vecuronium in the myasthenic patient. Anaesthesia 40: 848–853

Kim J-M, Mangold J 1989 Sensitivity to both vecuronium and neostigmine in a sero-negative myasthenic patient. British Journal of Anaesthesia 63: 497–500

Leventhal S R, Orkin F K, Hirsch R A 1980 Prediction of the need for postoperative mechanical ventilation in myasthenia gravis. Anesthesiology 53: 26–30

Lumb A B, Calder I 1989 'Cured' myasthenia gravis and neuromuscular blockade. Anaesthesia 44: 828–830

MacDonald A M, Keen R I, Pugh N D 1984 Myasthenia gravis and atracurium. British Journal of Anaesthesia 56: 651–654

Nilsson E, Meretoja O A 1990 Vecuronium dose-response and maintenance requirements in patients with myasthenia gravis. Anesthesiology 73: 28–32

Nilsson E, Muller K 1990 Neuromuscular effects of isoflurane in patients with myasthenia gravis. Acta Anaesthesiologica Scandinavica 34: 126–131

Pollard B J, Harper N J N, Doran B R H 1989 Use of continuous prolonged administration of atracurium in the ITU to a patient with myasthenia gravis. British Journal of Anaesthesia 62: 95–97

Smith C E, Donati F, Bevan D R 1989 Cumulative dose-response curves for atracurium in patients with myasthenia gravis. Canadian Journal of Anaesthesia 36: 402–406

Wainwrtight A P Broderick P M 1987 Suxamethonium in myasthenia gravis. Anaesthesia 42: 950–957

Ward S, Wright D J 1984 Neuromuscular blockade in myasthenia gravis with atracurium besylate. Anaesthesia 39: 51–53

MYASTHENIC SYNDROME
(see EATON–LAMBERT SYNDROME)

MYELOMA, MULTIPLE

This plasma cell neoplasm is one of the paraproteinaemias, whose peak incidence is in the seventh decade. It erodes bone and infiltrates bone marrow. The diagnosis requires two of the three following criteria: plasma cells in the bone marrow to be >20% of marrow nucleated cells, a paraprotein to be present in the serum and/or urine, and lytic bone lesions.

Preoperative abnormalities

1. Myeloma may present with bone pain, pathological fractures, anaemia, renal disease or hypercalcaemia. Hypercalcaemia causes drowsiness, vomiting, constipation, dehydration, confusion and

coma. Punched-out lytic lesions may occur anywhere in the skeleton, but are most frequent in the skull, vertebrae, ribs and long bones. Peripheral neuropathy may occur, or paraplegia may arise due to an extradural plasmacytoma or vertebral collapse.

2. The hyperviscosity syndrome produces neurological (confusion, vertigo, headaches, fits), ocular (visual disturbances and blindness), and haematological (bleeding) problems and cardiac failure.

3. There is usually anaemia, a high ESR, excretion of Bence–Jones protein in the urine, and abnormal protein electrophoresis. Bone marrow is infiltrated with plasma cells. The diagnosis requires plasma cells to be >20% of total marrow nucleated cells.

4. Patients may be taking corticosteroids or a variety of cytotoxic agents.

5. Renal impairment occurs in 50% of patients during the course of the disease, secondary to difficulties in salt and water conservation, to hypercalcaemia or to renal amyloid. Hydration and chemotherapy may reverse this (Alexanian et al 1990).

Anaesthetic problems

1. Bone involvement may result in rib fracture or vertebral collapse either spontaneously or with relatively minor trauma.

2. Urgent treatment may be required for spinal cord compression, hyperviscosity, or hypercalcaemia, all of which may be life-threatening. Hypercalcaemia, which results from widespread bone disease, is present in about 30% of cases and may be associated with severe dehydration.

3. Renal impairment occurs in almost half of the cases, and actual renal failure in 25% (McIntyre 1980).

4. There is an increased susceptibility to infection as a result of impairment of the normal production of IgG.

5. Thrombocytopenia or coagulation defects occasionally occur.

6. Hyperviscosity may produce vascular and CNS problems, which include headaches, visual disturbances and retinopathy (McIntyre 1980).

7. A high-output cardiac state may occur and result in cardiac failure (McBride et al 1990). Its occurrence was shown in eight out of 36 patients, and was thought to be related to extensive bone disease.

Management

1. Hb, WCC and platelets should be checked. Coagulation screening tests should be performed if there is any suggestion of abnormal bleeding.

2. Dehydration should be prevented and early renal impairment treated with a high fluid intake.

3. Hypercalcaemia >3.2 mmol/l is dangerous and requires urgent treatment. Initially this should be with intravenous saline 0.9%, 6–8

litres in the first 48 hours, which should reduce the level by 0.04 mmol/l. In patients susceptible to the effects of a fluid load, CVP monitoring may be required. Biphosphonates, given intravenously, reduce serum calcium by inhibiting bone resorption. Disodium pamidronate (as a single treatment), disodium etidronate (daily for 5 days), and sodium clodronate (daily for 5 days) are all licenced in the UK (Drugs and Therapeutics Bulletin 1990).

4. Patients should be moved and positioned particularly carefully during anaesthesia to prevent pathological fractures.

5. Regional anaesthesia should be avoided if a neuropathy or a coagulation abnormality is suspected.

6. Steroid supplements may be required.

BIBLIOGRAPHY
Alexanian R, Barlogie B, Dixon D 1990 Renal failure in multiple myeloma. Archives of Internal Medicine 150: 1693–1695
Drugs and Therapeutics Bulletin 1990 Treating cancer-associated hypercalcaemia. Drugs and Therapeutics Bulletin 28: 85–87
McBride W, Jackman J D, Grayburn PA 1990 Prevalence and clinical characteristics of a high output cardiac state in patients with multiple myeloma. American Journal of Medicine 89: 21–24.
McIntyre O R 1980 Current concepts in cancer: multiple myeloma. New England Journal of Medicine 301: 193–196
Winfield D A 1992 Multiple myeloma. British Journal of Hospital Medicine 47: 30–37

MYOGLOBINURIA
(see RHABDOMYOLYSIS)

MYXOEDEMA
(see HYPOTHYROIDISM)

MYXOMA

A benign cardiac tumour, often rapidly growing, which accounts for about one-third of primary intracardiac tumours. It occurs more frequently in females than in males, and in the age range 20–50 years. It most commonly arises in the left atrium (75%), from the rim of the fossa ovalis, and is usually pedunculated; 20–25% originate in the right atrium; the ventricle is rarely involved. Symptoms are protean and myxomas mimic other, much more common, diseases.

The tumour may cause intracardiac obstruction, valvular dysfunction or emboli of thrombus or myxomatous tissue. Syncope may occur as a result of sudden obstruction to intracardiac blood flow and its effects may be life-threatening. The advent of echocardiography has increased the number of tumours diagnosed (Sutton et al 1980).

Preoperative abnormalities

1. Increasing dyspnoea is the commonest symptom. Intracardiac obstruction may produce pulmonary oedema or right heart failure. Cardiac failure was the commonest presenting feature in one series and occurred in 24 out of 33 cases (Hanson et al 1985). Obstruction may be positional in nature and can also cause syncope or sudden death.
2. The pedunculated tumour may move through the mitral valve during diastole; thus there may be intermittent signs of mitral valve disease of sudden onset, again, sometimes positionally related.
3. Tachyarrhythmias such as atrial fibrillation may be the presenting sign.
4. Hypoxia, which may also be positional, can occur secondary to low cardiac output, a right-to-left shunt or tumour embolization.
5. Systemic embolization of myxomatous material or thrombi from tumour surface can occur, most commonly to the cerebral or coronary circulations. The diagnosis should be suspected when embolic disease occurs in young people.
6. Pulmonary hypertension may occur with left-sided lesions.
7. A small proportion of patients have systemic, constitutional symptoms such as fever, anaemia, raised ESR, and hyperglobulinaemia.
8. The possibility that myxomas produce hormones or vasoactive substances has been raised (Johns et al 1988). High levels of VIP, a potent vasodilator were found in one atrial myxoma.
9. An augmented first heart is common, and apical pansystolic and early diastolic sounds are often present. However, both auscultatory and CXR findings are, in general, unhelpful in making the diagnosis.
10. Investigations include 2-D echocardiography, which is now the investigation of choice (Fyke et al 1985), cardiac catheterization, or MRI.

Anaesthetic problems

1. Ventricular filling may be compromised by outflow obstruction. Cardiovascular collapse occurred on induction of anaesthesia in one patient who had a right atrial myxoma (Moritz & Azad 1989) and in another with a right ventricular myxoma (Lebovic et al 1991). However, even patients with large tumours may be asymptomatic. Three uneventful anaesthetics occurred in a woman subsequently found to have a large atrial myxoma (Carr et al 1988). The absence of problems was attributed to the fact that all operations had been carried out with the patient in the Trendelenberg position. However, rapid growth of a myxoma over 8 months has been shown (Roudaut et al 1987), so it might not necessarily have been present at the previous surgery.

2. Surgery may cause conduction defects, particularly complete heart block.
3. Valvular dysfunction.
4. A tachycardia in the presence of a large atrial myxoma may increase the pressure gradient across the mitral valve and also increase pulmonary artery pressure.
5. In the presence of a right atrial myxoma, pulmonary artery catheterization may be contraindicated. Tumour embolization or passage of the catheter through a right-to-left shunt may occur.
6. Supraventricular arrhythmias may occur during anaesthesia (Carr et al 1988), and have been reported in the postoperative period in up to 70% of cases.

Management

1. Diagnosis may be made with 2–D echocardiography, cardiac catheterization, or MRI.
2. If atrial fibrillation is present, the ventricular response should be controlled.
3. If there is positional dyspnoea, give oxygen.
4. The haemodynamic management depends upon the location of the tumour. In the presence of a left atrial myxoma, a tachycardia must be avoided, the rate of AF controlled, preload should be maintained, and vasodilators used cautiously (Moritz & Azad 1989). Anaesthesia for lung biopsy in the presence of a large right atrial myxoma which extended into the ventricle has been described (Kay & Koch 1989). The patient was intubated awake and the effect of IPPV tested before anaesthesia was induced. Maintenance was with ketamine, pancuronium and nitrous oxide.

BIBLIOGRAPHY
Carr C M E, Waller D A, Ettles D F 1988 Repeated general anaesthetics in the presence of a large undiagnosed left atrial myxoma. Anaesthesia 43: 1058
Fyke F E, Sward J B, Edwards W D et al 1985 Primary cardiac tumors: experience with 30 consecutive patients since introduction of two-dimensional echocardiography. Journal of the American College of Cardiology 5: 1465–1473
Hanson E C, Gill C C, Razavi M et al 1985 The surgical treatrnent of atrial myxomas. Journal of Thoracic and Cardiovascular Surgery 89: 298–303
Griffiths B 1987 Cardiac myxomas. Hospital Update 13: 280–294
Johns R A, Kron O L, Carey R M et al 1988 Atrial myxoma: case report, brief review, and recommendations for anesthestic management. Journal of Cardiothoracic Anesthesia 2: 207–212
Kay J, Koch J-P 1989 Anesthesia for open lung biopsy in a patient with intracardiac turnour. Anesthesiology 71: 607–610
Lebovic S, Koorn R, Reich D L 1991 Role of two-dimensional transoesophageal echocardiography in the management of a right ventricular tumour. Canadian Journal of Anaesthesia 38: 1050–1054
Moritz H A, Azad S S 1989 Right atrial myxoma: case report and anaesthetic considerations. Canadian Journal of Anaesthesia 36: 212–214
Roudaut R, Gosse P, Dallocchio M 1987 Rapid growth of a left atrial myxoma shown by echocardiography. British Heart Journal 58: 413–416

Sutton M G St J, Mercier L A, Guiliani E R et al 1980 Atrial myxomas. A review of clinical experience in 40 cases. Mayo Clinic Proceedings 55: 371–376

NEMALINE ROD MYOPATHY

An autosomal dominant congenital myopathy associated with the presence in skeletal muscle of rod-like structures composed, in part, of alpha-actinin. Recent linkage studies have assigned the gene for nemaline rod myopathy to chromosome 1 (Laing et al 1992). The condition affects all skeletal muscle, including the diaphragm.

Preoperative abnormalities

1. Weakness and hypotonia presenting in early childhood.
2. Swallowing difficulty, aspiration of food and weakness of respiratory muscles.
3. Skeletal abnormalities, including scoliosis, dislocation of the hip, pes cavus and pectus excavatum.
4. Micrognathia, hypertelorism and high arched palate.
5. Cardiac abnormalities, including septal defects, aortic regurgitation and patent ductus arteriosus.
6. Increased serum CK, aldolase and LDH levels.

Anaesthetic problems

1. Possible difficulties in tracheal intubation.
2. Patients are prone to pulmonary aspiration.
3. Recurrent respiratory tract infections and poor pulmonary reserve. Lung complications are the most frequent cause of death.
4. Bradycardias on tracheal intubation were reported in three patients undergoing cardiac surgery (Asai et al 1992). Mild temperature increases were also reported.
5. Abnormal resistance to suxamethonium has been demonstrated on a chart recorder, although there was no difficulty with tracheal intubation (Heard & Kaplan 1983).

Management

1. It has been suggested that neuromuscular blocking agents should be avoided if possible (Cunliffe & Burrows 1985). However, their uneventful use has been reported (Heard & Kaplan 1983, Asai et al 1992).
2. Atropine should be immediately available to treat bradycardias.
3. After major surgery, particularly for cardiac lesion, postoperative IPPV may be required. Chest infections should be treated vigorously.

BIBLIOGRAPHY
Asai T, Fujise K, Uchida M 1992 Anaesthesia for cardiac surgery in children with
    nemaline myopathy. Anaesthesia 47: 405–408
Cunliffe M, Burrows F A 1985 Anaesthetic implications of nemaline rod myopathy.
    Canadian Anaesthetists' Society Journal 32: 543–547
Heard S O, Kaplan R F 1983 Neuromuscular blockade in a patient with nemaline
    myopathy. Anesthesiology 59: 588–590
Laing N G, Majda B T, Akkari P A et al 1992 Assignment of a gene (NEMI) for
    autosomal dominant nemaline myopathy to chromosome 1. American Journal of
    Human Genetics 50: 576–583

NEUROFIBROMATOSIS

A term for at least two separate autosomal dominant inherited
conditions associated with the occurrence of neurofibromas, but in
which there is involvement of genes on different chromosomes;
neurofibromatosis 1 (NF-1, formerly known as von Recklinghausen's
disease), which accounts for 90% of cases, and neurofibromatosis-2.
There are now strict criteria for the diagnosis of each, and this is
important because of the differences in prognosis (Mulvihill et al 1990,
Riccardi 1991).

Neurofibromas may occur anywhere in the body and can cause a
variety of symptoms. A wide spectrum of associated abnormalities has
been described. The conditions are progressive and the effects vary from
mild to very severe. There is an increased incidence of malignancies.
The exact aetiology of the conditions is unknown, but the abnormalities
may originate from neural crest defects.

Preoperative abnormalities

1. The major features are the café au lait spots, the peripheral
   neurofibromas and the Lisch nodules. Short stature and
   macrocephaly may also occur. There is now consensus on the
   diagnostic criteria for each condition.
2. For neurofibromatosis-1 there should be two or more of the
   following:
   a. café au lait spots, at least six, having one diameter of more than
      1.5 cm in adults, or 5 mm before puberty, should be present
   b. freckling in the inguinal or axillary regions
   c. two or more neurofibromas or one plexiform neurofibroma
   d. optic glioma
   e. two or more iris hamartomas (Lisch nodules)
   f. a distinctive osseous lesion such as sphenoid dysplasia or
      thinning of long bone cortex with or without pseudoarthrosis
   g. a first-degree relative who fulfils the same criteria for NF-1.
3. The complications of NF-1 can affect any system in the body:
   a. Nervous system. In one series, two-thirds of cases had some
      neurological involvement (Riccardi 1981). Neurofibromas may

appear in the vertebral foramina and cause dumb-bell tumours. Cerebral tumours such as optic path gliomas and meningiomas occur in 5–15% of patients with NF-1. There is some intellectual impairment in 40% of cases, 2–5% of patients have frank mental retardation, and epilepsy is common. MRI is now used for localizing nervous system lesions.

b. Pulmonary. An associated fibrosing alveolitis may occur in up to 20% of cases.

c. Skeletal. Kyphoscoliosis develops in 2% patients and bone sarcoma can occur. Pseudoarthrosis of the tibia and fibula.

d. Endocrine. Phaeochromocytomas are present in 1–2% of patients and medullary thyroid carcinomas have been described.

e. Renal. There may be renal artery stenosis and hypertension.

f. Airway. Oral and upper airway tumours have been reported.

4. For neurofibromatosis-2 there are:

a. bilateral VIIIth nerve masses on imaging, or

b. a first degree relative with the condition and either a unilateral VIIIth nerve mass, or

c. two of the following: neurofibroma, meningioma, glioma, schwannoma or acoustic neuromas, a juvenile posterior subcapsular lens opacity.

5. The complications of NF-2 depend on the progression of the acoustic neuroma. In a rapidly progressive lesion, deafness may proceed to cerebellar ataxia, visual disturbances, and eventually death from brain stem compression

Anaesthetic problems

1. Airway difficulties can occur with neurofibromas in the upper respiratory tract. A laryngeal tumour caused these during laryngoscopy in a 13-year-old boy (Fisher 1975). Such tumours are very rare. Emergency cricothyroidotomy had to be performed in one patient, whose lungs could not be ventilated after induction of anaesthesia for, stabilisation of a mandibular fracture (Crozier 1987). Subsequently a large neurofibroma of the tongue was removed. Oral lesions are said to be present in 5% of cases (Baden et al 1955, Gutteridge 1991).

2. Difficulty in performing regional anaesthesia, thought to be due to the presence of a neurofibroma in the needle path, has been reported (Fisher 1975).

3. If kyphoscoliosis and pulmonary disease coexist, they may contribute to postoperative respiratory complications.

4. There is 10-fold greater incidence of phaeochromocytoma than in the normal population, so signs of this should be sought, particularly if hypertension is also present (Kallf et al 1982). In a study of 18 patients with both conditions, all phaeochromocytomas were associated with the adrenal glands, and each secreted both

adrenaline and noradrenaline. Convulsions, cardiovascular collapse and death occurred in late pregnancy in a patient with neurofibromatosis who, at autopsy, was found to have a phaeochromocytoma (Harper et al 1989).

5. Pregnancy is likely to be complicated by hypertensive disorders, and fetal outcome is poor (Sharma et al 1991).

6. A small number of patients have been reported to have prolonged neuromuscular blockade in response to neuromuscular blocking agents (Nagao et al 1983, Baraka 1974). However, normal responses have also been shown (McCarthy et al 1990).

Management

1. Careful preoperarive assessment is essential, with particular attention being paid to mouth and airway lesions, chest, and neurological complications.

2. If there is hypertension and phaeochromocytoma is suspected, urinary catecholamine estimation should be performed.

3. Neuromuscular monitoring is essential.

BIBLIOGRAPHY

Baraka A 1974 Myasthenic response to muscle relaxants in von Recklinghausen's disease. British Journal of Anaesthesia 46: 701–703

Baden E, Pierce H E, Jackson W F 1955 Multiple neurofibromatosis with oral lesions; review of the literature. Oral Surgery 8: 263–280

Crozier W C 1987 Upper airway obstruction in neurofibromatosis. Anaesthesia 42: 1209–1211

Fisher M McD 1975 Anaesthetic difficulties in neurofibromatosis. Anaesthesia 30: 648–650

Gutteridge D L 1991 Neurofibromatosis: an unusual oral manifestation. British Dental Journal 170: 303–304

Harper M A, Murnaghan G A, Kennedy L et al 1989 Phaeochromocytoma in pregnancy. Five cases and a review of the literature. British Journal of Obstetrics and Gynaecology 96: 594–606

Kalff V, Shapiro B, Lloyd R 1982 The spectrum of phaeochromocytoma in hypertensive patients with neurofibromatosis. Archives of Internal Medicine 142: 2092–2098

McCarthy G J, McLoughlin C, Mirakhur R K 1990 Neuromuscular blockade in von Recklinghausen's disease. Anaesthesia 45: 340–341

Mulvihill J J, Parry D M, Sherman J L et al 1990 NIH conference. Neurofibromatosis 1 (Recklinghausen disease) and neurofibrormatosis 2 (bilateral acoustic neurofibromatosis). An update. Annals of Internal Medicine 113: 39–52

Nagao H, Yamashita M, Shinozaki Y et al 1983 Hypersensitivity to pancuronium in a patient with von Recklinghausen's disease. British Journal of Anaesthesia 55: 253

Riccardi V M 1981 Von Recklinghausen neurofibromatosis. New England Journal of Medicine 305: 1617–1627

Riccardi V M 1991 Neurofibromatosis: past, present and future. New England Journal of Medicine 324: 1283–1285

Sharma J B, Gulati N, Malik S 1991 Maternal and perinatal complications in neurofibromatosis during pregnancy. Internal Journal of Gynaecology and Obstetrics 34: 221–227

NEUROGENIC PULMONARY OEDEMA
(SEE PULMONARY OEDEMA)

NEUROLEPTIC MALIGNANT SYNDROME
(NMS)

A rare but serious, idiosyncratic complication of treatment with
neuroleptic drugs, characterized by the development of catatonic,
extrapyramidal, and autonomic effects. Its aetiology is unknown, but
appears to be related to the antidopaminergic activity of the precipitating
drug on dopamine receptors in the striatum and hypothalamus. Its
occurrence in a patient after a tricyclic antidepressant has led to the
suggestion that the syndrome involves a central imbalance between
noradrenaline and dopamine, rather than dopamine depletion alone
(Baca & Martinelli 1990). Brain-damaged individuals are thought to be
more susceptible to NMS (Turk & Lask 1991). Its occurrence in
Parkinsonian patients after L-dopa withdrawal (Gibb 1988), and its
spontaneous appearance in a patient with Hallervorden–Spatz disease
(Hayashi et al 1993), both of which disorders involve the striatonigral
systems of the basal ganglia, is of interest.

Clinical features include hyperthermia, muscle rigidity, sympathetic
overactivity and a variable conscious level. A mortality of 20% has been
reported (Caroff et al 1983). The concept that NMS is related to
anaesthetic-induced malignant hyperthermia is supported in some
quarters (Caroff et al 1983, Denborough et al 1985), but others suggest
that, despite the superficial clinical similarities, MN and NMS are two
distinct and unrelated entities. When the criteria of the European MH
Group for muscle testing were applied to six NMS survivors, five were
found to be normal and one was equivocal (Krivosic-Horber et al 1987).
In addition, a retrospective study of 20 patients with NMS suggested no
cross vulnerability (Hermesh et al 1989).

Presentation

1. Haloperidol and fluphenazine are the drugs most frequently
   reported as being associated with NMS (Szabadi 1984). Others
   include chlorpromazine, trifluoperazine, droperidol, thioridazine,
   thiapride and metoclopramide. In most cases, these drugs have been
   given for a variety of psychiatric disorders. NMS has also occurred
   with tetrabenazine, desipramine, a tricyclic antidepressant, and after
   stopping treatment with levodopa in a patient with striatonigral
   degeneration (Gibb 1988). The condition may occur within hours of
   starting the drug, or after some months of treatment. Concurrent
   lithium therapy may facilitate its development. The episode may
   occur after normal doses, but sometimes after an overdose of the

drug. A probable case has been described which was associated with anaesthesia, in a young man given normal doses of droperidol and metoclopramide (Patel & Bristow 1987). Another patient developed NMS while receiving chlorpromazine suppositories when he was undergoing IPPV on the ITU (Montgomery & Ironside 1990). A schizophrenic who took an overdose of perphenazine and cyclizine was admitted with hyperthermia, thrombocytopenia, disseminated intravascular coagulation and rhabdomyolysis, which rapidly progressed to renal failure and death (Lenler-Petersen et al 1990).

2. Clinical features include catatonia, hyperthermia, sweating, stupor, tremor, muscle rigidity, akinesia, autonomic dysfunction, incontinence and renal failure.

3. Rhabdomyolysis may occur. The serum CK is usually increased and levels in excess of 10 000 iu/l have been reported. LFTs may be abnormal and leucocytosis often occurs.

4. In the cases in which muscle biopsy has been performed, areas of necrosis and hypercontraction have been seen, but with muscle fibres of normal size and normal fibre type distribution (Montgomery & Ironside 1990).

Management

1. The relevant medication is discontinued.

2. The patient is cooled.

3. The role of specific drugs in the management is controversial. There have been a large number of individual case reports advocating the use of dantrolene sodium and bromocriptine to accelerate recovery. Dantrolene sodium, 50 mg q.d.s. for 5 days and bromocriptine mesylate, 5 mg t.d.s. increasing to 10 mg t.d.s., are typical regimens recommended to treat NMS (Mueller et al 1983). However, there have been dissenting voices. Rosebush et al (1991) claimed that there was no evidence that dantrolene and bromocriptine were useful, and even suggested that they might prolong the course of the illness and increase the likelihood of sequelae. They prospectively studied 20 patients with their first episode of NMS, some of whom were treated with dantrolene, bromocriptine, or both. However, the treatments were not randomized and depended on the individual physician's familiarity with the literature. Resolution of the issue must await a properly controlled trial.

4. In severe cases, IPPV, fluid replacement, and intensive care facilities will be required.

5. Whether or not a survivor of NMS who requires an anaesthetic should be treated as MH-susceptible is arguable. Two papers have reported positive MH testing in NMS survivors (Denborough et al 1985, Caroff et al 1987), whereas two others could not confirm any

association between the two conditions (Krivosic-Horber et al 1987 Hermesh et al 1989).

BIBLIOGRAPHY

Baca L, Martinelli L 1990 Neuroleptic malignant syndrome: a unique association with a tricyclic antidepressant. Neurology 40: 1797–1798

Caroff S, Rosenberg H, Gerber J C 1983 Neuroleptic malignant syndrome and malignant hyperpyrexia. Lancet i: 244

Caroff S N, Rosenberg H, Fletcher J E et al 1987 Malignant hyperthermia susceptibility in neuroleptic malignant syndrome. Anesthesiology 67: 20–25

Denborough M A, Collins S P, Hopkinson K C 1985 Rhabdomyolysis and malignant hyperpyrexia. British Medical Journal 288: 1878–1879

Gibb W R G 1988 Neuroleptic malignant syndrome in striatonigral degeneration. British Journal of Psychiatry 153: 254–255

Hayashi K, Chihara E, Sawa T et al 1993 Clinical features of neuroleptic syndrome in basal ganglia disease. Spontaneous presentation in a patient with Hallervorden-Spatz syndrome in the absence of neuroleptic drugs. Anaesthesia 48: 499–502

Hermesh H, Aizenberg D, Lapidot M et al 1989 The relationship between malignant hyperthermia and neuroleptic malignant syndrome. Anesthesiology 70: 171

Krivosic-Horber R, Adnet P, Guevart E et al 1987 Neuroleptic malignant syndrome and malignant hypertherrnia. British Journal of Anaesthesia 59: 1554–1556

Lenler-Petersen P, Hansen B D, Hasselstrom L 1990 A rapidly progressing case of neuroleptic malignant syndrome. Intensive Care Medicine 16: 267–268

Montgomery J N, Ironside J W 1990 Neuroleptic malignant syndrome in the intensive care unit. Anaesthesia 45: 311–313

Mueller P S, Vester J W, Fermaglich J 1983 Neuroleptic malignant syndrome: successful treatment with bromocriptine. Journal of the American Medical Association 249: 386–388

Patel P, Bristow G 1987 Postoperative neuroleptic malignant syndrome. A case report. Canadian Journal of Anaesthesia 34: 515–518

Rosebush P I, Stewart T, Mazurek M F 1991 The treatment of neuroleptic malignant syndrome. Are dantrolene and bromocriptine useful adjuncts to supportive care? British Journal of Psychiatry 159: 709–712

Szabadi E 1984 Neuroleptic malignant syndrome. British Medical Journal 288: 1399–1400

Turk J, Lask B 1991 Neuroleptic malignant syndrome. Archives of Disease in Childhood 66: 91–92

NOONAN'S SYNDROME

A hereditary condition inherited as autosomal dominant, which is similar to Turner's syndrome, except that it affects both males and females and chromosornes are normal (Editorial 1992). It is associated with characteristic facial features. The child is usually mentally retarded and under height and weight for age. Right-sided cardiac lesions predominate, most commonly pulmonary stenosis with or without septal defects, and some patients have a hypertrophic cardiomyopathy. Musculoskeletal abnormalities are common and there is abnormal bleeding, especially in childhood. Undescended testis occurs in 77% of males. Anaesthesia may be required for orchidopexy, orthopaedic abnormalities, cardiac investigation, or corrective cardiac surgery.

Preoperative abnormalities

1. Facial features include hypertelorism, high-arched eyebrows, downward slanting palpebral fissures and low-set ears. Severe ptosis is present in 42%, webbing of the neck in 23% and dental malocclusion is common.
2. Cardiac abnormalities. In a recent study of 151 cases (Sharland et al 1992a), only 12.5% had normal echocardiographic findings. Sixty two per cent had pulmonary stenosis, which was sometimes associated with septal defects. A hypertrophic obstructive cardiomyopathy was present in 20% in this particular series, but others quote higher percentages of cardiac muscle abnormalities; however, the cardiomyopathy is not always obstructive or symptomatic.
3. Hepatosplenomegaly is present in 50% and undescended testis occurs in 77% of males.
4. Musculoskeletal abnormalities are common. There is short stature and short neck with webbing. Sternal defects occur, with pectus excavatus inferiorly, and pectus carinatus superiorly. There may be a narrow spinal canal, a lumbar lordosis and kyphoscoliosis. General hypotonia is present, with abnormal joint hyperextensibility.
5. Although fertility in females is normal, males frequently do not reproduce. This may be because of the high incidence of cryptorchism and the greater severity of the cardiac lesions, which may determine survival to adulthood (Collins & Turner 1973).

Anaesthetic problems

1. Webbed neck, micrognathia, high-arched palate, and dental malocclusion may contribute to intubation difficulties (Schwartz & Eisenkraft 1992).
2. Problems of anaesthesia in the presence of cardiac disease (Schwartz & Eisenkraft 1992, Campbell & Bousfield 1992).
3. A history of easy bruising and bleeding has been elicited from 65% of 72 patients with Noonan's syndrome, and 50% had specific abnormalities of the intrinsic coagulation pathway (partial factor XI:C, XII:C and VIII:C). However, there was a lack of correlation between the history of bleeding and the coagulation abnormalities, which makes prediction of bleeding in any individual patient difficult (Sharland et al 1992b). The possibility of impairment of platelet activation or aggregation has been suggested (Emmerich et al 1992).
4. If spinal canal stenosis is a feature, care should be taken when performing regional anaesthetic techniques.

Management

1. Cardiovascular assessment to determine the extent of any cardiac lesions.
2. Evaluation of airway and anticipation of difficult intubation. Cervical spine X-rays may be required if neck movements are a problem (Schwartz & Eisenkraft 1992).
3. Management of hypertrophic cardiomyopathy if present (see Cardiomyopathy). In such patients, outlet obstruction is worsened by tachycardia, increased contractility, arterial vasodilatation and decreased pre-load. Anaesthetic management should be directed towards minimizing these (Campbell & Bousfield 1992). A child with hypertrophic cardiomyopathy was treated with an esmolol infusion, a preinduction fluid load, inhalational induction with halothane, and intubation under deep anaesthesia (Schwartz & Eisenkraft 1992).
4. Management for Caesarean section under extradural anaesthesia has been described (Dadabhoy & Winnie 1988).

BIBLIOGRAPHY

Campbell A M, Bousfield J D 1992 Anaesthesia in a patient with Noonan's syndrome and cardiomyopathy. Anaesthesia 47: 131–133

Collins E, Turner G 1973 The Noonan syndrome – a review of the clinical and genetic features of 27 cases. Journal of Pediatrics 83: 941–950

Dadabhoy Z P Winnie A P 1988 Regional anesthesia for cesarean section in a parturient with Noonan's syndrome. Anesthesiology 68: 636–638

Editorial 1992 Noonan's syndrome. Lancet 340: 22–23

Emmerich J, Aiach M, Capron L et al 1992 Noonan's syndrome and coagulation factor deficiencies. Lancet 339: 431

Sharland M, Burch M, McKenna W M et al 1992a A clinical study of Noonan's syndrome. Archives of Diseases in Childhood 67: 178–183

Sharland M, Patton M A, Talbot S et al 1992b Coagulation-factor deficiencies and abnormal bleeding in Noonan's syndrome. Lancet 339: 19–21

Schwartz N, Eisenkraft J B 1992 Anesthetic management of a child with Noonan's syndrome and idiopathic hypertrophic subaortic stenosis. Anesthesia and Analgesia 74: 464–466

OBESITY

Morbid obesity has been defined as occurring when a subject's weight is more than 70% greater than the ideal weight for his or her age and height. Insurance statistics show a greatly increased mortality rate for such patients, and surgery and anaesthesia carry a number of risks. In addition to incidental procedures, the obese patient may be subjected to weight-reducing intestinal bypass operations, particularly in North America. A number of studies have been undertaken to identify the problems and determine the best method of anaesthesia.

Preoperative abnormalities

1. **Respiratory.** FRC is reduced, mainly due to a decrease in expiratory reserve volume. Tidal ventilation occurs below the closing volume, particularly in the supine position. The Pao_2 may be reduced, and the work and oxygen cost of respiration are increased.
2. **Cardiovascular.** An increased incidence of hypertension and coronary artery disease.
3. Increased glucose intolerance and diabetes.
4. The Pickwickian syndrome, characterized by hypoventilation, somnolence, cor pulmonale and hypoxia, is rare.

Anaesthetic problems

1. Difficulties with venous access.
2. Mechanical problems resulting from the size and weight of the patient.
3. Difficulties in locating the extradural or subarachnoid spaces. Standard length needles may be too short.
4. There is a more extensive spread of local anaesthetic solutions in the subarachnoid space when compared with patients of normal weight (Taivainen et al 1990).
5. Tracheal intubation problems. Obesity is a significant risk factor, particularly in obstetric anaesthesia (Rocke et al 1992).
6. Cyanosis occurs rapidly, especially in the supine position, due to a reduced FRC. The tidal volume may approach or fall within the closing volume. There is a 50% reduction in FRC at the onset of anaesthesia (Damia et al 1988). Apnoea is associated with an increased risk of hypoxia (Jense et al 1991), the effectiveness of preoxygenation is considerably reduced and desaturation may occur before tracheal intubation has been achieved (Berthoud et al 1991).
7. Rapid dehydration and poor tolerance of hypovolaemia results from a reduced blood volume per unit weight.
8. Reliable indirect blood pressure monitoring is difficult to achieve.
9. Difficulties in maintaining an airway during mask anaesthesia.
10. Problems with intraoperative oxygenation during abdominal surgery, particularly when in the head-down position, or when intra-abdominal packs are in place.
11. For the first 48 postoperative hours, the supine position is associated with a significant decrease in Pao_2 Vaughan et al 1976).
12. Sensitivity to postoperative analgesia may occur. Respiratory failure occurred after nephrectomy in an obese patient who was receiving patient-controlled analgesia together with a background infusion of morphine (VanDercar et al 1991). Following episodes of obstructive apnoea, periods of hyperpnoea associated with arousal were interpreted by the nursing staff as pain, and supplementary analgesia was given.

13. Increased incidence of postoperative respiratory problems.
14. Venous thrombosis and pulmonary embolism.
15. An increased risk of wound infection (8–28%).

Management

1. Detailed cardiovascular and respiratory assessment is required. If there is pre-existing hypoxia or hypercarbia, then some weight loss is advisable before elective surgery. Mandibular wiring has been suggested as an aid for this, before abdominal weight-reducing surgery.
2. If intubation difficulties are anticipated, awake intubation may be advisable. The incidence of difficult intubation under general anaesthesia lies between 6 and 13%. Even if difficulties are not anticipated, the ineffectiveness of preoxygenation may be another indication for awake intubation (Berthoud et al 1991). Little difference was found between preoxygenation with 3 minutes of 100% oxygen or 4 vital capacity breaths of 100% oxygen (Goldberg et al 1989). With the former technique, slight carbon dioxide retention was found.
3. Thoracic extradural anaesthesia has been recommended as an adjunct to general anaesthesia. The rationale is that, as a consequence of the block, only light general anaesthesia is required, good postoperative pain relief is provided, and early extubation and mobilization are permitted. Extradural analgesia was given to 70 patients in a series of 110 undergoing weight-reducing surgery (Fox et al 1981). There was an incidence of postoperative lung collapse of 18.5% in these patients, compared with 27.5% for those only receiving pethidine i.m.. However, there was a suggestion that pulmonary emboli might be slightly more common in the extradural group.

   Others do not consider that extradural analgesia offers significant advantages. Thoracic extradurals are technically difficult to perform in the grossly obese patient and there was a 20% failure rate in one series (Buckley et al 1983). Some improvement in cardiovascular function, as evidenced by a decrease in left ventricular stroke volume and myocardial oxygen requirement, was reported in patients with a thoracic extradural block and general anaesthesia, when compared with opiates and general anaesthesia (Gelman et al 1980). However it was found to be no better than i.v. morphine in terms of postoperative pain relief, vital capacity and gas exchange. A lesser number of pulmonary complications was experienced with extradural analgesia, but a greater incidence of intraoperative hypotension and bradycardia (Buckley et al 1983).

   Care must be taken to avoid giving an excessive volume of local anaesthetic to the morbidly obese. The reduced dose of bupivacaine required for extradural anaesthesia in obese pregnant patients

(Hodgkinson & Husain 1980) has been confirmed by others (Buckley et al 1983). This is probably as a result of venous engorgement in the extradural space.

4. The use of antacids and H2 receptor antagonists as a precaution against acid aspiration syndrome is recommended.

5. A comparison of adjuvants with IPPV were made in 67 patients for gastric stapling (Cork et al 1981). There was no difference between halothane, enflurane or fentanyl in terms of early postoperative recovery. However, the use of isoflurane, which is the least metabolized, would seem rational. The use of a ketamine infusion as sole anaesthetic for gastroplasty in 19 out of 24 patients has been reported (Strong et al 1989). After induction with ketamine 1 mg/kg, an infusion of 20–60 μg/kg per min was maintained.

6. During abdominal surgery, frequent blood gas sampling is advisable and an increased inspired oxygen concentration is required when the head-down position is employed. The use of subdiaphragmatic intra-abdominal packs may produce severe hypoxia and should be avoided if possible. Oxygenation in otherwise healthy obese subjects having abdominal surgery was studied (Vaughan & Wise 1976). Fourteen per cent of patients in the supine position, and 77% with a 15° head-down tilt, had a Pao_2 of <10.6 kPa 40% oxygen. In 23% of those in the latter group, the Pao_2 decreased to <8.0 kPa. Four patients in whom subdiaphragmatic packs were used all had a Pao_2 of <8.6 kPa.

7. Whilst patient-controlled analgesia may be valuable in the obese, the avoidance of a background infusion, the use of smaller bolus doses and the setting of 4-hourly dose limits would seem to be wise precautions (Levin et al 1992).

BIBLIOGRAPHY

Berthoud M C, Peacock JE, Reilly CS 1991 Effectiveness of preoxygenation in morbidly obese patients. British Journal of Anaesthesia 67: 464–466

Buckley F P Robinson N B, Simonowitz D A et al 1983 Anaesthesia in the morbidly obese. Anaesthesia 38: 840–851

Cork R C, Vaughan R W, Bentley J B 1981 General anesthesia for morbidly obese patients: an examination of postoperative outcomes. Anesthesiology 54: 310–313

Damia G, Mascheroni D, Croci M et al 1988 Perioperative changes in functional residual capacity in morbidly obese patients. British Journal of Anaesthesia 60: 574–578

Fisher A, Waterhouse T D, Adams A P 1975 Obesity: its relation to anaesthesia. Anaesthesia 30: 633–647

Fox G S, Whalley D G, Bevan D R 1981 Anaesthesia for the morbidly obese, experience with 110 patients. British Journal of Anaesthesia 53: 811–816

Gelman S, Laws H L, Potzick J et al 1980 Thoracic epidural versus balanced anesthesia in morbid obesity. An intraoperative and postoperative hernodynamic study. Anesthesia and Analgesia 59: 902–908

Goldberg M E, Norris M C, Larijani G E et al 1989 Preoxygenation in the morbidly obese: a comparison of two techniques. Anesthesia and Analgesia 68: 520–522

Hodgkinson R, Husain F J 1980 Obesity and the cephalad spread of analgesia following epidural administration of bupivacaine for Cesarean section. Anesthesia and Analgesia 59: 89–92

Jense H G, Dubin S A, Silverstein P I et al 1991 Effect of obesity on safe duration of apnoea in anaesthetized humans. Anesthesia and Analgesia 72: 89–93

Levin A, Klein S L, Brolin R E et al 1992 Patient-controlled analgesia for morbidly obese patients: an effective modality if used correctly. Anesthesiology 76: 857–858

Rocke D A, Murray W B, Rout C C et al 1992 Relative risk analysis of factors associated with difficult intubation in obstetric anesthesia. Anesthesiology 77: 67–73

Strong W E, Rubin A S, Reynolds W J et al 1989 Ketamine infusion: an alternative anesthetic technique. Anesthesia and Analgesia 68: S282

Taivainen T, Tuominen M, Rosenberg P H 1990 Influence of obesity on the spread of spinal analgesia after injection of plain 0.5% bupivacaine at the L3–4 or L 4–5 interspace. British Journal of Anaesthesia 64: 542–546

Vaughan R W, Bauer S, Wise L 1976 Effect of position (semirecumbent versus supine) on postoperative oxygenation in markedly obese subjects. Anesthesia and Analgesia 55: 37–41

Vaughan R W, Wise L 1976 Intraoperative arterial oxygenation in obese patients. Annals of Surgery 184: 35–42

VanDercar D H, Martinez A P, DeLisser E A 1991 Sleep apnea syndromes: a potential contraindication for patient-controlled analgesia. Anesthesiology 74: 623–624

OBSTRUCTIVE SLEEP APNOEA

A term used for recurrent hypoxaemic respiratory disturbances during sleep which result from varying combinations of anatomical airway obstruction, functional control of airway musculature, and central apnoea. A variety of definitions have been used. One definition of obstructive sleep apnoea (OSA) is a 10-second pause in respiration during sleep. The sleep apnoea syndrome is said to occur when more than 30 of these episodes occur during 7 hours of sleep (Hanning 1989), or more than 10 episodes in each hour (Hoffstein & Zamel 1990).

It is a common condition, although frequently undiagnosed, and up to 2% of the adult population may be affected. The multiplicity of contributing factors presumably accounts for the fact that OSA has been associated with a wide variety of conditions.

Contributing factors

1. The area of the pharynx is reduced compared with that of normal individuals. Increased adipose tissue, thickened pharyngeal mucosa, large tonsils and adenoids and mandibular hypoplasia may all contribute. The small pharyngeal space in the awake patient is reduced even further during sleep and in the supine posture. Thus, in the anaesthetized patient total obstruction often occurs.
   Obstruction in the supine posture is also related to FRC. The actual site of obstruction may vary (see Pierre Robin syndrome) and can be single or multiple. The pharynx is the commonest site and the larynx is the least common (Wilms et al 1982).
2. Impairment of muscle function. Muscular function depends on neurological control and coordination, particularly of the genioglossus, geniohyoid and tensor palati muscles. The pharynx

has a tendency to collapse and this is associated with a decrease in activity of the pharyngeal muscles. During inspiration the subatmospheric pressure may abolish muscle splinting, so that the pharynx is obliterated. There is also a lack of coordination between the pharyngeal and thoracic muscles and an associated reduction in FRC.

3. Central control. Obstructive sleep apnoea is made worse by diseases in which there is CNS involvement.

Preoperative abnormalities

1. Snoring, vividly described by the patient's partner, obesity, nocturnal sleep disturbance and often excessive daytime sleepiness.
2. Decreased nocturnal, and sometimes diurnal, saturation and secondary polycythaemia (Messinezy et al 1991).
3. Diagnosis can be made by polysomnography and continuous oxygen saturation measurements.
4. An increased neck circumference has been found in patients with OSA compared with non-apnoeic, snoring controls (Katz et al 1990). Increased mass loading of the upper airway was thought to contribute to the pathogenesis of the condition.
5. Systemic and pulmonary hypertension. There is an increased incidence of OSA in the hypertensive population.
6. Cardiac arrhythmias can be a feature.

Anaesthetic problems

1. Periods of apnoea and desaturation during normal sleep, which are worse and more frequent in the postoperative period. Such episodes are increased in incidence and severity during REM sleep. REM sleep is almost completely abolished for the first 1–3 days after surgery but a rebound occurs on night 5 following surgery (Knill et al 1990). Physiological accompaniments of REM sleep are episodic breathing disturbances, with hypoxia and fluctuations in heart rate and blood pressure. These factors may account for delayed cardiovascular and cerebrovascular complications following surgery. During such episodes, oxygen saturation may decrease to below 50%. In one patient, even before surgery, 33 minutes of the night were spent with oxygen saturations of less than 85% (Reeder et al 1991). Subsequent computer studies of his postoperative nights showed three types of respiratory events, each ranging in duration from 10–30 seconds. 'Obstructive', 'mixed' (cycles beginning with central apnoea, then obstruction with increasing respiratory effort, and finally sudden awakening) and 'apnoeic'. The last event was the least common. Patients having nasal surgery followed by nasal packing are particularly at risk from these problems (Tierney et al 1989).

2. Periodic fluctuations in heart rate and blood pressure associated with episodes of obstruction and the resultant major swings in intrathoracic pressure (Reeder et al 1991). The obstructive phase was associated with decrease in systemic pressure, whereas hypertension tended to be associated with arousal and relief of obstruction.

3. Sensitivity to postoperative analgesia may occur. Respiratory failure occurred after nephrectomy in an obese patient who was receiving a combination of PCA and a background infusion of morphine (VanDercar et al 1991). Nursing staff tend to interpret periods of hyperpnoea, associated with arousal and relief of obstruction, as pain, and consequently give supplementary analgesia.

4. Wound healing is reduced and infection more likely when wound oxygen tension is low.

5. Patients with severe OSA may die during sleep, secondary to hypoxaemia or arrhythmias.

6. The problems of the airway do not end following surgery. Acute obstruction occurred during emergence from anaesthesia after uvulopalatopharyngoplasty (Gabrielczyk 1988). The patient pulled out his own tracheal tube while still on the operating table and divested himself of cannulae and monitoring. The ensuing hypoxia necessitated emergency tracheostomy. This episode underlines the importance of retaining key personnel and equipment close to the patient until successful extubation has been accomplished.

Management

1. Monitoring with apnoea alarms or pulse oximetry.

2. Supplementary oxygen at night, particularly in the perioperative period.

3. Treatment of the underlying cause, e.g. obesity, by weight loss. Obesity is a major contributing factor in at least 70% of patients.

4. Avoidance, or at least the cautious use, of sedatives and narcotics during the perioperative period. If PCA is used, a background continuous infusion may be unwise, unless there is continuous observation of the patient at the same time.

5. Local anaesthetic blocks may help to reduce the need for opioid analgesics, but are more difficult to perform and may have a higher complication rate in the obese.

6. Nasal continuous positive airway pressure (CPAP) given by nasal mask abolished obstructive episodes and decreased blood pressure postoperatively in a surgical patient in whom preoperative obstructive sleep apnoea and desaturation had been demonstrated (Reeder et al 1991). Thomas et al (1992) describe one such system. These systems can generate pressures of 2.5–20 cmH$_2$O and improve sleep disturbance, hypoxia and cardiovascular changes. The probable effect of CPAP is to open up the airway and prevent collapse, but

the positive pressure may cause reflex activation of pharyngeal muscles.

7. Nasopharyngeal airways or other mechanical devices are of limited value.

8. Surgery. Detailed discussion is beyond the scope of this book. However, if palatal surgery is considered, direct measurements of intra-airway pressure to locate the sites of obstruction beforehand are essential.

   a. Tracheostomy is effective, but limited by side effects, particularly in the obese.

   b. Minitracheotomy was used for 4 months as a temporary measure in a patient with OSA awaiting tonsillectomy (Hassan et al 1989). This allowed resolution of cor pulmonale and papilloedema, and weight loss.

   c. Uvulopalatoplasty, the commonest definitive procedure, involves removal of uvula tonsils, part of soft palate and excess pharyngeal tissue. Complications are not insignificant and at the present time the benefits are questionable.

9. Associated conditions, such as respiratory disease, obesity, heart failure and pulmonary hypertension, must be treated before surgery.

10. Drugs are of limited value, but protryptiline may reduce REM sleep in which most of the apnoeic episodes occur.

BIBLIOGRAPHY

Gabrielczyk M R 1988 Acute airway ohstruction after uvulopharyngoplasty for obstructive sleep apnea syndrome. Anesthesiology 69: 941–943

Hanning C D 1989 Obstructive sleep apnoea. British Journal of Anaesthesia 63: 477–488

Hassan A, Mcguigan J, Morgan M D L et al 1989 Minitracheotomy: a simple alternative to tracheostomy in obestrvctive sleep apnoea. Thorax 44: 224–225

Hoffstein V, Zamel N 1990 Sleep apnoea and the upper airway. British Journal of Anaesthesia 65: 139–150

Katz I, Stradling J R, Slutsky A S et al 1990 Do patients with obstructive sleep apnea have fat necks? American Review of Respiratory Disease 141: 1228–1231

Knill R L, Moote C A, Skinner M I et al 1990 Anesthesia with abdominal surgery leads to intense REM sleep during the first postoperative week. Anesthesiology 73: 52–61

Messinezy M, Aubry S, O'Connell G et al 1991 Oxygen desaturation in apparent and relative polycythaemia. British Medical Journal 302: 216–217

Rafferty T D, Ruskis A, Sasaki C et al 1980 Perioperative considerations in the management of tracheotomy for the sleep apnoea patient. British Journal of Anaesthesia 52: 619–622

Reeder M K, Goldman M D, Loh L et al 1991 Postoperative obstructive sleep apnoea. Haemodynamic effects of treatment with nasal CPAP. Anaesthesia 46: 849–853

Rosenberg J, Kehlet H 1991 Postoperative episodic oxygen desaturation in the sleep apnoea syndrome. Acta Anaesthesiologica Scandinavica 35: 368–369

Thomas A N, Ryan J P, Jaran B et al 1992 A nasal CPAP system. Description and comparison with facemask CPAP. Anaesthesia 47: 311–315.

Tierney N M, Pollard B J, Bran B R H 1989 Obstructive sleep apnoea. Anaesthesia 44: 235–237

VanDercar D H, Martinez A P, De Lisser E A 1991 Sleep apnea syndrome: a potential contraindication for patient-controlled analgesia. Anesthesiology 74: 623–624

Wilms D, Popovich J, Conway W et al 1982 Anatomic abnormalities in obstuctive
  sleep apnoea. Annals of Otology, Rhinology and Laryngology 91: 595–596

OPIATE ADDICTION

Dependence on opiates is present when a physical withdrawal state
occurs on abrupt cessation of the drug, and when tolerance to the drug
develops. Psychological dependence can also occur. The anaesthetist
may be involved, either because a dependent patient requires surgery, or
for resuscitation when accidental or deliberate overdosage occurs. The
problem may be either admitted or concealed by the patient. He may or
may not be registered as an addict. Occasionally, a cured addict may
come for surgery. Opiates should be scrupulously avoided in these
patients. Alternatives, such as continuous extradural analgesia, should be
considered for postoperative pain.

In the absence of a history of drug abuse, bizarre behaviour,
malnutrition, or social deterioration in a patient under 40, should prompt
the search for injection marks.

Preoperative abnormalities

1. Malnutrition, skin infection, superficial venous thrombosis, anaemia
   or jaundice may be present.
2. There is a high incidence of liver disease. A 10% incidence of
   hepatitis has been reported. In one study of multiple attacks, 32% of
   cases were due to HAV, 42% to HBV and 25% to NANBV (Norkrans
   et al 1980). Malnutrition may contribute to liver disease. There is a
   significant risk of transmission of hepatitis and possibly AIDS.
3. An increased risk of bacterial or fungal endocarditis, most frequently
   due to *Staphylococcus aureus*, but sometimes to pseudomonas. Arterial
   emboli, sometimes septic, can result.
4. Pulmonary infection, infarction and atelectasis are common.
   Pulmonary hypertension or oedema can occur.
5. Tetanus may be seen, in part due to additives such as quinine
   which allow the growth of anaerobes (McGoldrick 1980).
6. Acrenocortical function is suppressed.

Anaesthetic problems

1. Venous access may be difficult.
2. Problems of management of HBV- or HIV-positive patients.
3. Physical dependence and withdrawal symptoms. These include
   tachycardia, tremor, acute anxiety, sweating, piloerection, mydriasis,
   nausea, and vomiting. There is evidence to suggest that brain
   catecholamines play some part in the aetiology of this syndrome
   (McGoldrick 1980).

The time course of the individual abstinence syndromes has been described (McCammon 1986):

Drug	Onset	Peak	Duration
Pethidine	3h	8–12h	4–5 days
Morphine	8–12 h	36–48 h	7–10 days
Heroin	8–12h	36–48 h	7–10 days
Methadone	1–2 days	3–6 days	2–3 weeks

4. Tolerance to all the effects of opiates occurs. Anaesthetic techniques relying on opioids are therefore unsuitable, since very high doses will be required to suppress sympathetic responses to surgical stimulation.
5. The administration of partial or pure narcotic antagonists may precipitate a withdrawal state.
6. Hypotension may occur.
7. Problems of the pregnant opiate user who appears for care in late pregnancy (Gerada et al 1990).

Management

1. A careful history should be taken and a thorough examination made. If the patient is registered, then the drug centre or his psychiatrist should be contacted to verify details. Expert advice on management may be necessary (DHS 1991). If doubt exists, urine may be tested for the presence of drugs. Belongings should be checked for concealed drugs.
2. Patients should be presumed to be HBV- and HIV-positive unless proved otherwise.
3. Most authorities are agreed that the perioperative period is not the correct time to institute detoxification. Opiates will therefore need to be given. This may be the preparation already being used, or the equivalent dose of methadone might be substituted.
    Approximately equivalent dosages (DHSS 1984) are reported as:
    a. Methadone: 10 mg (some authorities quote 5 mg).
    b. Morphine: 10 mg.
    c. Pethidine: 100 mg.
    d. Dextromoramide: 5 mg.
    e. Heroin: 10 mg.
    f. Dipipanone: 20 mg.
    g. Buprenorphine: 0.8 mg.
    h. Pentazocine: 125 mg.

    If genuine organic pain does exist then, as a result of tolerance, higher than normal doses of opiates will be required.
4. If there is venous thrombosis, internal jugular or subclavian venous cannulation, or a venous cutdown, may be required.

5. Partial opiate antagonists such as pentazocine, or pure antagonists such as naloxone, may produce severe withdrawal symptoms and should not be used.

6. The use of other drugs with addictive potential, such as the benzodiazepines, should be avoided.

7. Hypotension has been described preoperatively in opiate addicts. When it occurs during surgery, responses to various forms of treatment including opiates, fluids, vasoconstrictors or hydrocortisone have been reported.

8. For labour, there is little evidence that opiates are harmful to the fetus already exposed to opiates during pregnancy, and respiratory depression is thought not to be a feature. There is no contraindication to extradural analgesia.

BIBLIOGRAPHY

Caldwell T B 1990 Anesthesia for patients with behavioral and environmental disorders. In: Katz J, Benumof J, Kadis L (eds) Anesthesia and uncommon diseases. WB Saunders, Philadelphia

DHSS 1984 Guidelines of good clinical practice in the treatment of drug misuse. Report of the Medical Working Group on Drug Dependence. HMSO, London

DHSS 1991 Drug misuse and dependence. Guidelines on clinical management. NMSO, London

Gerada C, Dawe S, Farrell M 1990 Management of the pregnant opiate user. British Journal of Hospital Medicine 43: 138–141

McCammon R L 1986 Anesthesia for the chemically dependent patient. Anesthesia and Analgesia Review Course Lectures 47–55

McGoldrick K E 1980 Anesthetic implications of drug abuse. Anesthesiology Review 7: 12–17

Norkrans G, Frosner G, Hermodsson S et al 1980 Multiple hepatitis attacks in drug addicts. Journal of the American Medical Association. 243: 1056–1058

OPITZ-FRIAS SYNDROME

A rare congenital disorder whose features include craniofacial and genital abnormalities, and functional swallowing and laryngeal problems. Males are more severely affected than females.

Preoperative abnormalities

1. Hypertelorism, prominent parietal and occipital areas, micrognathia and a high-arched palate.

2. Hypospadias and bifid scrotum.

3. Dysphagia, probably of neuromuscular origin, oesophageal achalasia, hiatus hernia, gastric aspiration and pulmonary problems. There may be wheezing and inspiratory stridor, with a hoarse cry.

Anaesthetic problems

1. Recurrent gastric aspiration may cause cyanotic episodes, apnoea and asystole.

2. Craniofacial abnormalities can lead to intubation problems.

Management

Anaesthetic management of a 9-month-old child for fundoplication and feeding jejunostomy has been reported (Bolsin & Gilbe 1985). Several episodes of cyanosis and CXR changes had occurred after birth. A scan of an isotopic milk feed demonstrated reflux, and the child was fed through a nasogastric tube. Prior to surgery two admissions for respiratory distress and inhalation had been required. Some intubation difficulty was reported due to an immature larynx.

BIBLIOGRAPHY
Bolsin S N, Gillbe C 1985 Opitz-Frias syndrome. A case with potentially hazardous anaesthetic implications. Anaesthesia 40: 1189–1193

OSLER-WEBER-RENDU DISEASE
(HEREDITARY HAEMORRHAGIC TELANGIECTASIA)

An autosomal dominant disease, sometimes known as hereditary haemorrhagic telangiectasia, in which there are cutaneous, mucosal, and visceral vascular anomalies, accompanied by a family history of the disorder. Affected individuals may present with epistaxis or gastrointestinal bleeding, often after the fourth decade. Pulmonary arteriovenous fistulae are present in about 15% of patients. These fistulae can cause hypoxia and, if untreated, they carry a mortality which exceeds that of treatment. Anaesthesia may be required for control of epistaxis, for gastrointestinal bleeding, or for coil spring embolization or surgery to pulmonary arteriovenous fistulae.

Preoperative abnormalities

1. Telangiectasia, systemic or pulmonary arteriovenous malformations (PAVM) and aneurysms constitute the three forms of angiodysplasia.
2. Recurrent epistaxis from nasal telangiectasia is an early marker of the disease. In 90% of patients, recurrent epistaxis started before the age of 21.
3. Bleeding from gastrointestinal lesions may occur, usually from diffuse angiodysplasia and particularly in the older age group of patients. This is difficult to treat.
4. Patients with pulmonary arteriovenous fistulae may have exertional dyspnoea, cyanosis, clubbing, palpitations and pulmonary vascular bruits. Right-to-left shunting occurs, with blood flowing directly from a pulmonary artery into a pulmonary vein, since the lesions have no intervening capillary bed. There may be secondary polycythaemia. The bruit is increased by inspiration. In the majority of cases in which there is an arteriovenous fistula, the CXR is

abnormal. Often the abnormality shows as a peripherally placed dense area which is attached to the hilum by vascular markings (Burke et al 1986), or there may be isolated 'coin' lesions. Pulmonary angiography will confirm the diagnosis. Haemothorax may occur and is occasionally life-threatening. If the fistulae are large, the patient may develop high-output cardiac failure. One-third of patients who present with a single pulmonary vascular malformation will have Osler-Weber-Rendu disease. If these are multiple, the incidence of the condition increases to more than 50%.

5. Similar lesions in the brain may cause intracranial haemorrhage, neurological deficits and seizures.
6. Haematuria may occur as a result of bladder lesions.
7. Brain abscess formation is well documented and probably secondary to paradoxical embolus of infected material unfiltered by the lung capillaries.
8. Hepatic arteriovenous malformations may lead to fibrosis or cirrhosis. Arteriovenous and portosystemic shunts may occur.
9. Cardiac valvular disease has been reported although the reason for this is not known.

Anaesthetic problems

1. Pulmonary arteriovenous fistulae may be associated with hypoxia secondary to right-to-left shunting of blood. Fistulae may increase in size, or can produce paradoxical emboli of any type, including septic emboli. Hepatic arteriovenous shunts can also occur, with cardiac failure and pulmonary hypertension. High-output cardiac failure during pregnancy has occurred in association with a hepatic arteriovenous fistula. The diagnosis was confirmed by echocardiography and MRI (Gong et al 1988).
2. Hypoxaemia followed the onset of IPPV in a patient with a pulmonary arteriovenous fistula (Friedman et al 1992). This resolved when spontaneous respiration was resumed and was thought to have resulted from a deterioration of the right-to-left shunt caused by IPPV.
3. There may be recurrent admissions for control of epistaxis (Siegel et al 1991). In a study of 73 patients, the incidence of epistaxis was 93%; the mean age of onset was 12 years; the mean frequency of bleeding was 18 per month, and the mean duration of haemorrhage 7.5 minutes (Aassar et al 1991).
4. Abscess formation, particularly in the brain, may occur spontaneously or in association with surgery or dental treatment (Mohler et al 1991). The lesions are usually solitary and sited above the tentorium (Peery 1987). Osler-Weber-Rendu disease may be unrecognized before the presentation of the abscess (Gelfand et al 1988). Evidence of the presence of this condition should be sought when a solitary abscess occurs.

5. There is a risk of paradoxical embolism of any type because microemboli bypass the pulmonary capillary filter.
6. Spontaneous haemothorax has been reported (Karnik et al 1983).
7. Pregnancy may increase the rate of growth of pulmonary fistulae (Swinburne et al 1986), probably secondary to hormonal and cardiovascular changes (Chanatry 1992) and new fistula formation. Spontaneous haemothorax and hypoxaemia in the midtrimester may necessitate embolization of the fistulae (Gammon et al 1990, Waring et al 1990).
8. Although bleeding usually occurs secondary to vascular abnormalities and, in the absence of coagulation defects, there is an association between Osler-Weber-Rendu disease and von Willebrand's disease. Defects in the endothelial cells may result in impaired production of Factor VIII and vWF factor (Quitt et al 1990).

Management

1. Complications of the disease should be sought, particularly the presence of pulmonary arteriovenous malformations and resultant hypoxaemia.
2. Take care to avoid causing paradoxical emboli via sites of intravenous access. If extradural anaesthesia is performed, loss of resistance to saline, rather than air, should be used to identify the extradural space.
3. Although an extradural infusion for labour has been described in a patient with Osler-Weber-Rendu disease and rheumatic heart disease, this technique should be used cautiously and the patient monitored closely for the development of an extradural haematoma. There is a possibility of abnormal extradural vessels, and a small risk of coagulation problems if there are vWF or Factor VIII abnormalities.
4. Incidence of readmission for epistaxis was found to be reduced if treatment with laser therapy combined with septodermoplasty was undertaken (Siegel et al 1991).
5. In view of the risks of abscess formation, the use of antibacterial prophylaxis, similar to those with cardiac lesions, has been suggested (Swanson & Dahl 1991).
6. Desmopressin has been used to treat gastrointestinal bleeding which was unresponsive to cryoprecipitate, in a patient with decreased. vWF and also in those patients without a known deficiency (Quitt et al 1990). Oestrogen-progesterone therapy has also been used.

BIBLIOGRAPHY

Aassar O S, Friedman C M, White R I Jr 1991 The natural history of epistaxis in hereditary telangiectasia. Laryngoscope 101: 977–980
Burke C M, Safai C, Nelson D P et al 1986 Pulmonary arteriovenous malformations: a

critical update. American Review of Respiratory Disease 134: 334–339

Chanatry B J 1992 Acute hemothorax owing to pulmonary arteriovenous malformation in pregnancy. Anesthesia and Analgesia 74: 613–615

Friedman B C, McGrath B J, Willlams J F 1992 Pulmonary arteriovenous fistula: mechanical ventilation and hypoxemia. Canadian Journal of Anaesthesia 39: 963–965

Gammon R B, Miksa A K, Keller F S 1990 Osler–Weber–Rendu disease and pulmonary arteriovenous fistulas. Deterioration and embolotherapy during pregnancy. Chest 98: 1522–1524

Gelfand M S, Stephens D S, Howell E I et al 1988 Brain abscess: association with pulmonary arteriovenous fistula and hereditary hemorrhagic telangiectasia: report of three cases. American Journal of Medicine 85: 718–720

Gong B, Baken L, Julian T et al 1988 High-output heart failure due to hepatic arteriovenous fistula during pregnancy: a case report. Obstetrics and Gynecology 72: 440–442

Karnik A M, Sughayer A, Fenech F F 1983 Spontaneous haemothorax in Osler–Weber–Rendu disease. Postgraduate Medical Journal 59: 512–513

Mohler E R, Monahan B, Canty M D et al 1991 Cerebral abscess associated with dental procedure in hereditary haemorrhagic telangiectasia. Lancet 338: 508–509

Peery W H 1987 Clinical spectrum of hereditary hemorrhagic telangiectasia (Osler–Weber–Rendu disease). American Journal of Medicine 82: 989–997

Quitt M, Froom P, Veisler A et al 1990 The effect of desmopressin on massive gastrointestinal bleeding in hereditary telangiectasia unresponsive to treatment with cryoprecipitate. Archives of Internal Medicine 150: 1744–1746

Siegel M B, Keane W M, Atkins J F Jr et al 1991 Control of epistaxis in patients with hereditary hemorrhagic telangiectasia. Otolaryngology and Head and Neck Surgery 105: 675–679

Swanson D L, Dahl M V 1991 Embolic abscesses in hereditary hemorrhagic telangiectasia. Journal of the American Academy of Dermatology 24: 580–583

Swinburne A J, Fedullo A J, Bangemi R et al 1986 Hereditary telangiectasia and multiple arteriovenous fistulas. Clinical deterioration during pregnancy. Chest 89: 459–460

Waring P H, Shaw D B, Brumfield C G 1990 Anesthetic management of a parturient with Osler–Weber–Rendu syndrome and rheumatic heart disease. Anesthesia and Analgesia 71: 96–99

OSTEOGENESIS IMPERFECTA

The general term given to a heterogeneous group of inherited disorders of collagen, thought to involve a defect in type I collagen. Four broad types have been identified (Smith 1984), but increased knowledge of the large number of genetic mutations suggests that further expansion of groupings will be needed (Cole & Cohen 1991). In less severe cases, diagnosis may be delayed, but the resultant bony fragility and propensity to fractures may result in the mistaken diagnosis of child abuse (Gahagan & Rimsza 1991). Anaesthesia may be required for reduction of fractures, scoliosis surgery, neurosurgery and other corrections of skeletal deformities.

Type I is of autosomal dominant inheritance and present in 80% of cases. Extraskeletal tissues are mainly involved and the bone disease is mild. Fractures mainly occur in childhood but become less common after puberty. The joints are hypermobile and the tendons susceptible to rupture. Patients are almost normal in stature. The sclera are blue, there is early-onset deafness and some children have dental problems. The aortic valve is thin, and sometimes incompetent.

Type II have severe skeletal abnormalities and usually die in the perinatal period.

Type III have severe skeletal deformities which are progressive. Chest deformity, with kyphoscoliosis and prominent sternum, often results in respiratory problems. Long bones are narrow and bent. The skull is large and asymmetrical and there may be cortical atrophy. Patients with this type have white sclera.

Type IV is similar to type I, but with more bone abnormalities and some dwarfing. Teeth may be involved. Sclera are white.

Preoperative abnormalities

1. Individual features have been described. A number of other defects may occur in addition. Dentinogenesis imperfecta occurs in about 50% of patients.
2. Severe skeletal injuries may be associated with minor traumatic events, often in the absence of physical signs of bruising, swelling or contusion. A UK survey showed that out of 804 patients, in 113 the diagnosis of non-accidental injury had been made at some stage (Patterson 1990).
3. Hearing loss is common. Thirty one out of 57 patients with osteogenesis imperfecta had conductive or mixed loss. Anaesthesia may be required for middle-ear surgery (Bergstrom 1977).
4. There is some evidence of hypermetabolism, with excessive sweating and metabolic acidosis. Half of the patients have increased serum thyroxine levels.
5. Platelet dysfunction may occur and produce a mild bleeding tendency, although the platelet count may be normal.
6. Cardiovascular involvement may occur but is often clinically inapparent. Aortic root dilatation has been described in 12% of patients in one survey, but, unlike that seen in Marfan's syndrome, it is mild and non progressive (Hortop et al 1986). However, congenital cardiac lesions have been reported.
7. Kidney stones and renal papillary calcification may occur and dietary supplementation with calcium and vitamin D may predispose to this.
8. Cranial developmental defects (platybasia) may cause brain stem compression and hydrocephalus. Patients with severe type III osteogenesis imperfecta associated with macrocephaly and cortical atrophy have been reported.
9. Those patients with kyphoscoliosis may have restrictive pulmonary defects.

Anaesthetic problem

1. Bones and teeth are easy to break. The mandible is prone to fracture, but the facial bones are less so. Inadvertent rib fractures were followed by fatal haemorrhage in a young girl during spinal fusion surgery (Sperry 1989).
2. In the severest form, forcible extension of the head during intubation carries a risk of vertebral fracture.
3. Airway problems may occur if the head is large, if there is macroglossia, or if the skeletal deformities are severe.
4. Perioperative hyperthermia, metabolic disturbances, cardiovascular instability and excess sweating have been reported (Masuda et al 1990). An MH-like syndrome, which was terminated with dantrolene, was described in a young man who subsequently refused further investigation. His sister had died aged 14 years after a prolonged mask anaesthetic for reduction of a fracture (Rampton et al 1984). Postoperative hyperthermia, hypoxaemia, and acidosis without hypercarbia, which responded to active cooling, occurred in a child (Ryan et al 1989). There was biochemical evidence of mild rhabdomyolysis. Although one patient with osteogensis imperfecta and MH susceptibility on muscle testing has been reported (Rosenberg 1988), it is assumed that the hyperthermia associated with osteogenesis irnperfecta is a separate entity.
5. Multiple general anaesthetics may be required for orthopaedic or ENT procedures.
6. Violent suxamethonium fasciculations can produce fractures.

Management

1. Patients should be positioned on the operating table and handled with extreme care. Padding should be used. If the head is large, a pillow placed under the chest may assist tracheal intubation.
2. Surgery should be avoided in the pyrexial patient. Core temperature, oxygen saturation and ET_{CO2} should be monitored throughout surgery. Hyperthermia is reported to have responded to cooling alone (Cho et al 1992).
3. In the severe types of the disease, concern has been expressed that a blood pressure cuff may damage the humerus. Direct arterial monitoring has been suggested as an alternative (Libman 1981).
4. Suxamethonium should be avoided when the risk of fractures is high.
5. The use of ketamine has been reported (Oliverio 1973, Robison & Wright 1986). This offers a convenient method of avoiding mask and intubation anaesthesia.
6. Although skeletal deformity may make regional anaesthesia technically difficult, extradural anaesthesia has been used for the management of a Caesarean section (Cunningham et al 1984). In this

patient, platelet studies were normal. However, this is not a suitable technique if serious intubation difficulties are anticipated. In one patient for Caesarean section who refused regional anaesthesia, neuromuscular block was achieved with vecuronium (Cho et al 1992).

BIBLIOGRAPHY
Bergstrom L 1977 Osteogenesis imperfecta. Otological and maxillofacial aspects. Laryngoscope 87 (suppl 6): 1–42
Cho E, Dayan S S, Marx G F 1992 Anaesthesia in a parturient with osteogenesis imperfecta. British Journal of Anaesthesia 68: 422–423
Cole D E C, Cohen M M 1991 Osteogenesis imperfecta: an update. Journal of Pediatrics 119: 73–74
Cunningham A J, Donnelly M, Comerford J 1984 Osteogenesis imperfecta: Anesthetic management of a patient for Cesarean section. Anesthesiology 61: 91–93
Gahagan S, Rimsza M E 1991 Child abuse or osteogenesis imperfecta: how can we tell? Pediatrics 88: 987–992
Hortop J, Tsipouras P, Hanley J A et al 1986 Cardiovascular involvement in osteogenesis imperfecta. Circulation 73: 54–61
Libman R H 1981 Anaesthetic considerations for the patient with osteogenesis imperfecta. Clinical Orthopaedics and Related Research 159: 123–125
Masuda Y, Harada Y, Honma E et al 1990 Anesthetic management of a patient with osteogenesis imperfecta congenita (English abstr). Masui 39: 383–387
Oliverio R O 1973 Anesthetic management of intramedullary nailing in osteogenesis imperfecta. Anesthesia and Analgesia 52: 232–236
Patterson C R 1990 Osteogenesis imperfecta and other bone disorders in the differential diagnosis of unexplained fractures. Journal of the Royal Society of Medicine 83: 72–74
Rampton A J, Kelly D A, Shanahan E C et al 1984 Occurrence of malignant hyperpyrexia in a patient with osteogenesis imperfecta. British Journal of Anaesthesia 56: 1443–1446
Robison C, Wright D J 1986 Anaesthesia for osteogenesis irnperfecta. Today's Anaesthetist 1, 2: 22–23
Rosenberg H 1988 Clinical presentation of malignant hyperthermia. British Journal of Anaesthesia 60: 268–273
Ryan C A, Al-Ghamdi A S, Gayle M et al 1989 Osteogenesis imperfecta and hyperthermia. Anesthesia and Analgesia 68: 811–814
Smith R 1984 Osteogenesis imperfecta. British Medical Journal 289: 394–396
Sperry K 1989 Fatal intraoperative haernorrhage during spinal fusion surgery for osteogenesis irnperfecta. American Journal of Forensic Medicine and Pathology 10: 54–59

PACEMAKERS
(see HEART BLOCK)

PAGET'S DISEASE

A metabolic bone disease which may be either focal or diffuse. The aetiology is unknown, but epidemiological studies and the presence of inclusion bodies in osteoclasts suggest a viral origin. The primary process appears to be unusually active resorption of bone by abnormal osteoclasts, and although osteoblasts replace it, the architecture is disorganized and mineralization defective. There is fibrosis of the marrow, and both marrow and bone are very vascular. In the later, sclerotic stage, vascularity decreases and the bone becomes dense and hard.

Preoperative abnormalities

1. The patient may be asymptomatic, or have bone pain. Affected bones may be enlarged and deformed, and the overlying skin warm. The pelvis, femur, tibia, skull, and spine are the most commonly involved.
2. The bone is more vulnerable to fractures than is normal bone. About 1% of patients develop bone sarcoma.
3. Bone enlargement and deformity may cause a variety of neurological symptoms. Deafness, paraplegia, brainstem compression and hydrocephalus have been described.
4. If the disease is widespread, the vascular stage may be associated with a high cardiac output. Cardiac failure, secondary to the disease itself, occurs rarely.
5. Most patients require no treatment or mild analgesics only. Specific treatment is indicated in those with bone pain, complications of deformity, neurological symptoms or heart failure. Mithramycin has been used for the rapid relief of pain and in spinal cord compression. Calcitonin (i.m. or i.v.) reduces the vascularity of bone before orthopaedic procedures, and is used for bone pain and in osteolytic disease. Etidronate is increasingly used. It reduces bone turnover and may interfere with mineralization. Treatment is usually limited to 6 months, but the effect may be prolonged.

Anaesthetic problems

1. Bone fracture is a common complication of Paget's disease (Guyer 1980).
2. In view of the marked vascularity of the bone, there may be considerable blood loss during orthopaedic procedures. A spontaneous extradural haematoma has been reported. It was thought to be secondary to increased vascularity of bone resulting in greater than normal blood flow through the extradural veins (Hanna et al 1989).
3. Paget's disease may affect the atlas and axis (Brown et al 1971). Cervical spine disease can be associated with serious neurological complications. Bone hypertrophy and narrowing of the spinal canal may cause cord compression, or interference with the blood supply. Vertebral displacement can occur due to fracture or subluxation. Invagination of the foramen magnum into the posterior fossa is present in one-third of patients with Paget's disease of the skull (Guyer 1980).

4. If the lumbar spine is involved, regional anaesthesia may be technically difficult.

Management

1. To avoid fractures, patients should be moved and positioned very gently under anaesthesia Limbs should be supported and padded.
2. Treatment with calcitonin may decrease the bone vascularity. However, its effect is maximal in the early stages of treatment but may progressively diminish after the first 3 months.
3. Patients with cervical spine and skull disease should be treated with extreme care. Neurological symptoms and signs should be sought and documented in advance. Atlantoaxial subluxation must be excluded.
4. Cardiac failure, if present, should be treated.

BIBLIOGRAPHY

Brown H P, LaRocca H, Wickstrom J K 1971 Paget's disease of the atlas and axis. Journal of Bone and Joint Surgery 53B: 1441–1444
Guyer P B 1980 Radiology in Paget's disease. Hospital Update 6: 1079–1091
Hanna J W, Ball M R, Lee K S 1989 Spontaneous hematoma complicating Paget's disease of the spine. Spine 14: 900–902

PAPILLOMATOSIS
(see *LARYNGEAL PAPILLOMATOSIS*)

PARKINSON'S DISEASE

A disorder of the extrapyramidal motor system of unknown aetiology. Onset is gradual, and usually occurs after the age of 50. Pathological changes include degeneration of cells and loss of pigmented neurones in the substantia nigra. Biochemical abnormalities in brain neurotransmitters, and in particular a deficiency of dopamine in the striatum and substantia nigra, have been demonstrated. Parkinsonism has also occurred following insults to the brain such as encephalitis lethargica, trauma, certain chemicals, major psychotropic drugs, cerebrovascular disease or hypoxia. Parkinsonian features may occur in other degenerative CNS diseases (Editorial 1992), which may exhibit additional signs such as autonomic failure (e.g. Shy-Drager).

The aim of drug treatment is to increase dopamine concentrations in the basal ganglia, or to decrease the effects of acetylcholine – that is, to establish a balance between central dopaminergic and cholinergic activity. The introduction of levodopa, which increases the dopamine levels in the striatum, has produced a considerable improvement in the quality of life for many patients, although long-term therapy may cause a deterioration in response, resulting in fluctuations in mobility. Dopamine agonists such as bromocriptine, lisuride and pergolide are also used. Monoamine oxidase B inhibitors, such as selegeline hydrochloride, improve duration of action of brain dopamine. This latter drug has been shown to have a protective effect in early Parkinson's disease. Symptomatic relief and side-effects have to be balanced to find the optimum dosage. Improvements in drug therapy have decreased the requirement for stereotactic surgery. A number of patients have undergone autologous adrenal medulla transplants (Hyman et al 1988). However, any benefits produced by adrenal implants are thought to be outweighed by the risks of surgery (Marsden 1990), and the future of embryonic brain tissue transplants is at present unknown. In addition, significant ethical considerations are raised by such surgery (Editorial 1988).

Preoperative abnormalities

1. The main features are progressive akinesia, increased muscle tone with 'cogwheel' rigidity, and a tremor which is increased with stress, decreased during action, and absent during sleep. Postural changes involve flexion of the head and body. Symptoms may be asymmetrical. The facies becomes expressionless, giving a false impression of disinterest or poor cerebral function. However, the subject is usually intellectually unimpaired, although dementia or depression may occur in the later stages of the disease.
2. Drug therapy depends on the symptoms and stage of the disease. In the early stages, anticholinergics may ameliorate tremor and rigidity. Levodopa is appropriate when postural changes and akinesia develop, but large doses have to be given because only 5% of the drug crosses the blood-brain barrier, and the rest is broken down by dopa decarboxylase. However, the dose, and hence the side-effects resulting from high peripheral levels of levodopa metabolites, can be reduced by as much as 75% when it is combined with an inhibitor of extracerebral dopa decarboxylase, such as carbidopa or benserazide.
3. Gastrointestinal function is abnormal, and defects in deglutition, oesophageal motility, and colonic movement occur (Edwards et al 1992).

Anaesthetic problems

1. Abnormalities of swallowing have been demonstrated in 92% of Parkinsonian patients studied using videofluoroscopy, and tracheal aspiration occurred in 46% (Stroudley & Walsh 1991). This has implications for the perioperative period.
2. Arrhythmias may occur in patients taking high doses of levodopa alone without a decarboxylase inhibitor, because of its metabolism

to dopamine. However, the half-life is only 4 hours. The concomitant use of carbidopa reduces dopaminergic side-effects.

3. Orthostatic hypotension may occur in patients on chronic levodopa therapy. A combination of decreased intravascular volume, decreased noradrenaline production, and reduction of noradrenaline stores may be responsible.

4. Intraoperative exacerbation of the disease in a patient whose levodopa had been given 5 hours before has been described (Reed & Han 1992). The artefact produced on the ECG resembled coarse ventricular fibrillation.

5. If levodopa is stopped completely in the perioperative period, the patient will become rigid and immobile. Maintenance of adequate ventilation may be difficult. The risks of venous thrombosis and respiratory restriction are then increased.

6. Phenothiazines and butyrophenones antagonize levodopa and may cause a deterioration in the Parkinson's disease.

7. Levodopa can interact with direct-acting sympathomimetic amines and monoamine oxidase inhibitors to cause severe hypertension.

8. Autonomic dysfunction has been described in advanced disease.

9. Suxamethonium-induced hyperkalaemia (4.2–7.6 mmol/l) occurred in a patient with poorly controlled Parkinsonism (Gravlee 1980). This took place during induction of anaesthesia for CABG, when a number of drugs had been given. Levodopa had been stopped for 5 days. However, there is little evidence that this is generally a problem (Muzzi et al 1989, Ho 1989).

10. The theoretical possibility that high-dose opioid/nitrous oxide anaesthesia might be dangerous, on the grounds that opioid-induced rigidity resembles Parkinson's disease, has been suggested (Severn 1988). An acute dystonia occurred after the use of alfentanil 1 mg in a patient with untreated Parkinson's disease (Mets 1991). This was thought to result from decreased central dopaminergic transmission.

11. The suitability of local anaesthetic techniques may be limited by the extrapyramidal movements.

12. Sedatives such as the phenothiazines and butyrophenones should be avoided because they block central dopaminergic receptors.

Management

1. The patient's current drug therapy must be known. If levodopa alone is being given, then it should be stopped 12–24 hours before surgery. If, as in most cases, it is being given in combination with a dopa decarboxylase inhibitor, then the drugs can be given up to the time of surgery. In order to prevent exacerbation of the disease, it has been suggested that the oral preparation should be given 20 minutes before surgery (Reed & Han 1992). Medication should be continued after surgery, by nasogastric tube if necessary.

2. Evidence of autonomic neuropathy should be sought.
3. Careful cardiovascular monitoring for arrhythmias, hypotension, and hypertension. If intravascular volume is decreased, colloids may be required.
4. Regional anaesthesia may be inadvisable in certain patients, if they are receiving complex drug regimens, or if there is a suggestion of autonomic neuropathy.
5. The use of ketamine in one patient with severe disease, taking levodopa, was reported to have greatly improved tremor and rigidity for several hours (Hetherington & Rosenblatt 1980).
6. Diphenhydramine, which possesses central anticholinergic effects, has been used during ophthalmic surgery under local anaesthesia. It was found to produce sedation with minimal tremor (Stone & DiFazio 1988).

BIBLIOGRAPHY
Editorial 1988 Embryos and Parkinson's disease. Lancet i: 1087
Editorial 1992 Parkinson's disease: one illness or many syndromes? Lancet 339: 1263–1264
Edwards L L, Quigley E M, Pfeiffer R F 1992 Gastrointestinal function in Parkinson's disease: frequency and pathophysiology. Neurology 42: 726–732
Gravlee G P 1980 Succinlycholine-induced hyperkalemia in a patient with Parkinson's disease. Anesthesia and Analgesia 59: 444–446
Hetherington A, Rosenblatt R M 1980 Ketamine and paralysis agitans. Anesthesiology 52: 527
Ho AM-H 1989 Parkinsonism and the anaesthetist. British Journal of Anaesthesia 62: 580
Hyman S A, Rogers W D, Smith W et al 1988 Perioperative management for transplant of autologous adrenal medulla to the brain for Parkinsonism. Anesthesiology 69: 618–622
Marsden C D 1990 Parkinson's disease. Lancet 335: 948–952
Mets B 1991 Acute dystonia after alfentanil in untreated Parkinson's disease. Anesthesia and Analgesia 72: 557–558
Muzzi D A, Black S, Cucchiara R F 1989 The lack of effect of succinylcholine on serum potassium in patients with Parkinson's disease. Anesthesiology 71: 322
Reed A P, Han D G 1992 Intraoperative exacerbation of Parkinson's disease. Anesthesia and Analgesia 75: 850–853
Severn A 1988 Parkinsonism and the anaesthetist. British Journal of Anaesthesia 61: 761–770
Stone D J, DiFazio C A 1988 Sedation for patients with Parkinson's disease undergoing ophthalmic surgery. Anesthesiology 68: 821
Stroudley J, Walsh M 1991 Radiological assessment of dysphagia in Parkinson's disease. British Journal of Radiology 64: 890–893

PAROXYSMAL NOCTURNAL HAEMOGLOBINURIA

An acquired, clonal disorder of stem cells involving erythrocytes, leucocytes and platelets, which results in abnormal haematopoiesis, a reduction in life-span of cells, and haemolytic anaemia. Various biochemical abnormalities have been noted, including deficiencies in a number of membrane proteins which interact with complement (Editorial 1992), but the precise defect is not yet known. Cells of the paroxysmal nocturnal haemoglobinuria (PNH) clone are vulnerable to the haemolytic action of complement, acting either by the classic or the alternative pathways. Cyclical lysis of PNH cells occurs, resulting in a reduction in the life-span of the cell, although there is also usually a population of normal cells present. Sometimes, bone marrow aplasia develops, producing aplastic anaemia. The presentations of PNH are extremely variable, attacks ranging from mild and intermittent to severe. It is mainly a disease of adults, but sometimes it occurs in children, in whom the disease tends to be more severe (Ware et al 1991). Gallstones are common and patients may present for open or laparoscopic cholecystectomy, or sometimes bone marrow transplantation.

Preoperative abnormalities

1. Irregular episodes in which reddish-brown urine is passed. This may be precipitated by exercise, surgery or infections, pregnancy and drugs. There may be recurrent attacks of abdominal pain, symptoms of anaemia, recurrent infection and headaches.
2. Haematological abnormalities include haemolytic anaemia, nocturnal haemoglobinuria, variable but mild jaundice, haemosiderin in the urine leading to iron deficiency, leucopenia, thrombocytopenia, and reticulocytosis. Sometimes aplastic anaemia develops.
3. Isolated venous thrombosis may occur, possibly triggered by platelet activation. Hepatic venous thrombosis (Budd-Chiari syndrome) is found in about 20% patients with PNH. Intestinal thromboses and renal infarcts may also occur (see Budd-Chiari syndrome).
4. Patients are prone to recurrent infections because of leucopenia and defective leucocyte function.
5. Even in the presence of a normal glomerular filtration rate, there are defects in urinary concentrating ability.
6. Diagnosis may be suspected if haemosiderin is present in the urine. The Ham acid haemolysis test is used for the definitive diagnosis.
7. Supportive treatment includes transfusion, iron therapy, antibiotics or anticoagulants, and occasionally steroids. In some patients there may be indication for bone marrow transplant.

Anaesthetic problems

1. There is an increased incidence of postoperative venous thrombosis.
2. Pregnancy may be complicated. In a study of 38 pregnancies, both during pregnancy and peripartum, acute haemolysis and haemorrhage were the commonest complications. Nearly one-third of pregnancies ended in miscarriage (De Gramont et al 1987).
3. Reactions that involve complement are more serious than usual, because of the vulnerability of the red cells to lysis (Taylor et al 1987).
4. Severe haemolysis and renal failure has been precipitated by ABO-incompatible plasma in pooled platelets (Jackson et al 1992).

Management

1. The importance of cooperation between the surgeon, haematologist and anaesthetist has been emphasized (Braren et al 1981).
2. Treatment of infection.
3. Prevention of dehydration by intravenous infusion the night prior to surgery. Saline or dextrose saline, with or without potassium, (but not Ringer lactate solution) can be used. A urine output in excess of 100 ml/h should be maintained. Acidosis must be prevented because it may enhance haemolysis. For major surgery, a catheter should be inserted to monitor the urine for haemoglobinuria (Ogin 1990).
4. If blood transfusion is required, the use of washed red cells reduces the chance of reactions (Jackson et al 1992). In anaemic patients, blood transfusion will decrease the proportion of abnormal cells.
5. All i.v. drugs should be given cautiously. It has been suggested that those with a low incidence of anaphylactoid reactions should be used (Taylor et al 1987).
6. Should hepatic venous thrombosis develop, anticoagulants or thrombolytic therapy may be required. However, heparin protamine complexes activate the classical complement pathway, therefore protamine should be avoided.
7. Corticosteroids may abort haemolytic episodes in some patients (Rosse 1982), but they should only be given for short intervals. Prednisone given at 6 p.m. can prevent the nocturnal haemolytic episode in responders. Hydration should be maintained, and transfusion may suppress the production of complement-sensitive cells.
8. In pregnancy regular haematological monitoring is essential, because transfusions of red cells or platelets may be needed.

BIBLIOGRAPHY

Braren V, Jenkins D E, Phythyon J M et al 1981 Perioperative management of patients with paroxysmal nocturnal hemoglobinuria. Surgery, Gynecology and Obstetrics 153: 515–520

De Gramont A, Krulik M, Debray J 1987 Paroxysmal nocturnal haemoglobinuria and pregnancy. Lancet i: 868

Editorial 1992 Paroxysmal nocturnal haemoglobinuria. Lancet 339: 395–396

Jackson G H, Noble R S, Maung Z T et al 1992 Severe haemolysis and renal failure in a patient with paroxysmal nocturnal haemoglobinuria. Journal of Clinical Pathology 45: 176–177

Ogin G A 1990 Cholecystectomy in a patient with paroxysmal nocturnal haemoglobinuria. Anesthetic implications and management in the perioperative period. Anesthesiology 72: 761–764

Rosse W F 1982 Treatment of paroxsmal nocturnal hemoglobinuria. Blood 60: 20–23

Taylor M B, Whitwam J G, Worsley A 1987 Paroxysmal nocturnal haemoglobinuria. Perioperative management of a patient with Budd-Chiari syndrome. Anaesthesia 42: 639–642

Ware R E, Hall S E, Rosse W F 1991 Paroxysmal nocturnal hemoglobinuria with onset in childhood and adolescence. New England Journal of Medicine 325: 991–996

PERICARDIAL DISEASE
(see CARDIAC TAMPONADE)

PHAEOCHROMOCYTOMA
(see also Section 2)

A rare catecholamine-secreting tumour, which usually originates in the adrenal gland, but may arise from anywhere in the sympathetic chain. Secretion of noradrenaline is more common than adrenaline. Extra-adrenal phaeochromocytomas are usually below the diaphragm, most commonly in the superior para-aortic region (Goldfarb et al 1989).

Diagnosis may be made preoperatively, in which case adrenoceptor blockade must be instituted before surgery, or as soon as the diagnosis is made. Rarely, it may present unexpectedly during operation, or in labour as a life-threatening crisis (see Section 2). In these cases, presenting features include tachycardia, hypertension, pulmonary oedema and sudden death. Phaeochromocytomas may feature in a number of rare syndromes, which include neurofibromatosis, von Hippel–Lindau syndrome and the multiple endocrine neoplasias.

The existence of a catecholamine-induced myocarditis is increasingly being recognized (Editorial 1990). Initially the myocardium is infiltrated with acute inflammatory cells, but this may be succeeded by a frank cardiomyopathy. The precise aetiology is unknown, but changes in cardiac adrenoceptors, the chronic effects of catecholamines on lipids, and direct tissue damage from free radicals, are possible contributing factors.

Preoperative abnormalities

1. Episodes of headache, sweating and palpitations are the commonest presenting symptoms. The majority of patients have two or more of these complaints. If none of the three is present, or if flushing is a feature, then phaeochromocytoma is almost certainly not the cause (Bravo & Gifford 1984). Other useful markers are flank pain, visual symptoms and pallor (Stein & Black 1991).
2. Persistent hypertension occurs in 50% cases. In most of the remaining patients it is episodic.
3. Patients are frequently thin, appear anxious and may be peripherally vasoconstricted. Preoperative adrenoceptor blockade, with the accompanying expansion of the vascular volume, often causes the patient's face to fill out.
4. A number of cases have been reported in which cardiac failure has occurred in association with a phaeochromocytoma. Sometimes cardiac failure may occur in normotensive patients (Sardesai et al 1990). Six patients were reported, five of whom died of pulmonary

oedema. It has been suggested that a cardiomyopathy, secondary to the chronic high levels of catecholamines, occurs more frequently than has been recognized (Gilsanz et al 1983). The reversibility of cardiomyopathy, first by treatment with alpha-methyl-para-tyrosine, and subsequently by surgery, has been demonstrated (Imperato-McGinley et al 1987).

5. Biochemical diagnosis involves the initial screening of at least three 24-hour urine collections for catecholamine metabolites. Measurement of urinary HMMA (3-hydroxy 4-methoxy mandelic acid, sometimes called VMA or vanillylmandelic acid), or urinary metadrenalines can be performed. The latter is more accurate. Levels may be mildly increased in a proportion of individuals without a phaeochromocytoma. However, if the values are 1.5–2 times above the upper limit of normal, this suggests that a phaeochromocytoma is present (Stein & Black 1991).

Should the screening tests prove positive, then direct plasma adrenaline and noradrenaline estimations can be performed, but special laboratory facilities may be required. If the levels are only slightly elevated in the presence of hypertension, then the diagnosis is unlikely. Patients with phaeochromocytomas become less sensitive than normal patients to catecholamines. Thus, in a patient with a phaeochromocytoma who has hypertension, plasma catecholamines are likely to be at least twice normal levels (Brown 1987).

A number of drugs, including levodopa, methyl dopa and MAOIs, may interfere with the biochemical tests.

Several provocation and suppression tests have been described for cases in which the diagnosis is in doubt. However, the provocation tests are dangerous and should not be used. Suppression of plasma catecholamine levels with pentolinium and clonidine will occur with physiologically increased levels, but not when the catecholamines are tumour generated.

6. Ninety per cent of tumours are adrenal in origin, and are bilateral in 10% of cases. If adrenaline constitutes at least 20% of the total plasma catecholamines, then the tumour is likely to be in the adrenal (Brown 1987). This is so because the synthesis of adrenaline from noradrenaline is dependent on the presence of high levels of glucocorticoids, which are carried to the medulla in blood from the cortex.

For accurate localization, a CT scan is now the first line of investigation. Provided that the tumours are more than 1 cm in diameter, more than 90% of tumours will be identified.

Radioisotope meta-iodobenzylguanidine (mIBG) scanning may assist in both diagnosis and treatment of malignant tumours. mIBG is similar to noradrenaline in structure and is taken up and concentrated in the storage granules of chromaffin tissue. Imaging takes place at 24, 48 and 72 hours. Adrenergic tissue is thus located

(Editorial 1984). In cases in which the site is still in doubt, selective venous sampling from the inferior vena cava, or arteriography, may be necessary. Adrenoceptors must be blocked before any invasive investigation.

Anaesthetic problems

1. Problems during anaesthesia in the untreated patient.
   The undiagnosed, or the diagnosed but unblocked patient, is greatly at risk from hypertensive crises, particularly during arteriography, anaesthesia, surgery, or delivery. In the past, before the introduction of preoperative adrenoceptor blocking, the mortality from surgery was 25–40%. The risks in the undiagnosed patient undergoing incidental surgery (Sutton et al 1981) or of crises occurring in association with pregnancy (Mitchell et al 1987) remain high. The mortality in pregnancy for 1980–1987 was reported to be 17% (Harper et al 1989). Major problems are:
   a. Severe hypertension, with the dangers of cerebral haemorrhage, encephalopathy, pulmonary oedema, myocardial infarction, ventricular fibrillation and renal failure. This may occur at induction and intubation, during handling of the tumour, or in labour during uterine contractions. A hypertensive crisis can also be precipitated if a beta blocker is administered alone, before alpha blockade has been established. This is because removal of the beta vasodilator effects leaves the vasoconstrictor alpha effects totally unopposed.
   b. Severe hypotension following removal of the tumour, from a combination of hypovolaemia and the sudden decrease in circulating catecholamines. Before the era of adrenoceptor blockade, this was usually treated with noradrenaline or adrenaline infusions, and the patient frequently died in a state of profound vasoconstriction, hypovolaemia and hypotension.
   c. Severe and protracted hypoglycaemia following removal of the tumour has been reported (Levin & Heifetz 1990). The sudden cessation of catecholamine output may be associated with an increase in insulin output.
2. Formerly, a request for only partial preoperative blockade was often made by the surgeon, in order to assess, after initial tumour removal, whether or not a second was present. Improved methods of tumour location have now made this much less necessary. In practice, however, some hypertensive response to tumour handling often occurs.

Management

1. Diagnosis of the phaeochromocytoma and location of tumour.
2. Pharmacological treatment with adrenoceptor blocking agents.
   This is the most crucial part of the patient's management.

Preparation with oral drugs should be undertaken for at least 10–14 days to allow gradual re-expansion of vascular volume. Postural hypotension often indicates that the patient is volume-depleted. Thus, during the period of vasodilatation, i.v. repletion may be necessary. Criteria for the adequacy of blockade have been specified (Roizen et al 1982). These require that there must be control of blood pressure without undue postural hypotension, control of major symptoms, and 2 weeks' freedom from ST- and T-wave changes on ECG. A number of regimens have been described. The choice will depend upon individual preference.

a. Phenoxybenzamine oral 10 mg b.d. initially, increasing gradually until hypertension is controlled. Between 80 and 200 mg may be required. At least 10 days' treatment will be needed.

b. If a tachycardia develops, then a beta blocker, propranolol 40–80 mg daily, increasing gradually if necessary, should be given.

If ischaemic heart disease is present, blocking should be instituted very cautiously to prevent sudden hypotension or tachycardia.

Occasionally, intravenous blocking may be required. This should take a minimum of 3 days. There should be close monitoring by medical staff throughout the procedure, particularly in patients with a degree of myocardial ischaemia.

Day 1:
Phenoxybenzamine 1 mg/kg in 500 ml 5% dextrose over 2 hours.
Propranolol orally if pulse rate above 120/min.

Day 2:
Phenoxybenzamine 1–1.5 mg/kg over 2 hours.
Propranolol to keep pulse rate below 100/min.

Day 3:
Phenoxybenzamine 1–2 mg/kg over 2 hours.
Propranolol as necessary.

Day of operation:
Phenoxybenzamine 50 mg.
Propranolol as necessary.

At this stage the BP should be 110/70 and pulse rate <90/min.

c. Other suggested methods of preoperative adrenoceptor blocking:

i. Prazosin, an alpha-1 receptor antagonist. Recent work has shown that there is more than one alpha adrenoceptor site. Alpha-1 receptors are postsynaptic whereas alpha-2 are presynaptic. It appears that stimulation of the alpha-2 receptors has an inhibiting effect on the release of noradrenaline from the nerve terminal. Blocking of these receptors will therefore enhance the release of noradrenaline (Hoffman & Lefkowitz 1980). Phentolamine and phenoxybenzamine block both types of receptor, and the resultant tachycardia from the use of these drugs is said to result from cardiac beta receptor stimulation.

Prazosin is a selective alpha-1 blocker and does not usually produce a tachycardia. Its use for preoperative preparation has been reported in four patients (Nicholson et al 1983). An initial test dose of prazosin 1 mg only was given, because sudden hypotension has been described in some subjects (Wallace & Gill 1978). On the basis of the response to this, further doses were prescribed. Satisfactory preoperative stabilization was produced with between 6 and 16 mg prazosin. However, all four patients had marked hypertensive responses during surgery, which required phentolamine infusion, and in one case, surgery was abandoned to allow treatment with phenoxybenzamine for 2 weeks. Prazosin alone therefore may not provide the best protection from the effects of high catecholamine levels produced during surgery.

ii. Labetalol, a combined alpha and beta blocker. Its beta effects are 3–7 times those of its alpha effects and it is therefore potentially dangerous in patients with phaeochromocytomas. Paradoxical severe hypertension has been reported following its use (Navaratnarajah & White 1984).

iii. Seventeen cases have been reported of management of phaeochromocytoma with magnesium sulphate (James 1989).

vi. Alpha methylparatyrosine has been used to achieve blockade by generation of a false transmitter.

3. Anaesthetic technique

A wide variety of techniques and drugs have been recommended. After a randomized trial of four anaesthetic methods, it was concluded that the choice of technique was not the crucial factor in patient outcome (Roizen et al 1982). Adequacy of preoperative adrenoceptor blockade was probably of more importance.

The aim is to provide conditions under which catecholamine release by the tumour, or the effect of any catecholamines released, is kept to a mimimum. Intubation, handling of the tumour, and certain drugs are known stimuli. A sedative premedication and a quiet, unhurried induction of anaesthesia are essential.

Both morphine and pethidine release histamine, and atropine may produce a tachycardia. Droperidol has its advocates, but there have been reports of pressor responses, possibly secondary to inhibition of catecholamine uptake (Sumikawa & Amakata 1977). Suxamethonium is traditionally avoided, since fasciculations increase intra-abdominal pressure.

Although several cases have been reported in which extradural anaesthesia has been combined with general anaesthesia (Cousins & Rubin 1974, Hopkins et al 1989), it does add a further uncontrollable factor to the already complicated pharmacophysiological situation. Patients with extradural blockade are often extremely sensitive to circulating catecholamines (Hull 1986) and extradural anaesthesia does not suppress the release of catecholamines (Liem et al 1991). Tonnesen et al (1989) measured killer cell activity during surgery in a patient who had not received preoperative adrenoceptor blocking drugs, and showed a strong relationship between plasma catecholamines and natural killer cell activity. In this patient, despite the use of extradural anaesthesia, nitroglycerine, and phentolamine to control blood pressure during surgery, mean arterial pressures of up to 155 mmHg occurred during tumour handling.

Pancuronium has been used on many occasions in the past but hypertension has been reported (Jones & Hill 1981). Vecuronium is a more logical substitute since it avoids the hypertension and tachycardia produced by pancuronium.

Halothane sensitizes the heart to the effect of catecholamines.

4. Monitoring
Direct arterial monitoring should begin in the anaesthetic room. Measurement of central venous pressure. ET_{CO_2}, urine output and neuromuscular monitoring are required.

5. Treatment of intraoperative complications
   a. Hypertension
   Phentolamine, sodium nitroprusside and nitroglycerin have all been used. The choice again depends on individual preference. Phentolamine causes a tachycardia, whereas sodium nitroprusside may produce swings in blood pressure, with hypotension occurring when tumour stimulation stops. Magnesium sulphate has been used to control the blood pressure in a pregnant patient (James et al 1988) and for intraoperative blood pressure control in 17 anaesthetics for phaeochromocytoma (James 1989). Magnesium sulphate 40–60 mg/kg was given at induction, followed by infusions of 1–2 g/h throughout surgery to maintain blood pressure control. In five patients, sodium nitroprusside was required in addition. Magnesium inhibits the release of catecholamines from the adrenal medulla, decreases the sensitivity of alpha adrenergic receptors, and causes direct vasodilatation. The therapeutic range is thought to be 2–4 mmol/l.
   b. Tachycardia
   This usually responds to beta adrenoceptor blockers, propranolol i.v. 1–2 mg being the most frequently used. Bronchospasm has been noted in one non-asthmatic patient, occurring 2 hours after operation (personal observation). In asthmatic patients, a cardioselective blocker, such as practolol or atenolol, may be more appropriate. Esmolol, a short-acting beta blocker is increasingly being used for control of tachycardia (Zakowski et al 1989, Ryan

et al 1993). Loading doses of 500 μg/kg over 1 minute were followed by infusions of 300 μg/kg/min to maintain the pulse rate between 90 and 110 b.p.m.

If there is heart failure, beta blockers may not be suitable. Amiodarone has been used to treat a tachycardia in a patient with phaeochromocytoma and a cardiomyopathy (Solares et al 1986).

c. Hypotension

May occur after ligation of the main veins from the tumour. Sudden reduction in catecholamine output by the tumour is in part responsible, but hypovolaemia may contribute. Patients with adrenoceptor blockade are particularly sensitive to changes in blood volume. Rapid infusion and CVP monitoring will usually correct the hypotension. If this fails, the use of phenylephrine or dopamine has been suggested (Roizen et al 1982). An infusion of angiotensin II (2.5 mg in 100–1000 ml saline at a rate of 1–20 μg/min) has been used (Sommerville & McKellar 1989). Angiotensin II is an octapeptide produced by the breakdown of angiotensin I, with a half life of 1–2 minutes, and it has a powerful vasoconstrictor action.

6. Phaeochromocytoma during pregnancy

If phaeochromocytoma is diagnosed before delivery, frequently its removal is combined with Caesarean section (Hopkins et al 1989). Antepartum diagnosis reduces the mortality, but unfortunately is only made in about half of the patients (Harper et al 1989).

BIBLIOGRAPHY

Bravo E L, Gifford R W 1984 Pheochromocytoma: diagnosis, localisation and management. New England Journal of Medicine 311: 1298–1303

Brown M J 1987 The measurement of autonomic function in clinical practice. Journal of the Royal College of Physicians 21: 206–209

Cousins M J, Rubin R B 1974 The intraoperative management of phaeochromocytoma with total epidural sympathetic blockade. British Journal of Anaesthesia 46: 78–81

Crowley K J, Cunningham A J, Conroy B et al 1988 Phaeochromocytoma – a presentation mimicking malignant hyperthermia. Anaesthesia 43: 1031–1032

Editorial 1984 Iodobenzylguanidine for location and treatment of phaeochromocytoma. Lancet ii: 905–907

Editorial 1990 Phaeochromocytoma still surprises. Lancet 335: 1189–1190

Gilsanz F J, Luengo C, Conejero P et al 1983 Cardiomyopathy and phaeochromocytoma. Anaesthesia 38: 888–891

Goldfarb D A, Novick A C, Bravo E L et al 1989 Experience with extra-adrenal pheochromocytoma. Journal of Urology 142: 931–936

Harper M A, Murnaghan G A, Kennedy L et al 1989 Phaeochromocytoma in pregnancy. Five cases and a review of the literature. British Journal of Obstetrics and Gynaecology 96: 594–606

Hoffman B B, Lefkowitz R J 1980 Alpha-adrenergic receptor subtypes. New England Journal of Medicine 302: 1390–1396

Hopkins P M, Macdonald R, Lyons G 1989 Caesarean section at 27 weeks gestation with removal of phaeochromocytoma. British Journal of Anaesthesia 63: 121–124

Hull C J 1986 Phaeochromocytoma. Diagnosis, preoperative preparation and management. British Journal of Anaesthesia 58: 1453–1468

Imperato-McGinley J, Gautier T, Ehlers K et al 1987 Reversibility of catecholamine-induced dilated cardiomyopathy in a child with pheochromocytoma. New England Journal of Medicine 316: 793–797

James M F M 1989 Use of magnesium sulphate in the management of phaeochromocytoma: a review of 17 anaesthetics. British Journal of Anaesthesia 62: 616–623

James M F M, Huddle K R L, Owen A D et al 1988 Use of magnesium sulphate in the anaesthetic management of phaeochromocytoma. Canadian Journal of Anaesthesia 35: 178–182

Jones R M, Hill A B 1981 Severe hypertension associated with pancuronium in a patient with phaeochromocytoma. Canadian Anaesthetists' Society Journal 28: 394–396

Levin H, Heifetz M 1990 Phaeochromocytoma and severe protracted hypoglycaemia. Canadian Journal of Anaesthesia 37: 477–478

Liem T H, Moll J E, Booij L H D J 1991 Thoracic epidural analgesia in a patient with bilateral phaeochromocytoma undergoing coronary artery bypass grafting. Anaesthesia 46: 654–658

Mitchell S Z, Freilich J D, Brant D et al 1987 Anesthetic management of pheochromocytoma resection during pregnancy. Anesthesia and Analgesia 66: 478–480

Navaratnarajah M, White D C 1984 Labetalol and phaeochromocytoma. British Journal of Anaesthesia 56: 1179

Nicholson J P, Vaughn E D, Pickering T G et al 1983 Pheochromocytoma and prazosin. Annals of Internal Medicine 99: 477–479

Roizen M F, Horrigan R W, Koike M et al 1982 A prospective randomised trial of four anaesthetic techniques for resection of pheochromocytoma. Anesthesiology 57: A43

Ryan T, Timoney A, Cunningham A J 1993 Use of transoesophageal echocardiography to manage beta-adrenoceptor block and assess left ventricular function in a patient with a phaeochromocytoma. British Journal of Anaesthesia 70: 101–103

Sardesai S H, Mourant A J, Sivathandon Y et al 1990 Phaeochromocytoma and catecholamine-induced cardiomyopathy presenting as heart failure. British Heart Journal 63: 234–237

Solares G, Ramos F, Martin-Duran R et al 1986 Amiodarone, phaeochromocytoma and cardiomyopathy. Anaesthesia 41; 186–190

Sommerville K J, McKellar J B M 1989 Angiotensin II in the management of excision of phaeochromocytoma. Anaesthesia 44: 128–129

Stein P P, Black H R 1991 A simplified diagnostic approach to pheochromocytoma. Medicine 70: 46–66

Sumikawa K, Amakata Y 1977 The pressor effect of droperidol on a patient with pheochromocytoma. Anesthesiology 46: 359–361

Sutton M St J, Sheps S G, Lie J T 1981 Prevalence of clinically unsuspected pheochromocytoma. Mayo Clinic Proceedings 56: 354–360

Tonnesen E, Knudsen F, Nielsen H K et al 1989 Natural killer cell activity in a patient undergoing resection of phaeochromocytoma. British Journal of Anaesthesia 62: 327–330

Wallace J M, Gill D P 1978 Prazosin in diagnosis and treatment of pheochromocytoma. Journal of the American Medical Association 240: 2752–2753

Zakowski M, Kaufman B, Berguson P et al 1989 Esmolol use during resection of pheochromocytoma: report of three cases. Anesthesiology 70: 857–875

PHENYLKETONURIA

One of a group of inborn errors of amino acid metabolism of autosomal recessive inheritance, that involves the essential amino acid, phenylalanine. There is an absence of phenylalanine hydroxylase which catalyzes the conversion of phenylalanine to tyrosine, a reaction which only takes place in the liver, kidney, and pancreas. Protein synthesis is impaired, and the accumulation of phenylalanine in the blood and urine inhibits a number of enzyme systems. There are decreased catecholamine levels, alterations in the metabolism of 5-hydroxytryptamine and interference with melanin synthesis. Early diagnosis and treatment is essential, otherwise irreversible brain damage occurs. Mental retardation is not present at birth, but the metabolic defect becomes evident soon afterwards and, if untreated, brain damage ensues. Nowadays, mass screening means that the majority of cases will have been diagnosed and treated before the onset of brain damage.

Preoperative abnormalities

1. In the undiagnosed or untreated patient there is diffuse and focal demyelination. Clinical features include hyper-reflexia, hypertonia, seizures, behavioural problems, decreased pigmentation secondary to inhibition of melanin synthesis, eczematous skin, progressive loss of hair, and a musty smell. The maxilla is prominent, with gaps between the teeth and enamel abnormalities.
2. The diagnosed patient will have a dietary regimen that includes protein restriction, and the administration of supplementary amino acids with extra tyrosine, together with essential amino acids apart from phenylalanine (Editorial 1991a). A blood phenylalanine level of 100–400 μmol/l is aimed at and this requires close monitoring. However, excessive restriction of phenylalanine will result in protein catabolism, delayed growth, hypoglycaemia and neurological damage. The diet is relaxed, but not stopped, after the age of 8 years but a strict diet must be re-established during pregnancy (Phenylketonuria Symposium 1989).
3. There is evidence that performance on neuropsychological tests and blood phenylalanine levels are inversely correlated (Scriver et al 1989).

Anaesthetic problems

1. If the patient was not diagnosed early, seizures and mental retardation may be a problem.
2. Prolonged perioperative fasting may stimulate catabolism.
3. High blood levels of phenylalanine predispose to fits and behavioural abnormalities.
4. The fragile skin is vulnerable to pressure and friction stresses.

Management

1. Blood phenylalanine levels should be checked within 72 hours of elective surgery to assess adequacy of dietary therapy (Jackson & Millar 1990).
2. The patient should be first on the operating theatre list. A glucose infusion must be started in advance to prevent a catabolic state and a resultant increased phenylalanine levels.

3. If delayed diagnosis has resulted in cerebral impairment, the management is that of a retarded child with a seizure disorder.

BIBLIOGRAPHY
Editorial 1991a Phenylketonuria grows up. Lancet 337: 1256–1257
Editorial 1991b Phenylketonuria – genotypes and phenotpes. New England Journal of Medicine 324: 1280–1281
Jackson S H, Millar W M 1990 Genetic and metabolic diseases. In: Katz J, Benumof J, Kadis L (eds) Anesthesia and uncommon diseases. W B Saunders, Philadelphia
Phenylketonuria Symposium 1989 Phenylketonuria: diagnosis and management. Poceedings of symposium. Postgraduate Medical Journal 65 (suppl 2): S1–26
Scriver C R, Kaufman S, Woo S L C 1989 The hyperphenylalaninemias. In: Scriver et al. (eds) The metabolic basis of inherited disease. McGraw Hill, New York, p. 495– 546

PIERRE ROBIN SYNDROME
(and the ROBIN SEQUENCE)

A rare syndrome in which the combination of severe micrognathia and posterior prolapse of the tongue results in respiratory obstruction in infancy, failure to thrive and, occasionally, cor pulmonale. Other congenital abnormalities such as cleft palate and oesophageal atresia may occur. The 'Robin sequence', a term that is increasingly being used in the specialist surgical literature, describes a spectrum of anomalies, the common features of which include mandibular hypoplasia, glossoptosis and incomplete cleft palate, although all three are not necessarily present. The Robin sequence may be an isolated abnormality, or it may be part of a syndrome. Since there may be airway and intubation problems in any of these patients, several authors have considered them together.

Preoperative abnormalities

1. Many present as difficult or failed intubation at resuscitation following delivery. Hypoxic brain damage may be sustained at this stage. The remainder usually present within a few hours of birth when the micrognathia and glossoptosis cause breathing and feeding difficulties, with episodes of cyanosis when the child is in the supine position. Subsequently there is failure to thrive.
2. Cleft palate occurs in 60%, and eye problems in 40% of patients with the Pierre Robin syndrome.
3. Chronic upper airway obstruction can result in cor pulmonale (Mallory & Paradise 1979). An increased pulmonary artery pressure may produce right-to-left shunting through a patent foramen ovale or a persistent ductus arteriosus. Anaesthesia for cardiac catheterization in an infant with cor pulmonale, and subsequent management of the airway obstruction for a month by means of a nasopharyngeal tube, has been described (Freeman & Manners 1980).

4. Obstructive sleep apnoea has been reported (Brouillette et at 1982).
5. A sequence of strategies is recommended in an attempt to minimize
   respiratory obstruction and allow safe feeding. The treatment
   required depends upon severity. Initially, the infant is nursed in the
   prone position. If this fails, prolonged nasopharyngeal intubation
   may help to protect the airway (Sher 1992). Should respiratory
   distress and failure to thrive persist, and lateral X-ray of the neck in
   the supine position shows upper airway obstruction, suturing of the
   tongue to the lower gum or lip (tongue-to-lip adhesion) may be
   needed (Augarten et al 1990). Feeding may be undertaken via a
   nasogastric tube or a gastrostomy. Respiration and oxygen saturation
   are monitored, and appropriate oxygen supplementation given.
   Occasionally tracheostomy is required, although previously there has
   been reluctance to resort to this. Benjamin & Walker (1991), in a
   10-year retrospective study of 26 patients, classified them into three
   groups according to treatment required: mild (needing posture
   alone), moderate (needing nasopharyngeal tube), and severe
   (needing tracheal intubation or tracheostomy). All of the deaths
   occurred in this latter group (5 out of 11), one from hypoxic brain
   damage at birth, 2 whilst still intubated and 2 others who had
   tracheostomies.

As the child grows, the obstruction tends to improve, partly from
growth of the mandible and the size of the airway, and partly as a result
of better neurological control of the tongue muscles. Problems mainly
seem to resolve by the time the child is 6 months old. In one series
(Benjamin & Walker 1991), mild cases could be nursed supine from 3–6
months (mean 5.6 months). In the moderate group, nasopharyngeal
intubation was required for between 14 days and 14 weeks, after which
infants were nursed prone. All could sleep supine by 6 months.

Anaesthetic problems

1. Even in the unanaesthetized infant, during the first few months of
   life, respiratory obstruction occurs in the supine position.
   Glossoptosis, the prolapse of the tongue backwards, was thought to
   be the main mechanism for this, but the aetiology is now
   appreciated to be multifactorial. Sher (1992) believes the obstruction
   to be related to a combination of the anatomical abnormalities of the
   mandible, with functional impairment of the genioglossus and other
   pharyngeal muscles that are concerned with maintenance of the
   airway. Varying degrees of obstruction exist, ranging from none at
   all, to obstruction when the infant is asleep and, in the worst cases,
   obstruction in the awake state. In any infant, obstruction is
   exacerbated by an upper respiratory tract infection, and during
   feeding or crying. In addition, studies suggest that the site of

obstruction varies from patient to patient. From endoscopic observations, these have been classified (Sher 1992) as:

Type 1: A true glossoptosis in which the dorsum of the tongue is apposed to the posterior pharyngeal wall.

Type 2: The tongue compresses the soft palate against the posterior pharyngeal wall, so that all three structures meet in the upper oropharynx.

Type 3: Medial apposition of the lateral pharyngeal walls.

Type 4: A sphincteric constriction of the pharynx

2. Oxygen desaturation and obstructive sleep apnoea, detected by pulse oximetry and polysonography, occurs in the majority of infants and contributes to the mortality from obstruction (Bull et al 1990).
3. Gastro-oesophageal reflux may be present (Bull et al 1990).
4. The unusual facial configuration, in particular, the receding lower jaw, makes it difficult to maintain an airtight fit with an anaesthetic mask.
5. Difficulties in tracheal intubation result from a combination of micrognathia, and prolapse or inward sucking of the posteriorly attached, and often enlarged, tongue.
6. Pulmonary oedema has occurred after relief of airway obstruction following palatal repair in an 8-month-old baby (Lynch & Underwood 1991).

Management

1. Monitoring by pulse oximetry, to detect airway obstruction, is crucial.
2. The importance of an individualized approach to airway management for assessment or surgery has been stressed (Benjamin & Walker 1991). A number of methods to overcome the problem of difficult intubation have been proposed, some under general anaesthesia and some in the awake patient. The consensus of opinion now seems to favour awake techniques.
   a. Asleep technique with a special laryngoscope. Handler and Keon (1983) describe a technique for intubation for the anaesthetized spontaneously breathing patient, in which a Jackson anterior commissure laryngoscope is used. The head is elevated above the shoulders, with flexion of the lower cervical vertebrae and extension at the atlanto-occipital joint. The laryngoscope is introduced into the right side of the mouth. Only the tip is directed towards the midline, the proximal end remaining laterally, so that a further 30° of anterior angulation can be obtained. The narrow closed blade prevents the tongue from falling in and obscuring the view of the larynx. When visualized, the epiglottis is elevated, and the larynx entered. Intubation is then achieved by passing a lubricated tube, without its adaptor,

down the laryngoscope. It is then held in place with alligator forceps whilst the laryngoscope is withdrawn.

b. Asleep technique in the prone position. The appreciation of the problems in the supine position led to the description of a successful blind nasal intubation with the patient prone (Populaire et al 1985). This position allows the tongue and mandible to fall forward under the effect of gravity and leave the larynx exposed.

c. Fibreoptic bronchoscopic techniques. A variety of fibreoptic techniques have been described (Howardy-Hansen & Berthelsen 1988, Sher 1992). In small infants, the 'tube over bronchoscope' technique is not always possible because of the small size of the tube, therefore a Seldinger type approach may be necessary. Paediatric bronchoscopes of 2.5 mm diameter are now available, but their very fineness makes them less easy to handle than the 4 mm bronchoscopes. After the administration of atropine, ketamine i.m. and topical lignocaine, a fibreoptic bronchoscope (OD 3.6 mm, L 60 cm and suction channel 1.2 mm) was passed through one nostril. The tongue was held forward with Magill forceps until the vocal cords were seen, but not entered, because of the risk of total obstruction. Under direct vision, a Teflon-coated guide wire with a flexible tip was passed via the suction channel into the trachea. The bronchoscope was carefully removed leaving the wire in place, and a 3-mm nasotracheal tube then passed over it into the trachea.

d. Awake intubation techniques using a special laryngoscope. The use of a special purpose slotted laryngoscope (Holiger paediatric anterior commissure laryngoscope Karl Storz, Tuttlingen, FRG) has been described (Benjamin & Walker 1991).

e. Laryngeal mask techniques. The use of a laryngeal mask airway in an emergency, to guide an introducer for subsequent intubation, has been reported (Chadd et al 1992). Elective placement of the laryngeal mask airway following topical anaesthesia in three awake infants has also been described (Markakis et al 1992).

BIBLIOGRAPHY

Augarten A, Sagy M, Yahav J, et al 1990 Management of upper airway obstruction in the Pierre Robin syndrome. British Journal of Oral and Maxillofacial Surgery 28: 105–108.

Beniamin B, Walker P 1991 Management of airway obstruction in the Pierre Robin sequence. Internal Journal of Pediatric Otorhinolaryngology 22: 29–37

Brouillette R T, Fernbach S K, Hunt C E 1982 Obstructive sleep apnea in infants and children. Journal of Pediatrics 100: 31–40

Bull M J, Givan D C, Sadove A M, et al 1990 Improved outcome in Pierre Robin sequence: effect of multidisciplinary evaluation and management. Pediatrics 86: 294–301

Chadd G D, Crane D L, Phillips P M et al 1992 Extubation and reintubation guided by the laryngeal mask airway in a child with Pierr–Robin syndrome. Anesthesiology 76: 640–641

Freeman M K Manners J M 1980 Cor pulmonale and the Pierre Robin anomaly. Anaesthesia 35: 282–286

Handler S D, Keon T P 1983 Difficult laryngoscopy/intubation: the child with mandibular hypoplasia. Annals of Otology, Rhinology and Laryngology 92: 401–404

Howardy-Hansen P, Berthelsen P 1988 Fibreoptic bronchoscopic nasotracheal intubation of a neonate with Pierre Robin syndrome. Anaesthesia 43: 121–122

Lynch M, Underwood S 1991 Pulmonary oedema following the relief of upper airway obstruction in the Pierre-Robin syndrome. British Journal of Anaesthesia 66: 391–393

Mallory S B, Paradise J L 1979 Glossoptosis revisited: on the development and resolution of airway obstruction in the Pierre-Robin syndrome. Pediatrics 64: 946–948

Markakis D A, Sayson S C, Schreiner M S 1992 Insertion of the laryngeal mask airway in awake infants with the Robin sequence. Anesthesia and Analgesia 75: 822–824

Populaire C, Lundi J N, Pinaud M et al 1985 Elective tracheal intubation in the prone position for a neonate with Pierre-Robin syndrome. Anesthesioiogy 62: 214–215

Sher A E 1992 Mechanisms of airway obstruction in Robin sequence: implications for treatment. Cleft Palat-Craniofacial Journal 29: 224–231

PITUITARY APOPLEXY

A term used to describe a complication of a pituitary adenoma. Sudden enlargement secondary to haemorrhage, infarction, or both, in a previously undiagnosed tumour, results in symptoms and signs of compression of adjacent intracranial structures. The optic chiasma and cranial nerves, in particular the third, fourth, fifth and sixth cranial nerves, may be involved. Pituitary apoplexy can be of sudden onset and life-threatening in nature, or symptoms and signs may evolve gradually over a couple of weeks. A number of predisposing factors have been suggested. Sometimes pituitary apoplexy has followed surgery, mostly after cardiopulmonary bypass.

Preoperative abnormalities

1. Headache, ophthalmoplegia and visual disturbances may be associated with meningism, vomiting and impaired conscious level. The clinical picture can be suggestive of subarachnoid haemorrhage.
2. There may be a varying pattern of associated endocrine disorders. However, these are usually mild and previously unnoticed.
3. Radiological signs might suggest an expanded pituitary fossa or an empty sella turcica (Editorial 1986).
4. The differential diagnosis includes intracranial or subarachnoid haemorrhage, brain abscess or cavernous sinus thrombosis.
5. Diagnosis may be made by CT scan, which is most helpful in the early days after haemorrhage, or MRI, which is more sensitive in the subacute or chronic stages (Ostrov et al 1989).
6. There may be predisposing factors such as trauma, anticoagulation, radiotherapy, IPPV or cardiac surgery.

Anaesthetic problems

1. Pituitary apoplexy has presented with a variety of neurological symptoms and signs following surgery. The majority of cases have been associated with cardiac surgery (Cooper et al 1986, Shapiro 1990) although on one occasion it occurred after cholecystectomy performed under combined general and extradural anaesthesia (Yahagi et al 1992). The exact sequence of events is unknown, but the adenoma may have a relatively compromised blood supply (Cooper et al 1986), possibly secondary to tumour compression or pathological abnormalities of the vessels. It is thus susceptible to ischaemia secondary to reduced perfusion pressure during surgery, to the effects of microemboli, or to haemorrhage occurring as a result of incomplete reversal of anticoagulants.

2. The problems of making a differential diagnosis when cerebral symptoms and signs of sudden onset, including deterioration in conscious level, follow surgery.

3. Hormone abnormalities may be present. These include panhypopituitarism with amenorrhoea, galactorrhoea and elevated prolactin levels, and hypothyroidism.

Management

1. If neurological symptoms and signs follow surgery, a neurosurgeon or neurologist should be consulted. Urgent CT or MRI scans may be necessary to establish the diagnosis.

2. If there is evidence of an expanding adenoma, pituitary decompression surgery may be required (Yahagi et al 1992, Shapiro 1990). Initially corticosteroids should be given in an attempt to reduce any associated oedema.

3. Pituitary hormone function should be investigated since hormonal replacement with thyroxine or steroids may be required.

BIBLIOGRAPHY

Cardoso E R, Peterson E W 1984 Pituitary apoplexy: a review. Neurosurgery 14: 363–373

Cooper D M, Bazaral M G, Furlan A J et al 1986 Pituitary apoplexy: a complication of cardiac surgery. Annals of Thoracic Surgery 41: 547–550

Editorial 1986 Pituitary tumours and the empty sella syndrome. Lancet ii: 1371–1372

Fraioli B, Exposito V, Palam L et al 1990 Hemorrhagic pituitary adenomas: clinicopathological features and surgical treatment. Neurosurgery 27: 741–748

Lewin I G, Mohan J, Norman P F et al 1988 Pituitary apoplexy. British Medical Journal 297: 1526–1527

McFadzean R M, Doyle D, Rampling R et al 1991 Pituitary apoplexy and its effect on vision. Neurosurgery 29: 669–675

Ostrov S G, Quencer R M, Hoffman J C, et al 1989 Hemorrhage within pituitary adenomas: how often associated with pituitary apoplexy syndrome? American Journal of Roentgenology 153: 153–160

Shapiro L M 1990 Pituitary apoplexy following coronary artery by pass surgery. Journal of Surgical Oncology 44: 66–68

Yahagi N, Nishikawa A, Matsui S et al 1992 Pituitary apoplexy following
cholecystectomy. Anaesthesia 47: 234–236.

PLASMA CHOLINESTERASE ABNORMALITIES
(see also Section 2)

Plasma cholinesterase (ChE) is present in plasma and most other tissues, apart from erythrocytes, and is an enzyme capable of hydrolyzing many esters. It must be distinguished from acetylcholinesterase (AChE), which is found in erythrocytes and at the neuromuscular junction. ChE is a protein manufactured in the liver and its half-life is thought to be approximately 8–12 days. No physiological role for the enzyme has as yet been unequivocally demonstrated.

Its anaesthetic significance lies in the fact that it hydrolyzes the depolarizing neuromuscular blocker suxamethonium, thus terminating its action after 1–5 minutes. In the presence of normal ChE activity, a two-stage hydrolysis of suxamethonium occurs.

$$succinyl\ dicholine + water \rightarrow succinyl\ monocholine + choline$$
$$\downarrow$$
$$succinic\ acid + choline$$

If there is a low level of normal plasma cholinesterase (normal level = 3700–11 500 iu/l), or if the cholinesterase is abnormal, prolonged apnoea may occur. In either case, following suxamethonium administration, the duration of muscle paralysis can vary from about 10 minutes to 2 hours. Decreased ChE activity may be due to genetic variants of the enzyme, pre-existing disease, or iatrogenic causes.

Genetic variants

Plasma cholinesterase synthesis is controlled by two allelic genes, the normal genotype being designated $E_1^u\ E_1^u$. There are several genetic defects which result in an individual having a diminished ability to metabolize suxamethonium (Whittaker 1980).

Differentiation between the normal and an atypical cholinesterase was first demonstrated by comparing the rates at which each hydrolyzed benzoylcholine, in the presence of varying concentrations of an inhibitor, dibucaine. The percentage inhibition by a 10^{-5} molar concentration of dibucaine is known as the dibucaine number. Homozygous individuals for the atypical (or dibucaine-resistant) genotype ($E_1^a\ E_1^a$) have a dibucaine number of about 20, heterozygotes ($E_1^u\ E_1^a$) about 60, and those with normal enzyme, about 80. Further genetic variants have subsequently been found. These include a 'silent' gene, E_1^s, which has little or no enzymic activity, and a fluoride-resistant gene, E_1^f. The fluoride number is determined in a similar way to the dibucaine number, but sodium fluoride is used as the inhibitor.

The distribution of the genotypes in suxamethonium-sensitive individuals has been studied by Whittaker and Britten (1987). So far, more than 12 genotypes have been recognized. Since ChE is a large molecule of four polypeptide chains, it is likely that further variants will be described.

The main categories of subjects sensitive to suxamethonium have the genotypes $E_1^a E_1^a$ and $E_1^a E_1^s$ and their frequency is about 1 in 1800.

Disease states

Low levels of normal enzyme have been reported in association with a number of pathological conditions. These include severe liver disease, malnutrition, renal failure, malignant disease, tetanus, Huntington's chorea and collagen disorders. It has also been described in Churg-Strauss syndrome (Taylor et al 1990), although in the cases reported, it may have been associated with the immunosuppressive therapy.

Pregnancy

In late pregnancy, there may also be decreased ChE activity, although not necessarily to such a degree as to produce clinical problems. However, two circumstances have been reported in which problems may arise.

1. The use of plasmapheresis in the treatment of rhesus isoimmunization is associated with marked reduction in maternal ChE activity (Whittaker et al 1988). A patient with a normal phenotype was reported to have been apnoeic for 50 minutes following suxamethonium 75 mg. This was given during a Caesarean section undertaken 2 days after the seventh plasmapheresis, and was associated with extremely low ChE activity (Evans et al 1980).

2. The heterozygous patient. Pregnancy can also cause clinically detectable apnoea in a heterozygous patient, which would not normally be manifested in the non-pregnant state, and especially if a suxamethonium infusion is used (Whittaker et al 1988).

Iatrogenic causes

Reported iatrogenic associations include radiotherapy, renal dialysis, plasmapheresis, cardiac bypass, ecothiopate eye drops, oral contraceptives, propanidid, neostigmine, pyridostigmine chlorpromazine, pancuronium, metoclopramide and exposure to organophosphorus compounds. Cancer patients undergoing chemotherapy may have ChE levels that are low enough to prolong neuromuscular blockade if suxamethonium is used (Ragasa et al 1989).

Anaesthetic problems

1. In individuals with suxamethonium sensitivity, varying lengths of apnoea can follow the administration of suxamethonium. Apnoea from this cause may be distinguished from that due to other causes, by the use of a peripheral nerve stimulator. A cumulative dose-response curve in a patient with low plasma cholinesterase activity showed the increased potency of the drug to be four to seven times that of a normal individual (Smith et al 1989).
2. There are changes in plasma cholinesterase levels during pregnancy, so that heterozygous individuals may become sensitive to suxamethonium. There is evidence that metoclopramide is a powerful inhibitor of plasma cholinesterase, therefore patients receiving both this and suxamethonium should be carefully monitored (Kao et al 1990).
3. If suxamethonium sensitivity is confirmed, subsequent investigation of the patient, and if possible his close relatives, is required.

Management

1. When spontaneous respiration fails to return after the administration of suxamethonium, IPPV should be continued. Light anaesthesia must be maintained to prevent the patient becoming distressed. The presence of a neuromuscular blockade should be confirmed with a peripheral nerve stimulator. This is most important because about 30% of patients referred to the Cholinesterase Research Unit have a normal phenotype. The routine use of a nerve stimulator might influence this figure. IPPV should be continued until adequate respiration can be maintained. Treatment with fresh frozen plasma (Gill et al 1991) and a purified form of human cholinesterase (Benzer et al 1992) have been reported but their use is controversial.
2. When the patient has recovered, detailed anaesthetic, family, and drug histories should be taken. A simple explanation of the need for further investigation should be given.
3. Plasma cholinesterase activity, and dibucaine and fluoride numbers should be investigated. Whilst this may be done in a local laboratory, there are advantages of using the service provided by the Cholinesterase Research Unit.

   A rapid service can be obtained, by sending 10 ml heparinized or whole blood, or separated plasma or serum, by first-class post, to Dr J Britten, Cholinesterase Research Unit, Royal Postgraduate Medical School, Hammersmith Hospital, London (Whittaker & Britten 1987).
4. If the results are abnormal, the patient's notes should be clearly marked and the general practitioner informed.

Section 1

Plasma
Cholinesterase
Abnormalities

BIBLIOGRAPHY
Benzer A, Luz G, Oswald E, Schmoigl C, Menardi G 1992 Succinylcholine-induced

prolonged apnea in a 3-week-old newborn: treatment with human plasma cholinesterase. Anesthesia and Analgesia 74: 137–138

Evans R T, MacDonald R, Robinson A 1980 Suxamethonium apnoea associated with plasmaphoresis. Anaesthesia 35: 198–201.

Gill R S, O'Connell N, Scott R P F 1991 Reversal of prolonged suxamethonium opnoea with fresh frozen plasma in a six-week-old infant. Anaesthesia 46: 1036–1038

Kao Y J, Tellez J, Turner D R 1990 Dose-dependent effect of metoclopramide on cholinesterases and suxamethonium metabolism. British Journal of Anaesthesia 65: 220–224

Ragasa J, Shah N K, Crystal D et al 1989 Plasma cholinesterase levels in cancer patients treated with chemotherapy. Anesthesia and Analgesia 68: S229

Smith C E, Lewis G, Donati F et al 1989 Dose-response relationship for succinylcholine in a patient with genetically determined low plasma cholinesterase activiry Anesthesiology 70: 156–158

Taylor B L, Whittaker M, Van Heerden V et al 1990 Cholinesterase deficiency and the Churg–Strauss syndrome. Anaesthesia 45: 649–652

Whittaker M 1980 Plasma cholinesterase variants and the anaesthetist. Anaesthesia 35: 174–197

Whittaker M, Britten J J 1987 Phenotyping of individuals sensitive to suxamethonium. British Journal of Anaesthesia 59: 1052–1055

Whittaker M, Crawford I S, Lewis M 1988 Some observations of levels of plasma cholinesterase activity within an obstetric population. Anaesthesia 43: 42–45

POLYCYTHAEMIA VERA

Polycythaemia is a general term for an increased haemoglobin (Hb>17 g/dl in men and >16 g/dl in women), an increased red cell count, or packed cell volume (>0.51 in men and >0.47 in women). It can be relative, (in which there is an increased Hb and PCV, a normal red cell mass but a reduction in plasma volume), apparent (an increased Hb and PCV, a normal red cell mass and normal plasma volume) or absolute (in which the increased Hb and PCV is associated with an increased red cell mass). Absolute polycythaemia can be primary or secondary. Causes of secondary polycythaemia include pulmonary disease, cyanotic heart disease and inappropriate production of erythropoietin. The primary disease, polycythaemia vera, is a neoplastic condition and is one of the chronic myeloproliferative disorders. It is associated with abnormal haemostasis, abnormal platelet function, hyperviscosity and reduced organ blood flow. As a result of these abnormalities, surgery in untreated polycythaemia vera carries a high risk of either thrombotic or bleeding complications.

Preoperative abnormalities

1. Occurs most commonly in men, usually over 50 years of age. Patients can present with a range of symptoms due to hyperviscosity, a thrombotic or a bleeding episode, or a high haemoglobin level found on routine testing.
2. Splenomegaly, hepatomegaly, and hypertension are common.
3. Haematological abnormalities include a raised haemoglobin level, an increased red cell mass and packed cell volume (50–70%), and often

a leucocytosis and thrombocythaemia. A venous haematocrit of >0.50 in males and >0.47 in females should warrant further investigation (Pearson 1980). A higher incidence of vascular occlusion is found when the platelet count is $>400 \times 10^9/l$ (Pearson 1980). The diagnosis should also be considered in patients with a normal haemoglobin but a microcytosis. This may be secondary to slow blood loss from the gastrointestinal tract, resulting in severe iron deficiency.

4. Platelet function may be abnormal.
5. Hyperuricaemia and secondary gout is common.
6. The method of treatment is controversial. It may involve venesection to keep the PCV below 50%, radioactive phosphorus, busulphan or hydroxyurea.

Anaesthetic problems

1. Polycythaemia carries an increased surgical and anaesthetic risk. The level at which this risk begins is debatable, but it has been suggested that levels above 17 g/dl for men and 16 g/dl for women require an explanation (Irving 1991). An early study showed that 79% of untreated patients whose haemoglobin was greater than 17 g/dl had postoperative thrombotic or haemorrhagic problems, with a 43% morbidity and a 36% mortality (Wasserman & Gilbert 1964). These figures contrasted with a group whose polycythaemia had been controlled for more than 4 months, in whom there was a morbidity of only 5% and no deaths.

2. Polycythaemia vera is associated with thrombotic complications, and the patient's first presentation may be for emergency surgery. In a study involving 200 patients, nearly 50% presented with vascular complications (Barabas 1980). Seventy-eight arterial complications occurred in 68 patients, 66 venous complications in 57 patients, and there were 27 patients who had both. Distal arterial disease is more common than that involving major vessels.

3. Despite the fact that polycythaemia vera is primarily a thrombotic condition, bleeding can also occur as a result of abnormal platelet function. A history of recurrent epistaxis is common, and gastrointestinal haemorrhage may occur. One patient presented with a spontaneous retropharyngeal haematoma, and emergency tracheal intubation for airway obstruction was required (Mackenzie & Jellicoe 1986). Patients with polycythaemia may occasionally be anaemic, secondary to bleeding, in which case the diagnosis may not be immediately obvious.

4. Increases in total blood volume and the presence of a high blood viscosity increase both the cardiac output, and the work of the heart. Cerebral blood flow is low, and this contributes to the high incidence of cerebrovascular occlusion.

5. Cyanosis occurs readily.

6. In the emergency case, the main problem is to decide whether or not a patient with a high haemoglobin and a raised haematocrit has the primary condition, or a polycythaemia secondary to respiratory disease. In the first case cerebral blood flow will be low, and venesection is appropriate, while in the second, cerebral blood flow may actually be increased. One hundred patients with Hb>16 g/dl resulting from chronic obstructive pulmonary disease and 100 matched controls were compared for thrombotic and haemorrhagic complications in the first postoperative month (Lubarsky et al 1991). No differences were found between the groups and it was concluded that secondary polycythaemia did not increase postoperative risk, although the authors acknowledged that the study was retrospective, the groups were small, and few patients with extreme Hb values were included. However, these results might have been expected simply on consideration of the basic pathological processes. Secondary polycythaemia is not accompanied by abnormal haemostasis or reduced cerebral blood flow, both of which are characteristics of polycythaemia vera and are most probably responsible for the complications.

7. However, secondary polycythaemia may be associated with other problems, since it may result from daytime and nocturnal hypoxaemia. More recently, it has been shown that nocturnal oxygen desaturation can also occur in some patients with apparent and relative polycythaemia (Messinezy et al 1991). Sixteen patients were studied and in the four who had nocturnal desaturation, supine daytime oximetry showed an oxygen saturation of less than 92% on air.

Management

1. If a high haemoglobin level and an increased haematocrit is found, arterial blood gases may assist in the diagnosis. The presence of hypoxia or hypercarbia suggests a respiratory cause. Other causes of secondary polycythaemia should be sought. Nocturnal oximetry may indicate obstructive sleep apnoea, and correction of hypoxia may abolish polycythaemia. If polycythaemia vera is likely, elective surgery should be postponed until there is medical control of the condition. It has been suggested that the peripheral blood picture and the blood volume should be normal for at least 4 months preoperatively (Barabas 1980).

2. If emergency surgery is required, venesection should be performed and the blood replaced with the same volume of PPF or colloid. Cerebral blood flow is increased as the venous haematocrit is reduced (Pearson 1980).

3. Prevention of venous stasis.

4. Extremes of hypotension and hypertension should be avoided.
5. Anticoagulants are inadvisable, since bleeding may occur.

BIBLIOGRAPHY
Barabas A P 1980 Surgical problems associated with polycythaemia. British Journal of Hospital Medicine 23: 289–294
Irving G 1991 Polycythaemia and the anaesthetist. South African Medical Journal 80: 418–419
Lubarsky D A, Gallagher C J, Berend J L 1991 Secondary polycythemia does not increase the risk of perioperative hemorrhagic or thrombotic complications. Journal of Clinical Anesthesia 3: 99–103
Mackenzie J W, Jellicoe J A 1986 Acute upper airway obstruction. Spontaneous retropharyngeal haemorrhage in a patient with polycythaemia rubra vera. Anaesthesia 41: 57–59
Messinezy M, Aubry S, O'Connell G, et al 1991 Oxygen desaturation in apparent and relative polycythaemia. British Medical Journal 302: 216–217
Pearson T C 1980 Who should you treat for polycythaemia? British Journal of Hospital Medicine 24: 66–73
Wasserman L R, Gilbert H S 1964 Surgery in polycythemia vera. New England Journal of Medicine 269: 1226–1230

POMPE'S DISEASE

A glycogen storage disease, type IIa, in which there is a deficiency of alpha-1,4-glucosidase (acid maltase). This enzyme is present in lysosomes and involved in glycogen breakdown. Glycogen deposits are found in cardiac, skeletal and smooth muscle, kidney, liver, spleen, brain, spinal cord and tongue. Three different modes of presentation are now recognized (Hers et al 1989). The most severely affected patients present with cardiac failure in the first 3 months of life, and usually die in the first year. There is a less severe form appearing in infancy, with death before adulthood. A third form presents as a myopathy in the 20–40 year age group. Anaesthesia may be required for diagnostic muscle biopsy, cardiac catheterization or bronchoscopy.

Preoperative abnormalities

1. There is generalized hypotonia and muscle weakness, although muscle mass is normal.
2. The heart is greatly enlarged as a result of a hypertrophic cardiomyopathy. Outflow obstruction secondary to enlargement of the interventricular septum occurs in 50% of patients. Murmurs are usually absent. Cardiac failure rapidly supervenes.
3. CXR shows massive biventricular hypertrophy. Lobar collapse is common due to bronchial obstruction.
4. ECG shows a short PR interval (>0.09 seconds) and massive, wide QRS complexes.
5. Glucose, lactate and lipid levels are normal. Muscle enzymes are moderately increased.

6. In the most severe form of the disease, cardiorespiratory failure, pulmonary aspiration, and pneumonia all contribute towards death.

Anaesthetic problems

1. Problems associated with cardiomyopathies and cardiac failure. Inhalational induction with halothane resulted in bradycardia and ventricular fibrillation in a 5-month-old baby (McFarlane & Soni 1986) and cardiac arrest occurred in a child having a muscle biopsy (Ellis 1980). In the latter case, the diagnosis of Pompe's disease was only made at postmortem examination. Outflow tract obstruction often occurs, and the diseased muscle of the ventricles cannot compensate by hypertrophy and increased contractility. Massive cardiomegaly may produce lobar collapse by bronchial compression.
2. Muscle weakness can predispose to respiratory failure.
3. Macroglossia may occur and can cause upper airway obstruction and difficult intubation. Protrusion of the tongue secondary to respiratory distress can give a false impression of macroglossia (McFarlane & Soni 1986).
4. Impaired neurological function depresses cough and swallowing reflexes and predisposes to aspiration, atelectasis, and pneumonia. All these factors may contribute to hypoxia.
5. Patients are sensitive to respiratory depressants.

Management

1. If there is a hypertrophic cardiomyopathy, appropriate management should be undertaken (see Cardiomyopathies). It is important to monitor the patient carefully and avoid hypoxia (McFarlane & Soni 1986). Two anaesthetics were given to the same patient a week apart. The first, a halothane induction, began without monitoring and ended with ventricular fibrillation and abandonment of the procedure. In the second, uneventful anaesthetic, there was direct arterial monitoring. Subsequent induction was established with ketamine and vecuronium and the patient's lungs were ventilated.

    Ketamine, halothane, and suxamethonium were used successfully on different occasions in two patients (Kaplan 1980). However, on the evidence of a limited number of case reports, induction with halothane in these patients may be hazardous. Whether this was associated with the effect of halothane on the myocardium, or with hypoxia secondary to airway obstruction, is impossible to judge. Undoubtedly, if tracheal intubation and control of respiration are rapidly achieved, this will reduce the potential for hypoxia and the need for high concentrations of inhalation agents.
2. In view of the risk of hyperkalaemia or rhabdomyolysis, doubts have been cast on the wisdom of using suxamethonium in a patient with any myopathy.

3. It has been suggested that neuromuscular blockers may not be required, since muscle hypotonia facilitates IPPV.
4. A local anaesthetic technique should be considered. Diagnostic muscle biopsy has been described using a modified femoral nerve block and a peripheral nerve stimulator. Ketamine was used for sedation (Rosen & Broadman 1986). Caudal anaesthesia has also been suggested as a suitable technique (Kaplan 1980).
5. If macroglossia is present, and the possibility of difficult intubation exists, awake intubation may be advisable.

BIBLIOGRAPHY
Ellis F R 1980 Inherited muscle disease. British Journal of Anaesthesia 52: 153–164
Hers H G van Hoof F, de Barsy T 1989 Glycogen storage diseases. In: Scriver C R, Beaudet A L, Sly W S, Valle D (eds) The metabolic basis of inherited disease. McGraw Hill, New York
Kaplan R 1980 Pompe's disease presenting for anesthesia. Anesthesiology Review 7: 21–28
McFarlane H J, Soni N 1986 Pompe's disease and anaesthesia. Anaesthesia 41: 1219–1224
Rosen K R, Broadman L M 1986 Anaesthesia for diagnostic muscle biopsy in an infant with Pompe's disease. Canadian Anaesthetists' Society Journal 33: 790–794

PORPHYRIA

A group of disorders of porphyrin metabolism resulting from defects in certain enzymes involved in the synthesis of haem. They may be inherited or acquired. Although porphyria is very rare in the UK, one type variegate porphyria (VP), is common in certain regions of South Africa, whilst in Sweden and Finland both acute intermittent porphyria (AIP) and VP are relatively common. As a result, much of the clinical and experimental work on the subject originates from these countries.

Haem, which is synthesized in the liver, bone marrow, and erythrocytes, is required for the manufacture of haemoglobin, myoglobin and a number of other respiratory pigments, such as the cytochrome enzymes.

In the hepatic porphyrias, only the liver is involved in the abnormality of haem synthesis. It is this group of porphyrias which is of particular concern to the anaesthetist, and only they are discussed here. In each of these, there is a different relative deficiency of one of the enzymes involved in the hepatic synthesis of haem. The majority of haem manufactured by the liver is used in the biosynthesis of the cytochrome P–450 enzyme system. This system is important for drug metabolism.

The administration of certain drugs to patients with porphyria can, on occasions, result in serious neurological defects. Most of the drugs which are potentially dangerous in porphyria can increase delta-aminolaevulinic acid (ALA) synthase activity. This is the first enzyme required to initiate the sequence which results in the manufacture of haem. These drugs are usually lipid soluble, and to assist their excretion by the kidneys, they require transformation into water-soluble compounds by the cytochrome P-450 enzyme system. The presence of any of these drugs can therefore increase the activity of this system. In other words, they share the common property of being enzyme inducers of the cytochrome P-450 system. A demand for haem secondary to this induction of cytochrome P-450, results in a feedback mechanism stimulating further production of ALA synthase. The hepatic haem metabolic pathway is thus stimulated, but because the underlying enzyme deficiencies cannot fully cope with this extra activity, there is an accumulation of certain porphyrins or precursors at specific levels in the metabolic chain. These levels will vary according to the particular relative enzyme deficiency.

The exact relationship between the biochemistry, and the clinical features of the porphyric crises and neurological deficits, is not known. However, there are characteristic pathological lesions in the central nervous system, the spinal cord, and the autonomic ganglia. Axon degeneration and demyelination are particular features. It has been suggested that the signs and symptoms of porphyria can be entirely attributed to neurological damage (Laiwah et al 1987). However, porphyrin precursors do not seem to be the main cause of the neurotoxicity, as has been previously postulated. Existing evidence suggests that the nervous system lesions are primarily due to a deficiency of haem, whilst neurotoxicity secondary to increased levels of ALA may be an additional factor in their evolution.

Although some patients still die during acute attacks, recent long-term studies show that the frequency of attacks is less common than before 1967, and the mortality lower (Kauppinen & Mustajoki 1992). Morbidity and mortality are most often associated with delay in diagnosis or failure of treatment. Porphyria has been associated with an increased incidence of hepatocellular carcinoma, hypertension, and acute renal failure

Preoperative abnormalities

1. The clinical and biochemical features of the hepatic porphyrias rarely appear before puberty, and some patients remain permanently asymptomatic. Symptoms, which depend on the particular type of porphyria, may involve the gastrointestinal tract, the nervous system, and the skin. Intermittent acute crises, which may result in severe neurological deficits and occasionally death, may be precipitated by a variety of drugs including alcohol. Crises may also be associated with menstruation, acute infection, fasting, and pregnancy (Harrison & McAuley 1992).
2. Clinical features of the individual types of porphyria
   a. Acute intermittent porphyria (AIP) is an autosomal dominant condition in which there is a reduction in porphobilinogen

deaminase. During an attack there are increased amounts of ALA and porphobilinogen produced and excreted. AIP often presents with episodes of acute abdominal pain, vomiting and pyrexia in adult life. Peripheral sensory and motor deficits, cranial nerve palsies, and autonomic disturbances may occur. There may be severe neuropsychiatric manifestations, including hallucinations, mental changes, and epilepsy. In adults with AIP, the risk of attacks has been found to correlate with the excretion of porphobilinogen in the urine. A low excretion of porphyrins predicted low risk (Kauppinen & Mustajoki 1992).

b. Hereditary coproporphyria (HC) is a rare condition which is similar to AIP. There is a deficiency of coproporphyrinogen oxidase, so that coproporphyrin levels may be elevated, in addition to those of ALA and porphobilinogen.

c. Variegate porphyria (VP) results from a deficiency of protoporphyrinogen oxidase; the enzymatic block is therefore one step further on from that in HC. Cutaneous lesions are also present in this condition, commonly on the hands and face. Photosensitivity causing blisters is due to the presence of certain porphyrins in the skin.

3. In the screening test for porphobilinogen the patient's urine turns dark red on the addition of Ehrlich's aldehyde. Specific tests exist for different precursors and/or porphyrins to elicit the exact type of porphyria.

4. Acute crises can vary in length from hours to days. Tachycardia and hypertension may occur during an attack.

5. Haematin, which suppresses ALA synthase activity, has been used to relieve the symptoms of porphyria.

Anaesthetic problems

1. Drug porphyrinogenicity

   A wide range of drugs possess a potential for increasing the production of porphyrins or their precursors, thus precipitating an acute attack. The use of any of these drugs may result in severe neurological deficits, including paraplegia or quadriplegia. In a survey of Finnish patients with AIP, 2% of surgical operations and 4% of pregnancies were associated with acute attacks (Kauppinen & Mustajoki 1992).

   Since the overall number of patients with porphyria presenting for anaesthesia is small, experience with any individual anaesthetic drug is limited. In addition, a patient's response to a particular drug will vary according to the state of their porphyria. A retrospective analysis of 78 anaesthetics given to 47 patients, suggested that if the patient was in a latent period, the risks of using thiopentone were small. In contrast, 7 out of 10 patients given thiopentone during an acute episode had a deterioration of porphyric symptoms (Mustajoki & Heinonen 1980). However, with such potentially devastating complications, the scope for prospective human 'studies' is limited.

For this reason, experimental models are being used to assess the porphyrinogenicity of certain anaesthetic drugs. Rats primed with 3,5-dicarbethoxy-1,4-dihydrocolidine (DDC) provide a model for latent variegate porphyria. With this system, various drugs have been tested for their ability to increase hepatic ALA-synthase activity and produce intermediate porphyrins (Blekkenhorst et al 1980, Harrison et al 1985). Although animal studies cannot necessarily be extrapolated to man, additional testing with known safe and unsafe drugs have provided some measure of control (Blekkenhorst et al 1980).

A simple method of drug classification has been suggested as a clinical guide to therapy in porphyria (Disler et al 1982):

Category A: drugs reported in terms of clinical experience as dangerous or safe by three or more authorities.

Category B: as Category A, but reported by only two or fewer authorities.

Categories A and B are usually associated with corroborated experimental animal data.

Category C: drugs evaluated only in the experimental rat model.

Category D: drugs evaluated in chick embryo liver cell culture or 'in ovo'.

Neither Categories C nor D have corroborative reports of human cases.

In some drugs the data is conflicting.

For detailed information on general prescribing, Disler's article is recommended.

Probably dangerous drugs include: barbiturates, carbamazepine, carbromal, chloramphenicol, chlordiazepoxide, cimetidine, ergot alkaloids, erythromycin, flunitrazepam, frusemide, glutethimide, griseofulvin, hydantoins, imipramine, meprobamate, methyl dopa, metoclopramide, nalidixic acid, nikethimide, nitrazepam, pargyline, pentazocine, phenoxybenzamine, steroids, sulphonamides, sulphonylurea antidiabetic agents, theophylline and tranylcypromine.

Possibly dangerous drugs. A number of drugs have often been used without complication, but a single case report or set of experimental data exists, implicating it as being porphyrinogenic. This group includes: corticosteroids, diazepam, enflurane*, etomidate*, fentanyl*, halothane*, hydralazine, ketamine*,

---

*Specific reference to these drugs is made below.

lignocaine*, pancuronium*, pethidine*, paraldehyde, and the sex hormones.

Although a single dose of etomidate produced equivocal results using the DDC-primed rat model, a continuous infusion of etomidate caused an increase in ALA synthase, coproporphyrin and protoporphyrin levels. The authors of this study believed it should be considered as category C, and thus potentially porphyrinogenic (Harrison et al 1985). In this same study, ketamine did not produce any change. A single case report has implicated ketamine as porphyrinogenic but there is clinical and experimental evidence suggesting that it is safe (Rizk et al 1977, Blekkenhorst et al 1980, Capouet et al 1987).

Halothane, lignocaine, fentanyl, pethidine and pancuronium have been implicated in single case reports only, and have been used on other occasions without complication (Disler et al 1982).

2. Acute abdominal crises can cause undiagnosed porphyrics to be subjected to surgery. There may be an accompanying tachycardia and hypertension.
3. A porphyric crisis may last for several days and result in dehydration, hyponatraemia and hypokalaemia.
4. Fasting prior to surgery induces cytochrome P-450 enzyme activity.

Management

1. All drugs known to precipitate acute crises should be avoided. Individual clinical judgements must be made about the controversial ones, taking into account the presence or absence of an acute attack (see above).
2. Drugs which are reported to be safe in porphyrics (Disler et al 1982, Magnus 1984) include: adrenaline, aminoglycosides, aspirin atropine, beta blockers, biguanides, bupivacaine, buprenorphine, cephalosporins, chlorpheniramine, chlorpromazine, codeine, coumarins, diazoxide, digitalis, droperidol, d-tubocurarine, erythromycin, ether, heparin, hyoscine, insulin, labetalol, lorazepam, morphine, neostigmine, nitroglycerin, nitrous oxide, paracetamol, penicillins, procaine, prochlorperazine, promazine, promethazine, propranolol, sodium nitroprusside, suxamethonium, thyroxine and trifluoperazine.
3. Clinical and experimental reports have suggested that propofol may be safe for anaesthesia (Mitterschiffthaler et al 1988, Meissner et al 1991, Christian 1991) and for sedation on the ITU (Harrison & McAuley 1992). Propofol following extradural blockade with lignocaine and fentanyl produced urinary porphobilinogen levels above the upper limit of normal but with no porphyric symptoms (Kantor & Rolbin 1992). The clinical use of atracurium has been

reported but no porphyrin metabolites were measured (Lin & Chen 1990). The safety of alcuronium and vecuronium is not yet known.

4. A careful history and examination must be made, to document existing neurological deficits.

5. A patient admitted in a porphyric crisis may require correction of fluid and electrolyte balance. Tachycardia and hypertension may be treated with beta blockers.

6. Glucose administration inhibits enzyme induction and fasting increases it. Administration of dextrose should therefore begin before a period of starvation.

7. Haematin has been reported to be effective in aborting clinical episodes of porphyria, by decreasing ALA synthase activity. A haematin infusion has been used to treat increased urinary porphobilinogen levels in a patient following cardiopulmonary bypass (Roby & Harrison 1982).

8. Regional anaesthesia may be appropriate on occasions. Caesarean section under both spinal and extradural anaesthesia using bupivacaine has been described (McNeill & Bennet 1990, Brennan et al 1990). However, the importance of early antenatal assessment is emphasized so that a plan for the emergency situation can be written into the patient's notes.

9. Additional advice can be obtained from the Porphyria Research Unit, Western Infirmary, Glasgow G11 6NT. Tel: 041 339 8822 ext 4150.

BIBLIOGRAPHY

Blekkenhorst G H, Harrison G G, Cook E S, et al 1980 Screening of certain anaesthetic agents for their ability to elicit acute porphyric phases in susceptible patients. British Journal of Anaesthesia 52: 759–762

Brennan L, Halfacre J A, Woods S D 1990 Regional anaesthesia in porphyria. British Journal of Anaesthesia 65: 594

Capouet V, Dernovoi B, Azagra J S 1987 Induction of anaesthesia with ketamine during an acute crisis of hereditary coproporphyria. Canadian Journal of Anaesthesia 34: 388–390

Christian A S 1991 Safe use of propofol in a child with acute intermittent porphyria. Anaesthesia 46: 423–424

Disler P B, Blekkenhorst G H, Eales L et al 1982 Guidelines for drug prescription in patients with the acute porphyrias. South African Medical Journal 61: 656–660

Harrison G G, Moore M R, Meissner P N 1985 Porphyrinogenicity of etomidate and ketamine as continuous infusions. British Journal of Anaesthesia 57: 420–423

Harrison J C. McAuley F T 1992 Propofol sedation in intensive care in a patient with an acute porphyric attack. Anaesthesia 47: 355–356

Kantor G, Rolbin S H 1992 Acute intermittent porphyria and caesarean delivery. Canadian Journal of Anaesthesia 39: 282–285

Kauppinen R, Mustajoki P 1992 Prognosis of acute porphyria: occurrence of acute attacks, precipitating factors, and associated diseases. Medicine 74: 1–13

Laiwah A C Y Moore M R, Goldberg A 1987 Pathogenesis of acute porphyria. Quarterly Journal of Medicine 63: 377–392

Lin Y, Chen L 1990 Atracurium in a patient with acute intermittent porphyria. Anesthesia and Analgesia 71: 440–445

McNeill M J, Bennet A 1990 Use of regional anaesthesia in a patient with acute porphyria. British Journal of Anaesthesia 64: 371–373

Magnus I A 1984 Drugs and porphyria. British Medical Journal 288: 1474–1475
Meissner P N, Harrison G G, Hift R J 1991 Propofol as an i.v. induction agent in variegate porphyria. British Journal of Anaesthesia 66: 60–65.
Mitterschiffthaler G, Theiner A, Hetzel H et al 1988 Safe use of propofol in a patient with acute intermittent porphyria. British Journal of Anaesthesia 60: 109–111
Mustajoki P, Heinonen J 1980 General anesthesia in 'inducible' porphyrias. Anesthesiology 53: 15–20
Rizk S K, Jacobsen J H, Silva G 1977 Ketamine as an induction agent for acute intermittent porphyria. Anesthesiology 46: 305–306
Roby H P, Harrison G A 1982 Anaesthesia for coronary artery by pass in a patient with porphyria variegata. Anaesthesia and Intensive Care 10: 276–278.

PRADER-WILLI SYNDROME

A syndrome of unknown aetiology, in which obesity is associated with disturbances of carbohydrate and fat metabolism. Abnormalities of chromosome 15 are thought to be involved. It usually presents in infancy with hypotonia, and feeding and respiratory difficulties. Despite the hypotonia, no histological, biochemical or neurophysiological abnormalities of the muscle have been demonstrated, and a hypothalamic lesion has been postulated. Obesity develops by the age of 3 years, and a non-insulin-dependent diabetes around 10 years. Orchidopexy is commonly required for undescended testes. Dental and orthopaedic surgery may also be needed.

Preoperative abnormalities

1. Initially, the infant is hypotonic, feeds poorly, coughs and has episodes of asphysia. Obesity and hyperphagia develop from about the age of 3 years. Children are of small stature with hypermobile joints. Mental retardation is usual. Amongst other features which assist diagnosis at an early stage are an abnormal cry, genital hypoplasia and alveolar ridge abnormalities (Aughton & Cassidy 1990).
2. Abnormal glucose tolerance curves are recorded and episodes of hypoglycaemia may occur. A mild non-insulin-dependent diabetes develops around the age of 10 years. This may be secondary to obesity.
3. Enamel defects and dental caries are common.
4. Skeletal abnormalities include kyphosis, scoliosis, narrow bifrontal diameter, small hands and feet, a straight ulnar border, and hand and finger anomalies. In one child, kyphosis and spinal canal stenosis resulted in cervical myelopathy (Tsuji et al 1991).

Anaesthetic problems

There have been at least 15 reports of anaesthetics given to these patients (Milliken & Weintraub 1975, Mayhew & Taylor 1983, Palmer & Atlee 1976, Yamashita et al 1983, Mackenzie 1991). Some have been uneventful, in others a variety of complications have been described.

1. The general problems of obesity.
2. Disturbances of thermoregulation may occur. Two cases had fever and acidosis during anaesthesia, and in six, fever occurred in the postoperative period (Yamashita et al 1983). In one child, intubation difficulty was experienced after suxamethonium (Mayhew & Taylor 1983). The anaesthetic was continued with halothane and curare, but was terminated because the patient's temperature increased. However, the postoperative serum CK was only 240 u/l. A subsequent anaesthetic, in which pancuronium, nitrous oxide and fentanyl were used, was uneventful. Although comparisons with MH patients have been made, there is nothing to suggest that the episodes of fever originate from abnormal muscle metabolism. A hypothalamic mechanism would seem more likely.
3. Cardiac arrhythmias were reported in five cases. A sixth, an 8-year-old child, was having a pacemaker implanted for sick sinus syndrome.
4. Difficulty in intubation was reported in two patients, but its origins were not stated. Mild micrognathia, high-arched palate, and large head circumference are features in these infants that may contribute (Aughton & Cassidy 1990).
5. Regurgitation of gastric secretions and rumination has been observed (Sloan & Kaye 1991). These may contribute to the development of dental caries and aspiration pneumonitis.
6. Snoring, obstructive sleep apnoea, hypersomnolence, and daytime hypoventilation have been described, although polysomnography in five patients indicated that the disorder was mild (Kaplan et al 1991).
7. Episodes of hypoglycaemia have been reported.
8. Scoliosis is sometimes associated.
9. Convulsions have been recorded.
10. Hypotonia has been noted. The cause has not been elucidated, but it is said to improve with age.

Management

1. Blood glucose should be monitored carefully, and a glucose infusion even pre- and intraoperatively.
2. ECG, core temperature and ET_{CO_2} should be monitored from the beginning of the anaesthetic.
3. In view of the obesity, a technique using IPPV is advisable. No prolongation of response to muscle relaxants has been reported, despite depolarizing and non-depolarizing drugs having been used.
4. Patients should be assumed to be at high risk from aspiration of gastric contents (Sloan & Kaye 1991), and appropriate precautions should be taken to reduce and neutralize acid secretions and to secure the airway rapidly.

BIBLIOGRAPHY
Aughton D J, Cassidy S B 1990 Physical features of Prader-Willi syndrome in neonates. American Journal of Diseases in Children 144: 1251–1254
Kaplan J, Frederickson P A, Richardson J W 1991 Sleep and breathing in patients with the Prader-Willi syndrome. Mayo Clinic Proceedings 66: 1124–1126
Mackenzie J W 1991 Anaesthesia and the Prader-Willi syndrome. Journal of the Royal Society of Medicine 84: 239
Mayhew J F, Taylor B 1983 Anaesthetic considerations in the Prader-Willi syndrome. Canadian Anaesthetists' Society Journal 30: 565–566
Milliken R A, Weintraub D M 1975 Cardiac abnormalities during anesthesia in a child with Prader-Willi syndrome. Anesthesiology 43: 590–592
Palmer S K, Atlee J L 1976 Anesthetic management of the Prader-Willi syndrome. Anesthesiology 44: 161–163
Sloan T B, Kaye C I 1991 Rumination risk of aspiration of gastric contents in the Prader-Willi syndrome. Anesthesia and Analgesia 73: 492–495
Tsuji M, Kurihara A, Uratsuji M et al 1991 Cervical myelopathy with Prader-Willi syndrome in a 13-year-old boy. A case report. Spine 16: 1342–1344
Yamashita M, Koishi K, Yamaya R et al 1983 Anaesthetic considerations in the Prader-Willi syndrome. Canadian Anaesthetists' Society Journal 30: 179–184

PROTEIN C DEFICIENCY

In the normal subject, protein C is an essential anticoagulant. It acts by selective inhibition of activated factors V and VIII, and by stimulation of fibrinolysis. Synthesis occurs in the liver and is vitamin K dependent. Inherited and acquired deficiencies may occur. Since the first report in 1981 by Griffin et al, a number of families have been described in which relatively young members have had recurrent spontaneous venous thromboses in association with reduced levels (between 35 and 65% of normal) of protein C.

However, the situation has proved to be more complicated than was initially thought. When attempting to define the normal range of values of protein C, it was found that 1 in 60 of healthy adults had levels of 55–65% and, conversely, that 1 in 200–300 patients with heterozygous protein C deficiency had no history of venous thrombosis (Miletich et al 1986). It was therefore thought that heterozygous subjects with venous thromboses had some additional predisposing abnormality, or conversely, heterozygous subjects without venous thrombosis had some compensating mechanism. However, a recently developed technique for functional assay has helped to detect patients who have reduced protein C activity but normal levels of protein C as measured by immunological assay. It appears now that there are two types of the condition, one in which there is an absence, or reduced levels, of protein C, and the other in which there is a functional defect.

Severe congenital homozygous protein C deficiency (often with no detectable levels) has been described in infants of parents who both had heterozygous deficiency. These babies presented with widespread skin lesions and necrosis secondary to thrombosis of small veins.

Levels of protein C may also be reduced in liver disease, ARDS, and following surgery. They may be very low or undetectable in DIC states.

Preoperative abnormalities

1. When the condition presents in infancy, it is usually homozygous, and often fatal, since it is associated with purpura fulminans, cutaneous necrosis and extensive venous thrombosis.
2. There is a high risk of deep venous thrombosis and pulmonary embolism. In adults or children with the familial heterozygous deficiency, the first thrombotic event may be in association with another predisposing factor. Thus, pulmonary embolism may occur in the perioperative period (Sternberg et al 1991), during pregnancy (Morrison et al 1989), or in association with oral contraceptives and infection.
3. Warfarin-induced skin necrosis has been reported in a small number of patients, secondary to capillary thrombosis.
4. Patients may present with conditions that are secondary to thromboses at unusual sites. Mesenteric (peritonitis), cerebral, axillary, hepatic venous (Budd-Chiari syndrome) and penile thromboses (priapism) have been recorded.
5. Patients known to have the condition, and who have already had venous thromboses, will usually be taking permanent coumarin therapy. Warfarin, despite one of its actions being to lower protein C levels, has been found to be beneficial in preventing recurrent venous thromboembolism in protein C deficiency (Broekmans et al 1983). Occasionally, warfarin-induced skin necrosis, particularly in skin overlying fatty areas, may occur.
6. In a young patient who has had a previous spontaneous venous thrombosis, or who has a family history of thromboses, the possibility of this condition should be considered (Melissari & Kakkar 1989). It is said to account for 5–8% of such cases. Other inherited thrombophilias to be considered include antithrombin III deficiency, dysfibrinogenaemia, and plasminogen abnormalities (Schafer 1985).

Anaesthetic problems

1. Homozygous infant
   a. Skin necrosis over pressure points.
   b. There is a theoretical risk of tracheal damage during the period of tracheal intubation.
2. Heterozygous adult or child
   a. The problems of the management of a patient for anaesthesia and surgery who is anticoagulated.
   b. The risk of venous thrombosis and pulmonary embolism. Fatal perioperative pulmonary embolism occurred in an 8-year-old child following laparotomy (Sternberg et al 1991) and in a 19-year-old man after knee surgery (Rick 1990).

c. The problems of management during pregnancy, a state which constitutes a risk factor for venous thrombosis in these patients (Morrison et al 1989). In addition, pregnancy appears to be associated with a poor fetal outcome (Bertault et al 1991) with intrauterine growth retardation probably secondary to insufficiency of the uteroplacental circulation.

Management

1. Homozygous infant
   a. The anaesthetic literature is very limited. Three consecutive anaesthetics were reported for partial omentectomy and insertion of Tenkhoff catheter, in a homozygous infant with renal failure (Wetzel et al 1986). Despite the theoretical risks, tracheal intubation was employed, using a small tube to reduce tracheal pressure. The trachea was examined with a flexible laryngoscope at the subsequent anaesthetics and no damage was found.
   b. The advice of a haematologist should be sought for the correction of the protein C deficiency. Current treatment includes fresh frozen plasma and Factor IX concentrate. There are recent reports of use of a purifed protein C concentrate (Dreyfus et al 1991).
2. Heterozygous adult or child
   a. If the patient is taking warfarin, heparin should be substituted to obtain more flexible control. Normally, when therapy is initiated for acute thrombosis, heparin should be given for 4–6 days before warfarin is started, to prevent skin necrosis. Anticoagulants should be restarted as soon as the surgery allows.
   b. If the patient is not anticoagulated, low-dose heparin should be started preoperatively.
3. Pregnancy
   a. In pregnancy, management will have to be decided in each individual case. A patient presenting for the first time with venous thrombosis will initially require full anticoagulation with heparin.
   b. Those without venous thrombosis are increasingly being managed on subcutaneous low-dose heparin (Bertault et al 1991). Low molecular weight heparin 7500 u daily was given in one patient from 4 months' gestation until postpartum.

BIBLIOGRAPHY

Bertault D, Mandelbrot L, Tchobroutsky C et al 1991 Unfavourable pregnancy outcome associated with congenital protein C deficiency. Case reports. British Journal of Obstetrics and Gynaecology 98: 934–936

Broekmans A W, Veltkamp J J, Bertina R M 1983 Congenital protein C deficiency and venous thromboemholism. New England Journal of Medicine 309: 340–344

Dreyfus M, Magny J F, Bridey F et al 1991 Treatment of homozygous protein C deficiency and neonatal purpura fulminans with a purified protein C concentrate. New England Journal of Medicine 325: 1565–1568

Eason J D, Mills J L, Beckett W C 1992 Hypercoagulable states in arterial thromboembolism. Surgery, Gynecology and Obstetrics 174: 211–215

Freed J A 1991 Hypercoagulability. Should every patient with venous thrombosis be tested? Postgraduate Medicine 90: 157–160

Griffin J H, Evatt B, Zimmerman T S, Kleiss A J, Widerman C 1981 Deficiency of protein C in congenital thrombotic disease. Journal of Clinical Investigation 68: 1370–1373

Melissari E, Kakkar V V 1989 Congenital severe protein C deficiency in adults. British Journal of Haematology 72: 222–228

Miletich J, Sherman L, Broze G 1986 Absence of thrombosis in subjects with heterozygous protein C deficiency. New England Journal of Medicine 317: 991–996

Morrison A E, Walker I D, Black W P 1989 Protein C deficiency presenting as deep venous thrombosis in pregnancy. Case report. British Journal of Obstetrics and Gynaecology 95: 1077–1080

Rick M E 1990 Protein C and Protein S. Vitamin K-dependent inhibitors of blood coagulation. Journal of the American Medical Association 263: 701–703

Schafer A I 1985 The hypercoagulable states. Annals of Internal Medicine 102: 814–828

Sternberg T L, Bailey M K, Lazarchick J et al 1991 Protein C deficiency as a cause of pulmonary embolism in the perioperative period. Anesthesiology 74: 364–366

Wetzel R C, Marsh B R, Yaster M et al 1986 Anesthetic implications of protein C deficiency. Anesthesia and Analgesia 65: 982–984

PULMONARY HYPERTENSION

Can be applied to any condition in which the pulmonary artery pressure is increased to 35/15 mmHg or higher, or a mean of 15–18 mmHg (N = 15–30/5–12 mmHg). Can be primary or secondary. Secondary pulmonary hypertension may be due to pulmonary emboli, chronic hypoxic lung disease, left-to-right shunts, sickle cell anaemia, increased left ventricular filling pressures, left atrial outflow obstruction and vasculitis.

Primary pulmonary hypertension (PPH) is a rare disease of the pulmonary vasculature and of unknown aetiology. After elimination of other causes, the diagnosis is one of exclusion. It is more common in women than in men and there may be a family history. There is an increased pulmonary artery pressure and pulmonary vascular resistance. The mortality in PPH is high and the average survival time is 2 years (Rich & Brundage 1984). Heart-lung transplantation has been successful. Work on pulmonary vasodilators is under investigation. This includes the use of nitric oxide (Pepke-Zaba et al 1991). The prognosis is poor. Sudden death and deaths secondary to right ventricular failure, are common.

Preoperative abnormalities

1. Increasing dyspnoea and intense fatigue occurs, initially on exertion but later at rest. Chest pain and haemoptysis may feature. In advanced disease, hypoxaemia occurs at rest.

2. Signs of a low cardiac output, signs of the original disease, an elevated JVP, and a right ventricular heave. A loud pulmonary second sound, right ventricular gallop (loud third sound at the left

sternal edge) and possibly an early diastolic murmur of pulmonary regurgitation. Right heart failure will develop, with hepatomegaly, and peripheral oedema Tricuspid regurgitation may occur.
3. ECG shows right axis deviation, right ventricular hypertrophy and right atrial hypertrophy (P pulmonale). Right bundle branch block is common.
4. CXR shows a prominent pulmonary artery and an increased cardiothoracic ratio at a later stage. There are oligaemic lung fields, except when the secondary disease is a result of increased blood flow, in which case the lung fields are plethoric,
5. Certain conditions are more commonly associated with PPH. These include collagen vascular disorders, Raynaud's disease, hepatic cirrhosis, and sickle cell anaemia.
6. Patients may be taking prophylactic anticoagulants.
7. Although vasodilators have been used for treatment, there is as yet no evidence that they improve long-term survival. Calcium antagonists in high doses are currently being used (Rich et al 1992).
8. Mortality was closely associated with right ventricular function as characterized by pulmonary artery pressure, right atrial pressure and cardiac index (D'Alonzo et al 1991). Right ventricular failure indicated a poor prognosis.

Anaesthetic problems

1. The pre-existing high pulmonary vascular resistance (PVR) may be further increased by hypoxaemia, acidosis, hypercarbia, cold, alpha adrenoceptor stimulation, nitrous oxide, anxiety, and PEEP.
2. A further elevation of PVR during anaesthesia can increase the degree of right ventricular failure or decrease venous return to the left heart, thus causing systemic hypotension. Sudden hypotension and hypoxaemia occurred on induction of anaesthesia in a child undergoing ventriculoatrial shunt. Subsequent investigation showed pulmonary hypertension secondary to recurrent pulmonary thromboembolism (Butler et al 1990).
3. There is a poor correlation between RAP and LAP, therefore PAP and PCWP measurement has been recommended for severe cases. However, there is an increased risk of pulmonary vessel perforation during PAWP measurement in patients with acute pulmonary hypertension (Kranz & Viljoen 1979).
4. The patient is often receiving anticoagulants, and the cardiologists may press to resume treatment soon after surgery. However, death from haemorrhage occurred in a patient in whom heparin was restarted within hours of a Caesarean section performed using the classical approach (Roessler & Lambert 1986).
5. Childbirth is associated with a high mortality, and death often occurred not during labour but early in the postpartum period.

Management

1. The cause should be established, since this influences the therapy. For example, PPH secondary to chronic hypoxic lung disease responds to reversal of airway obstruction, anticholinergics, oxygen, and steroids, rather than to vasodilators (Peacock 1990). The severity of the pulmonary hypertension must also be assessed. Hypoxaemia on air suggests advanced disease. Cardiac catheterization and pulmonary angiography produce the best information on the degree of pulmonary hypertension and the effect of vasodilators.

2. The risks of surgery must be weighed against the benefits. There are relatively few case reports of anaesthesia in patients with PPH. In those that exist, the perioperative mortality was high, especially in the pregnant patient, for whom the prognosis is poor (Nelson et al 1983, Roberts & Keast 1990).

3. For the pregnant patient, a multidisciplinary team of obstetrician, cardiologist, anaesthetist and paediatrician is required. Roberts and Keast (1990) suggest that assessment of disease severity, plans for the mode and timing of delivery, management of circulatory stability and provision of analgesia or anaesthesia all need to be discussed and agreed early in pregnancy. Such a policy would require frequent review. Vaginal delivery is associated with a better chance of maternal survival. Extradural analgesia with an infusion of low-dose bupivacaine and fentanyl has been reported (Power & Avery 1989).

4. An adequate preoperative assessment of the degree of cardiorespiratory impairment. Treatment is difficult. Although diuretics improve peripheral oedema, they produce a fall in right ventricular, and hence cardiac, output. Pulmonary vasodilators are not very effective.

5. Pulmonary artery, pulmonary capillary wedge, and systemic artery pressures need to be monitored with care to avoid pulmonary vessel perforation. Monitoring of pulmonary pressures, particularly pulmonary vascular resistance, allows rational treatment of perioperative pressure changes with appropriate vasodilators, or fluid replacement.

6. Factors known to increase pulmonary vascular resistance are avoided. A sedative premedication relieves anxiety. Oxygenation should be maintained, and hypercarbia and acidosis avoided. The theatre should be warm, and a heated mattress and blood warmer used. Nitrous oxide produces a significant elevation of PAP in patients with pre-existing high levels, but not in those with normal PAP (Schulte-Sasse et al 1982).

7. Pulmonary vasodilators may be required during anaesthesia. It has been suggested that patients should be admitted to the ITU before

surgery or delivery to assess the effect of various forms of therapy on the above parameters (Roessler & Lambert 1986). A patient due for Caesarean section under extradural anaesthesia was tested for the haemodynamic effects of a fluid load, changes in inspired oxygen percentage, tolazoline, sodium nitroprusside, and glyceryl nitrate. In this patient, sodium nitroprusside was the most effective in reducing pulmonary artery pressure but achieved this at the expense of systemic hypotension. Similar management in another parturient demonstrated a reduction in PAP and PVR with an isoprenaline infusion of 0.2 mg/h (Slomka et al 1988). In this patient, a double catheter extradural analgesia technique was used for vaginal delivery. Extradural anaesthesia was also reported in a patient undergoing vascular surgery (Davies & Beavis 1984). Although hypotension responded to colloid and metaraminol, a simultaneous moderate increase in PAP occurred. Isoflurane may have a beneficial effect on pulmonary vascular pressures (Cheng & Edelist 1988). A young man with primary pulmonary hypertension, whose pre-induction PAP was equal to his systemic pressure, showed a marked decrease in PVR and PAP during oxygen/isoflurane anaesthesia. Recently, the acute effects of nitric oxide (NO) have been compared with prostacyclin (24 μg/h) in 8 patients with severe pulmonary hypertension, and 10 patients with cardiac disease but without pulmonary hypertension (Pepke-Zaba et al 1991). Inhaled NO (40 p.p.m. in air) reduced PVR in the patients with pulmonary hypertension but had no effect on systemic vascular resistance in any of the patients or volunteers, whereas prostacyclin led to decreases in both parameters. Nitric oxide appears to be a selective and effective pulmonary vasodilator and has been identified as the powerful endothelium-derived relaxing factor.

8. If an inotropic agent is required, noradrenaline may be suitable. It increases systemic vascular resistance without causing a tachycardia and in animal studies has been shown to decrease pulmonary vascular resistance.

9. Adequate pain relief is important and a thoracic extradural block for intraoperative and postoperative analgesia has been used (Armstrong 1992).

BIBLIOGRAPHY

Armstrong P 1992 Thoracic epidural anaesthesia and primary pulmonary hypertension. Anaesthesia 47: 496–499

Butler P J, Wheeler R A, Spargo P M 1990 Life-threatening complications during anaesthesia in a patient with ventriculo-atrial shunt and pulmonary hypertension. Anaesthesia 45: 946–948

Cheng D C H, Edelist G 1988 Isoflurane and primary pulmonary hypertension. Anaesthesia 43: 22–24

D'Alonzo G E, Barst R J, Ayres S M et al 1991 Survival in patients with primary pulmonary hypertension: results from a National Prospective Registry. Annals of Internal Medicine 115: 343–349

Section 1

Pulmonary
Hypertension

Davies M J, Beavis R E 1984 Epidural anaesthesia for vascular surgery in a patient with primary pulmonary hypertension. Anaesthesia and Intensive Care 12: 165–167

Kranz E M, Viljoen J F 1979 Haemoptysis following insertion of a Swan-Ganz catheter. British Journal of Anaesthesia 51: 457–459

Nelson D M, Main E, Crafford W et al 1983 Peripartum heart failure due to primary pulmonary hypertension. Obstetrics and Gynecology 62: 58S–62S.

Peacock A 1990 Pulmonary hypertension due to chronic hypoxia. Treat the lung not the pressure. British Medical Journal 300: 763

Pepke-Zaba J, Higenbottam T W, Dinh-Xuan A T et al 1991 Inhaled nitric oxide as a cause of selective pulmonary vasodilation in pulmonary hypertension. Lancet 338: 1173–1174

Power K. Avery A F 1989 Extradural analgesia in the intrapartum management of a patient with pulmonary hypertension. British Journal of Anaesthesia 63: 116–120

Rich S, Brundage B H 1984 Primary pulmonary hypertension. Journal of the American Medical Association 251: 2252–2254

Rich S, Kaufmann E, Levy P S 1992 The effect of high doses of calcium channel blockers on survival in primary pulmonary hypertension. New England Journal of Medicine 327: 76–81

Roberts N V, Keast P J 1990 Pulmonary hypertension and pregnancy – a lethal combination. Anaesthesia and Intensive Care 18: 366–374

Roessler P, Lambert T F 1986 Anaesthesia for Caesarean section in the presence of primary pulmonary hypertension. Anaesthesia and Intensive Care 14: 317–320

Schulte-Sasse U, Hess W Tarnow J 1982 Pulmonary vascular responses to nitrous oxide in patients with normal and high pulmonary vascular resistance. Anesthesiology 57: 9–13

Slomka F, Salmeron S, Zetlaoui P et al 1988 Primary pulmonary hypertension and pregnancy: anesthetic management for delivery. Anesthesiology 69: 959–961

PULMONARY OEDEMA

Causes of acute pulmonary oedema occurring in the perioperative period can be broadly divided into two groups; those of cardiogenic, and those of non-cardiogenic, origin. There are some cases in which the aetiology may not be clearly defined, and in which a number of factors may contribute. Broadly, one of two basic abnormalities may develop to produce pulmonary oedema. The first is an increase in the gradient between hydrostatic and colloid osmotic pressure across the pulmonary capillary wall, and the second is an increase in capillary permeability.

1. Increased pulmonary hydrostatic pressure may be due to:
   a. Increase in right atrial pressure or preload from fluid retention or fluid overload.
   b. Decreased myocardial contractility secondary to myocardial infarction or cardiomyopathy.
   c. Increase in left atrial pressure, e.g. in mitral stenosis.
   d. Increased afterload as a result of severe hypertension, peripheral vasoconstriction, or anatomical or pathological obstruction.
2. Increased capillary permeability may result from:
   a. Pulmonary aspiration of acid gastric contents.
   b. Air, gas, or amniotic fluid embolism.
   c. Allergic reactions to drugs or blood products.
   d. Poisoning with higher oxides of nitrogen.

e. Pneumonias and septicaemias

f. Shock lung or ARDS

There are a number of specific types of non-cardiogenic pulmonary oedema whose mechanisms have not been completely elucidated, but which may present in the perioperative period. These include: neurogenic pulmonary oedema; oedema associated with the relief of severe upper airway obstruction or re-expansion of a collapsed lung; the therapeutic use of beta 2 adrenoceptor stimulators for premature labour, or of naloxone for opiate antagonism; and gas or amniotic fluid embolism. Since the treatment required may differ, these conditions will be considered separately.

Differentiation between cardiogenic and permeability pulmonary oedema

1. History

   In many cases the diagnosis will be obvious. There may be history of previous myocardial infarction, hypertension, valvular heart disease, or episodes of cardiac failure. The sudden onset of an arrhythmia, such as atrial fibrillation, may cause rapid cardiac decompensation. If none of these is found, the presence of a known precipitating factor for non-cardiogenic oedema should be sought.

2. Clinical examination

   Physical signs tend to be similar. Tachycardia, cool peripheries, respiratory distress, frothy sputum, cyanosis and basal and parasternal crepitations feature in both. In primary cardiac disease there may be obvious cardiac enlargement, murmurs or an arrhythmia. An added third sound points to a cardiac cause.

3. CXR may show cardiac enlargement, in addition to the pulmonary oedema.

4. ECG may show evidence of infarction, an arrhythmia or chamber hypertrophy.

5. In difficult cases, measurement of PAP and PCWP may be required.

6. Measurement of protein levels in pulmonary oedema fluid

   This can only be done when there is copious, uncontaminated fluid for sampling.

   A number of studies have shown that, depending on the cause, the protein content in oedema fluid varies. When caused by an increased hydrostatic pressure, i.e. when it is cardiogenic, there is a low protein content, whereas when secondary to permeability problems the protein content tends to be high.

   A study of 21 patients showed that all patients with a PCWP of <20 mmHg had an oedema fluid to plasma protein ratio >0.6, whereas the mean ratio in four patients with cardiogenic oedema was 0.46 (Fein et al 1979). When permeability problems exist, large protein molecules such as globulins will be present in oedema fluid and the protein content will approach that of blood. It has been suggested that the use of globulin ratios in conjunction with total protein ratios gives a more clear-cut differentiation between cardiac and non-cardiac causes (Sprung et al 1981).

If oedema protein levels are high, and pulmonary artery catheterization is unavailable, it is reasonable to assume that the cause is likely to be a permeability problem.

BIBLIOGRAPHY
Fein A, Grossman R F, Jones J G et al 1979 The value of edema fluid protein measurement in patients with pulmonary edema. American Journal of Medicine 67: 32–38
Sprung C L, Rackow E C, Fein A et al 1981 The spectrum of pulmonary oedema. American Review of Respiratory Diseases 124: 718–722

CARDIOGENIC PULMONARY OEDEMA

This results from an increase in pulmonary capillary pressure secondary to a high left atrial pressure. As a consequence, the lung water content increases. Cardiogenic pulmonary oedema may originate from: left atrial outflow obstruction (mitral valve disease, cardiac myxoma); left ventricular dysfunction (ischaemic or myopathic); left ventricular outflow obstruction; or an increased afterload. It may be associated with a fluid overload, or with normovolaemia.

Presentation
In a patient with cardiac disease, pulmonary oedema may occur at any time during the perioperative period.

1. Preoperatively, it presents as a sudden onset of dyspnoea, tachycardia, a third heart sound (gallop rhythm), sweating and hypertension, with bilateral basal or parasternal crepitations on auscultation. It is most likely to occur in a patient with known ischaemic, hypertensive, or rheumatic heart disease and may be associated with overenthusiastic fluid therapy instituted before emergency surgery.
2. Pulmonary oedema is relatively rare during surgery, because the combination of IPPV and decreased peripheral vascular resistance during anaesthesia tend to oppose the hydrostatic forces and reduce the afterload. Early signs are tachycardia, decreased pulmonary compliance and reduced oxygen saturation. The patient may try to breathe against the ventilator. In severe cases, pulmonary oedema fluid may emerge from the tracheal tube.
3. In the postoperative period, a combination of factors may precipitate a patient from a borderline state into florid pulmonary oedema, usually within the first half hour of the recovery period. Redistribution of fluid from the peripheral into the pulmonary circulation is probably a major factor. At this stage, systemic

vasoconstriction from pain or cold coincides with the vasodilator effects of the anaesthetic receding. In addition, intravenous fluids administered during the operation may compound the problem. In obstetric practice, the use of ergometrine in patients with cardiac lesions has, in the past, sometimes been associated with pulmonary oedema.

Differential diagnosis

1. Inhalation of gastric contents.
2. Oedema following the relief of upper airway obstruction.
3. Neurogenic pulmonary oedema.
4. Pulmonary oedema associated with naloxone administration.

Management

1. If the patient is conscious, he should be placed in an upright position and oxygen administered. If not, IPPV should be continued or started.
2. Morphine i.v., should be given in 2 mg increments at 2-minute intervals to a total of 10 mg. This reduces preload by venodilatation and relieves agitation.
3. Frusemide i.v. or i.m. 20–50 mg, especially if there is fluid overload. Acute venodilatation and subsequent diuresis results.
4. A vasodilator, such as isosorbide dinitrate, nitroglycerin, or nitroprusside may be used. An isosorbide infusion (diluted) can be given at a rate of 2–10 mg/h.
5. If the patient is in fast AF, control of the heart rate with verapamil or digoxin is required. With ECG control, verapamil 5–10 mg i.v. is given slowly.
   N.B. Verapamil i.v. is contraindicated if the patient is taking beta adrenoceptor blockers.
6. In severe myocardial dysfunction, a dilating inotrope such as dobutamine may be required.

NEUROGENIC PULMONARY OEDEMA (NPO)

A rare complication associated with intracranial damage, which may be secondary to head injury, tumour, or vascular accident. It is postulated that the primary brain insult increases intracranial pressure and causes a secondary disturbance in hypothalamic function. A massive sympathetic neuronal discharge results in pronounced systemic vasoconstriction, diverting blood from the systemic to the pulmonary circulation (Theodore & Robin 1975). Pulmonary oedema results from the sequential increase in left heart pressures, as the left ventricle attempts to eject blood against a greatly elevated systemic vascular resistance (i.e.

increased LVEDP, LAP and pulmonary venous pressures), together with an increased pulmonary blood volume. Both factors will result in increased pulmonary capillary pressure. There is some evidence that altered pulmonary capillary permeability, resulting from capillary damage, may subsequently contribute to the oedema. Cases of NPO have been reported in which pulmonary oedema persisted after pulmonary pressures returned to normal, and in which the oedema protein content was similar to that of plasma (Harari et al 1976). There is a suggestion that the onset of NPO may be precipitated by noxious stimuli such as tracheal intubation, particularly if it is performed in a semiconscious patient. In the past, NPO has been associated with a high mortality (Casey 1983). However, with the better understanding of the pathophysiology of the condition, and the general improvement in intensive care facilities, this may change.

Presentation

1. The patient, (often a young adult or child who is unconscious after a head injury), develops sudden dyspnoea, cyanosis, a pronounced tachycardia or bradycardia, and hypertension, intraoperatively or postoperatively. This occurred during induction of anaesthesia in a patient with a malfunctioning ventriculo-peritoneal shunt, in whom the intraventricular pressure was subsequently found to be >300 mmH$_2$O (22.8 mmHg) (Braude & Ludgrove 1989).
2. Clinical signs of intense systemic vasoconstriction occur, with pallor, sweating and cold extremities.
3. If the patient's trachea is intubated, profuse frothy pink pulmonary secretions will pour from the tube. If the patient is undergoing IPPV, there will be a sudden decrease in lung compliance, and, unless fully paralyzed, the patient will attempt to breathe against the ventilator. Oxygen saturation decreases rapidly.

Differential diagnosis

1. Inhalation of gastric contents.
2. Fluid overload during resuscitation.

Management

1. Maintenance of oxygenation
   If not already instituted, IPPV with a high inspired oxygen is required. PEEP may be needed.
2. Manoeuvres to reduce intracranial pressure (if raised)
   a. Pa_{CO_2} should be maintained at about 3–4 kPa. A Pa_{CO_2} of 3.4 kPa reduces cerebral blood flow by 33%.
   b. An infusion of thiopentone.
   c. Surgical decompression, if necessary.

d. High dose steroids. Dexamethasone is often used, but its value is doubtful.

3. Reduction of peripheral vasoconstriction
   a. Diuretics will assist in reducing the overall blood volume, especially if large quantities of crystalloid solution have been used for resuscitation. Frusemide 2 mg/kg may be used. Mannitol is usually only indicated immediately before surgical decompression, since it causes a subsequent rebound increase in intracranial pressure.
   b. Alpha adrenoceptor blockers such as phenoxybenzamine 0.5–2 mg/kg in 300 ml 5% dextrose have been recommended on the assumption that the syndrome is associated with massive sympathetic neuronal discharge. Experimentally, neurogenic pulmonary oedema can be produced in certain animals by the inflation of a balloon in the extradural space to produce a sudden increase in intracranial pressure. Pretreatment with alpha blockers can prevent the occurrence of pulmonary oedema. Large doses of chlorpromazine were used successfully in a 17-month-old child with NPO following a head injury (Wauchob et al 1984). Other drugs which have been used are droperidol i.v. 200–300µg/kg or a phentolamine infusion 30 µg/kg per min.
   c. Vasodilators, such as sodium nitroprusside, 1-8 µg/kg per min as a short-term infusion, have also been recommended to reduce peripheral vascular resistance. Direct arterial monitoring is essential. The haemodynamic responses of a patient with intractable neurogenic pulmonary oedema were assessed using sodium nitroprusside and isoprenaline in turn (Loughnan et al 1980). Both drugs transiently reduced PCWP and LVEDP, although the Pao_2 was not improved. However, when phenoxybenzamine was given (see b), the Pao_2 improved and the pulmonary oedema resolved rapidly.
4. Inotropic support may occasionally be required. Isoprenaline and dobutamine are both suitable, since neither has alpha adrenoceptor stimulating properties.
5. Control of fits with benzodiazepines or thiopentone.

BIBLIOGRAPHY
Braude N, Ludgrove T 1989 Neurogenic pulmonary oedema precipitated by induction of anaesthesia. British Journal of Anaesthesia 62: 101–103
Casey W F 1983 Neurogenic pulmonary oedema. Anaesthesia 38: 985–988
Harari A, Rapin M, Regnier B et al 1976 Normal pulmonary capillary pressures in the late stage of neurogenic pulmonary oedema. lancet i: 494
Loughnan P M, Brown T C K, Edis B et al 1980 Neurogenic pulmonary oedema in man: aetiology and management with vasodilators based upon haemodynamic studies. Anaesthesia and Intensive Care 8: 65–71
Theodore J, Robin E D 1975 Pathogenesis of neurogenic pulmonary oedema. Lancet ii: 749–751
Wauchob T D, Brooks R D, Harrison K M 1984 Neurogenic pulmonary oedema. Anaesthesia 39: 529–534

Section 1

Pulmonary Oedema
Pulmonary Oedema
associated with the relief
of severe upper airway
obstruction

PULMONARY OEDEMA ASSOCIATED WITH THE RELIEF OF SEVERE
UPPER AIRWAY OBSTRUCTION

A well-recognized complication of acute upper airway obstruction, and
in more than 50% of reported cases, the onset of clinical pulmonary
oedema followed relief of the obstruction (Barin et al 1986). The exact
mechanism is not known, but it has been suggested that the marked
negative pressures produced by attempted inspiration against a closed
glottis may permit either transudation of fluid into the alveoli, or
increased capillary permeability (Weissman et al 1984). Other factors such
as pulmonary aspiration and hypoxic pulmonary vasoconstriction may
contribute. Although potentially dangerous because of the hypoxaemia
produced, this type of pulmonary oedema is usually relatively shortlived.
Croup in children, and laryngospasm and upper airway lesions in adults,
account for more than 50% of the cases
reported (Lang et al 1990).

Unilateral pulmonary oedema associated with lung re-expansion will
also be considered here, since increases in capillary permeability are also
involved.

Presentation

1. The onset of pulmonary oedema is preceded by an episode of
   severe upper respiratory tract obstruction. Recognized causes include
   laryngeal spasm or oedema (Barin et al 1986), epiglottitis (Galvis et al
   1980, Lang et al 1990), bilateral vocal cord paralysis (Dohi et al
   1991), malignancy and attempted strangulation. Unilateral
   pulmonary oedema may occur after sudden re-expansion of a lung
   which has been compressed by a pneumothorax, a pulmonary
   effusion, or a tumour (Khoo & Chen 1988, Matsumiya et al 1991).
   Re-expansion pulmonary oedema is thought to be associated with
   increased pulmonary capillary permeability and may be related both
   to the duration of the collapse and to the rate and force with which
   the lung is re-expanded. Unilateral pulmonary oedema, possibly
   secondary to amiodarone pulmonary toxicity, may occur (Herndon et
   al 1992).
2. Relief of the airway obstruction or re-expansion of a collapsed lung
   is usually accompanied by the outpouring of large amounts of pink,
   frothy oedema fluid. There is cyanosis and respiratory distress.

Diagnosis

1. Bilateral basal crepitations are heard on auscultation.
2. CXR shows diffuse, or unilateral, pulmonary oedema. The heart size
   is usually normal.
3. Blood gases show a large arterial/alveolar PO_2 difference.

Management

Section 1

Pulmonary Oedema

Pulmonary Oedema
associated with beta-2
adrenoceptor stimulants
for premature labour

1. Oxygenation, either via a mask or a tracheal tube. A review of cases
   showed that more than 50% of patients had a Pao_2 of <8 kPa at
   the time of intubation or soon after (Barin et al 1986).
2. IPPV or PEEP may be required to improve oxygenation. A
   pneumothorax may occur as a complication of this.
3. The use of diuretics has been suggested. However, in cases in which
   intracardiac pressures have been measured, these have not, in
   general, been found to be elevated (Weissman et al 1984).
4. Prevention of re-expansion pulmonary oedema. It is suggested that
   a lung which has been collapsed for more then 3 days should be
   re-expanded gradually and that, in the case of an effusion, not more
   than 1.5 litres of fluid should be removed at one time (Khoo &
   Chen 1988).

BIBLIOGRAPHY

Barin E S, Stevenson I F, Donnelly G L 1986 Pulmonary oedema following acute
  airway ohstruction. Anaesthesia and Intensive Care 14: 54–57
Dohi S, Okuho N, Kondo Y 1991 Pulmonary oedema after airway obstruction due to
  bilateral vocal cord paralysis. Canadian Journal of Anaesthesia 38: 492–495
Galvis A G, Stool S E, Bluestone C D 1980 Pulmonary edema following relief of acute
  upper airway obstruction. Annals of Otology, Rinology and Laryngology 89: 124–
  128
Herndon J C, Cook A O, Ramsay M A E et al 1992 Postoperative unilateral
  pulmonary edema: possible amiodarone toxicity. Anesthesiology 76: 308–311
Khoo S T, Chen F G 1988 Acute localized pulmonary oedema. Re-expansion
  pulmonary oedema following the surgical repair of a ruptured hemidiaphragrn.
  Anaesthesia 43: 486–489
Lang S A, Duncan P G, Shephard D A et al 1990 Pulmonary oedema associated with
  airway obstruction. Canadian Journal of Anaesthesia 37: 210–218
Matsumiya N, Dohi S, Kimura T et al 1991 Reexpansion pulmonary edema after
  mediastinal tumor removal. Anesthesia and Analgesia 73: 646–648
Weissman C, Damask: M C, Yang J 1984 Non-cardiogenic pulmonary edema following
  laryngeal obstruction. Anesthesiology 60: 163–165

PULMONARY OEDEMA ASSOCIATED WITH BETA-2 ADRENOCEPTOR STIMULANTS FOR PREMATURE LABOUR

Seventy-three case reports of pulmonary oedema associated with the use
of beta 2 adrenoceptor stimulants to suppress premature labour have
been reviewed (Hawker 1984a). There were seven deaths. The fetal and
maternal benefits of their use for suppression of labour have therefore
been questioned.

The exact aetiology is unknown, although a number of mechanisms
have been considered as possibly contributing. The few haemodynamic
studies reported in patients with pulmonary oedema following tocolytics,
are consistent with the oedema being primarily of a non-cardiogenic,
permeability type (Hawker 1984a,b, Brown & Mullis 1985). However,
there is evidence to suggest that fluid overload and persistent
adrenoceptor stimulation are potent contributing factors (Hawker 1984a).

Section 1

Pulmonary Oedema
Pulmonary Oedema
associated with beta-2
adrenoceptor stimulants
for premature labour

Predisposing factors

1. Drugs thought to be linked with this type of pulmonary oedema include terbutaline, ritodrine, isoxuprine, salbutamol and fenoterol. Tachycardia is a prominent feature.

   It is known that the beta 2 agonists do have inotropic effects on the heart via beta 1 receptors. Indeed, tachycardia can be a very common and troublesome side-effect of the tocolytics. A further contributing feature may be a 'down-grading' of the beta adrenoceptors during continued stimulation. After chronic exposure to catecholamines, cardiac beta receptors may become 'down-regulated', resulting in a decreased adrenergic support for the heart. This has been suggested to occur in severe heart failure, and is supported by the discovery of a decreased beta adrenoceptor population in failing hearts (Bristow et al 1982). Myocardial changes have been found to occur with chronic administration of catecholamines both experimentally and clinically. Patients with phaeochromocytoma can develop a cardiomyopathy, which is usually reversible after removal of the tumour.

2. Pulmonary oedema has been reported with oral, subcutaneous, and intravenous routes of administration. The duration of treatment prior to its onset varied from 6 to 96 hours (Hawker 1984a). The rates of infusion were similarly variable. Of those cases in which information was adequate, pulmonary oedema occurred in 29 before delivery, and in 17, within a further 11 hours. In one patient it developed at 5 days and she died at home on day 60. Late development may suggest a cardiomyopathy. Thirty-three per cent of cases involved twin pregnancy and in 63% of patients, steroids were given in addition. In the four cases in which haemodynamic monitoring was undertaken, three had a normal or low PAWP.

3. In 21 patients in whom fluid balance was recorded, 15 had a positive balance of at least 1 litre. Fluid overload can easily occur. In normal pregnancy blood volume is already increased by 45%. Tocolytics, which are often given in large volumes of diluent, can increase ADH secretion. Fluid retention is a feature of treatment with steroids and indomethacin, both of which may be prescribed in premature labour.

4. Acute redistribution of vascular volumes can sometimes be the precipitating factor in the development of pulmonary oedema, when volume overload is present. Ergometrine has been known to cause pulmonary oedema secondary to vasoconstrictor effects. During recovery from anaesthesia, vasoconstriction as a result of cold or pain can also cause movement of fluid from the peripheral into the central circulation.

Presentation

1. A history of a sudden onset of dyspnoea, cyanosis and expectoration of pink frothy sputum, during or after suppression of premature labour with beta 2 tocolytics. There is a pre-existing tachycardia and the patient is usually in positive fluid balance.
2. On auscultation, bilateral basal crepitations are heard. CXR shows pulmonary oedema, and blood gases, hypoxaemia.

Management

1. The justification for the use of tocolytics should be considered before instituting such treatment. The patient will require careful observation for the detection of a positive fluid balance. A persistent tachycardia during therapy may be a warning sign of impending pulmonary oedema.
2. If evidence of early pulmonary oedema occurs, the infusion should be stopped.
3. Oxygen should be administered and, if necessary, IPPV established.
4. Diuretics are required.

BIBLIOGRAPHY

Bristow M R, Ginsberg R, Minobe W et al 1982 Decreased catecholamine sensitivity and beta adrenergic receptor density in failing human hearts. New England Journal of Medicine 307: 205–211

Brown M, Mullis S 1985 Pulmonary oedema associated with tocolytic therapy. Anaesthesia and Intensive Care 13: 102–103

Hawker F 1984a Pulmonary oedema associated with beta 2 sympathomimetic treatment of premature labour. Anaesthesia and Intensive Care 12: 143–151

Hawker F 1984b Five cases of pulmonary oedema associated with beta 2 sympathomimetic treatment of premature labour. Anaesthesia and Intensive Care 12: 159–171

PULMONARY OEDEMA ASSOCIATED WITH NALOXONE REVERSAL OF OPIATES

Naloxone was originally thought to be a pure opiate antagonist, with no agonist action, and no side-effects. This does not appear to be correct. A few cases have occurred in which opiate reversal with naloxone has been associated with a state of acute central adrenergic stimulation, resulting in cardiovascular complications. Pulmonary oedema is one of these, and appears to most closely resemble neurogenic pulmonary oedema.

In view of suggestions that opiates may in some way modulate the release of catecholamines, the report that a large dose (10 mg) of naloxone caused catecholamine release in a patient with a proven phaeochromocytoma is of interest (Mannelli et al 1983).

Section 1

Q–T Interval
Syndrome, Prolonged
(Romano-Ward,
Jervell and
Lange-Nielsen
Syndromes, Familial
Ventricular
Tachycardia)

Presentation

The onset of pulmonary oedema has been reported in close association with the administration of naloxone to reverse the effect of opiates in the recovery period. It was first described in a 70-year-old man after cardiac surgery in which high-dose morphine was used (Flacke et al 1977). In view of the patient's pre-existing cardiac disease, this might not be considered to be remarkable. However, pulmonary oedema has also been reported after small doses of naloxone in four healthy patients having elective surgery (Andree 1980, Taff 1983, Prough et al 1984) and one having emergency surgery (Wride et al 1989). Two patients died.

Management

Oxygenation, and IPPV if necessary.

BIBLIOGRAPHY

Andree R A 1980 Sudden death following naloxone administration. Anesthesia and Analgesia 59: 782–788

Flacke J W, Flacke W E, Williams S G D 1977 Acute pulmonary edema following naloxone reversal of high dose morphine anesthesia. Anesthesiology 47: 376–378

Mannelli M, Maggi M, DeFeo M L et al 1983 Naloxone administration releases catecholamines in a patient with pheochromocytoma. New England Journal of Medicine 308: 654–655

Partridge B L, Ward C F 1986 Pulmonary edema following low-dose naloxone administration. Anesthesiology 65: 709–710

Prough D S, Roy R, Bumgarner J et al 1984 Acute pulmonary edema in healthy teenagers following conservative doses of i.v. naloxone. Anesthesiology 60: 485–486

Taff R H 1983 Pulmonary edema following naloxone administration in a patient without heart disease. Anesthesiology 59: 576–577

Wride S R N, Smith R E R, Courtney P G 1989 A fatal case of pulmonary oedema in a healthy young male following naloxone administration. Anaesthesia and Intensive Care 17: 374–377

Q–T INTERVAL SYNDROME, PROLONGED
(ROMANO–WARD, JERVELL AND LANGE–NIELSEN SYNDROMES, FAMILIAL VENTRICULAR TACHYCARDIA)

The Q–T interval represents depolarization and repolarization of the ventricle; that is, one complete ventricular contraction. The long Q–T syndrome (LQTS) describes a group of inherited disorders in which there are repolarization abnormalities which result in a long Q–T interval on ECG together with other unusual features. Affected individuals may have episodes of syncope associated with serious ventricular arrhythmias, and those who are untreated have a high incidence of sudden death.

In two of these rare inherited conditions the Q–T interval is prolonged, and in the third it is normal at rest but prolonged on exercise. The first, described by Jervell and Lange-Nielsen, is recessive and associated with nerve deafness, but the second, the Romano-Ward syndrome, a dominant condition, is not. The third, familial ventricular tachycardia, is also autosomal dominant.

Section 1

Q–T Interval
Syndrome, Prolonged
(Romano-Ward,
Jervell and
Lange-Nielsen
Syndromes, Familial
Ventricular
Tachycardia)

The cause of the long Q–T interval is thought to be an imbalance between the sympathetic supply to the right and left sides of the heart. Ventricular tachyarrhythmias can be precipitated by sudden increases in sympathetic activity, mostly mediated by the left stellate ganglion (Schwartz et al 1991). More recently, a high incidence of echocardiographic abnormalities has been demonstrated in patients with LQTS compared with matched healthy controls (Nador et al 1991). These consisted of unusual ventricular wall motion abnormalities, which were more likely to be found in the patients who were symptomatic. In addition, right stellate ganglionectomy in dogs produced the same abnormality.

In any of the conditions, emotion or exercise can provoke syncopal attacks which are associated with either VT or VF, and can result in death. There is often a family history of sudden deaths, but the degree of Q–Tc (the Q–T interval corrected for heart rate) prolongation is not an independent predictor of risk.

International studies of LQTS have helped to increase the understanding of the pathophysiology, and the prognosis has improved with active management. The effects of long-term therapy on mortality in the long Q–T syndrome were examined in 203 patients (Schwartz et al 1975). Untreated patients had a mortality of 73%, while in those treated with beta adrenoceptor blockers it was only 6%. A third group, who were treated, but not with beta blockers, had a mortality of 64%. In some patients, left cervical sympathectomy has shortened the Q–T interval and reduced the incidence of syncopal attacks (Yanagida et al 1976). Other drugs which have been used for treatment include phenytoin, verapamil, bretylium and primidone. However, beta blockers prevent syncope in about 75–80% of patients. In those patients refractory to treatment with beta blockers other measures such as left cervicothoracic ganglionectomy (Schwartz et al 1991), permanent pacing (Moss et al 1991), and the use of automatic implanted cardioverter defibrillators have been shown to reduce the incidence of syncope and tachyarrhythmias. Children are particularly likely to be refractory to treatment (Weintraub et al 1990), therefore it has been suggested that the children that survive into adulthood are the least severely affected.

The condition, and its treatment, has considerable anaesthetic significance. There have been a number of case reports in which VT, VF or cardiac arrest have occurred during anaesthesia in otherwise fit young patients. Most patients have been of the age at which preoperative ECGs are unlikely to have been performed, or even if they have, the condition may not have been recognized. A history of recurrent syncope (which may be diagnosed as epilepsy), congenital deafness, or a family history of sudden deaths, should alert the anaesthetist to the possibility of this condition (Adu-Gyamfi et al 1991, Holland 1993). Although the

Section 1

Q–T Interval
Syndrome, Prolonged
(Romano-Ward,
Jervell and
Lange-Nielsen
Syndromes, Familial
Ventricular
Tachycardia)

condition is rare, its mere existence illustrates the importance of initiating ECG monitoring from the start of the anaesthetic, whatever the age of the patient.

Preoperative abnormalities

1. There may be a known family history of the condition, or a history of sudden and unexpected deaths in young members of a family. Congenital sensorineural deafness may be associated.

2. The patient may give a history of syncopal attacks or, as sometimes happens, may be diagnosed as being epileptic (Ponte & Lund 1981) or hysterical. In a study of 23 children, the mean age of diagnosis was 10 years (range 4 days to 19 years) and initial symptoms included syncope, aborted sudden death and near drowning (Weintraub et al 1990).

3. ECG abnormalities. The Q–T interval is measured from the beginning of the QRS complex to the end of the T wave. It varies with heart rate, shortening as heart rate increases, and therefore must be corrected for rate (see below). In general, the normal Q–T interval should be less than 0.42 seconds, whilst in the prolonged Q–T interval syndrome it may be as long as 0.6 seconds. T waves are also usually abnormal, being broad and diphasic or altering in polarity. There is often a bradycardia, a feature that is unusual in children.

   Approximate relationship between heart rate and Q–T interval in a normal subject.

50 b.p.m.	0.38–0.42 s
60 b.p.m.	0.35–0.41 s
70 b.p.m.	0.33–0.39 s
80 b.p.m.	0.29–0.37 s
90 b.p.m.	0.28–0.36 s
100 b.p.m.	0.26–0.34 s

4. Treadmill testing in children has shown that the QTc interval is significantly prolonged during exercise (Weintraub et al 1990).

5. An abnormal ventricular contraction pattern was seen on echocardiography in 55% LQTS patients and consisted of a rapid early contraction and a prolonged phase of slow ventricular thickening before rapid relaxation (Nador et al 1991). This feature may provide a non-invasive marker for screening patients with stress-induced syncope.

6. Some patients with long Q–T syndrome have a prolapsed mitral valve (Forbes & Morton 1979).

Anaesthetic problems

1. VT, VF or cardiac arrest can occur during anaesthesia. Thirteen anaesthetic papers describe a total of 17 anaesthetics given to

patients with congenital long Q–T interval syndrome. In nine anaesthetics, the patients were treated with propranolol (Owitz et al 1979, O'Callaghan et al 1982, Medak & Benumof 1983, Carlock et al 1984, Galloway & Glass 1985), whilst one patient had a left cervical sympathetic block (Callaghan et al 1977). None of these had complications. In the eight anaesthetics in which the diagnosis had not been made (therefore no beta blocker had been given) there were three episodes of VF, four of VT and one of asystole. (Forbes & Morton 1979, Wig et al 1979, Ponte & Lund 1981, Brown et al 1981, Medak & Benumof 1985, Adu-Gyamfi et al 1991, Richardson et al 1992, Holland 1993). One patient died, the others were resuscitated.

Section 1

Q–T Interval
Syndrome, Prolonged
(Romano-Ward,
Jervell and
Lange-Nielsen
Syndromes, Familial
Ventricular
Tachycardia)

2. The risk of transient attacks of VT or VF is increased by sympathetic stimulation, emotion, exercise, or alcohol.

3. Some drugs, including halothane, isoflurane and enflurane, when used for slow inhalation induction, caused significant increases in Q–Tc interval, suggesting that they directly affected ventricular repolarization (Schmeling et al 1991). Thiopentone (Martineau & Nadeau 1987), and large doses of opiates, may also prolong the Q–T interval. Propofol was found to produce less prolongation than thiopentone (McConachie et al 1989, Giraud et al 1991). In one child, the use of adrenaline (for caudal anaesthesia and infiltration by the surgeon) resulted in torsade de pointes tachycardia. Treatment with lignocaine produced VF (Richardson et al 1992).

4. Pregnancy in patients with LQTS has occasionally been described. Problems arose in interpretation of cardiotocography, particularly because of maternal beta adrenoceptor blockade and the possibility of a fetal conduction defect. In this case, both twins were found to have congenital LQTS (Wilkinson et al 1991). In Jervell and Lange-Nielsen syndrome, profound deafness proved to be a problem in two women requiring Caesarean section, one under general anaesthesia (Freshwater 1984), the other under extradural anaesthesia (Ryan 1988).

5. Communication problems other than deafness may prevent a significant family history being unearthed before anaesthesia. Ventricular fibrillation occurred at the end of anaesthesia in a deaf, Sikh child, whose parents spoke little English (Holland 1993). Later, a family history of unexplained deaths was discovered. Consanguinity of parents may predispose to the syndrome and another Sikh patient has been described (Freshwater 1984).

Management

1. Preoperative family history taking is important. In a child with sensorineural deafness, a history of syncope or a family history of sudden deaths should alert the anaesthetist to the possibility of the Jervell, Lange-Nielsen syndrome.

Section 1

Q-T Interval
Syndrome, Prolonged
(Romano-Ward,
Jervell and
Lange-Nielsen
Syndromes, Familial
Ventricular
Tachycardia)

2. If the patient has congenital LQTS, he should have full beta adrenoceptor blockade, usually with propranolol, before anaesthesia. It has been suggested that pindolol and oxprenolol should be avoided, in view of their intrinsic sympathetic activity (Galloway & Glass 1985).

3. ECG monitoring should be continued through the perioperative period or during labour, and a defibrillator should be available.

4. A good premedication and reassurance helps to relieve anxiety.

5. Left stellate ganglion block may shorten the Q-T interval and increase the threshold for ventricular fibrillation.

6. Tracheal intubation and extubation cause sympathetic stimulation, and should not be performed during very light anaesthesia.

7. Any drug known to produce a tachycardia, or to prolong the Q-T interval, should be avoided. Drugs in these categories include pancuronium, atropine, thiopentone, halothane and high-dose opiates.

8. Isoflurane has been suggested as a suitable inhalation agent (Carlock et al 1984).

BIBLIOGRAPHY

Adu-Gyamfi Y, Said A, Chawdhury U M et al 1991 Anaesthetic-induced ventricular tachyarrhythmias in Jewell and Lange-Nielsen syndrome. Canadian Journal of Anaesthesia 38: 345–346

Brown M, Liberthson R R, Ali H A et al 1981 Perioperative management of a patient with long Q-T interval syndrome. Anesthesiology 55: 586–589

Callaghan M L, Nichols A B, Sweet R B 1977 Anesthetic management of prolonged Q-T interval syndrome. Anesthesiology 47: 67–69

Carlock F J, Brown M, Brown E M 1984 Isoflurane anaesthesia for a patient with long Q-T syndrome. Canadian Anaesthetists' Society Journal 31: 83–85

Forbes R B, Morton G H 1979 Ventricular fibrillation in a patient with unsuspected mitral valve prolapse and prolonged Q-T interval. Canadian Anaesthetists' Society Journal 26: 424–427

Freshwater J V 1984 Anaesthesia for Caesarean section and the Jervell, Lange-Nielsen syndrome (prolonged Q-T interval syndrome). British Journal of Anaesthesia 56: 655–657

Galloway P A, Glass P S A 1985 Anesthetic implications of prolonged Q-T interval syndrome. Anesthesia and Analgesia 64: 612–620

Giraud M, Chassard D, Gelas P et al 1991 QT interval during intubation with propofol or thiopental. Anesthesiology 75: A83

Holland R R 1993 Cardiac arrest under anaesthesia in a child with previously undiagnosed Jervell and Lange-Nielsen syndrome. Anaesthesia 48: 149–151

McConachie I, Keaveny J P, Healy T E J et al 1989 Effect of anaesthesia on the QT interval. British Journal of Anaesthesia 63: 558–560

Martineau R J, Nadeau S G 1987 Q-Tc interval changes during induction of anaesthesia. Canadian Journal of Anaesthesia 34: S61–62

Medak R, Benumof J L 1985 Perioperative management of the prolonged Q-T interval syndrome. British Journal of Anaesthesia 55: 361–364

Moss A J, Liu J E, Gottlieb S et al 1991 Efficacy of permanent pacing in the management of high risk patients with long QT syndrome. Circulation 84: 1524–1529

Nador F, Beria G, De Ferrari G M et al 1991 Unsuspected echocardiographic abnormality in the long QT syndrome. Circulation 84: 1530–1542

O'Callaghan A C, Normandale J P, Lowenstein E 1982 The prolonged Q-T syndrome. A review with anaesthetic implications and the report of two cases. Anaesthesia and Intensive Care 10: 50–55

Owitz S, Pratilas V, Pratila M G et al 1979 Anaesthetic considerations in the
    prolonged Q–T interval (LQTS). Canadian Anaesthetists' Society Journal 26: 50–54
Ponte J, Lund J 1981 Prolongation of the Q–T interval (Romano Ward syndrome):
    anaesthetic management. British Journal of Anaesthesia 53: 1347–1350
Richardson M G, Roark G L, Helfaer M A 1992 Intraoperative epinephrine-induced
    torsade de pointes in a child with long QT syndrome. Anesthesiology 76: 647–649
Ryan H 1988 Anaesthesia for Caesarean section in a patient with Jervell, Lange-
    Nielsen syndrome. Canadian Journal of Anaesthesia 35: 422–424
Schmeling W T, Warltier D C, McDonald D J et al 1991 Prolongation of the QT
    interval by enflurane, isoflurane and halothane in humans. Anesthesia and
    Analgesia 72: 137–142
Schwartz P J, Locati E, Moss A J et al 1991 Left cardiac sympathetic denervation in
    the therapy of congenital long QT syndrome. Circulation 84: 503–511
Schwartz J, Periti M, Malliani A 1975 The long Q–T syndrome. American Heart
    Journal 89: 378–390
Weintraub R G, Cow R M, Wilkinson J L 1990 The congenital long QT syndromes in
    childhood. Journal of the American College of Cardiology 16: 674–680
Wilkinson C, Gyaneshwar R, McCusker C 1991 Twin pregnancy in a patient with
    idiopathic long QT syndrome. Case report. British Journal of Obstetrics and
    Gynaecology 98: 1300–1302
Wig J, Bali I M, Singh R G et al 1979 Prolonged Q–T interval syndrome. Sudden
    cardiac arrest during anaesthesia. Anaesthesia 34: 37–40
Yanagida H, Kemi C, Suwa K 1976 The effects of stellate ganglion block on the
    idiopathic prolongation of the Q–T interval with cardiac arrhythmia (The Romano-
    Ward syndrome). Anesthesia and Analgesia 55: 782–787

RABIES

An infectious acute neurological disease caused by a rhabdovirus,
transmitted through saliva from the bite of a rabid animal. The virus
accumulates locally and then ascends via the peripheral nerves to the
central nervous system, where it replicates in the neural cells. Peripheral
dissemination then occurs via the nerves to a number of different organ
sites (Morrison & Wenzel 1985). Recovery is rare. Animals reported to
transmit rabies include dogs, foxes, badgers, bats, skunks and racoons.
Rabies is not yet endemic in Britain, although its relentless spread
through Europe is such that its appearance is inevitable. Prophylaxis is
crucial, and the new human diploid cell strain vaccines are very
effective. No case of rabies has been reported in anyone given the
vaccine correctly, with the hyperimmune serum, on the day of contact
with the rabid animal (Editorial 1988). Present controls are directed
towards parenteral vaccination of domestic animals and oral vaccination
of foxes (Tyrell & Nicholson 1990, Muller & Blancou 1992).

Presentation

1. A patient who develops an acute neurological condition, and who
   has a history of an animal bite sustained in an endemic area, is
   suspect. Sensory changes may occur at the site of the bite.
2. Presentation may include acute hydrophobic spasms, opisthotonos,
   flaccid paralysis, and coma. When the subject tries to drink water,

there are painful inspiratory, pharyngeal and laryngeal muscle spasms (hydrophobia). Asphyxia may occur during a spasm. Autonomic involvement and haematemesis may occur. Those surviving this stage of 'furious rabies' may progress to a paralytic phase.

3. Recovery from the disease is extremely rare.

Anaesthetic problems

1. Although the outlook is poor in the established disease, intensive care provides the only hope for the patient (Cundy 1980, Udwadia et al 1989). The three survivors of clinical rabies required intensive care facilities and prolonged hospitalization (Morrison & Wenzel 1985).
2. Management of the airway in hydrophobic spasms, or respiratory support if paralysis occurs, may be required.
3. Serious cardiac arrhythmias may occur with autonomic involvement.
4. Other complications include cardiac and renal failure, increased intracranial pressure, ARDS, hyperthermia, hypothermia, and diabetes insipidus (Udwadia et al 1989).

Management

The admission of rabid patients to British hospitals is rare, but the occasional case appears. The isolation and management of such a case for 12 days on a British ITU has been described (Cundy 1980). Consultation with microbiological and clinical experts is essential. An outline of management is given but the bibliography offers more detailed advice.

1. A microbiologist must be consulted. Rabies prophylaxis requires local wound care and both passive and active rabies immunization. Animal studies have shown the importance of scrubbing the wound with soap, iodine or alcohol. Tetanus prophylaxis should also be even.
2. Barrier nursing, by a limited special staff who may be offered vaccination. Airborne transmission of rabies has been reported, so mask, gown and gloves should always be worn (Morrison & Wenzel 1985).
3. IPPV, sedation and treatment to control spasms.
4. Monitoring of cerebral and cardiovascular function.
5. The standard support required by an ITU patient requiring IPPV.

BIBLIOGRAPHY

Chavenet P, Grebert C, Waldner A et al 1990 Abbreviated schedule for rabies postexposure prophylaxis. Lancet 335: 1462

Cundy J M 1980 Rabies encephalitis: management in a district general hospital ICU. Anaesthesia 35: 35–41

Editorial 1988 Rabies vaccine failures. Lancet 1: 917–918

Morrison A J, Wenzel R P 1985 Rabies: A review and current approach for the clinician. Southern Medical Journal 78: 1211–1218
Muller W W, Blancou J 1992 Rabies in Europe. Now possible to confine and eliminate. British Medical Journal 305: 725–726
Tyrrell D A, Nicholson F G 1990 Rabies in Britain. British Medical Journal 300: 137–138
Udwadia Z F, Udwadia F E, Katrak S M et al 1989 Human rabies: clinical features, diagnosis, complications, and management. Critical Care Medicine 17: 834–836

RELAPSING POLYCHONDRITIS

A rare systemic inflammatory disease in which there is gradual destruction of the cartilage of the nose, ears, joints, larynx and trachea. Inflammation, oedema, and scarring of the tracheal rings results in tracheal narrowing and dynamic airway obstruction. The condition usually presents between the ages of 40 and 60 years. Early onset, anaemia, laryngotracheal stricture, saddle nose and systemic vasculitis are associated with a poor prognosis (McAdam et al 1976, Michet et al 1986). Anaesthesia may be required for surgical reconstruction of the nose or ear, or occasionally for treatment of airway collapse.

Preoperative abnormalities

1. The most common features are nasal and auricular chondritis, with saddle nose and cauliflower ears, and polyarthritis. Ocular inflammation and audiovestibular damage may also occur.
2. Cutaneous vasculitis and systemic symptoms such as fever and anaemia.
3. In a study of airway complications of relapsing polychondritis, symptoms included breathlessness, cough, stridor, wheezing, hoarseness, and tenderness over the laryngotracheal cartilages (Eng & Sabanathan 1991). Although respiratory involvement is uncommon early in the disease, up to 50% patients are eventually affected. Respiratory complications are responsible for significant morbidity and mortality. A detailed study of five patients showed that expiratory obstruction usually resulted from airway abnormalities rather than loss of lung elastic forces (Krell et al 1986).
4. The incidence of cardiovascular involvement is 15–46% and includes aortic and mitral regurgitation and myocarditis (VanDecker & Panidis 1988). Aortic regurgitation is probably secondary to dilatation of the aortic root and annulus as a result of degenerative changes, therefore the improvement after valve replacement may be shortlived. Valve thickening and myxomatous degeneration may also contribute to the problem.
5. CXR and CT scan may show tracheal narrowing, although if the obstruction is dynamic these may be normal. Inspiratory and

expiratory flow-volume loops will show dynamic obstruction and whether it is primarily intrathoracic or extrathoracic. Intrathoracic obstruction is worse during expiration, and extrathoracic obstruction worse on inspiration (Eng & Sabanathan 1991).

6. Increased ESR and the presence of fetal cartilage antibodies.
7. Biopsy of cartilage involved will confirm the diagnosis.

Anaesthetic problems

1. Tracheomalacia results in tracheal collapse on forced inspiration and expiration. Since the obstruction is dynamic, it may be difficult to demonstrate on conventional static investigations. A CT scan does not reliably predict the degree of airway obstruction and the airway may be reported to be normal. Thus, inspiratory and expiratory flow-volume curves may be needed.

2. The diagnosis may sometimes be missed. A pregnant patient whose dyspnoea had been attributed to chronic asthma was found to have tracheal narrowing and stenosis of the left main bronchus (Gimovsky & Nishiyama 1989). Biopsy of the auricular cartilage confirmed relapsing polychondritis.

3. Anaesthesia may precipitate airway obstruction. During bronchoscopy, the tracheal lumen was observed to collapse almost completely on each inspiration (Burgess et al 1990).

4. There is a high incidence of subglottic stenosis. In one patient during general anaesthesia for tracheostomy a size 3-mm tube was passed with the aid of a metal introducer (Hayward & Al-Shaikh 1988). Later the tracheostomy tube became dislodged, and on this occasion when anaesthesia was required, the larynx would only admit a 14-gauge Harris catheter.

5. The tracheal and laryngeal disease may result in difficulty in clearing secretions; one patient had a respiratory arrest immediately after reconstruction of his nose and subsequent bronchoscopy showed thick secretions and inflammation of the tracheal mucosa (Eng & Sabanathan 1991).

6. Sudden death may occur following tracheal cartilage collapse, in association with endoscopy or intubation.

7. The use of intratracheal stents may be associated with displacement and respiratory obstruction. Death has occurred secondary to obstruction of the stent by a mucus plug (Goddard et al 1991).

Management

1. If airway problems exist, assessment of their extent with CXR, CT scan, bronchoscopy and flow-volume loops.

2. Corticosteroids are the first line of treatment, particularly when the disease is active. Other treatment includes immunosuppressives and NSAIDs. Plasmapheresis may have a role.

3. Surgery may occasionally be required for respiratory complications, but experience is limited and results uncertain. Posterior membrane fixation of the bronchial tree or internal stenting with a tracheal prosthesis, such as a Montgomery tube, have been performed (Neville et al 1990). However, intratracheal stents may be associated with asphyxia secondary to displacement and obstruction.

4. Intensive physiotherapy, humidification and suction are necessary in the perioperative period.

5. Tracheostomy may be needed, but is only of assistance when there are isolated subglottic problems.

BIBLIOGRAPHY

Burgess F W, Whitlock W, Davis M J et al 1990 Anesthetic implications of relapsing polychondritis: a case report. Anesthesiology 73: 570–572

Eng J, Sabanathan S 1991 Airway complications in relapsing polychondritis. Annals of Thoracic Surgery 51: 686–692

Gimovsky M L, Nishiyama M 1989 Relapsing polychondritis in pregnancy: a case report and review. American Journal of Obstetrics and Gynecology 161: 332–334

Goddard P, Cook P, Laszlo G et al 1991 Relapsing polychondritis: report of an unusual case and a review of the literature. British Journal of Radiology 64: 1064–1067

Hayward A W, Al-Shaikh B 1988 Relapsing polychrondritis and the anaesthetist. Anaesthesia 43: 573–577

Krell W S, Staats B A, Hyatt R E 1986 Pulmonary function in relapsing polychondritis. American Review of Respiratory Disease 133: 1120–1123

McAdam L P, O'Hanlan M A, Bluestone R et al 1976 Relapsing polychondritis: prospective study of 23 patients and review of the literature. Medicine 55: 193–215

Michet C J, McKenna C H, Luthra H S et al 1986 Relapsing polychondritis. Survival and predictive role of early disease manifestations. Annals of Internal Medicine 104: 74–78

Neville W E, Bolanowski P J P, Kotia G G 1990 Clinical experience with the silicone tracheal prosthesis. Journal of Thoracic and Cardiovascular Surgery 99: 604–613

VanDecker W, Panidis I P 1988 Relapsing polychondritis and cardiovascular involvement. Annals of Internal Medicine 109: 340–341

RENAL FAILURE, CHRONIC

This term is intended to encompass a progressive reduction of glomerular filtration rate, from decreased renal reserve, to renal insufficiency, and finally to end-stage renal failure. In all cases an acute reduction in function can be superimposed on the chronic disease. The anaesthetist must ensure that neither omissions nor commissions worsen renal function, cause drug-induced nephrotoxicity, or seriously interfere with the patient's compensatory mechanism for his disease. The hyperbolic relationship between serum creatinine or urea, and GFR, means that more than 50% of excretory function may be lost without change in the serum chemistry outside the normal range. Many of the patients will be on some form of dialysis. Dialysis provides the means by which the most serious abnormalities of hyperkalaemia, circulatory overload and acidosis can be corrected in the 12–24 hours before surgery. Renal failure has a profound effect on all systems of the body. Some of the abnormalities seen will be due to the renal disease itself, others are associated with long-term dialysis.

Anaesthesia may be required for renal transplantation, insertion of Tenckhoff catheters, CAPO, creation of arteriovenous (A-V) fistulae, or for parathyroid or incidental surgery.

Preoperative abnormalities

1. In contrast to acute renal failure, when the causes are principally pre-renal, the causes of chronic renal failure are primarily a result of intrinsic renal disease. These include glomerulonephritis, hypertension, diabetes, chronic pyelonephritis, hereditary renal disease including polycystic disease and Alport's disease, the systemic vasculitides including SLE, PAN and Wegener's granulomatosis, the paraproteinaemias and amyloid. Postrenal (obstructive) causes must also be considered, and include prostatic hypertrophy, bladder and other pelvic tumours, calculus disease, retroperitoneal fibrosis and tumours.
2. Renal failure has widespread systemic effects:
   a. Cardiovascular
   Hypertension is common, either from retention of water and sodium, or secondary to increased renin secretion by the kidney. Left ventricular failure may be due to this, to the high cardiac output secondary to anaemia, or to uraemic cardiomyopathy. Occasionally, high blood flow through the arteriovenous fistula may contribute. Pericardial effusions can be associated either with terminal uraemia or with dialysis. Tamponade occasionally occurs. Cardiovascular lesions are numerically by far the most important cause of death in the dialysis population, with an increased incidence of atheroma, coronary artery disease, and cerebrovascular accidents. Conduction defects may be associated with hyperkalaemia Cardiovascular instability can occur during or after dialysis, or may be secondary to autonomic neuropathy.
   b. Pulmonary
   Pulmonary venous congestion or frank pulmonary oedema may occur. On CXR there is a typical symmetrical bat-wing appearance radiating from the lung hila. There is an increased susceptibility to lung infection. A low Pa_{CO_2} results from respiratory compensation for the metabolic acidosis.
   c. Nervous system
   There may be peripheral or autonomic neuropathies. Loss of nerve fibres and demyelination occur. Neuropathies are usually reversed after successful renal transplantation. Mental changes may be associated with chronic dialysis. Uraemic encephalopathy may reflect underdialysis, or be associated with disequilibrium

(with probable elevated ICP) related to dialysis. A characteristic encephalopathy (associated with bone disease and anaemia) has been attributed to aluminium intoxication. Aluminium is excreted by the normal body, but accumulates during maintenance therapy, being derived from the softened waters (in certain geographical areas) used to make dialysate, or by ingestion of aluminium compounds used to chelate and inhibit gastrointestinal absorption of dietary phosphate. There are now stringent EEC recommendations limiting the concentration of aluminium in dialysate fluids. Some success in its removal has been achieved by desferrioxamine.

d. Gastrointestinal

Delayed gastric emptying and increased acid secretion occurs. There is a high incidence of gastrointestinal inflammation and bleeding. Liver function may be abnormal. An increased carrier rate for HBsAg occurs.

e. Bone disease

Renal bone disease may include elements of osteomalacia, osteitis fibrocystica and osteosclerosis. Failure of phosphate excretion is associated with increased serum phosphate levels, and hypocalcaemia. The latter induces secondary hyperparathyroidism and PTH secretion may then become autonomous.

3. Biochemical abnormalities

Nephron loss is associated with failure of hydrogen ion excretion and a metabolic acidosis ensues. Serum bicarbonate is further reduced by compensatory respiratory alkalosis.

4. Haematological abnormalities

A normochromic, normocytic, hypoproliferative anaemia occurs, in part due to inadequate production of erythropoietin. Anaemia starts as the creatinine level increases above 250 μmol/l, and a haemoglobin between 3 and 9 g/dl results. Repeated blood transfusion carries the danger of iron overload and may require therapy with desferrioxamine. Erythropoietin can now be manufactured by a recombinant DNA technique. There are criteria for selection for treatment (MacDougall et al 1990), which is is aimed at partial correction of the anaemia to a level of 10–12 g/dl. Complete correction may carry the risk of increased blood viscosity, thrombosis of the A-V fistula and hypertension (Cotes 1988, MacDougall et al 1990). Treatment three times a week corrected the anaemia, reduced iron overload, and improved the quality of life (Eschbach et al 1989). In untreated anaemia, compensation occurs by an increase in cardiac output and a shift of the oxygen dissociation curve. Uraemia causes a prolonged bleeding time as a result of platelet dysfunction, but this improves on dialysis.

5. Treatment for end-stage renal failure may involve regular haemodialysis, continuous ambulatory peritoneal dialysis or renal transplantation.
6. The patient may have a permanent A-V fistula for vascular access.

Anaesthetic problems

1. Delayed gastric emptying occurs, which is further prolonged by haemodialysis. Gastric acidity is increased.
2. The incidence of hepatitis in patients on dialysis was high (up to 25%), and a percentage of patients become chronic HBsAg carriers. With the advent of regular screening this has been greatly reduced. There is an increased risk to staff. Impaired liver function is common, secondary to hepatic venous congestion.
3. Hypertension and cardiovascular instability may be a problem. There is a decreased tolerance to variations in fluid balance. Both fluid overload and dehydration readily occur.
4. Drug excretion
   Although gallamine is the only anaesthetic drug which is entirely excreted by the kidney, the excretion of many drugs will be delayed. Accumulation of either the parent drug, or its metabolites may occur, especially if repeated doses are given (Drayer 1977).
   a. Benzodiazepines
      The majority of benzodiazepines are relatively long acting and many have active metabolites. Lorazepam, oxazepam and diazepam all have increased half-lives in renal failure. This is not so with the shorter acting ones such as temazepam and midazolam (Vinik et al 1983).
   b. Opiates
      i. There is increased sensitivity to morphine, which is in part due to decreased binding by plasma proteins, especially in the presence of an acidosis.
      ii. Pethidine has CNS-depressant effects and has a short half-life, but one of its metabolites, norpethidine, has excitatory effects and a long half-life. With chronic administration or multiple doses of pethidine, norpethidine accumulates. Two cases were reported in which twitching and irritability were associated with high ratios of norpethidine to pethidine (Szeto et al 1977). One of these patients had impaired renal function.
   c. Neuromuscular blocking agents
      i. In renal failure, a single dose of suxamethonium will normally only produce an increase in serum potassium of 0.5–0.7 mmol/l. However, an increase of 2.8 mmol/l occurred following a second dose of suxamethonium in a patient with uraemic neuropathy (Walton & Farman 1973).
      ii. Early reports suggested that dialysis was associated with low

plasma cholinesterase levels. A later study of 81 patients having renal transplants did not confirm this (Ryan 1977). Improvements in dialysis membranes may explain these discrepancies.

iii. d-Tubocurarine, alcuronium and, in particular, pancuronium have all been shown to produce prolonged neuromuscular blockade (McCleod et al 1976). The half-life of neostigmine is also prolonged (Cronnelly et al 1979) but that of vecuronium is only slightly longer than normal (Meistelman et al 1983).

d. Inhalation agents

Isoflurane, halothane and enflurane have all been used in renal failure. Although there have been a small number of reports of deterioration of renal function following enflurane, the levels of inorganic fluoride produced are usually well below those associated with renal toxicity. When halothane and enflurane were given to patients with mild to moderate renal failure, all showed a slight improvement in renal function (Mazze et al 1984).

5. Regional anaesthesia

A reduction in duration of brachial plexus block has been reported and attributed to an increased cardiac output (Bromage & Gertel 1972). However, this finding has been disputed (Martin et al 1988, Rice et al 1991). The presence of acidosis may increase CNS toxicity of local anaesthetics.

6. A-V fistula patency

There are risks of occluding the A-V fistula during surgery. Mechanical pressure, hypotension, cold, and hypercoagulability will predispose to this.

7. Hypercarbia and acidosis increase serum potassium levels. Both hypercarbia and hypocarbia reduce renal blood flow.

Management

1. Correction of fluid overload and electrolyte (particularly potassium) abnormalities. Dialysis should take place within 12–36 hours of surgery.
2. A coagulation screen, LFTs and HBsAg should be reviewed.
3. Prophylactic treatment for acid aspiration syndrome should be given, with antacid and H2 receptor antagonists. The half-life of cimetidine is increased to 3–4 hours, so doses should be reduced.
4. Only short-acting benzodiazepines such as temazepam or midazolam should be used.
5. The hypertensive response to intubation may be reduced by treatment with propranolol, lignocaine, fentanyl or alfentanil.
6. Monitoring.
   The fistula arm should not be used for the blood pressure cuff, nor

for i.v. infusions. Direct arterial monitoring should be avoided, so as to preserve arteries for subsequent vascular access. If monitoring of vascular volume is required, a CVP is preferred to a pulmonary artery catheter, which carries an increased risk of infection. Normocarbia is maintained by use of a capnograph. Serious increases in serum potassium can be detected by ECG monitoring of T-wave changes. Neuromuscular monitoring is essential. Pulse oximetry is a useful adjunct.

7. Venous access

Arteries and veins must be conserved, and the A-V fistula protected from potentially occlusive insults. A bruit over the fistula must be heard both before and after surgery. The fistula arm should not be used, and hypotension and cooling avoided. Occlusion of the fistula, if it occurs, is an indication for immediate thrombectomy. Wide-bore subclavian catheters are commonly employed as temporary access for haemodialysis and should not be used for routine intravenous purposes.

8. General anaesthesia

a. Thiopentone is a suitable induction agent, although etomidate may be indicated if there is significant cardiac disease. A study of 15 patients given midazolam 0.2 mg/kg showed that the elimination half-life was identical to that in normal patients (Vinik et al 1983). Bradycardia frequently occurs in renal failure, so the use of an anticholinergic is indicated.

b. Suxamethonium should be avoided if the serum potassium is >5.5 mmol/l, or if there is a uraemic neuropathy. If suxamethonium is used, a second dose may produce a variety of arrhythmias. The pharmacokinetics and pharmacodynamics of atracurium, which is spontaneously broken into inactive components (Hofmann elimination), are unaltered by renal failure (Fahey et al 1984, de Bros et al 1985). Animal experiments suggest that laudanosine is unlikely to reach high enough levels to produce adverse EEG effects (Ingram et al 1983). Only small increases in the half-life of vecuronium have been found (Meistelman et al 1983). The half-life of neostigmine is prolonged, but the changes are similar to those occurring with d-tubocurarine and pancuronium.

c. Fentanyl is probably the most suitable analgesic. However, caution should be used with repeated doses, since increases in plasma fentanyl, probably due to drug redistribution, have been reported 2–5 hours after injection (Gulden et al 1984).

9. Regional anaesthesia

In the absence of bleeding problems, the use of reigonal anaesthesia reduces the need for giving cumulative doses of drugs. Brachial plexus block has been used for vascular access, and local anaesthesia for insertion of Tenckhoff catheters for CAPD. Two diabetic patients had severe cardiovascular depression about 20 minutes after brachial plexus block for A-V fistula formation; this was attributed to autonomic neuropathy (Lucas & Tsueda 1990). Selective anaesthesia of the musculocutaneous and medial antebrachial cutaneous nerves of the forearm for A-V fistula creation has also been described (Eldredge et al 1992). A-V fistula blood flows were compared using four techniques of anaesthesia: brachial plexus block, local anaesthesia, isoflurane, and halothane (Mouquet et al 1989). All techniques were found to be satisfactory, but the flows in the brachial artery were significantly less when local anaesthesia was used.

High spinal anaesthesia has been reported to produce satisfactory conditions for renal transplantion (Linke & Merin 1976). A reduction in local anaesthetic dosage by 25% has been recommended (Weir & Chung 1984) and severe hypertension, or uraemic neuropathy are contraindications to regional techniques.

10. Maintenance of cardiac output and blood pressure are essential.

BIBLIOGRAPHY

Bromage P R, Gertel M 1972 Brachial plexus anesthesia in chronic renal failure. Anesthesiology 36: 488–493

Cotes P M 1988 Erythropoietin: the developing story. British Medical Journal 296: 805–806

Cronnelly R, Stanski D R, Miller R D et al 1979 Renal function and the pharmacokinetics of neostigmine in anesthetised man. Anesthesiology 51: 222–226

de Bros F M, Lai A, Scott R et al 1985 Pharmacokinetics and pharmacodynamics of atracurium under isoflurane anesthesia in normal and anephric patients. Anesthesia and Analgesia 64: 207

Drayer D E 1977 Active drug metabolites and renal failure. American Journal Medicine 62: 486–489

Eldredge S J, Sperry R J, Johnson J O 1992 Regional anesthesia for arteriovenous fistula creation in the forearm: a new approach. Anesthesiology 77: 1230–1231

Eschbach J W, Addulhadi M H, Browne J K et al 1989 Recombinant human erythropoietin in anemic patients with end-stage renal disease: results of a phase III multicenter clinical trial. Annals of Internal Medicine 111: 992–1000

Fahey M R, Rupp S M, Fisher D M et al 1984 The pharmacokinetics and pharmacodynamics of atracurium in patients with and without renal failure. Anesthesiology 61: 699–702

Graybar G B, Tarpey M 1987 Kidney transplantation. In: Gelman S (ed) Anesthesia and organ transplantation. W B Saunders, Philadelphia

Gulden D, Koehntop D, Rodman J et al 1984 Fentanyl pharmacokinetics during renal transplant. Anesthesiology 61: A243

Ingram M D, Sclabassi R J, Stiller R L et al 1985 Cardiovascular and electroencephalographic effects of laudanosine in 'nephrectomised' cats. Anesthesia and Analgesia 64: 232

Linke C L, Merin R G 1976 A regional anesthetic approach for renal transplantation. Anesthesia and Analgesia 55: 69–73

Lucas L F, Tsueda K 1990 Cardiovascular depression after brachial plexus block in two diabetic patients with renal failure. Anesthesiology 73: 1032–1035

MacDougall I C, Hutton R D, Cavill I et al 1990 Treating renal anaemia with recombinant human erythropoietin: practical guidelines and a clinical algorithm. British Medical Journal 300: 655–658

McLeod K, Watson M J, Rawlins M D 1976 Pharmacokinetics of pancuronium in patients with normal and impaired renal function. British Journal of Anaesthesia 48: 341–345

Maddern P J 1983 Anaesthesia for the patient with impaired renal function. Anaesthesia and Intensive Care 11: 321–328

Mazze R I, Sievenpiper T S, Stevenson J 1984 Renal effects of halothane and enflurane in patients with abnormal renal function. Anesthesiology 60: 161-163

Martin R, Beauregard L, Tetrault J P 1988 Brachial plexus block and chronic renal failure. Anesthesiology 69: 405–406

Meistelman C, Leinhart A, Leveque C et al 1983 Pharmacology of vecuronium in patients in end stage renal failure. Anesthesiology 59: A293

Mouquet C, Bitker M O, Bailliart O et al 1989 Anesthesia for creation of a forearm fistula in patients with endstage renal failure. Anesthesiology 70: 909–914

Rice A S C, Pither C E, Tucker G T 1991 Plasma concentrations of bupivacaine after supraclavicular brachial plexus blockade in patients with chronic renal failure. Anaesthesia 46: 354–357

Ryan D W 1977 Preoperative serum cholinesterase concentration chronic renal failure. British Journal of Anaesthesia 49: 945–949

Szeto H H, Inturrisi C E, Houde R et al 1977 Accumulation of normeperidine, an active metabolite of meperidine in patients with renal failure or cancer. Annals of Internal Medicine 86: 738–741

Vinik H R, Rever J G, Greenblatt D J et al 1983 The pharmacokinetics of midazolam in chronic renal failure. Anesthesiology 59: 390–394

Walton J D, Farman J V 1973 Suxamethonium hyperkalaemia in uraemic neuropathy. Anaesthesia 28: 666–668

Weir P H C, Chung F F 1984 Anaesthesia for chronic renal failure. Canadian Anaesthetist Society Journal 31: 468–480

RETROLENTAL FIBROPLASIA
(RLF)

A condition occurring in premature infants, or those with a birth weight <1500 g, in which an acute vascular retinopathy may progress to retinal scarring, detachment and possible blindness. Although originally attributed to exposure to high oxygen tensions in the neonatal period, it is now thought that there are many factors involved in the development of the severe form of the disease. Prematurity seems to be the most important of these, since approximately 45% neonates weighing <1000 g develop acute retinal changes at birth. Out of this group however, only 10–20% will progress to cicatricial changes, retinal detachment and impairment of vision. Oxygen is probably only one of the factors which determines this unpredictable progression. The increase in incidence of RLF, despite care to limit oxygen tensions, probably reflects in part the increasing ability of neonatal units to salvage the lower-birthweight infants.

Anaesthetic problems

1. The extent of risk to premature infants during major surgery is of concern. A twin (1140 g) who had surgery for duodenal atresia, and who had an increased inspired oxygen concentration for 4.5 hours, with the Pa_{O_2} varying from 8.5–43 kPa, developed the cicatricial form of RLF, whereas the other normal twin (1440 g) did not. No retinal examination had been made prior to surgery (Betts et al 1977).

2. The multifactorial elements of this disorder have been stressed in a description of the clinical course of a 1445-g infant who developed severe RLF (Merritt et al 1981). No oxygen was given at delivery, but on day 7 abdominal surgery was required. The FIo_2 varied between 25% and 30% for the 45-minute procedure, apart from three separate 5-minute periods when it was 50%. Air only was given in the recovery room. Bicarbonate was required for a persistent metabolic acidosis over an 11-day period, and packed red cells were given for anaemia on day 12. A patent ductus arteriosus was also present, but asymptomatic. At 16 months, the child was found to have severe RLF. It was suggested that the acidosis and the blood transfusion might have increased the oxygen delivery to the retinal tissues and hence the susceptibility of the immature vessels to damage.

3. The lack of data linking the development of RLF with concentrations of oxygen <50% has merited editorial comment (Flynn 1984). The view that a multiplicity of factors, including continual exposure to artificial light, might render the immature retinal vessels more susceptible to oxygen damage than normal, was accepted. In an analysis of 134 cases of RLF in 639 infants, it was concluded that those who had major surgery in the course of their care were at no greater risk of developing permanent retinal damage than those who did not have surgery.

Management

1. All premature infants are at risk of developing RLF, presumably until the retinal vessels are mature. If surgery is required in this period, it has been suggested that ophthalmological assessment of vascular maturity should be made. There are practical difficulties in this (Merritt et al 1981).

2. An attempt should be made to maintain a Pao_2 of not greater than 10.6–12 kPa. In the presence of a patent ductus arteriosus, the most significant measurement is that of preductal Pao_2, since this will reflect most accurately retinal exposure. Inspired concentration and trancutaneous Po_2 give indirect information.

BIBLIOGRAPHY
Betts E K, Downes J J, Schaffer D B et al 1977 Retrolental fibroplasia and oxygen administration during general anesthetia. Anesthesiology 47: 518–520
Flynn J T 1984 Oxygen and retrolental fibroplasia. Anesthesiology 60: 397–399
Merritt J C Sprague D H, Merritt W E et al 1981 Retrolental fibroplasia: a multifactorial disease. Anesthesia and Analgesia 60: 109–111

RHABDOMYOLYSIS

Injury to skeletal muscle producing myoglobinaemia and myoglobinuria, and associated with an increase, sometimes massive, of the creatine kinase (CK) levels. Free myoglobin appears in the blood soon after exposure to the cause. It may be detected in blood and urine almost immediately, but its transient appearance means it is frequently missed, whereas the plasma CK levels take several hours to increase. Renal damage may occur, but the exact mechanism is unclear. Rhabdomyolysis of varying degrees of severity can be precipitated by a wide range of conditions, including drug overdoses and the administration of certain anaesthetic drugs. It is more likely to occur when there is muscle disease, but drugs and drug overdoses may precipitate rhabdomyolysis in apparently normal muscle.

Rhabdomyolysis not associated with anaesthesia

1. Predisposing conditions for rhabdomyolysis not associated with anaesthesia include crush and burns injury, ischaemia, viral infections, polymyositis, heat stroke, marathon running, McArdle's syndrome (McMillan et al 1989), Taurius' syndrome, neuroleptic malignant syndrome and carnitine palmitoyl transferase deficiency (Kelly et al 1989). Occasionally it has occurred following status epilepticus accompanied by lactic acidosis (Winocour et al 1989).

2. Drug overdose may be associated with rhabdomyolysis, and reports have included theophylline (Parr & Willatts 1991), 'Ecstasy', 'Eve' and other related synthetic amphetamines (Singarah & Lavies 1992, Tehan et al 1993), cocaine, and beta 2 adrenoreceptor agonists. In a study of cocaine users presenting to an emergency department, 24% had rhabdomyolysis, defined as a serum CK of greater than 1000 u/l, although symptoms were often absent (Welch et al 1991). Massive rhabdomyolysis and acute renal failure have been reported. Rhabdomyolysis, acute renal failure and compartment syndrome have been described in young alcoholics undergoing treatment with benzodiazepines (Rutgers et al 1991). Rhabdomyolysis and acute renal failure also occurred after an overdose of terbutaline, a beta 2 adrenoreceptor agonist, secondary to intense beta adrenoceptor stimulation (Blake & Ryan 1989).

3. The passage of dark brown urine, positive for blood on reagent strip, but with no RBCs on microscopy, is suggestive of the diagnosis. Serum CK levels may sometimes be massively elevated.

4. The appearance of renal failure may be the first indication that rhabdomyolysis has occurred.

Anaesthetic problems

1. Rhabdomyolysis in association with anaesthesia is most frequently precipitated by suxamethonium and it may occasionally occur in an otherwise normal patient. Children are more susceptible to muscle injury after suxamethonium than are adults, particularly if halothane has been given first (McKishnie et al 1983). However, those

individuals who have a significant degree of muscle destruction are often subsequently found to have some underlying muscle disorder. In such patients, inhalational agents alone have been known to precipitate rhabdomyolysis.

2. Conditions in which there may be anaesthetic drug-induced muscle breakdown include malignant hyperthermia myopathy, Duchenne and Becker muscular dystrophy (Bush & Dubowitz 1991), myotonia congenita, spinal muscle atrophy, Guillain-Barré syndrome (Scott et al 1991), carnitine palmitoyl transferase deficiency (Katsuya et al 1988), McArdle's syndrome, polyneuropathy and burns.

3. Masseter muscle rigidity (MMR) is a term applied to severe spasm of the muscles of mastication lasting for 2–3 minutes following suxamethonium. This may be accompanied by varying degrees of rhabdomyolysis. About 50% of patients with severe MMR were reported to be susceptible to MH (Rosenberg & Fletcher 1986). However, it is now known that increased tension in the masseter muscle is a normal response to suxamethonium and MMR has been reported to occur in 1% of children, particularly when an inhalational agent has been given first (See also Section 2, Masseter muscle rigidity.)

4. Sometimes the first sign of muscle breakdown is the occurrence of a serious cardiac arrhythmia, secondary to acute hyperkalaemia. Early cardiac arrest has been reported in Guillain-Barré syndrome (Hawker et al 1985), Duchenne muscular dystrophy (Seay et al 1978, Linter et al 1982, Chalkiadis & Branch 1990), or non-specific myopathy (Schaer et al 1977).

5. Myoglobinuria may present unexpectedly in the postoperative period (Hool et al 1984, Rubiano et al 1987), and if severe, or untreated, may progress to renal failure. Postoperative myoglobinuria and renal failure after suxamethonium and halothane was reported in a 3-year-old with a strong family history of DMD (McKishnie et al 1983). The author has seen severe rhabdomyolysis in a 13-year-old boy after dental anaesthesia in whom the maximum serum CK, which occurred the next day, was 252 000 u/ml. A presumptive diagnosis of MH was made, but investigations undertaken 4 years later were negative for MH and showed an asymptomatic spinal muscular atrophy.

6. Rhabdomyolysis has been reported in several patients subjected to protracted surgery in the lithotomy (Lydon & Spielman 1984) or the lateral position (Targa et al 1991), and after a prolonged tourniquet time.

7. Postoperative muscle weakness or stiffness may occur.

Management

1. Anticipation of the problem. Suxamethonium is best avoided in patients with myopathic or neuropathic types of disease, in

particular those who are immobile. It should certainly not be given in DMD, Guillain-Barré syndrome, McArdle's syndrome, MH myopathy, or after thermal injury.

2. Should sudden cardiac arrest occur after suxamethonium, the possibility of hyperkalaemia should be urgently considered. Blood samples should be taken for serum potassium and if levels are high, treatment must be directed to emergency treatment. In myopathic muscle, it may take a long time to restore the serum potassium to normal (Chalkiadis & Branch 1990). In such cases, myoglobinaemia and myoglobinuria should be anticipated.

3. If myoglobinuria occurs, intravenous fluid therapy and an osmotic diuretic should be given to maintain an adequate urine flow. Urine output and serum CK, urea, creatinine, and electrolyte levels should be checked regularly in the acute phase.

4. If renal failure ensues, haemodialysis should be instituted until renal function recovers (Hool et al 1984, Hawker et al 1985).

5. Dantrolene has been used in the treatment of hyperthermia and rhabdomyolysis caused by theophylline overdose (Parr & Willatts 1991), that is secondary to the consumption of the synthetic amphetamines 'Ecstasy' (Singarajah & Lavies 1992), and 'Eve' (Tehan et al 1993), and in the neuroleptic malignant syndrome.

BIBLIOGRAPHY

Blake P G, Ryan F 1989 Rhabdomyolysis and acute renal failure after terbutaline overdose. Nephron 53: 76–77

Bush A, Dubowitz V 1991 Fatal rhabdomyolysis complicating general anaesthesia in a child with Becker muscular dystrophy. Neuromuscular Disorders 1: 201–204

Chalkiadis G A, Branch K G 1990 Cardiac arrest after isoflurane anaesthesia in a patient with Duchenne's muscular dystrophy. Anaesthesia 45: 22–25

Hawker F, Pearson I Y, Soni N et al 1985 Rhabdomyolytic renal failure and suxamethonium. Anaesthesia and Intensive Care 13: 208–209

Hool G J, Lawrence P J, Sivaneswaran N 1984 Acute rhabdomyolytic renal failure due to suxamethonium. Anaesthesia and Intensive Care 12: 360–364

Katsuya H, Misumi M, Ohtani Y et al 1988 Postanesthetic acute renal failure due to carnitine palmityl transferase deficiency. Anesthesiology 68: 945–948

Kelly K J, Garland J S, Tang T T et al 1989 Fatal rhabdomyolysis following influenza infection in a girl with familial carnitine palmityl transferase deficiency. Pediatrics 84: 312–316

Linter S P K, Thomas P R, Withington P S et al 1982 Suxamethonium hypertonicity and cardiac arrest in unsuspected pseudohypertrophic muscular dystrophy. British Journal of Anaesthesia 54: 1331–1333

Lydon J C, Spielman F J 1984 Bilateral compartment syndrome following prolonged surgery in the lithotomy position. Anesthesiology 60: 236–238

McKishnie J D Muir J M, Girvan D P 1983 Anaesthesia induced rhabdomyolysis. Canadian Anaesthetists' Society Journal 30: 295–298

McMillan M A, Hallworth M J, Doyle D et al 1989 Acute renal failure due to McArdle's disease. Renal Failure 11: 23–25

Parr M J A, Willatts S M 1991 Fatal theophylline poisoning with rhabdomyolysis. A potential role for dantrolene treatment. Anaesthesia 46: 557–559

Rosenberg H, Fletcher J E 1986 Masseter muscle rigidity and malignant hyperthermia susceptibility. Anesthesia and Analgesia 65: 161–164

Rubiano R, Chang J-L, Carroll J et al 1987 Acute rhabdomyolysis following halothane anesthesia without succinylcholine. Anesthesiology 67: 856–857

Rutgers P H, van der Harst E, Koumans R K 1991 Surgical implications of drug-induced rhabdomyolysis. British Journal of Surgery 78: 490–492

Schaer H, Steinmann B, Jerusalem S et al 1977 Rhabdomyolysis induced by anaesthesia with intraoperative cardiac arrest. British Journal of Anaesthesia 49: 495–499

Scott A J, Duncan R, Henderson L et al 1991 Acute rhabdomyolysis associated with atypical Guillain-Barré syndrome. Postgraduate Medical Journal 67: 73–74

Seay A R, Ziter F A, Thompson J A 1978 Cardiac arrest during induction of anaesthesia in Duchenne muscular dystrophy. Journal of Pediatrics 93: 88–90

Singarajah C, Lavies N G 1992 An overdose of ecstasy. A role for dantrolene. Anaesthesia 47: 686–687

Targa L, Droghetti I, Caggese G et al 1991 Rhabdomyolysis and operating position. Anaesthesia 46: 141–143

Tehan B, Hardem R, Bodenham A 1993 Hyperthermia associated with 3,4-methylene dioxyethamphetamine ('Eve'). Anaesthesia 48: 507–510

Welch R D, Todd K, Krause G S 1991 Incidence of cocaine-associated rhabdomyolysis. Annals of Emergency Medicine 20: 154–157

Winocour P H, Waise A, Young G et al 1989 Severe, self-limiting lactic acidosis and rhabdomyolysis accompanying convulsions. Postgraduate Medical Journal 65: 321–322

RHEUMATOID ARTHRITIS

A common autoimmune connective tissue disease, primarily involving the joints, but with widespread systemic effects. There is hypergammaglobulinaemia, and rheumatoid factors, which are autoantibodies of IgE, IgA and IgM classes, are present.

Preoperative abnormalities

1. The joint disease involves inflammation, the formation of granulation tissue, fibrosis, joint destruction and deformity. Any joint may be affected. Those of particular concern to the anaesthetist are the cervical, the temporomandibular and the cricoarytenoid joints.

2. Extra-articular problems occur in more than 50% patients.

   a. Lungs. May be affected by effusions, nodular lesions, diffuse interstitial fibrosis or Caplan's syndrome. This is a form of massive pulmonary fibrosis seen in coal miners with rheumatoid arthritis or positive rheumatoid factor, and probably represents an abnormal tissue response to inorganic dust. There may be a restrictive lung defect, with a contribution from reduced chest wall compliance.

   b. Kidney. Twenty-five per cent of patients eventually die from renal failure. Renal damage may be related to the disease process itself, from secondary amyloid disease, or from drug treatment.

   c. Heart. Is involved in up to 44% of cases. Small pericardial effusions are common, but are not usually of clinical significance. Rarely pericarditis and tamponade may occur, usually in seropositive patients and those with skin nodules (Burney et al 1979). Other problems include endocarditis or left ventricular failure. Occasionally, heart valve lesions occur and are of two types: rheumatoid granulomata involving the leaflets and ring, and non-granulomatous valvular inflammation with thickening and fibrosis of the leaflets.

d. Blood vessels

A widespread vasculitis can occur. Small arteries and arterioles are often involved, frequently in the presence of relatively disease-free main trunk vessels. Significant ischaemia may result, the actual effects depending on the tissue or organ supplied.

e. Swallowing problems and dysphagia were found in 8 out of 29 patients with classical rheumatoid arthritis compared with only one in a control group (Geterud et al 1991b). Oesophageal manometry showed upper oesophageal dysfunction in the rheumatoid group but there was no correlation between the results of manometry and the symptoms of dysphagia.

f. Peripheral neuropathy.

3. Chronic anaemia, which has been shown to respond to erythropoietin therapy, is common (Salvarani et al 1991).

Anaesthetic problems

1. Involvement of cervical vertebrae; possible damage to the cervical spinal cord associated with neck manipulation during anaesthesia and sedation.

   Cervical instability is reported to occur in 25% of patients with rheumatoid arthritis. Of these, one-quarter will have no neurological symptom to alert the physician (Norton & Ghanma 1982). The presenting symptoms of 31 patients with cervical myelopathy were analyzed (Marks & Sharp 1981). Sensory disturbances occurred in 74% but these were often dismissed and attributed to peripheral neuropathy. Weakness occurred in 19%, flexor spasms in 16% and incontinence in 6%. By the time the diagnosis was made, 77% had spastic paraparesis or quadriparesis. The problem of instability is not necessarily confined to those with longstanding disease.

   The commonest lesion is that of atlantoaxial subluxation, although subaxial subluxations may occur in addition. Destruction of bone and weakening of the ligaments allow the odontoid peg to migrate backwards and upwards, compressing the spinal cord against the posterior arch of the atlas. Thus, the main danger lies in cervical flexion. In an MRI study of 34 patients with atlantoaxial instability, the relationships between spinal cord diameter in the neutral and flexed positions, the clinical signs, and the latency of motor evoked potentials, were examined. Thickening of inflammatory tissue of greater than 3 mm behind the odontoid peg was observed in 22 patients and this contributed to a decreased spinal cord diameter when the neck was in the flexed position. A spinal cord diameter in flexion of less than 6 mm, severe pain and cranial migration of the axis, were suggested to indicate the need for surgical intervention (Dvorak et al 1989).

The potential dangers of anaesthesia and endoscopy have been emphasized. Flexion of the head and reduction in muscle tone may result in cervical cord damage (McConkey 1982, Norton & Ghanma 1982). Dislocation of the odontoid process and spinal cord damage was discovered in a patient undergoing postoperative IPPV on the ITU (Bollensen et al 1991). It was not known exactly when this had occurred. In an analysis of 113 rheumatoid patients having total hip or knee arthroplasty, cervical spine X-rays were examined for signs of atlantoaxial subluxation, atlantoaxial impaction and subaxial subluxation (Collins et al 1991). One or more of these findings were present in 61% of patients.

2. Patients who have previously undergone occipital cervical fusion may develop cervical instability below the level of the original arthrodesis (Kraus et al 1991). Two groups of patients were compared: one group had undergone occipitocervical fusion for atlantoaxial subluxation and superior migration of the odontoid; the other group had undergone atlantoaxial fusion for isolated axial subluxation. In the first group, 36% of patients developed subaxial subluxation requiring surgery at an average of 2.6 years, whereas in the second group 5.5% of patients developed subaxial subluxation requiring surgery after an average of 9 years. Occipital cervical fusion is thought to generate a greater force at lower cervical level, which in turn stresses the unfused facet joints.

3. Laryngeal problems. A constant pattern of laryngeal and tracheal deviation is reported to occur in some patients, particularly those with proximal migration of the odontoid peg (Keenan et al 1983). The larynx is tilted forwards, displaced anteriorly and laterally to the left and the vocal cords rotated clockwise. Involvement of the larynx in the rheumatoid process is more common than was previously thought. In a study of 29 females, one or more signs of laryngeal involvement were found in 69% of patients; physical signs were seen on fibreoptic examination in 59%; there was evidence of extrathoracic airway obstruction in 14%; and 10% had abnormal X-rays (Geterud et al 1991a). Although symptoms of breathing difficulty occurred in 75% of the group studied, cricoarytenoid joint involvement only rarely produces actual upper airway obstruction.

4. Limitation of mouth opening may occur secondary to arthritis of the temporomandibular joints. This is a particular problem in juvenile rheumatoid arthritis (Hodgkinson 1981).

5. A pericardial effusion and tamponade presented as an acute abdominal emergency in a young patient with seropositive rheumatoid arthritis (Bellamy et al 1990). Hypoxaemia and hypotension occurred at induction of anaesthesia. Laparotomy

showed gross hepatic congestion and ascites, CXR revealed cardiomegaly, and one litre of turbid fluid was drained at pericardial fenestration.

6. If there is rheumatoid aortic valve involvement, it may be more rapidly progressive than aortic valve disease from other causes, so that there is little time for compensatory hypertrophy of the ventricle to occur. Acute aortic regurgitation, which produced sudden cardiac failure in a young woman and required urgent valve replacement, has been described (Camilleri et al 1991).

7. Lung disease may cause reduced pulmonary reserve and hypoxaemia.

8. There may be an increased sensitivity to anaesthetic agents.

Management

1. Clinical assessment of neck and jaw mobility. The Sharp and Purser test gives some indication of cervical spine instability (Norton & Ghanma 1982). The patient should be upright, relaxed and with the neck flexed. With a finger on the spinous process of the axis, the forehead should be pressed backwards with the other hand. Normally there is minimal movement. If subluxation is present, the head moves backwards as reduction occurs.

2. A lateral view of the cervical spine in flexion and extension will show the distance between the odontoid peg and the posterior border of the anterior arch of the atlas. If subluxation is present, this distance is greater than 3 mm.

3. Cervical X-rays of patients who have previously undergone occipital spinal fusion should be examined for evidence of cervical instability at a lower level.

4. Cervical instability may be an indication for awake fibreoptic intubation and application of a collar or Crutchfield tongs to maintain rigidity during surgery. Since spinal instability is usually in flexion, some authors believe that safe tracheal intubation can be achieved under general anaesthesia by careful extension of the head, except in the rare instances of posterior atlantoaxial subluxation, when fibreoptic intubation is indicated (Heywood et al 1988). Emergency control of the airway has been described using a laryngeal mask airway in a patient who developed acute pulmonary oedema following occipitocervical fusion (Calder et al 1990).

5. Deviation of the larynx may make fibreoptic laryngoscopy more difficult in some patients (Keenan et al 1983). Examination of the orientation of the larynx by indirect laryngoscopy at preoperative assessment may be helpful. If there is cricoarytenoid involvement, care should be taken with the choice of tracheal tube size and tube insertion.

6. Assessment of pulmonary function and reserve.

7. Examination for other significant complications such as valvular disease or pericardial effusion.

8. The use of extradural or caudal anaesthesia may be unwise in patients in whom intubation difficulties are anticipated.

BIBLIOGRAPHY

Bellamy M C, Natarajan V, Lenz R J 1990 An unusual presentation of cardiac tamponade. Anaesthesia 45: 135–136

Bollensen E, Schonle P W, Braun U et al 1991 An unnoticed dislocation of the dens axis in a patient with primary chronic polyarthritis undergoing intensive therapy. (English abstr) Anaesthetist 40: 294–297

Burney D P, Martin C E, Thomas C S et al 1979 Rheumatoid pericarditis. Journal of Thoracic and Cardiovascular Surgery 77: 511–515

Calder I, Ordman A J, Jackowski A et al 1990 The Brain laryngeal mask airway. An alternative to emergency tracheal intubation. Anaesthesia 45: 137–139

Camilleri J P, Douglas-Jones A G, Pitchard M H 1991 Rapidly progressive aortic valve incompetence in a patient with rheumatoid arthritis. British Journal of Rheumatology 30: 379–381

Collins D N, Barnes C L, FitzRandolph R L 1991 Cervical spine instability in rheumatoid patients having total hip or knee arthroplasty. Clinical Orthopaedics 272: 127–135

Dvorak J, Grob D, Baumgartner H et al 1989 Functional evaluation of the spinal cord by magnetic resonance imaging in patients with rheumatoid arthritis and instability of the upper cervical spine. Spine 14: 1057–1064

Geterud A, Bake B, Berthelsen B et al 1991a Laryngeal involvement in rheumatoid arthritis. Acta Otolaryngologie (Stockholm) 111: 990–998

Geterud A, Bake B, Bjelle A et al 1991b Swallowing problems in rheumatoid arthritis. Acta Otolaryngologie (Stockholm) 111: 1153–1161

Heywood A W B, Learmonth I D, Thomas M 1988 Cervical spine instability in rheumatoid arthritis. Journal of Bone and Joint Surgery 70-B: 702–707

Hodgkinson R 1981 Anesthetic management of a parturient with severe juvenile rheumatoid arthritis. Anesthesia and Analgesia 60: 611–612

Keenan M A, Stiles C M, Kaufman R L 1983 Acquired laryngeal deviation associated with cervical spine disease in erosive polyarticular arthritis. Anesthesiology 58: 441–449

Kraus D R, Peppelman W C, Agarwal A K et al 1991 Incidence of subaxial subluxation in patients with generalized rheumatoid arthritis who have had previous occipital cervical fusions. Spine 16: S486–489

Marks J S, Sharp J 1981 Rheumatoid cervical myelopathy. Quarterly Journal of Medicine 50: 307–319

McConkey B 1982 Rheumatoid cervical myelopathy. British Medical Journal 284: 1731–1732

Norton M L, Ghanma M A 1982 Atlanto-axial instability revisited; an alert for endoscopists. Annals of Otology, Rhinology and Laryngology 91: 567–570

Salvarani C, Lasagni D, Casali B et al 1991 Recombinant human erythropoietin therapy in patients with rheumatoid arthritis with the anaemia of chronic disease. Journal of Rheumatology 18: 1168–1171

SARCOIDOSIS

A multisystem granulomatous disorder, of variable natural history and prognosis, most frequently presenting in young adults with bilateral hilar lymphadenopathy, pulmonary infiltration, cutaneous, and ocular lesion. In some, an acute onset may resolve spontaneously; in others slow onset may herald progressive disease with serious complications such as pulmonary fibrosis, blindness, cardiac involvement, and nephrocalcinosis.

Preoperative abnormalities

1. The patient may be asymptomatic, and about one-third of cases present because of an abnormality found on CXR. With more advanced disease there may be variable degrees of respiratory impairment, CXR usually shows bilateral hilar lymphadenopathy with increased reticular shadowing in the lung fields. Lung function tests may be impaired, Restrictive, gas transfer and obstructive defects may all occur at different stages of the disease. In advanced disease, pulmonary hypertension may develop.

2. Other more commonly involved organs are the skin, eyes, liver, spleen, and the bones of the hands and feet. Hypercalcaemia may occur which is secondary to the production of excess 1,25-dihydroxycholecalciferol. Nephrocalcinosis may result.

3. Cardiac disease, although rare, is more common than was previously thought (Fleming 1986) and carries a poor prognosis, Its diagnosis is of anaesthetic importance.

   The pathological lesions can be diffuse or focal. Localized granulomata and fibrous scarring most commonly occur in the basal portion of the ventricular septum and left ventricular wall (Valantine et al 1987). These lesions will be asymptomatic unless they happen to involve the conducting system, in which case arrhythmias or conduction defects occur. Less commonly, the distribution of granulomata may be widespread, and they may coalesce to produce diffuse interstitial fibrosis, The resulting hypokinesia and subsequent heart failure will be clinically indistinguishable from that of other cardiomyopathies (Fleming 1986).

   At autopsy on 84 patients with sarcoidosis, 27% were found to have myocardial granulomata, one-third of which had been unsuspected (Silverman et al 1978). In those patients diagnosed as having cardiac involvement, the signs in order of frequency of presentation were: complete heart block, ventricular ectopics or ventricular tachycardia, myocardial disease causing heart failure, sudden death, and first-degree heart block or bundle branch block. A further analysis of 57 patients with complete heart block and sarcoid revealed that in 72%, the heart block was the first sign of the disease (Perhsson & Tornling 1985). Sudden death had occurred in two-thirds of patients in an autopsy study of cardiac sarcoid (Roberts et al 1977). In approximately 18% of these, death was the initial manifestation of cardiac involvement, and in the majority death occurred during a period of exercise.

4. Central nervous system sarcoid also carries a poor prognosis, Presentation can vary widely and includes cranial nerve palsies, peripheral neuropathy, epilepsy and cerebellar ataxia.

5. Laryngeal sarcoidosis may occur. The commonest lesion reported is an oedematous, pale, diffuse enlargement of the supraglottic structures (Neel & McDonald 1982).
6. The diagnosis can be made on biopsy of a skin lesion, or lung and bronchial biopsy via a fibreoptic bronchoscope. The Kveim test has a high positivity in the active stages, but is lower in the chronic disease. Serum angiotensin-converting enzyme, serum calcium and 24-hour urinary calcium levels may be increased in active sarcoid.
7. Treatment of active disease may include corticosteroids, immunosuppressants, methotrexate, NSAIDS and calcium chelating agents.

Anaesthetic problems

1. In advanced disease, respiratory function may be considerably impaired.
2. Although rare, cardiac disease may be unexpected, and can occur in young, previously asymptomatic patients. The sudden onset of complete heart block during anaesthesia in an athletic young man with sarcoid was described (Thomas & Mason 1988). Permanent pacing was required after surgery. Difficulties with pacemaker management can be a feature of cardiac sarcoidosis (Lie et al 1974).
3. A case of upper airway obstruction secondary to laryngeal sarcoid has been described (Wills & Harris 1987).

Management

1. If there is widespread pulmonary involvement and the patient is symptomatic lung function tests, including blood gases, should be performed.
2. A preoperative ECG is essential, even in young patients. If there is evidence of a conduction defect, a temporary pacemaker should be inserted before anaesthesia.
3. Assessment and management of laryngeal sarcoid.
4. Corticosteroids may improve symptoms and signs of cardiac and pulmonary sarcoidosis (Schaedel et al 1991).

BIBLIOGRAPHY

Fleming H A 1986 Sarcoid heart disease. British Medical Journal 292: 1095–1096
Lie J T, Hunt D, Valentine P A 1974 Sudden death from cardiac sarcoidosis with involvement of the conduction system. American Journal of the Medical Sciences 267: 123–128
Neel H B, McDonald T J 1982 Laryngeal sarcoidosis: report of 13 patients. Annals of Otology, Rhinology and Laryngology 91: 359–362
Pehrsson S K, Tornling G 1985 Sarcoidosis associated with complete heart block. Sarcoidosis 2: 135–141
Roberts W C, McAllster H A, Ferrans V J 1977 Sarcoidosis of the heart. American Journal of Medicine 63: 86–108
Schaedel H, Kirsten D, Schmidt A et al 1991 Sarcoid heart disease: results of follow-up investigations. European Heart Journal 12 (Suppl D): 26–27

Silverman K J, Hutchins G M, Bulkley B H 1978 Cardiac sarcoid: a chinicopathologic study of 84 unselected patients with systemic sarcoidosis. Circulation 58: 1204–1211

Thomas D W, Mason R A 1988 Complete heart block during anaesthesia in a patient with sarcoidosis. Anaesthesia 43: 578–580

Valantine H, McKenna W J, Nihoyannopoulos P et al 1987 Sarcoidosis: a pattern of clinical and morphological presentation. British Heart Journal 57: 256–263

Wills M H, Harris M M 1987 An unusual airway complication with sarcoidosis. Anesthesiology 66: 554–555

SCLERODERMA

A spectrum of diseases involving abnormal collagen deposition and vascular changes in the skin and other organs. Various forms have been described, including a localized cutaneous form (morphoea), systemic sclerosis, and the CREST syndrome (Calcinosis, Raynaud's, (o)Esophageal problems, Sclerodactyly and Telangiectasia). Scleroderma occurs more commonly in women, often in the 30–50 years age group. Pregnancy may worsen the disease, and there is a high incidence of fetal loss. Pulmonary hypertension was found to be the most frequent cause of death, and renal, cardiac, and pulmonary involvement were features associated with reduced survival (Lee et al 1992).

Preoperative abnormalities

1. The skin becomes taut, shiny and waxy looking. Skin folds are lost and there is a non-pitting oedema. Contractures of the joints and the mouth may develop. Multiple telangiectasia may occur. Sweating is reduced.

2. Disease of the peripheral vessels is predominant and Raynaud's of the hands and feet is the presenting feature in 90% of cases.

3. Oesophageal involvement has been reported in up to 80% of patients and may produce dysphagia, reflux oesophagitis, and strictures. It has been suggested that the basis of the dysphagia lies in disturbances of motility, rather than structural changes in the oesophagus (Weisman & Calcaterra 1978).

4. The lungs are commonly involved. Pulmonary vascular disease, progressing to pulmonary hypertension, and interstitial lung disease are the two main lesions (Arroliga et al 1992). Weakness of the respiratory muscles and diaphragm may occur (Iliffe & Pettigrew 1983).

5. Cardiac lesions may occur in 50–90% of cases of the systemic disease. A study of 46 patients with systemic sclerosis showed that 56% had arrhythmias or conduction defects, and 28% had a pericardial effusion demonstrated by echocardiography (Clements et al 1981). Cardiac and pulmonary artery enlargement secondary to pulmonary vascular disease may be seen on CXR.

6. Gut involvement may cause malabsorption, and occasionally vitamin C deficiency. Intestinal obstruction can occur.
7. Renal disease and hypertension are common in the systemic form of the disease. Clinical and pathological features of an accelerated phase occur, and the loss of renal function may be abrupt.
8. Antinuclear antibodies are present in 40–90% cases.
9. Patients may be receiving steroids or immunosuppressants.

Anaesthetic problems

1. Skin changes may result in difficulties with venous access. The contractures of the mouth are susceptible to damage, and may result in poor access to the oral cavity. Two problems occurred in a case during dental extraction. Injection into a peripheral cannula produced local complications in the patient's hand, and insertion of the mouth prop caused a tear of the angle of the mouth (Davidson-Lamb & Finlayson 1977).
2. Oesophageal involvement may make the patient more prone to acid reflux and regurgitation. Abnormalities of oesophageal function can occur even in asymptomatic patients, and there is an inability of the oesophagus to empty without the aid of gravity.
3. There is evidence that impaired nerve conduction occurs in scleroderma, affecting most sensory modalities (Schady et al 1991). In addition, complications have been described in association with local anaesthetic techniques. Prolonged sensory loss, which may be due to reduced blood flow, has been reported (Eisele & Reitan 1971, Lewis 1974). Injection of a large volume of solution can produce a degree of tension in the skin sufficient to interfere with local blood supply. Sclerotic skin may conceal landmarks.
4. Tracheal intubation may be more difficult than usual if there are mouth and neck contractures. Telangiectasia in the mouth or nose may bleed. Involvement of the larynx has been described (Rapp et al 1991).
5. Problems associated with systemic or pulmonary hypertension. Left ventricular failure, arrhythmias or pericardial effusions may arise. A maternal death was reported associated with the development of pulmonary oedema and pulmonary hypertension following Caesarean section (Younker & Harrison 1985). Severe hypertension and pulmonary oedema causing a maternal death in the 32nd week of pregnancy has been seen by the author.
6. The combination of pulmonary abnormalities and contraction of the skin of the chest wall may contribute to postoperative respiratory inadequacy. Inflammatory alveolitis occurs in up to 50% of patients and it is possible that interstitial fibrosis is an end result of this process (Silver et al 1990).

Management

1. Assessment of respiratory function, including lung function tests and blood gases, if there is pulmonary involvement. There is a suggestion that bronchiolar lavage may help to identify patients with active alveolitis.
2. Adequate venous access may require the use of a central vein or a venous cutdown. Vasoconstriction can be reduced by keeping the theatre temperature high and by warming intravenous fluids.
3. Precautions should be taken against acid aspiration.
4. Potential difficulties posed by tracheal intubation should be assessed preoperatively. Under certain circumstances, the possibility of an awake intubation or tracheostomy under local anaesthesia will need consideration.
5. Problems in measuring the blood pressure may be overcome by the use of an ultrasonic blood pressure device. If direct monitoring is necessary, then a large artery should be chosen.
6. For Caesarean section, the choice between a general or regional technique may be difficult. Successful extradural anaesthesia was reported in a patient with advanced systemic sclerosis and the CREST syndrome (Thompson & Conklin 1983). A coagulation screen should be performed, and care taken with the dose of local anaesthetic used.

BIBLIOGRAPHY

Arroliga A C, Podell D N, Matthay R A 1992 Pulmonary manifestations of scleroderma. Journal of Thoracic Imaging 7: 30–45
Clements P J, Furst D E, Cabeen W et al 1981 The relationship of arrhythmias and conduction disturbances to other manifestations of cardiopulmonary disease in progressive systemic sclerosis. American Journal of Medicine 71: 38–46
Davidson-Lamb R W, Finlayson M C K 1977 Scleroderma: complications encountered during dental anaesthesia. Anaesthesia 32: 893–895
Eisele J H, Reitan J A 1971 Scleroderma, Raynaud's phenomenon, and local anesthesics. Anesthesiology 34: 386–387
Iliffe G D, Pettigrew N M 1983 Hypoventilatory respiratory failure in generalised scleroderma. British Medical Journal; 286: 337–338
Lee P, Langevitz P, Alderdice C A et al 1992 Mortality in systemic sclerosis (scleroderma). Quarterly Journal of Medicine 82: 139–148
Lewis G B 1974 Prolonged regional analgesia in scleroderma. Canadian Anaesthetists' Society Journal 21: 495–497
Rapp M F, Guram M, Konrad H R et al 1991 Laryngeal involvement in scleromyxedema: a case report. Otolaryngology and Head and Neck Surgery 104: 362–365
Schady W, Sheard A, Hassell A et al 1991 Peripheral nerve dysfunction in scleroderma. Quarterly Journal of Medicine 80: 661–675
Silver R M, Miller K S, Kinsella M B et al 1990 Evaluation and management of scleroderma lung disease using bronchiolar lavage. American Journal of Medicine 88: 470–476
Steen V D 1989 Pregnancy in women with systemic scleroderma. Arthritis and Rheumatism 32: 151–157
Thompson J, Conklin K A 1983 Anesthetic management of a pregnant patient with scleroderma. Anesthesiology 59: 69–71
Tuffanelli D L 1989 Systemic scleroderma. Medical Clinics of North America 73(5): 1167–1179

Weisman R A, Calcaterra J C 1978 Head and neck manifestations of scleroderma. Annals of Otology, Rhinology and Laryngology 87: 332–339
Younker D, Harrison B 1985 Scleroderma and pregnancy. Anaesthetic considerations. British Journal of Anaesthesia 57: 1136–1139

SCOLIOSIS

A lateral curvature of the spine occurring in association with actual rotation of the vertebral body and spine, in the direction of the concavity of the curve. There is wedging of the vertebral body and discs. The resulting prominence of the posterior part of the ribs on the side of the convexity may give a false impression of kyphosis.

Scoliosis can be broadly divided into three categories, the commonest of which is the idiopathic form. Otherwise, scotiosis may be congenital, or may develop as a secondary feature of a variety of neuromuscular or connective tissue disorders. Causes of secondary scoliosis include poliomyelitis, syringomyelia, Friedreich's ataxia, muscular dystrophy, neurofibromatosis, Marfan's syndrome and rheumatoid arthritis.

Scoliosis is described in terms of its angle. The greater the angle, the more severe the respiratory and subsequent cardiovascular impairment.

Preoperative abnormalities

1. Respiratory changes

   Respiratory impairment in scoliosis results from a number of factors. These include abnormalities in the development of the rib cage, the muscles of respiration, and in the distribution of the pulmonary vascular bed in relation to the alveoli. Respiratory impairment is usually restrictive, the vital capacity, total lung capacity and functional residual capacity being between 60 and 80% of that predicted. As the severity of the scoliosis increases, airway closure encroaches on the functional residual capacity. The greater the angle of scoliosis, the greater the abnormalities in lung function. Gas exchange is impaired as a result of ventilation/blood flow inequalities, and it has been suggested that the greater maldistribution is on the side the concavity. Pa_{O_2} reduction occurs initially, and may deteriorate further with increasing age. The respiratory response to CO_2 is abnormal and pulmonary vascular resistance maybe elevated. Subsequently, hypercapnoea may develop. Initially, the abnormalities may occur only during sleep, and studies have shown a decreased vital capacity, hypoxia and respiratory failure in some patients at night.

2. Cardiovascular changes

   In the more severe cases, increased pulmonary vascular resistance results from a combination of structural changes in the pulmonary vascular bed and the effects of hypoxia. An increased pulmonary vascular pressure results. In the later stages there will be ECG changes of right atrial dilatation (P wave >2.5 mm in height) and right ventricular hypertrophy (R>S in leads V1 and V2). Right ventricular failure secondary to pulmonary disease, may finally ensue.

3. Associated problems
   a. Neuropathic: poliomyelitis, Friedreich's ataxia, syringomyelia.
   b. Myopathic: muscular dystrophy, spinal muscle atrophy.
   c. Miscellaneous: neurofibromatosis, Marfan's syndrome, rheumatoid arthritis.

Anaesthetic problems

Surgery may be incidental, or directed towards correction of the scoliosis. In general, the prognosis for patients with secondary scoliosis is less good than for the idiopathic form. Death from cardiac failure occurred in the seventh hour of a scoliosis correction in a 13-year-old patient with DMD (Sethna et al 1988). Another death was reported in a retrospective review of nine cases of DMD and one Becker's muscle dystrophy, undergoing spinal fusion. The particular patient had a VC of only 12% of that predicted and could not be weaned off the ventilator (Milne & Rosales 1982).

Surgery in general

1. Problems attributable to the underlying cause, if the scoliosis is not idiopathic.
2. Respiratory problems depend upon the degree of existing impairment. An already decreased respiratory response to CO_2 may be made worse by the anaesthetic. Whilst mild hypoxia is common, the onset of hypercarbia, unless precipitated by an acute infection, is of bad prognostic significance. A biphasic carbon dioxide excretion waveform was demonstrated in a severe kyphoscoliotic during IPPV. This was thought to result from the patient having two lungs with entirely different mechanics. The early peak represented the appearance of exhaled gas from well-ventilated regions of the lung with low airway resistance having a relatively low CO_2 concentration, followed by that from poorly-ventilated areas with high airway resistance having high CO_2 concentrations (Nichols & Benumof 1989).
3. As a result of the anatomical changes, the respiratory muscles work at a mechanical disadvantage, so that postoperative respiratory inadequacy and retention of secretions may occur.
4. In advanced cases, there may be the problems of pulmonary hypertension and right ventricular failure. Cardiac abnormalities, including hypertrophic cardiomyopathy and conduction defects, occur in 90% of patients with Friedreich's ataxia.

In DMD there may be hypertrophic cardiomyopathy and diastolic failure. Mitral valve prolapse may occur in some patients. Marfan's syndrome can be associated with mitral or aortic regurgitation, dissecting aortic aneurysm, aortic or pulmonary dilatation, or coronary artery disease.

5. Hyperkalaemia following the use of suxamethonium has been reported in patients with neuromuscular problems, particularly in cases in which there is a motor deficit.
6. Rhabdomyolysis and myoglobinuria may occur following the use of suxamethonium and halothane in patients with myopathies (including McArdle's syndrome and spinal muscular atrophy).
7. Serious arrhythmias and cardiac arrest have been described following the use of halothane and suxamethonium in Duchenne muscular dystrophy (see also Duchenne muscular dystrophy).
8. Satisfactory regional anaesthesia, which is particularly indicated during labour, may be difficult to achieve because of anatomical distortion of the spinal column and uneven spread of local anaesthetic (Moran & Johnson 1990).

Surgery for scoliosis

1. Inadequate preoperative respiratory reserve has resulted in postoperative deaths in patients subjected to surgery for scoliosis.
2. Evaluation of spinal cord function may be required after spinal distraction with Harrington rods. It may be necessary to waken the patient during the procedure, so that motor deficits can be detected and the spinal distraction decreased. Evoked cortical responses may be used, although these have not always been reliable.
3. Blood loss may be substantial. Losses of up to 92% of the patient's blood volume have been recorded (Abott & Bentley 1980).
4. Deliberate hypotensive techniques have been associated with a decrease in blood supply to the spinal cord, and subsequent paraplegia.
5. The problems of surgery performed in the prone position.
6. Hypothermia may occur in prolonged procedures, and when extensive blood loss has been replaced.
7. Haemopneumothorax.
8. Two fatal cases of air embolism have been reported during posterior spinal fusion and instrumentation (McCarthy et al 1990).

Management

Surgery in general

1. In severe cases, respiratory assessment should include the VC measured in both seated and supine positions, FEV with and without bronchodilators, and blood gases (Kafer 1980).

2. Cardiovascular assessment. If the PVR and PAP are increased, and there are ECG changes and signs of RVH, then the prognosis is poor. Right ventricular failure must be treated.
3. In severe cases, a decision must be made as to whether or not elective surgery should be undertaken.
4. If possible, regional or local anaesthesia should be used.
5. Monitoring should include EGG, core temperature, ET_{CO_2}, and blood pressure, measured directly or indirectly. When indicated, urine output, central venous pressure, blood gases, and occasionally PAP monitoring may be required.
6. Regional anaesthesia should be considered (Sethna & Berde 1991), although technical difficulties may be a problem. Continuous spinal anaesthesia with combined hyperbaric and hypobaric bupivacaine was used after failed extradural anaesthesia during labour (Moran & Johnson 1990).

Surgery for scoliosis

1. A VC of at least 20 ml/kg or 30% of predicted, and an inspiratory capacity of 15 ml/kg, have been suggested as being essential for scoliosis surgery (Milne & Rosales 1982).
2. The tracheal tube must be firmly secured in place.
3. A wake-up test should be performed, provided that the patient is a suitable subject and the matter has been discussed in advance. Techniques described for this include N_2O/O_2/relaxants with morphine (Sudhir et al 1976, Abott & Bentley 1980), with fentanyl (McEwen et al 1975) and with alfentanil (Chamberlain & Bradshaw 1985). The use of hypnosis (Crawford et al 1976) has also been reported. Reversal at the appropriate time is achieved with neostigmine and atropine, and by the use of a narcotic antagonist if necessary.
4. Sensory evoked potentials have been used both alone, and in conjunction with the wake-up test, to detect neurological damage (Grundy et al 1982). The reliability of sensory evoked potentials alone in predicting cord damage has not yet been established.
5. Theatre temperature should be maintained at a higher than usual level and a warming blanket and blood warmer used.
6. The use of deliberate hypotension should be carefully considered (Grundy et al 1982).
7. If the anterior approach through the diaphragm is used, postoperative IPPV may be required.

BIBLIOGRAPHY
Abott T R, Bentley G 1980 Intro-operative awakening during scoliosis surgery. Anaesthesia 35: 298–302
Chamberlain M E, Bradhaw E G 1985 The 'wake-up test'. Anaesthesia 40: 780–782
Crawford A H, Jones C W Perisho J A et al 1976 Hypnosis for monitoring intraoperative spinal cord function. Anesthesia and Analgesia 55: 42–44

Grundy B L, Nash C L, Brown R H 1982 Deliberate hypotension for spinal fusion: prospective randomised study with evoked potential monitoring. Canadian Anaesthetists' Society Journal 29: 456–461

Kafer E R 1980 Respiratory and cardiovascular functions in scoliosis and the principles of anesthetic management. Anesthesiology 52: 339–351

McCarthy R E, Lonstein J E, Mertz J D et al 1990 Air embolism in spinal surgery. Journal of Spinal Disorders 3: 1–5

McEwen G D, Bunnell W P, Sriram K 1975 Acute neurological complications in the treatment of scoliosis. Journal of Bone and Joint Surgery 57A: 404–408

Milne B, Rosales J K 1982 Anaesthetic considerations in patients with muscular dystrophy undergoing spinal fusion and Harrington rod insertion. Canadian Anaesthetists' Society Journal 29: 250–254

Moran D H, Johnson M D 1990 Continuous spinal anesthesia with combined hyperbaric and hypobaric bupivacaine in a patient with scoliosis. Anesthesia and Analgesia 70: 445–447

Nichols K P, Benumof J L 1989 Biphasic carbon dioxide excretion waveform from a patient with severe kyphoscoliosis. Anesthesiology 71: 986–987

Phillips D P, Roye D P Jr, Fatty J-P C et al 1990 Surgical treatment of scoliosis in a spinal muscular atrophy population. Spine 15: 942–945

Sethna N F, Rockoff M A, Worthen M et al 1988 Anesthesia-related complications in children with Duchenne muscular dystrophy. Anesthesiology 68: 462–465

Sethna N F, Berde C B 1991 Continuous subarachnoid analgesia in two adolescents with severe scoliosis and impaired pulmonary function. Regional Anesthesia 16: 333–336

Sudhir K G, Smith R M, Hall J E et al 1976 Intraoperative awakening for early recognition of possible neurological sequelae during Harrington rod spinal fusion. Anesthesia and Analgesia 55: 526–528

SHY-DRAGER SYNDROME
(see also AUTONOMIC DYSFUNCTION)

A condition presenting in late life, In which autonomic failure or dysfunction is associated with, or precedes, the onset of widespread central neuronal degeneration. In particular, there is loss of cells in the intermediolateral nuclei of the lateral horn in the spinal cord, which are the preganglionic sympathetic neurones. Features of autonomic failure, Parkinsonism, and cerebellar ataxia are combined.

Preoperative abnormalities

1. Neurological symptoms and signs of widespread neuronal involvement, including cerebellar ataxia and Parkinsonism.
2. Postural hypotension and an inability, in response to stress, to produce the normal pressor response which depends on reflex vasoconstriction and tachycardia. There is reversal of the usual diurnal pattern of blood pressure and that normally produced by postural changes.
3. Anhidrosis, incontinence and impotence can occur.
4. Fluid and electrolyte homeostasis is disturbed, resulting in a failure to concentrate urine at night and producing a nocturnal diuresis and sodium loss.

5. Vocal cord paralysis secondary to abductor palsy may result in stridor and respiratory failure. In some cases, isolated palsy has preceded the disease by as much as 2 years (Kew et al 1990). Sudden deaths have been reported.
6. There may be a disordered respiratory pattern and obstructive sleep apnoea.
7. Denervation hypersensitivity has been reported.
8. Osteoporosis and aseptic necrosis of bone are thought to be a result of impaired periosteal vascular control. Orthopaedic surgery may therefore be required.

Anaesthetic problems

1. The inability of the cardiovascular system to respond to stress by vasoconstriction and tachycardia results in a pronounced cardiovascular instability. The heart rate may be relatively fixed, with lack of response to atropine. An inability to release catecholamines has been suggested (Bannister 1979). A lack of pressor response to painful stimuli under light anaesthesia has been noted (Sweeney et al 1985).
2. Decreased sensitivity of the respiratory system to increased carbon dioxide levels under anaesthesia may make techniques using spontaneous respiration difficult to achieve (Sweeney et al 1985). Pulmonary respiratory reflexes are impaired.
3. Defective lacrimation, decreased sweating, and sluggish pupillary reflexes may be present. The unreliability of these reflexes may cause difficulties in assessing the depth of anaesthesia.
4. A denervation hypersensitivity type of response to the infusion of catecholamines (Malan & Crago 1979) and a lack of response to indirectly acting amines such as ephedrine, methylamphetamine and tyramine have been reported. However, it has been suggested that these features should only be seen in conditions in which there is peripheral, not central, autonomic dysfunction (Stirt et al 1982).
5. Sensitivity to the cardiovascular effects of intravenous and volatile anaesthetics (Sweeney et al 1985).
6. Bilateral abductor vocal cord paralysis has contributed to the occurrence of postoperative respiratory failure, with subsequent difficulties in weaning from IPPV and removing the tracheostomy tube (Drury & Williams 1991). A neurologist was consulted and Shy–Drager syndrome diagnosed.

Management

1. If there is stridor, snoring or other signs suggestive of laryngeal abductor palsy, endoscopy should be undertaken. The presence of bilateral vocal cord paralysis should suggest the possibility of Shy–Drager syndrome. Tracheostomy may be the only effective long-term treatment.

2. Anaesthestic agents with minimal cardiovascular depression should
   be chosen.
3. Hypovolaemia should be corrected promptly (Bevan 1979).
4. Techniques using spontaneous respiration should probably be
   avoided.
5. Careful monitoring of blood pressure is essential for the correction
   of hypotension.
6. Postoperative observation to detect respiratory insufficiency.
7. Treatment with fludrocortisone may increase extracellular fluid
   volume (Watson 1987).

BIBLIOGRAPHY
Bannister R 1979 Chronic autonomic failure with postural hypotension. Lancet ii: 404–
   406
Bevan D R 1979 Shy-Drager syndrome. Anaesthesia 34: 866–873
Drury P M E, Williams E G N 1991 Vocal cord paralysis in the Shy-Drager syndrome.
   A cause of postoperative respiratory ohstruction. Anaesthesia 46: 466–468
Hutchinson R C, Sugden J C 1984 Anaesthesia for Shy-Drager syndrome. Anaesthesia
   39: 1229–1231
Kew J, Gross M, Chapman P 1990 Shy-Drager syndrome presenting as isolated
   paralysis of vocal cord abductors. British Medical Journal 300: 1441
McGlashan J A, Golding-Wood D G 1989 Snoring as a presenting feature of the Shy-
   Drager syndrome. Journal of Laryngology and Otology 103: 610–611
Malan M D, Crago R R 1979 Anaesthetic considerations in idiopathic orthostatic
   hypotension and the Shy-Drager syndrome. Canadian Anaesthetists' Society
   Journal 26: 322–327
Martinovits G, Leventon G, Goldhammer Y et al 1988 Vocal cord paralysis as a
   presenting sign in Shy-Drager syndrome. Journal of Laryngology and Otology 102:
   280–281
Stirt J A, Frantz R A, Gunz E F et al 1982 Anesthesia, catecholamines and
   haemodynamics in autonomic dysfunction. Anesthesia and Analgesia 61: 701–704
Sweeney B P, Jones S, Langford R M 1985 Anaesthesia in dysautonomia: further
   complications. Anaesthesia 40: 783–786
Watson R D S 1987 Treating postural hypotension. British Medical Journal 294: 390–
   391

SICK SINUS SYNDROME

A general term for various disorders of sino-atrial node function which
usually present in the elderly, but can sometimes occur in young people.
Patients may have a sinus bradycardia and periods of sinus arrest with
escape rhythms, and sometimes intermittent episodes of
tachyarrhythmias (the bradycardia/tachycardia syndrome). The sino–
atrial node is under autonomic control and is a small area of specialized
muscle situated at the junction of the superior vena cava and the base
of the right atrial appendage. Its arterial supply is variable, arising from
the right coronary artery in 65%, and the left circurnflex artery in 35%
of cases. Dysfunction of the node most commonly results from its
replacement by fibrous tissue. Other causes include coronary artery
disease, drugs and post cardiac surgery.

Preoperative abnormalities

1. A typical patient is commonly older than 60 years, and may complain of episodes of syncope, dizziness or palpitations, and extreme tiredness. A 24-hour ambulatory ECG may show episodes of brady- or tachyarrhythmias which may be asymptomatic, but may coincide with the symptoms. Occasionally young people are affected, and this form may be familial. A group of nine people below the age of 25 with sino-atrial disease has been studied (Mackintosh 1981). They were all male, taller than average, and ambulatory monitoring of close relatives revealed an increased incidence of conducting system disorders.

2. Episodes of arrhythmia may cause fatigue, faintness, or precipitate angina or cardiac failure.

3. There is an inappropriate heart rate in response to stress or drugs. Often, there is a sinus bradycardia of <60 b.p.m. during the awake state.

4. ECG may show alternate brady- and tachyarrhythmias. In sino-atrial block, P waves are dropped intermittently and the R–R intervals are multiples of cycle length.

Anaesthetic problems

1. The occurrence of brady- or tachyarrhythmias during anaesthesia may reduce cardiac output and compromise cerebral or coronary artery circulation. A number of such episodes have been reported under both spinal and general anaesthesia. Sinus bradycardias unresponsive to repeated doses of atropine or glycopyrronium (Pratila & Pratilas 1976, Levy 1990), recurrent episodes of sinus arrest with nodal escape (Burt 1982) and severe bradycardias (Levy 1990) have been reported. Asystole, which responded to cardiopulmonary resuscitation and atropine, occurred 10 minutes after administration of a spinal anaesthetic for prostatectomy in a patient with sinus bradycardia and RBBB (Cohen 1988). Several periods of asystole were reported in a 46-year-old lady, some hours after spinal anaesthesia for varicose vein surgery (Underwood & Glynn 1988). Sick sinus syndrome was diagnosed and a pacemaker inserted. Subsequent questioning revealed that the patient had a history of blackouts, usually related to vomiting.

2. A high incidence (15.3%) of systemic embolism has been reported in this syndrome. For this reason, the patient may already be taking anticoagulants.

3. Bradycardias associated with sick sinus syndrome, which do not respond to anticholinergics, should be distinguished from those secondary to drugs given during anaesthesia, or which sometimes occur during spinal anaesthesia (Corr & Thomas 1989). Sick sinus syndrome bradycardias are often precipitated by the use of drugs

such as fentanyl and vecuronium, and they do respond to normal doses of atropine or glycopyrronium.

Management

1. Twenty-four-hour ambulatory monitoring may be required to confirm the diagnosis. If there is inadequate time, and the diagnosis is in doubt, then the response of the patient to atropine may be tested. In a normal subject, atropine i.v. 0.02 mg/kg should increase the heart rate by more than 14 b.p.m.
2. If sick sinus syndrome is diagnosed, a temporary pacemaker should be inserted before anaesthesia. Halothane and eflurane may prolong conduction, and impair the ability of the myocardium to maintain cardiac output by increasing stroke volume. Under these circumstances there is no guarantee that cerebral or coronary perfusion will be adequate. Patients who are symptomatic are usually given a permanent pacemaker. Although this abolishes symptoms and improves the quality of life, studies have suggested that cardiac pacing does not affect long-term survival in the condition (Shaw et al 1980).
3. Anticoagulation may be required after surgery.

BIBLIOGRAPHY

Burt D E R 1982 The sick sinus syndrome. A complication during Anaesthesia. Anaesthesia 37: 1108–1111

Cohen L I 1988 Asystole during spinal anesthesia in a patient with sick sinus syndrome. Anesthesiology 68: 787–788

Corr C S, Thomas D A 1989 Sick sinus syndrome manifest after spinal anaesthesia. Anaesthesia 44: 179

Levy D M 1990 Recurrent bradycardia due to latent sick sinus syndrome. Anaesthesia 45: 488–489

Mackintosh A F 1981 Sinuatrial disease in young people. British Heart Journal 45: 62–66

Pratila M G, Pratilas V 1976 Sick-sinus syndrome manifest during anesthesia. Anesthesiology 44: 433–436

Shaw D B, Holman R R, Gowers J I 1980 Survival in sinoatrial disorders (sick-sinus syndrome). British Medical Journal 280: 139–141

Underwood S M, Glynn C J 1988 Sick sinus syndrome manifest after spinal anaesthesia. Anaesthesia 43: 307–309

SIPPLE'S SYNDROME
(MEN TYPE IIA)

An autosomal dominant condition in which medullary carcinoma of the thyroid is frequently associated with phaeochromocytoma and, less commonly, with a parathyroid adenoma. Sipple's syndrome is one of a group of three familial diseases, and is otherwise known as multiple endocrine neoplasia (MEN) type IIa (Bouloux 1987).

Preoperative abnormalities

1. A thyroid mass may be associated with symptoms of hoarseness, dysphagia, cough and cervical lymphadenopathy.
2. Fifty per cent of cases have a phaeochromocytoma; 70% of the phaeochromocytomas are bilateral. A parathyroid adenoma is present in 10% of cases.
3. The tumour may secrete a number of hormones including calcitonin, serotonin, prostaglandins and ACTH/MSH or insulin. Symptoms depend upon the hormone secreted.
4. Metastasis may occur to the liver, lungs and bone.

Anaesthetic problems

1. Those of a phaeochromocytoma, if present (Ishizaki et al 1991). Treatment of thyrotoxic symptoms with propranolol precipitated a hypertensive crisis in a patient who was found to have a phaeochromocytoma (Blodgett & Reasner 1990). The family history was later elicited. Extreme levels of catecholamines were thought to have been responsible for the increased levels of thyroid hormones. Management of a pregnant patient with Sipple's syndrome has been described (Palot et al 1991). Elective Caesarean section was combined with removal of phaeochromocytoma, whilst thyroidectomy with block dissection of the neck was carried out 3 weeks later.
2. Cardiovascular complications, if hormones such as serotonin or prostaglandins are secreted.

Management

Exclude the presence of a phaeochromocytoma. If present, preoperative preparation will be required (see Phaeochromocytoma).

BIBLIOGRAPHY

Blodgett J, Reasner C A 1990 Transient thyrotoxicosis associated with a pheochromocytoma in a patient with multiple endocrine neoplasia type IIa. American Journal of Medicine 88: 302–303

Bouloux P-M 1987 Multiple endocrine neoplasia. Surgery 50: 1180–1185

Ishizaki A, Kim S, Shiratsuchi T et al 1991 Anesthetic management of a patient with Sipple syndrome. (English Abstr). Masui 40: 821–825

Palot M, Burde A, Quereux C et al 1991 Anesthesia for cesarean section and excision of pheochromocytoma caused by Sipple's syndrome. (English abstr). Annales Francaises d'Anesthesie et de Reanimation 10: 84–87

Thakker R V, Ponder B A J 1988 Multiple endocrine neoplasia. Bailliere's Clinical Endocrinology and Metabolism 2: 1031–1067

SJOGREN'S SYNDROME

A chronic inflammatory autoimmune disease which results in drying of secretions, and involves a number of exocrine organs, in particular the lacrimal and salivary glands (Isenberg & Crisp 1985). Sjogren's may be primary or secondary. About 75% of cases are secondary to a connective tissue disorder, of which the commonest is rheumatoid arthritis. The glandular element is relatively mild in the secondary form, but in primary disease, infiltration of the salivary and lacrimal glands predominates and there may be considerable swelling, accompanied by striking dryness of the eyes and mouth. Occasionally, in association with lymphadenopathy, this type may proceed to malignant lymphoma.

Preoperative abnormalities

1. Symptoms of the sicca syndrome include dryness of the eyes, mouth, vagina and skin.
2. Conditions associated with the secondary form include rheumatoid arthritis, systemic lupus erythemotosus, scleroderma, the polymyositis/dermatomyositis complex, polyarteritis nodosa, chronic active hepatitis and Grave's disease.
3. Swelling of the salivary and lacrimal glands may be prominent.
4. Lung, kidney, liver, pancreas and lymphoid tissue are other major organs at risk of involvement. Either a sensory or motor neuropathy may occur, and central nervous system lesions have been described.
5. There may be a spectrum of pulmonary disease, of which the commonest features are tracheobronchial sicca and interstitial pulmonary fibrosis (Gardiner 1993).
6. The patient may be on corticosteroids or occasionally immunosuppressive agents.

Anaesthetic problems

1. Swelling of the salivary glands may make mask anaesthesia difficult (Eisele 1990).
2. Those of the primary disease (see under individual names).
3. Pulmonary disease, if present.
4. The dry eyes are susceptible to damage during anaesthesia.

Management

1. If the patient's Sjogren's syndrome is secondary to another disorder, there should be careful assessment of the primary disease and of any pulmonary involvement.
2. Dryng agents should be avoided if possible.
3. The eyes should be protected with pads.
4. Anaesthetic gases should be humidified.
5. Steroid supplements may be required.

BIBLIOGRAPHY
Eisele J H 1990 Connective tissue diseases. In: Katz J, Benumof J, Kadis L (eds) Anesthesia and uncommon diseases. W B Saunders, Philadelphia

Gardiner P 1993 Primary Sjogren's syndrome. Bailliere's Clinical Rheumatology 7(1): 59–71
Isenberg D, Crisp A 1985 Sjogren's syndrome. Hospital Update 11: 273–283

SNAKE BITES

The adder (*Vipera berus*) is the only poisonous snake in Britain and the majority of its bites are uncomplicated, requiring no more than immobilization of the affected part. It has however been suggested that hospital admission for 12 hours is advisable, for observation and early treatment of complications, should they occur (Reid 1980). Deaths, although rare, have occurred between 6 and 60 hours after the bite. The venom causes local swelling, probably secondary to changes in vascular permeability. Occasionally, systemic absorption may cause activation of the complement and kinin systems, producing a severe anaphylactoid response with hypotension, ECG changes, increased serum CK levels, and pulmonary oedema.

Presentation

1. Pain at the site of the bite.
2. Local swelling usually starts within 10 minutes, but may occur after an hour, and can last for 48–72 hours.
3. Regional lymph nodes draining the affected limb are enlarged.
4. Gastrointestinal symptoms. Vomiting can start within 5 minutes or up to several hours after the bite. Sweating, abdominal pain and diarrhoea may occur. Continuing symptoms suggest a serious reaction.
5. Rarely there may be cardiovascular collapse, hypotension, or peripheral vasoconstriction.
6. Angioneurotic oedema of the lips, face and tongue may develop at any time up to 48 hours after the event.
7. Bleeding is rare, although local bruising is common. Oozing from mucosal surfaces, such as the tooth sockets, is the first sign of generalized problems.

Management

1. The limb is immobilized and the patient reassured.
2. Monitor:
   a. Hourly pulse rate, blood pressure and respiratory rate.
   b. Any persistent symptoms. Continuing vomiting, diarrhoea and abdominal pain, or the onset of spontaneous bleeding, is suggestive of a serious reaction.
   c. Local swelling. The circumference should be measured at an identifiable level on the affected limb.

    d. WCC, serum CK levels, serum bicarbonate and ECG should be measured 12-hourly.

3. Zagreb antivenom should be given to reduce morbidity (Reid 1976) only if:

    a. Hypotension and peripheral vasoconstriction persist.

    b. There is a leucocytosis of >20 × 10^9/l.

    c. An adult has swelling which extends up the forearm or the leg within 2 hours of a bite.

Antivenom regimen

Zagreb antivenom 2 ampoules diluted with saline 0.9% 100 ml and given i.v., and repeated in 1–2 hours if no clinical improvement occurs.

    N.B. Adrenaline 1 in 1000, 0.5 ml diluted to 10 ml, must be immediately available at the patient's side.

    A known allergic history is an absolute contraindication to the use of antivenom.

Antivenoms for foreign venomous snakes

Contact either:

    a. Pharmacy Department, Walton Hospital, Liverpool, UK. (Tel: 051-525-3611), or

    b. Poisons Unit, Guy's Hospital, London, UK. (Tel: 071-407-7600)

BIBLIOGRAPHY

Reid H A 1976 Adder bites in Britain. British Medical Journal 12: 153–156
Reid H A 1980 Poisoning caused by snake bite. Hospital Update 6: 675–682

SOLVENT ABUSE

The incidence of solvent abuse is increasing in Britain. An epidemiological study reported 282 deaths in the period 1971–1983 and 80 deaths in 1983 (Anderson et al 1985). The latter represented 2% of all deaths in males between the ages of 10 and 19 years. Fifty-one per cent of the deaths were attributed to direct toxic effects, 21% to plastic bag asphyxia, 18% to inhaled gastric contents, and 11% to trauma.

    Sudden death during 'sniffing' or 'huffing' is thought to result from arrhythmias associated with the sensitization of the heart to the effect of endogenous catecholamines by the inhaled volatile hydrocarbon (Cunningham et al 1987). Death is therefore likely to occur more commonly during periods of intense cardiac stimulation, such as exercise. Animal studies with inhaled hydrocarbons would seem to confirm this. Serious ventricular arrhythmias can be provoked by both exogenous and endogenous catecholamines. However, asystolic cardiac arrest has also been documented following butane inhalation (Roberts et al 1990). Once an arrhythmia develops, the victim's heart becomes more resistant to resuscitation and the risk of a sudden arrhythmia remains for some hours after inhalation has taken place (Ashton 1990).

Volatile hydrocarbons also have chronic effects on the liver, kidney, lung, and brain. Chronic cardiotoxicity may also occur (Boon 1987, Marjot 1989).

It has been suggested that interactions may occur with halothane, whose chemical structure closely resembles that of 1,1,1-trichloroethane (McCleod et al 1987).

Typical products inhaled include glues, dry-cleaning agents, nail polish, paint thinners, antifreeze, lighter fuel, propellants for spray cans, and degreasing agents.

Preoperative abnormalities

1. Agents most frequently encountered:
   a. Toluene ($C_6H_5CH_3$)
      A solvent in cements and glues. Cardiac arrhythmias are common during inhalation, and the most frequent cause of death is cardiac arrest precipitated by exercise.
   b. 1,1,1-trichloroethane
      An industrial cleaning solvent and paint remover. Is present in Tippex fluid thinner, audiovisual equipment cleaners, glues, adhesive plaster removers, and degreasing agents used in steel welding. Sudden deaths can occur either with solvent abuse or following industrial accidents. Cardiac arrhythmias can occur at the time of abuse, but may also persist for up to 2 weeks after the exposure. It has now been shown that this agent can cause chronic cardiac damage, and that there may be provocation of symptoms of cardiac toxicity when re-exposure to the agent, or to chemically similar substances, occurs.
   c. Butane from lighter fuel.
   d. Fluorocarbons used as propellants in spray cans.
2. The abuser is most likely to be a teenager, 13–15 years being the peak age. There is a high incidence of users from social class V, and from the armed forces (Anderson et al 1985). Perioral eczema, erythematous spots around the nose, and chronic inflammation of the upper respiratory tract may suggest repeated contact with a solvent or indicate the use of a plastic bag.
3. Cardiac arrhythmias may be noticed preoperatively; the risk of sudden arrhythmias lasts for some hours after the episode of solvent abuse.
4. There is evidence that long-term abuse may result in damage to a number of organs including the kidney, liver, heart, and lung (Marjot & McLeod 1989). Toluene abuse is also associated with a number of neurological effects including chronic psychosis, temporal lobe epilepsy and a decreased IQ (Byrne et al 1991).

Anaesthetic and resuscitative problems

1. Cardiac arrhythmias
   Cardiac problems in two patients chronically exposed to 1,1,1-trichloroethane, were attributed to an interaction with halothane during anaesthesia (McLeod et al 1987). The first, a 14-year-old boy, developed multiple ventricular extrasystoles and ventricular tachycardia during tonsillectomy. The arrhythmias persisted postoperatively and needed treatment with a number of antiarrhythmic drugs. At one stage a pacemaker was required. Evidence of 1,1,1-trichloroethane abuse was subsequently found. The second was a 55-year-old man who had previously developed AF and cardiac failure. This was diagnosed as being due to industrial exposure to 1,1,1-trichloroethane in the steel industry. He was removed from exposure and his condition did not worsen. Two years later, and following an anaesthetic (halothane, but no details) he became symptomatic. Echocardiography and myocardial biopsy indicated a deterioration in cardiac function of recent onset. Since halothane is very similar in structure to 1,1,1-trichloroethane, it was postulated that this was reponsible for the cardiac problems encountered in both cases.
2. Documented cardiac arrest during abuse has also been reported (Roberts et al 1990).
3. A cardiomyopathy developed in a 15-year-old boy, who had a 2-year history of solvent abuse with toluene-containing substances. He subsequently required cardiac transplantation (Wiseman & Banim 1987).
4. Intractable vomiting occurs in about 25% of butane gas overdoses and may result in pulmonary aspiration (Roberts et al 1990).
5. Acute psychosis may occur in the recovery period after resuscitation following toxicity associated with cardiopulmonary arrest (Roberts et al 1990).
6. Fatal cerebral oedema and tonsillar herniation has been reported after trichloroethane abuse (D'Costa & Gunasekera 1990).
7. Toluene vapour abuse during pregnancy is associated with morbidity in both the mother and child (Wilkins-Haug & Gabow 1991). Renal tubular acidosis, hypokalaemia, arrhythmias and rhabdomyolysis occurred in the women, and prematurity, growth retardation and sometimes death amongst the infants.

Management

1. The occurrence of unexpected arrhythmias in a teenager, particularly in the presence of spots around the mouth and nose, should alert the anaesthetist to the possibility of solvent abuse.

2. Continuous ECG monitoring during anaesthesia. These case reports underline the importance of ECG monitoring from the start of the anaesthetic, even in apparently fit young patients.
3. It is suggested that during resuscitation from cardiopulmonary arrest associated with acute toxicity, tracheal intubation should be performed to protect the lungs from gastric aspiration.
4. If gross cerebral oedema is suspected, hyperventilation and treatment with dexamethasone and mannitol should be instituted (D'Costa & Gunasekera 1990).
5. The possibility of abuse of other substances should be considered. In one US population studied, solvent users were 5–10 times more likely to abuse opioids, stimulants, depressants and hallucinogens (Dinwiddie et al 1991).

BIBLIOGRAPHY
Anderson H R, Macnair R S, Ramsey J D 1985 Deaths from abuse of volatile substances: a national epidemiological study. British Medical Journal 290: 304–307
Ashton C H 1990 Solvent abuse. Little progress after 20 years. British Medical Journal 300: 135–136
Boon N A 1987 Solvent abuse and the heart. British Medical Journal 294: 722
Byrne A, Kirby B, Zibin T et al 1991 Psychiatric and neurological effects of chronic solvent abuse. Canadian Journal of Psychiatry 36: 735–738
Cunningham S R, Dalzell G W N, McGirr P et al 1987 Myocardial infarction and primary ventricular fibrillation after glue sniffing. British Medical Journal 294: 739–740
D'Costa D F, Gunasekera N P R 1990 Fatal cerebral oedema following trichloroethane abuse. Journal of the Royal Society of Medicine 83: 533–534
Dinwiddie S H, Reich T, Cloniger C R 1991 The relationship of solvent to other substance abuse. American Journal of Drug and Alcohol Abuse 17: 173–186
McLeod A A, Marjot R, Monaghan M J et al 1987 Chronic cardiac toxicity after inhalation of 1,1,1-trichloroethane. British Medical Journal 294: 727–729
Marjot R 1989 The relevance of volatile substance abuse to anaesthetists. Anaesthesia 44 162–163
Marjot R, McLeod A A 1989 Chronic non-neurological toxicity from volatile substance abuse. Human Toxicology 8: 301–306
Roberts M J D, McIvor R A, Adgey A A J 1990 Asystole following butane gas inhalation. British Journal of Hospital Medicine 44: 294
Wilkins-Haug L, Gabow P A 1991 Toluene abuse during pregnancy: obstetric complications and perinatal outcomes. Obstetrics and Gynecology 77: 504–509
Wiseman M N, Banim S 1987 'Glue sniffers' heart. British Medical Journal 294: 739

SPINAL MUSCULAR ATROPHY
(SEE ALSO WERDNIG-HOFFMANN DISEASE)

A group of diseases affecting peripheral motor neurones, usually hereditary, and associated with anterior horn degeneration. Type I is a rapidly progressive disease of infants (Werdnig-Hoffman disease). In type II the course is similar but death occurs more slowly. The onset of type II is later in childhood and runs a slower course. Type IV presents in the adult and gradually evolves (Editorial 1990). The genes affected have been mapped, but the underlying defect is unknown.

Preoperative abnormalities

1. The proximal muscles are involved more than those distally, and lower limbs more than upper. In mild disease, there is no arm involvement. Tongue fasciculation may be present.
2. Scoliosis occurs in all but the mildest cases and is progressive. Its onset is before puberty, at an average age of 8.8 years (Phillips et al 1990).

Anaesthetic problems

1. Suxamethonium may be hazardous in these patients. Severe rhabdomyolysis (CK 252 000 u/l) and myoglobinuria in a 13-year-old boy following suxamethonium, given during dental surgery, has been encountered by the author. A diagnosis of MH was assumed, but investigation 4 years later showed the patient not susceptible. Electron microscopy suggested a subclinical spinal muscular atrophy.
2. Increased sensitivity to non-depolarizing neuromuscular blockers may occur.
3. If there is bulbar muscle involvement, the risk of pulmonary aspiration exists.
4. Surgery for scoliosis will halt the progression of the deformity and improve sitting, but if respiratory reserve is poor, prolonged postoperative IPPV may be required (Phillips et al 1990).

Management

1. If major surgery is undertaken, careful respiratory assessment is crucial. Neuromuscular monitoring is essential and postoperative respiratory support may be required.
2. When there is bulbar involvement, precautions should be taken to prevent postoperative aspiration.
3. The use of suxamethonium is contraindicated.
4. Management of two parturients with spinal muscular atrophy has been described (Wilson et al 1992). Both received extradural anaesthesia, one for Caesarean section, the other for assisted vaginal delivery.

BIBLIOGRAPHY
Editorial 1990 Spinal muscular atrophies. Lancet 336: 280–281
Phillips D P, Roye D P Jr, Farcy J-P C et al 1990 Surgical treatment of scoliosis a spinal muscular atrophy population. Spine 15: 942–945
Wilson R D, Williams K P 1992 Spinal muscular atrophy and pregnancy. British Journal of Obstetrics and Gynaecology 99: 516–517

STURGE-WEBER SYNDROME

A congenital syndrome of unknown aetiology, in which a cavernous haemangioma of one side of the face is associated with an intracranial angioma. The angiomas, which become increasingly calcified, are usually surgically untreatable, although subtotal hemispherectomy has been performed to control intractable epilepsy. General anaesthesia may be required for the management of glaucoma, which is difficult to treat. Sturge-Weber may be associated with Klippel-Trenaunay syndrome (see Section 4). In this condition, haemangiomas on the trunk or limbs are associated with spinal cord malformations, which may bleed and result in paraplegia.

Preoperative abnormalities

1. A naevus (port wine stain) of one side of the face, which may involve one or more divisions of the trigeminal nerve. It is often associated with progressive mental retardation.
2. Epilepsy, and a hemiparesis involving the contralateral side. Fits may be refractory to drug control. Gum hypertrophy can develop from long-term phenytoin therapy.
3. There are variations in the full clinical picture. One side of the vault and the hemiparetic half of the body may be smaller than the other. There may be unilateral glaucoma, increased scalp vascularity and unilateral hypertrophy of the carotid artery.
4. A venous haemangioma usually involves the meninges of the occipitoparietal surface of the brain. The adjacent cortex is gradually destroyed, possibly as a result of pressure. Deeper arteriovenous malformations, which occur only rarely, may be fed by large arteries and increasingly large veins. If this happens, a considerable arteriovenous shunt may result in cardiac hypertrophy and failure. Angiomas bleed spontaneously at some time in 80% of cases.
5. Skull X-ray shows linear calcification of the underlying brain tissue.
6. Arteriography or DVI will demonstrate the extent of the lesion.

Anaesthetic problems

1. The patient may be severely retarded and uncooperative. Seizure disorders are usual.
2. Mask anaesthesia is often difficult because of gross vascular hypertrophy of the lips, buccal mucosa, gums, and tongue (de Leon-Casasola & Lema 1991). In addition, if there is a significant A-V shunt causing increased cardiac output, inhalational induction will be delayed. Airway obstruction occurred during inhalational induction in one patient (Aldridge 1987), but laryngoscopy and intubation are reported not to be difficult once induction is achieved (de Leon-Casasola & Lema 1991). The facial abnormalities have also caused airway obstruction in the recovery period.
3. Episodes of sudden hypertension, as may occur on tracheal intubation, may cause an angioma to bleed.
4. Small haemangiomas of the tracheal mucosa have been reported (de Leon-Casasola & Lema 1991).

5. The cerebral lesion is usually too large for operative intervention, but neurosurgery may be indicated for intractable seizures (Ito et al 1990). If undertaken, surgery may be associated with massive bleeding.
6. In patients with large cavernous haemangiomas, hypovolaemia may precipitate thrombocytopenia and hypofibrinogenaemia, which can progress to DIC.

Management

1. Assessment of the degree of significance of the arteriovenous shunt.
2. Management of the retarded patient with epilepsy.
3. Assessment of possible airway difficulties. Early laryngoscopy and intubation has been advised because of difficulties with mask anaesthesia.
4. Prevent sudden hypertension, particularly on tracheal intubation. Treat hypertension during surgery.
5. Extreme hyperventilation should be avoided.
6. Avoid hypovolaemia.
7. A hypotensive technique may be required for neurosurgical procedures.

BIBLIOGRAPHY

Aldridge L M 1987 An unusual case of upper airway obstruction. Anaesthesia 42: 1239–1240
de Leon-Casasola O A, Lema M J 1991 Anesthesia for patients with Sturge–Weber disease and Klippel-Trenaunay syndrome. Journal of Clinical Anesthesia 3: 409–413
Ito M, Sato K, Ohnuki A et al 1990 Sturge-Weber disease: operative indications and surgical results. Brain Development 12: 473–477

SUBACUTE BACTERIAL ENDOCARDITIS, PROPHYLAXIS DURING SURGERY
see ENDOCARDITIS, BACTERIAL

SYSTEMIC LUPUS ERYTHEMATOSUS
(SLE)

An autoimmune connective tissue disorder predominantly occurring in females between the ages of 20 and 50 years, and which involves type III immune complexes against nucleic acid antigens and phospholipids. Anaesthetists may be involved with the pregnant patient with SLE.

Preoperative abnormalities

1. Arthritis and cutaneous lesions are the commonest presenting features, and occur in 86–100% of patients (Bellamy et al 1984).

Skin lesions include the well-known, but often transient, butterfly facial rash, vasculitis, alopecia and a photosensitivity dermatitis. Other common features are nephritis (75% patients), central nervous system lesions (60%), myocarditis and pericarditis (20–30%). Pulmonary atelectasis is common and may be associated with lupus pneumonitis and, occasionally, fibrosing alveolitis. Pulmonary function tests may show a restrictive defect. The diaphragm may be elevated, and a diaphragmatic myopathy has been suggested as a cause of the 'vanishing lung' syndrome.

2. There may be anaemia, leucopenia, and occasionally thrombocytopenia. Laboratory tests show a variety of antibodies to nuclear and cytoplasmic components (Bellamy et al 1984). Anti-cardiolipin antibodies in SLE were found to be associated with venous thrombosis, thrombocytopenia, recurrent fetal loss, leg ulcers, transverse myelitis and pulmonary hypertension (Alarcon-Segovia et al 1989). Lupus antibody, as assessed by diluted APTT, is strongly associated with thrombosis.

3. There can be exacerbations and remissions. The condition may be made worse by stress, drugs, infection, and pregnancy. A significant proportion of the patients develop atherosclerotic disease in late life (Rubin et al 1985).

4. Medication may include corticosteroids, antimalarials, aspirin, and occasionally cytotoxics.

5. Circulating lupus anticoagulant occurs in up to 37% of patients with SLE (Malinow et al 1987). Paradoxically, this is an autoantibody associated with systemic vascular thromboses, which actually causes prolongation of some coagulation tests.

6. Although exacerbations of the disease may occur in pregnancy (Wong et al 1991) it has been found to be uncommon (Lockshin 1989). Relapses tend to be associated with disease activity in the early stages of pregnancy. Adverse fetal outcome has been reported (Editorial 1991), but was not shown in all series (Wong et al 1991). Pregnancies in the presence of a high titre of antiphospholipid antibodies usually result in fetal loss. The incidence of this may be reduced by corticosteroids or antiplatelet therapy. A small proportion of infants of patients with anti-Ro antibodies develop neonatal lupus syndrome, which is associated with congenital heart block (Editorial 1991).

Anaesthetic problems

1. Pulmonary involvement may result in a restrictive lung defect.
2. Thrombotic problems. Up to 28% of patients with lupus anticoagulant may have arterial or venous thrombotic episodes.
3. Coagulation tests in patients with lupus anticoagulant may show a prolonged PT, APTT or KCCT, or thrombocytopenia and platelet dysfunction.
4. Pregnancy complications.

Management

1. Assessment of pulmonary, cardiac, and renal function. Anaesthetic management will depend upon the affected organs (Davies 1991).
2. In labour, coagulation studies, including PT, PTT, platelets, and bleeding time, should be performed. If these are increased, extradural anaesthesia is contraindicated, except when there is isolated elevation of PTT in association with lupus anticoagulant (Davies 1991).
3. There should be a multidisciplinary approach to the patient in pregnancy (Davies 1991). The problems posed by the presence of lupus anticoagulant in the pregnant patient who is on aspirin therapy have been discussed (Malinow et al 1987). Both authors suggest that the benefits of extradural anaesthesia must be weighed against the possibility (but still very low risk) of an extradural haematoma developing.
4. If valvular lesions are present, antibiotic prophylaxis should be given, when appropriate.

BIBLIOGRAPHY
Alarcon-Segovia D, Deleze M, Oria C V et al 1989 Antiphospholipid antibodies and the antiphospholipid syndrome in systemic lupus erythematosus. Medicine 68: 353–365
Bellamy N, Kean W F, Buchanan W W 1984 Connective tissue diseases: systemic lupus erythematosus. Hospital Update 10: 65–76
Davies S R 1991 Systemic lupus erythematosus and the obstetrical patient – implications for the anaesthetist. Canadian Journal of Anaesthesia 38: 790–796
Editorial 1991 Systemic lupus erythematosus in pregnancy. Lancet 338: 87–88
Lockshin M D 1989 Pregnancy does not cause systemic erythematosus to worsen. Arthritis and Rheumatism 32: 665–670
Malinow A M, Rickford W J K, Mokriski B L K et al 1987 Lupus anticoagulant. Implication for obstetric anaesthetists. Anaesthesia 42: 1291–1293
Rubin L A, Urowitz M B, Gladman D D 1985 Mortality in systemic lupus erythematosus: the bimodal pattern revisited. Quarterly Journal of Medicine 55: 87–98
Wong K L, Chan F Y, Lee C P 1991 Outcome of pregnancy in patients with systemic lupus erythematosus. A prospective study. Archives of Internal Medicine 151: 269–273

TAKAYASU'S ARTERITIS

A non-specific chronic panarteritis, usually occurring in young women, and originally described in the Far East. In the early stages there is an inflammatory process in the large arteries which progresses to chronic arterial occlusion (Hall et al 1985). It is also known as 'pulseless disease', since there are usually reduced or absent pulses in the affected arteries.

Type 1   involves the aortic arch and its branches.
Type 2   involves the descending thoracic and abdominal aorta, without arch involvement.

Type 3   is a mixed picture of types 1 and 2.

Type 4   can consist of any of the above features in association with pulmonary artery involvement.

Preoperative abnormalities

1. There may be pulse deficits, depending upon the stage of the disease and the arteries involved in the condition. Bruits may be heard over stenosed arteries. There are also ectatic lesions of the aorta with aneurysm formation.
2. Possible cerebrovascular or retinal insufficiency.
3. Renal involvement occurs in 63% of patients.
4. Hypertension.
5. In type 4 (45%) there may be moderate pulmonary hypertension.
6. Heart failure can occur as a consequence of either systemic or pulmonary hypertension.
7. The ESR is related to the stage of the disease and is high in 78% of cases, notably in early inflammatory disease. There are ECG abnormalities in 40% and hypergammaglobulinaemia in 37%.
8. The patient may be taking corticosteroids.

Anaesthetic problems

1. There may be difficulties in haemodynamic monitoring because of an absence of palpable pulses (Ramanathan et al 1979, Warner et al 1983).
2. Pressure recording from one vessel does not necessarily reflect the pressure in another vessel.
3. Hypertension or pulmonary hypertension may be present, with or without heart failure. In a study of 54 patients, hypertension was found in 35 and congestive heart failure in 24; the results of myocardial biopsy suggested that many patients had an inflammatory myocarditis which might account for the development of heart failure (Talwar et al 1991).
4. The myocardium may be sensitive to drugs with negative inotropic effects (Thorburn & James 1986).
5. In the presence of pulmonary hypertension, high lung inflation pressures may be required.
6. Hyperextension of the neck during laryngoscopy and intubation may reduce carotid artery blood flow.
7. Pregnancy may be associated with a worsening of hypertension, cerebral haemorrhage and a hypercoagulable state. Anaesthesia may be required for termination of pregnancy (Gaida et al 1991), labour (Crofts & Wilson 1991) or tubal ligation (McKay & Dillard 1992). Extradural anaesthesia was given for Caesarean section in a patient with multiple aortic aneurysms (Beilin & Bernstein 1993).

Management

1. The nature and degree of organ involvement must be assessed. Particular evidence of cardiac, respiratory, cerebral, and renal insufficiency should be sought.
2. Hypertension or heart failure should be treated, if present.
3. For the purposes of blood pressure monitoring, the arteries involved in the disease process must be fully assessed.
4. The degree of monitoring depends upon the state of the patient, the accessibility of the arteries, and the magnitude of the surgery.
   a. Care must be taken to monitor an artery representative of true arterial pressure (Thorburn & James 1986).
   b. The use of a Doppler ultrasonic probe and a sphygmomanometer cuff, which permitted blood pressure recording despite an impalpable pulse, has been suggested (Warner et al 1983). The flow from a Doppler flow probe can also be displayed on an oscilloscope and recorded on a multichannel recorder (Ramanathan et al 1979).
   c. The use of oximetry in combination with a mercury manometer to assess arterial blood pressure has been described (Chawla et al 1992), and the technique was successfully employed in two patients without arm pulses (Chawla et al 1990). The oximeter can still show a pulsatile plethysmographic waveform even when arteries are not easily palpable (Ramanathan et al 1979).
   d. A cutdown onto the dorsalis pedis or superficial temporal arteries may be required for direct arterial monitoring. The appropriateness of these techniques will depend on the degree and distribution of the underlying ischaemia and the nature of the surgery being performed. On occasions the surgeon can be requested to place a cannula in the aorta during surgery.
   e. If pulmonary hypertension is present, a pulmonary artery catheter may be needed to measure PAP (Ramanathan et al 1979, Warner et al 1983). However, it must be remembered that PAP may be unreliable.
   f. Measurement of cardiac stroke volume using an impedance cardiograph has been described (Ramanathan et al 1979).
   g. Urine output may need careful monitoring.
5. In a patient with pulmonary hypertension, invasive haemodynamic monitoring demonstrated that extradural anaesthesia had a more beneficial effect on blood pressure and afterload control than vasodilators (Thorburn & James 1986).
6. Before anaesthesia is induced, the head should be fixed in a position that does not produce symptoms of cerebral blood flow impairment. The use of a transcranial Doppler, and continuous measurement of jugular venous oxygen saturation to evaluate changes in cerebral

perfusion, has been reported (Kawaguchi et al 1993, Nakajima et al 1992).

7. The use of extradural anaesthesia for Caesarean section (Beilin & Bernstein 1993), labour and postpartum tubal ligation (McKay & Dillard 1992, Crofts & Wilson 1991) and paracervical block for therapeutic abortion (Gaida et al 1991), have been described.

BIBLIOGRAPHY

Beilin Y, Bernstein H 1993 Successful epidural anaesthesia for patient with Takayasu's arteritis presenting for Caesarean section. Canadian Journal of Anaesthesia 40: 64–66

Chawla R, Kumarvel V, Girdhar K K et al 1990 Oximetry in pulseless disease. Anaesthesia 45: 92–93

Chawla R, Kumarvel V, Girdhar K K et al 1992 Can pulse oximetry be used to measure systolic blood pressure? Anesthesia and Analgesia 74: 196–200

Crofts S L, Wilson E 1991 Epidural analgesia for labour in Takayasu's arteritis. Case report. British Journal of Obstetrics and Gynaecology 98: 408–409

Gaida B J, Gervais H W, Mauer D et al 1991 Anesthesiology problems in Takayasu's syndrome. (English abstr.) Anaesthesist 40: 1–6

Hall S, Barr W, Lie J T et al 1985 Takayasu arteritis. Medicine 64: 89–99

Kawaguchi M, Ohsumi H, Nakajima T et al 1993 Intraoperative monitoring of cerebral hemodynamics in a patient with Takayasu's arteritis. Anaesthesia 48: 496–498

McKay R S F, Dillard S R 1992 Management of epidural anesthesia in a patient with Takayasu's disease. Anesthesia and Analgesia 74: 297–299

Nakajima T, Kuro M, Hayashi Y et al 1992 Clinical evaluation of cerebral oxygen balance during cardiopulmonary bypass: on-line continuous monitoring of jugular venous oxyhemoglobin saturation. Anesthesia and Analgesia 74: 630–635

Ramanathan S, Gupta U, Chalon J et al 1979 Anesthetic considerations in Takayasu arteritis. Anesthesia and Analgesia 58: 247–249

Talwar K K, Kumar K, Chopra P et al 1991 Cardiac involvement in nonspecific aortoarteritis (Takayasu's arteritis). American Heart Journal 122: 1666–1670

Thorburn J R, James M F M 1986 Anaesthetic management of Takayasu's arteritis. Anaesthesia 41: 734–738

Warner M A, Hughes D R, Messick J M 1983 Anesthetic management of a patient with pulseless disease. Anesthesia and Analgesia 62: 532–535

TETANUS

An infection caused by *Clostridium tetani*, an anaerobic bacillus present in soil and gut. It is able to survive for long periods outside the body. Under anaerobic conditions it multiplies and produces a potent neurotoxin which can travel up nerves into the spinal cord and medulla. The primary effect is on the spinal cord, with a lesser effect on the peripheral nerves. Tetanus neurotoxin is a high-molecular-weight protein, so its long half-life allows time for neural penetration (Flowers 1988). Tetanospasmin prevents transmission at inhibitory synapses in the CNS, therefore causes disinhibition of the motor system. The incubation period of the disease is 3–21 days. In about 60–65% of cases there is a history of a wound, but it is often trivial. Several cases have occurred following surgery, the commonest operation reported being cholecystectomy (Crokaert et al 1984, Lennard et al 1984, Farling et al

1989). Cases may be classified (Edmondson & Flowers 1979) as:

Grade 1   Mild
Grade 2   Moderate
Grade 3a   Severe
Grade 3b   Very severe

In their report of 100 cases treated in Leeds, the mortality was 10%.

There is an increased risk of tetanus in heroin addicts, in part due to additives such as quinine, which provide anaerobic conditions for multiplication of the bacillus. The mortality is higher in severe disease, the elderly, and in drug addicts.

Presentation

1. General muscle hypertonicity.
2. Muscle spasm resulting in trismus (lockjaw), rigidity of the facial muscles (risus sardonicus), neck stiffness, or opisthotonos. Intermittent muscle spasms are superimposed on hypertonicity. Breathing difficulties can occur from spasm of the laryngeal or intercostal muscles, and respiratory failure may ensue. Dysphagia may sometimes be the major symptom, with pooling of saliva and episodes of pharyngeal spasm (Kasanew et al 1989).
3. Occasionally, wounds in the head and neck may produce cephalic tetanus, which can result in a variety of cranial nerve palsies.
4. A small number of patients have localized tetanus only.
5. Sympathetic disturbances occur in 23–60% of severe cases probably as a result of the action of tetanospasmin on brainstem and autonomic interneurones causing increased circulating catecholamine levels. These consist of episodes of hypertension, tachycardia, arrhythmias, systemic vasoconstriction, sweating, salivation, and pyrexia.
6. Episodes of hypotension and bradycardia have been reported, particularly after tracheal suction. These may be secondary to parasympathetic autonomic dysfunction.

Diagnosis

1. Is generally made on clinical grounds.
2. Tetanus is not an immunizing disease, therefore it is possible to contract it on more than one occasion. This is probably because the toxin travels up the nerves and thus may not come into contact with gamma globulin. The blood level of tetanus antibody cannot be used as a diagnostic test for the disease (Stoddart 1979a).
3. Differentiation must be made from other causes which mimic tetanus. These include hysteria, and treatment with drugs, such as the phenothiazines and butyrophenones, which can produce dyskinetic symptoms (Stoddart 1979b).

Anaesthetic (or intensive care) problems

1. Any strong external stimulus can precipitate severe muscle spasm. Death may occur because ventilation impairment coincides with a greatly increased oxygen consumption by the muscles. In one patient, the diagnosis was only made when severe, recurrent pharyngeal spasm occurred after removal of the tracheal tube, following oesophagoscopy for dysphagia (Baronia et al 1991).
2. Cardiovascular instability, with episodes of hypertension and tachycardia, is often associated with increased circulating catecholamine levels (Domenighetti et al 1984).
3. Hypotension and bradycardia may occur, particularly after tracheal suction (Edmondson & Flowers 1979). There are several reports which suggest that treatment of sympathetic disturbances with beta adrenoceptor blockers may predispose to bradycardias, and in one case, cardiac arrest occurred (Buchanan et al 1978).
4. Reduced serum cholinesterase levels have been reported, the level often correlating with the severity of the disease. In one report, there was no enzymic activity for the first 3 days after admission (Porath et al 1977).
5. The use of suxamethonium in the later stages of the disease may cause cardiac arrest from hyperkalaemia.
6. Hypovolaemia occurs readily, from a combination of sweating, excessive salivation, and gastrointestinal losses. Hyponatraemia may occur secondary to inappropriate ADH secretion.
7. Gastrointestinal stasis is a problem.
8. Pyrexia may be secondary to infection, or it sometimes occurs as a result of autonomic dysfunction.
9. One patient is reported who required surgery during active tetanus (Farling et al 1989).
10. In patients who need IPPV for long periods, there is an increased risk of deep venous thrombosis and pulmonary embolism. In the Leeds series of 100 cases, nine venous thromboses, three pulmonary emboli and one death occurred (Edmondson & Flowers 1979). Another embolic death has been reported, despite the use of low-dose heparin (Jenkins & Keep 1976).

Management

1. Initial management
   a. Antitetanus immunoglobulin 30 mg/kg i.m.
   b. Antibiotic: benzylpenicillin 600 mg i.m. 6 hrly
   c. Tetanus toxoid course is started.
   d. The wound should be excised and cleaned, and tissue sent for microscopy and bacterial culture. It has been suggested that this should be delayed for several hours after the immunoglobulin

has been given. so that any neurotoxin released can be neutralized. Mutilating surgery is not justified (Flowers 1988).

2. Management of spasm and hypertonus

Grade 1	Usually diazepam only.
Grade 2	Diazepam, tracheostomy and nasogastric tube.
Grade 3a and 3b	IPPV, sedatives, neuromuscular blockers and analgesics.

More recently other drugs have been used for both sedation and reduction in spasms. These include:

a. Propofol (Borgeat et al 1991) or midazolam and propofol (Orko et al 1988).

b. Inhaled isoflurane (Stevens et al 1993). The prolonged use of isoflurane was associated with potentially toxic concentrations of serum inorganic fluoride, although serum urea and creatinine levels remained within normal limits.

c. Intrathecal baclofen (Muller et al 1987) for tetanus-induced spinal and supraspinal spasticity. Baclofen, a GABA agonist, may produce central depression, hypotonia, sedation and coma, and the central effects have been reversed using flumazenil followed by a flumazenil infusion, thus preserving its spinal action (Saissy et al 1992).

d. Dantrolene has been suggested to decrease the necessity for IPPV in patients with severe tetanus (Checketts & White 1993).

3. Fluid replacement is required for sweating, salivation, and gastrointestinal losses. The latter depend on measured loss, but may amount to as much as 6–8 l/day. Nutrition is also needed, which may have to be given parenterally if there is gastrointestinal failure.

4. Sympathetic disturbances have been treated in a number of ways. These have included:

a. Beta adrenoceptor blockade. However, the use of beta blockers is controversial, since profound bradycardia may occur. Extremely high catecholamine levels, equivalent to those encountered in a phaeochromocytoma were reported in one case (Domenighetti et al 1984). During convalescence, these levels returned to normal.

In this case, labetalol was used to treat sympathetic overactivity. The use of labetalol in 15 cases was reported to produce great variability of response and poor control of blood pressure (Wesley et al 1983). This is not surprising, since the beta blockade produced by labetalol is at least three to seven times greater than the alpha blockade. In addition, five of the treated patients had episodes of cardiac standstill. The death of a 4-year-old child was associated with the use of propranolol (Buchanan et al 1978). In the Leeds series (Edmondson & Flowers 1979), only two of the patients were treated with propanolol. Both had severe

bradycardias and cardiac standstill after tracheal suction. More recently an infusion of esmolol, a short-acting beta blocker, has been tried (King & Cave 1991). This produced stability with less hypotension than that produced by propranolol.
   b. Magnesium sulphate and clonidine (Sutton et al 1990).
   c. Morphine (5–30 mg in an infusion over 30 minutes every 2–8 hours) for hypertension and/or tachycardia or hypotension (Wright et al 1989).
   d. Atropine infusion 72–2756 mg/day (Dolar 1992),
   e. Sodium valproate.
   f. ACE inhibitors.
   g. Continuous extradural and spinal anaesthesia.
5. Patients should be preoxygenated before tracheal suction, to avoid hypoxia.
6. Low-dose heparin should be given to prevent venous thrombosis. A fatal embolism occurred in an obese lady despite low-dose heparin. The use of full anticoagulation has been suggested (Jenkins & Keep 1976).

BIBLIOGRAPHY

Baronia A K, Singh P K, Dhiman R K 1991 Intractable pharyngeal spasm following tracheal extubation in a patient with undiagnosed tetanus. Anesthesiology 75: 1111
Borgeat A, Popovic V, Schwander D 1991 Efficiency of a continuous infusion of propofol in a patient with tetanus. Critical Care Medicine 19: 295–297
Buchanan N, Smit L, Cane R D et al 1978 Death of a child with tetanus due to propranolol. British Medical Journal 2: 254–255
Checketts M R, White R J, 1993 Avoidance of intermittent positive pressure ventilation in tetanus with dantrolene therapy. Anaesthesia (in press)
Crokaert F, Glupczynaski Y, Fastrez R et al 1984 Postoperative tetanus. Lancet i: 1466
Dolar D 1992 The use of a continuous atropine infusion in the management of severe tetanus. Intensive Care Medicine 18: 26–31
Domenighetti G M, Savary G, Stricker H 1984 Hyperadrenergic syndrome in severe tetanus; extreme rise in catecholamines responsive to labetalol. British Medical Journal 288: 1483–1484
Edmondson R S, Flowers M W 1979 Intensive care in tetanus: management, complications, and mortality in 100 cases. British Medical Journal 1: 1401–1404
Farling P A, Sharpe T D, Gray R C 1989 Major thoracic surgery during active tetanus Anaesthesia 44: 125–127
Flowers M W 1988 Tetanus. Surgery 55: 1300–1303
Jenkins J, Keep P 1976 Fatal embolism despite low dose heparin. Lancet i: 541
Kasanew M, Browne B, Dawes P 1989 Tetanus presenting as dysphagia. Journal of Laryngology and Otology 103: 229–230
King W W, Cave D R 1991 Use of esmolol to control autonomic instability of tetanus. American Journal of Medicine 91: 425–428
Lennard J W, Gunn A, Sellars J et al 1984 Tetanus after elective cholecystectomy and exploration of the common bile duct. Lancet i: 1466–1467
Muller H, Borner U, Zierski J et al 1987 Intrathecal baclofen for treatment of tetanus-induced spasticity. Anesthesiology 66: 76–79
Orko R, Rosenberg P H, Himherg J-J 1988 Intravenous infusion of midazolam, propofol and vecuronium in a patient with severe tetanus. Acta Anaesthesiologica Scandinavica 32: 590–592
Porath A, Acker M, Perel A 1977 Serum cholinesterase in tetanus. Anaesthesia 32: 1009–1011
Saissy J M, Vitris M, Demaziere J et al 1992 Flumazenil counteracts intrathecal baclofen-induced CNS depression in tetanus. Anesthesiology 76: 1051–1053

Stevens J J W M, Griffin R M, Stow P J 1993 Prolonged use of isoflurane in a patient with tetanus. British Journal of Anaesthesia 70: 107–109

Stoddart J C 1979a The immunology of tetanus. Anaesthesia 34: 863–-65

Stoddart J C 1979b Pseudotetanus. Anaesthesia 34: 877–881

Sutton D N, Tremlett M R, Woodcock T E et al 1990 Management of autonomic dysfunction in severe tetanus: the use of magnesium sulphate and clonidine. Intensive Care Medicine 16: 75–80

Wesley A G, Hariparsad D, Pather M et al 1983 Labetalol in tetanus. Anaesthesia 38: 243–249

Wright D K, Lalloo U G, Nayiager S et al 1989 Autonomic nervous system dysfunction in severe tetanus: current perspectives. Critical Care Medicine 17: 371–375

THALASSAEMIA

An abnormality of haemoglobin resulting from an imbalance of globin chain synthesis, affecting the population in a wide geographical band from the Mediterranean area, through the Middle East, and into India and China.

In beta thalassaemia major (homozygous state) there is an absence, or a reduced production of beta chains, and therefore an increased production of alpha chains. The alpha chains precipitate in the red cell precursors, leading to ineffective erythropoiesis and shortened red cell survival. The haemolytic anaemia leads to tissue hypoxia and excess erythropoietin production, with marrow expansion and extramedullary erythropoiesis. Iron overload secondary to increased iron absorption and recurrent transfusion is another major clinical problem. Thalassaemia is therefore a quantitative haemoglobinopathy, as opposed to sickle cell anaemia, in which the defect is qualitative.

In alpha thalassaemia there is absent or deficient alpha chain synthesis. Excess beta chains produce HbH, which has a high affinity for oxygen, but will not release it. Excess gamma chains in fetal haemoglobin produces HbBarts. Both HbH and HbBarts are physiologically useless.

The prognosis in thalassaemia major has improved since more aggressive treatment has been undertaken. Multiple blood transfusions, to maintain the Hb at 10–12 g/dl, help to suppress erythropoiesis and reduce bone deformity. Simultaneous iron chelation with desferrioxamine decreases iron deposition in the body. The effects of starting treatment at an earlier age are being tried. Bone marrow transplantation to patients under 16 years of age can correct the disorder (Lucarelli et al 1990). Active treatment has reduced many of the problems previously associated with this condition.

Patients with thalassaemia minor (heterozygous state) are normally symptom free, except when exposed to stresses such as pregnancy, when they may become anaemic, usually as a result of folic acid deficiency.

Preoperative abnormalities

Homozygous disease

1. Haemolysis leads to gross anaemia.
2. In untreated disease, bony changes occur from marrow hyperplasia.
3. Iron deposition takes place, particularly in the liver and myocardium and the commonest complications are those associated with iron overload (Davies & Wonke 1991).
4. Hypothyroidism is seen in >17% of patients, diabetes mellitus in 8–15%, and hypocalcaemia in 7%.
5. There is gross hepatosplenomegaly.
6. A hyperdynamic circulation with an increase in the circulating blood volume results.
7. Neutropenia, and occasionally thrombocytopenia, secondary to hypersplenism or folate deficiency, may be seen.
8. There is an increased incidence of gall bladder stones.
9. Patients treated with desferrioxamine commonly develop infection with *Yersinia spp*, which may result in abdominal complaints.

Heterozygous beta thalassaemia

1. The haemoglobin level is normal, or there is only a mild anaemia, except during pregnancy.
2. The red cells are hypochromic and microcytic, therefore there is a low mean corpuscular haemoglobin and a low mean cellular volume.
3. The HbA_2 may be elevated to 4–6%. Fifty per cent of subjects have HbF levels of 1–5%.

Anaesthetic problems of homozygous disease

There are few case reports of anaesthesia in thalassaemia major. The management of open heart surgery in patients with haemoglobinopathies was described (de Laval et al 1974). No complications were experienced in the three patients with thalassaemia.

1. Anaemia, associated with a hyperdynamic circulation.
2. Intubation difficulties have been reported. In untreated patients, frontal bossing and maxillary bone enlargement may occur secondary to bone marrow hyperplasia. Intubation problems in an 11-year-old child were due to massive forward protrusion of the maxilla (Orr 1967). Marrow hyperplasia is now reduced by starting transfusion therapy at an earlier age.
3. An increased risk of transfusion reactions and the presence of irregular red-cell antibodies.
4. Increased risk of overwhelming infection in splenectomized patients, particularly those receiving desferrioxamine.

Management

1. Patients with homozygous disease will be having regular transfusions at 2-4-week intervals to maintain the Hb at about 12 g/dl, and desferrioxamine i.v. or s.c. to chelate iron. Those whose blood requirements exceeds 1.5 times the standard requirement of splenectomized patients undergo splenectomy (Rebulla & Modell 1991).
2. Transfusion reactions are reduced by the routine use of white-cell filters.
3. In untreated patients, the possible potential intubation difficulties should be considered.
4. Serum ferritin levels will indicate the iron status in patients with thalassaemia minor.
5. Bone marrow transplantation in suitable patients improves survival.

BIBLIOGRAPHY
Davies S C, Wonke B 1991 The management of haemoglobinopathies. Bailliere's Clinical Haematology 4(2): 361–389
de Laval M R, Taswell H F, Bowie E J W et al 1974 Open heart surgery in patients with inherited hemoglobinopathies, red cell dyscrasias and coagulopathies. Archives of Surgery 109: 618–622
Lucarelli G, Galimberti M, Polchi P et al 1990 Bone marrow transplantation in patients with thalassemia. New England Journal of Medicine 322: 417–421
Orr D 1967 Difficult intubation: a hazard in thalassaemia. British Journal of Anaesthesia 39: 585–587
Rebulla P, Modell B 1991 Transfusion requirements and effects in patients with thalassaemia major. Lancet 337: 277–280

THALIDOMIDE-RELATED DEFORMITIES

An association between the ingestion of thalidomide in early pregnancy and limb defects was suspected, and subsequently confirmed, in 1961 (Editorial 1981). About 450 individuals in the UK were affected and they are therefore now in their third decade. A number of the abnormalities have required surgery (Fletcher 1980).

Preoperative abnormalities

1. A range of defects, from the absence of a limb to minor anomalies of thumbs or toes. The upper limb is more commonly involved. Hands and feet, which are deformed and rotated, may grow directly out of shoulders or trunk. The head and trunk size is normal.
2. Other anomalies described include a depressed nasal bridge, ocular and facial palsies, Coloboma, spinal abnormalities, congenital heart defects, profuse sweating, absence of ears, or small ears, with deafness, bowel, urological and gynaecological defects (Quibell 1981).

Anaesthetic problems

1. Potential sites for venous access are limited and femoral or subclavian veins may be poorly formed. There may be problems in obtaining blood for pathological investigations.
2. Arterial blood pressure measurement may be extremely difficult.
3. The reduction in total body skeletal muscle mass of about 75% resulted in rapid induction of anaesthesia, followed by fluctuations in depth of anaesthesia, in a patient having inhalational anaesthesia for minor gynaecological surgery (McCrory 1988).
4. Spinal abnormalities appear to be more common than was first thought and particularly involve fusion of vertebrae in the dorsolumbar region.
5. Patients may present for obstetric interventions, particularly since uterine and vaginal abnormalities have been described. A high Caesarean section rate has been found in women with major malformations (Maouris & Hirsch 1988). Extradural anaesthesia for Caesarean section has been described (Grayling & Young 1989).
6. In those who are deaf and have speech impairment, there may be communication difficulties.

Management

1. May require jugular venous cannulation. A cannula of suitable length must be chosen.
2. The use of a paediatric sphygmomanometer cuff with a carbon microphone pulse meter on a rudimentary hand to measure blood pressure was described by Grayling & Young (1989).

BIBLIOGRAPHY
Editorial 1981 Thalidomide: 20 years on. Lancet 2: 510–511.
Fletcher I 1980 Review of the treatment of thalidomide children with limb deficiency in Great Britain. Clinical Orthopaedics and Related Research 148: 18–25
Grayling G W, Young P N 1989 Anaesthesia and thalidomide-related deformities. Anaesthesia 44: 69
Maouris P G, Hirsch P J 1988 Pregnancy in women with thalidomide-induced disabilities. Case report and a questionnaire. British Journal of Obstetrics and Gynaecology 95: 717–719
McCrory J W 1988 Anaesthesia and thalidomide-related deformities. Anaesthesia 43: 613–614
Quibell E P 1981 The thalidomide embryopathy. An analysis from the UK. Practitioner 225: 721–726

THYROTOXICOSIS
(see also Section 2 THYROTOXIC CRISIS)

A state of thyroid overactivity, which should be controlled before elective surgery, to avoid precipitating a thyroid crisis. If antithyroid drugs are used, preparation for thyroid surgery may take up to 2 months.

With beta adrenoceptor blockers and potassium iodide alone, control can be achieved within 2 weeks, but not all are agreed on the suitability of this method for patients who need surgery. Beta blockers only block the peripheral effects of the hormones. They do not affect their synthesis or release, and may obscure a crisis (Eriksson et al 1977). Since they are short acting, their omission in the perioperative period may lead to an unexpected crisis. Occasionally a thyrotoxic patient requires urgent surgery. Alternatively, surgery may be unwittingly undertaken in a thyrotoxic patient, because the diagnosis is obscured by other pathology. Thyrotoxicosis may also be precipitated by infections, labour, trauma, acute medical illness, and stress (Smallridge 1992). The diagnosis is most frequently missed in elderly patients, or during pregnancy when it is difficult to distinguish it from normal increases in metabolic rate.

Preoperative abnormalities

1. A history of weight loss, heat intolerance, tremor, sweating, palpitations, fatigue, diarrhoea and anxiety.
2. Tachycardia, in particular an increased sleeping pulse rate, atrial fibrillation in the elderly, and occasionally heart failure.
3. There may be thyroid swelling, exophthalmos and lid lag. Rarely, a goitre may cause tracheal compression.
4. The diagnosis is made on increased serum T4, free thyroxine index and T3 concentrations, with an undetectable TSH. The TRH test may be needed in difficult cases.
5. Clinically obvious myopathy is infrequent, but there is some degree of EMG abnormality in 90% of thyrotoxic patients.

Anaesthetic problems

1. Tachyarrhythmias are common during anaesthesia.
2. A hypermetabolic state may occur, which can resemble malignant hyperthermia (Stevens 1983, Peters et al 1981). Atrial fibrillation was precipitated by induction of anaesthesia in one patient (Bennett & Wainwright 1989).
3. Pulmonary oedema may develop intraoperatively. This can present as cyanosis, tachycardia and respiratory distress. It is caused by a combination of hypertension, tachycardia and increased blood volume. A case was reported in which an undiagnosed thyrotoxic patient with a fractured hip developed pulmonary oedema, pyrexia and tachycardia during surgery (Stevens 1983). Again, this hypermetabolic state was diagnosed and treated as malignant hyperthermia. The true diagnosis was only revealed during postoperative investigations.
4. A thyroid crisis, or storm, may rarely develop postoperatively and present with agitation, pyrexia, sweating, tachycardia, hypertension

and cardiac failure (Jamison & Dove 1979). Similarly this may occur during labour or Caesarean section (Halpern 1989).

5. The crisis can be masked by beta blockers, which do not block the output of thyroid hormones (Jones & Solomon 1981). In addition the negative inotropic effect may be disadvantageous. Circulatory collapse has been reported during the use of propranolol to control severe thyrotoxicosis in an elderly patient (Vijayakumar et al 1989).

6. Thyrotoxic myopathy occasionally results in delayed recovery from neuromuscular blockade. A case was described in which beta blockers masked the signs of thyrotoxicosis, but not the thyrotoxic myopathy (Uusitupa et al 1980).

7. When proptosis is present the eyes are more vulnerable to damage than normal.

8. Thyrotoxicosis may occur in pregnancy, but is more difficult to diagnose because the two states have common symptoms. Cardiac dysfunction may occur in thyrotoxicosis and has been reported in association with both Caesarean section (Clark et al 1985) and septic abortion (Hankins et al 1984).

9. Patients may occasionally present to the emergency department in coma (Gilbert et al 1992).

Management

1. The patient should be rendered euthyroid prior to surgery.
   a. Antithyroid drugs inhibit thyroid hormone synthesis and block T3 and T4, but will take 6–8 weeks to become fully effective. The physical size of the thyroid gland may significantly increase during this therapy.
   b. Potassium iodide will reduce the concentration of circulating hormone to well within the normal range, but its action only lasts for 10 days.
   c. Beta adrenoceptor blockers will block the peripheral effects of the hormones, but will not block hormone release. Thyroid hormone will therefore still be present, as will the catabolic state. For the small gland, beta blockers are effective in combination with potassium iodide but this is not so for the more toxic patients.
      i. Propranolol. 40–120 mg daily in divided doses for 2–3 weeks, with the addition of potassium iodide for the last 10 days. However, the systemic clearance of propranolol is increased by thyrotoxicosis, and in combination with the half-life of the already circulating thyroxine means that it needs to be continued for a week after operation. It may also produce hypoglycaemia in the perioperative period. If propranolol cannot be given orally, an infusion will be required. The dose required to maintain therapeutic blood levels has been suggested to be 1 mg/h (Prys-Roberts 1984) and 3 mg/h (Smulyan et al 1982).

ii. Nadolol. Is more slowly metabolized by the liver, more slowly eliminated, and its clearance not altered by thyrotoxicosis. It can be given in a single daily dose of 160 mg, which gives prolonged beta blockade and more satisfactory blood levels than propranolol (Peden et al 1982). Preoperative potassium iodide is added in the usual manner. Bradycardias have been more frequently noticed than with propranolol, and atropine has been recommended instead of hyoscine as a premedication.

iii. The use of esmolol to control the tachycardia in severe thyrotoxicosis that was refractory to treatment has been described (Thorne & Bedford 1989). Surgery was urgent because of airway compromise. An infusion was started in the anaesthetic room and continued for 10 hours after the end of surgery. On one occasion, a dose of 351 µg/kg per min was required, which exceeds the dose recommended by the manufacturer. In another patient, the use of propranolol had resulted in cardiovascular collapse (Vijayakumar et al 1989). The success of esmolol infusion was attributed to its more selective beta-1 adrenoceptor blocking action, its ease of titration and the lowered systemic vascular resistance.

2. Atrial fibrillation, heart failure or hypertension should be treated preoperatively.

3. The eyes should be carefully protected.

4. Treatment of a thyrotoxic crisis (see Section 2)

BIBLIOGRAPHY

Bennett M H, Wainwright A P 1989 Acute thyroid crisis on induction of anaesthesia. Anaesthesia 44: 28–30

Burger A G, Philippe J 1992 Thyroid emergencies. Bailliere's clinical Endocrinology and Metabolism 6:1 77–93

Clark S L, Phelan J P Montoro M et al 1985 Transient ventricular dysfunction associated with cesarean section in a patient with hyperthyroidism. American Journal of Obstetrics and Gynecology 151: 384–386

Eriksson M, Rubenfeld S, Garber A J et al 1977 Propranolol does not prevent thyroid storm. New England Journal of Medicine 296: 263–264

Gilbert R E, Thomas G W, Hope R N 1992 Coma and thyroid dysfunction. Anaesthesia and Intensive Care 20: 86–87

Halpern S 1989 Anaesthesia for Caesarean section in patients with uncontrolled hyperthyroidism. Canadian Journal of Anaesthesia 36: 454–459

Hankins G D V, Lowe T W, Cunningham F G 1984 Dilated cardiomyopathy and thyrotoxicosis complicated by septic abortion. American Journal of Obstetrics and Gynecology 149: 85–86

Jamison M H, Dove H J 1979 Postoperative thyrotoxic crisis in a patient prepared for thyroidectomy with propranolol. British Journal of Clinical Practice 32: 82–83

Jones D K, Solomon S 1981 Thyrotoxic crisis masked by treatment with beta blockers. British Medical Journal 283: 659

Peden N R, Gunn A, Browning M C K et al 1982 Nadolol and potassium iodide in combination in the surgical patient. British Journal of Surgery 69: 638–640

Peters K R, Nance P, Wingard D W 1981 Malignant hyperthyroidism or malignant hyperthermia. Anesthesia and Analgesia 60: 613–615

Prys-Roberts C 1984 Kinetics and dynamics of beta adrenoceptor antagonists. In: Prys-

Roberts C (ed) Pharmacokinetics of anaesthesia. Blackwell Scientific Publications, Oxford

Smallridge R C 1992 Metabolic and anatomic thyroid emergencies: a review. Critical Care Medicine 20: 276–291

Smulyan H, Weinberg S E, Howanitz P J 1982 Continuous propranolol infusion following abdominal surgery. Journal of the American Medical Association 247: 2539–2542

Stevens J J 1983 A case of thyrotoxic crisis that mimicked malignant hyperthermia. Anesthesiology 59: 263

Thorne A C, Bedford R F 1989 Esmolol for perioperative management of thyrotoxic goiter. Anesthesiology 71: 291–294

Uusitupa M, Aro A, Korhon E N T et al 1980 Beta blockade, myopathy and thyrotoxicosis. British Medical Journal 1: 183

Vijayakumar H R, Thomas W O, Ferrara J J 1989 Perioperative management of severe thyrotoxicosis with esmolol. Anaesthesia 44: 406–408

TORSADE DE POINTES
(ATYPICAL VENTRICULAR TACHYCARDIA)

An atypical paroxysmal ventricular tachycardia associated with delayed repolarization of the ventricle. It is frequently drug induced, but may also occur with metabolic abnormalities.

Presentation

1. The patient may complain of episodes of palpitations, faintness, or fatigue.
2. As an unusual type of ventricular tachycardia. Instead of a rapid succession of extrasystoles of identical configuration, the axis of the QRS complex appears to rotate around the baseline. Before the event there is a characteristic 'long-short' sequence (Raehl et al 1985) in which a premature ectopic beat is followed by a long pause, then another premature ectopic initiates the torsade de pointes.
3. The ventricular tachycardia is not resolved by conventional antiarrhythmic treatment.
4. Factors which predispose to the development of torsade de pointes include:
   a. Drug therapy
      i. Prenylamine.
      ii. Disopyramide.
      iii. Quinidine.
      iv. Tricyclic antidepressants.
   b. Conduction problems
      i. sick sinus syndrome.
      ii. Congenital prolonged Q–T interval (Richardson et al 1992).
      iii. Atrioventricular block.
   c. Electrolyte imbalance
      i. Hypokalaemia.

    ii. Hypomagnesaemia. Torsade de pointes has been reported after massive blood transfusion for severe postpartum haemorrhage (Kulkarni et al 1992). Magnesium infusion restored the Q–T interval to normal, and temporary ventricular pacing prevented further ventricular arrhythmias.

  d. Right radical neck dissection (Otteni et al 1983). Prolongation of the Q–T interval occurred in association with right-sided neck surgery, but not with left, and persisted in more than one-third of 32 patients studied. Three patients had episodes of torsade de pointes in the postoperative period.

Diagnosis

1. Is best made on a 12-lead ECG. A ventricular tachycardia is shown, with the QRS axis undulating over 5–6 beats and with a change in direction. The 'long-short' initiating sequence may be seen.
2. In between episodes of torsade de pointes the corrected Q–T interval (Q–Tc) may be prolonged.

Management

1. The underlying cause is corrected.
     a. Any potentially causative drug is stopped. A recurrent ventricular tachycardia appeared 6 hours after pleurectomy in a patient with severe lung disease (Alexander & Potgieter 1983). A further 20 hours of treatment with a number of drugs including lignocaine, disopyramide, digoxin procainamide, and propranolol, and DC shock was unsuccessful. A 12-lead ECG showed an undulating QRS axis and the Q–Tc in between episodes of tachycardia was 0.863 seconds. A diagnosis of atypical ventricular tachycardia was made. All drugs were stopped and the hypokalaemia was corrected. Review of earlier ECGs also demonstrated prolonged Q–Tc.
     b. Metabolic causes such as hypokalaemia, hypocalcaemia or hypomagnesaemia (Ramee et al 1985) are corrected.
     c. Patients with the long QT syndrome should remain permanently on beta adrenoceptor blocking drugs. The use of labetalol in a patient with recurrent torsade de pointes, refractory to treatment, has been described.
2. Avoid the use of class I antiarrhythmics, and those drugs already mentioned.
3. In cases in which the tachycardia persists, atrial pacing may be required.
4. If VF occurs, defibrillation will be necessary.
5. Treatment can be directed towards either shortening the action potential duration with beta agonists or vagolytic agents, or suppressing early after-depolarization (Rosen & Schwartz 1991).

6. Thus, isoprenaline may increase the heart rate and therefore shorten the Q–T interval. A dose of 1–2 μg/kg has been recommended (Raehl et al 1985). However, extreme caution is required. Contraindications include myocardial ischaemia and hypertensive heart disease.

7. Early after-depolarization can be suppressed with calcium channel blockers, magnesium sulphate (Ramee et al 1985), or beta adrenoceptor blockers.

BIBLIOGRAPHY

Alexander M G, Potgieter P D 1983 Atypical ventricular tachycardia (torsade de pointes). Anaesthesia 38: 269–274

Kulkarni P, Bhattacharya S, Petros A J 1992 Torsade de pointes and long QT syndrome following major blood transfusion. Anaesthesia 47: 125–127

Martinez R 1987 Torsade de pointes: atypical rhythm, atypical treatment. Annals of Emergency Medicine 16: 878–884

Otteni J C, Pottecher R T, Bronner G et al 1983 Prolongation of the Q–T interval and sudden cardiac arrest following right radical neck dissection. Anesthesiology 59: 358–361

Raehl C L, Patel A K, LeRoy M 1985 Drug-induced torsade de pointes. Clinical Pharmacy 4: 675–690

Ramee S R, White C J, Svinarich J T et al 1985 Torsade de pointes and magnesium deficiency. American Heart Journal 109: 164–167

Richardson M G, Roark G L, Helfaer M A 1992 Intraoperative epinephrine-induced torsade de pointes in a child with long QT syndrome. Anesthesiology 76: 647–649

Rosen M R, Schwartz P J 1991 The 'Sicilian Gambit'. A new approach to the classification of antiarrhythmics drugs based on their actions on arrhythmogenic mechanisms. Task Force of the Working Group on Arrhythmias of the European Society of Cardiology. European Heart Journal 12: 1112–1131

TREACHER COLLINS SYNDROME
(see also PIERRE ROBIN SYNDROME)

A craniofacial defect associated with developmental anomalies of the first arch. Abnormalities vary from minimal defects, to the complete syndrome. Patients may require anaesthesia for manoeuvres to temporarily improve upper airway obstruction, or for correction of some of the congenital defects.

Preoperative abnormalities

1. Features may include mandibular and malar hypoplasia, antimongoloid palpebral fissure, a large mouth and irregular maloccluded teeth, microphthalmia, lower lid defects, cleft palate, macroglossia, and auricular deformities.

2. Associated abnormalities include mental retardation, deafness, dwarfism, cardiac defects, and skeletal deformities.

3. The predominant problem is that of chronic upper respiratory tract obstruction, which in its severest form leads to retarded growth and occasionally cor pulmonale. If the child is failing to compensate for

his airway dysfunction, his growth will be well below the average percentile (Mallory & Paradise 1979).
4. Sleep apnoea has been described.

Anaesthetic problems

1. Airway obstruction. In the small baby this may require urgent temporary corrective manoeuvres, such as stitching the tongue to the lower lip.
2. Excess secretions may hamper induction of anaesthesia.
3. Inhalation induction may be difficult.
4. Difficult tracheal intubation. A number of papers have described difficult or failed intubation, (Sklar & King 1976, Miyabe et al 1985, Rasch et al 1986). One resulted in a near fatality (Ross 1963).
5. Obstructive sleep apnoea may occur postoperatively (Roa & Moss 1984).
6. Pulmonary oedema. Respiratory arrest and pulmonary oedema were reported in a 15-year-old boy 40 minutes after a N_2O/O_2/halothane anaesthetic (Roa & Moss 1984).

Management

1. Respiratory depressant agents should be avoided both for premedication, and postoperatively.
2. Drying agents should always be used.
3. A muscle relaxant must never be given until the airway has been secured.
4. Awake intubation or awake direct laryngoscopy to visualize the vocal cords, should be considered. A successful direct laryngoscopy, performed with the patient in the sitting position, and using a 5-gauge feeding tube taped to the side of the laryngoscope to give oxygen, has been described (Rasch et al 1986). The use of the fibreoptic bronchoscope or tracheostomy under local anaesthetic has been recommended in order to avoid the hazards of inhalational induction and failed intubation. In older children, some of whom are retarded, this may not be possible.
5. If general anaesthesia is essential, a number of techniques have been described to assist intubation.
   a. The use of an anterior commissure laryngoscope, which prevents the tongue from falling in on the laryngoscope, has been described (Handler & Keon 1983; see Pierre Robin syndrome for a full description).
   b. A tactile nasal intubation technique was used in a 4-year-old boy (Sklar & King 1976). Induction was with halothane followed by ether, and the tongue was pulled downwards and forwards. The tube was initially used as a nasal airway, while the index and middle finger were used to palpate the epiglottis, below which the tube was then passed.

   c. The use of an assistant to pull out the tongue with forceps, and at the same time to apply cricoid pressure, was found to assist laryngoscopy (Miyabe et al 1985).

   d. A 14-year-old boy was anaesthetized with incremental ketamine. A gum elastic bougie was inserted into the larynx and the tube was threaded over the top (MacLennan & Robertson 1981).

   e. A laryngeal mask was used in place of a tracheal tube in a patient undergoing tympanoplasty (Ebata et al 1991).

6. The tracheal tube should remain in place until the patient is fully awake. There have been a number of reports of airway obstruction occurring during the recovery period. These have necessitated reintubation and, in one case, a tracheostomy.

7. Patients should be nursed in a high-dependency area postoperatively. The combination of sleep apnoea and drugs with CNS depressant effects may make these children particularly susceptible to respiratory arrest. The use of an oximeter is essential.

BIBLIOGRAPHY

Ebata T, Nishiki S, Masuda A et al 1991 Anaesthesia for Treacher Collins syndrome using a larygeal mask airway. Canadian Journal of Anaesthesia 38: 1043–1045

Handler S D, Keon T P 1983 Difficult laryngoscopy/intubation: the child with mandibular hypoplasia. Annals of Otology, Rhinology and Laryngology 92: 401–404

MacLennan F, Robertson G S 1981 Ketamine for induction and intubation in Treacher-Collins syndrome. Anaesthesia 36: 196–198

Mallory S B, Paradise J L 1979 Glossoptosis revisited: on the development and resolution of airway obstruction in the Pierre-Robin syndrome. Pediatrics 64: 946–948

Miyabe M, Dohi S, Homma E 1985 Tracheal intubation in an infant with Treacher Collins syndrome – pulling out the tongue by a forceps. Anesthesiology 62: 213–214

Rasch D J, Browder F, Barr M et al 1986 Anaesthesia for Treacher-Collins and Pierre-Robin syndromes: a report of three cases. Canadian Anaesthetists' Society Journal 33: 364–370

Roa N L, Moss K S 1984 Treacher-Collins syndrome with sleep apnea: anesthetic considerations. Anesthesiology 60: 71–73

Ross E D 1963 Treacher-Collins syndrome. An anaesthetic hazard. Anaesthesia 18: 350–354

Sklar G S, King B D 1976 Endotracheal intubation and Treacher-Collins syndrome. Anesthesiology 44: 247–249

TURNER'S SYNDROME

A syndrome associated with a sex chromosome abnormality, which includes gonadal dysgenesis, primary amenorrhoea, skeletal, renal, and other anomalies.

Preoperative abnormalities

1. Skeletal abnormalities may include short stature, a short webbed neck with fusion of cervical vertebrae, a low hairline, cubitus

valgus, a high-arched palate, micrognathia, a shield chest, and a short fourth metacarpal.

2. Cardiac defects include partial anomalous pulmonary venous drainage, coarctation of the aorta and aortic stenosis (Moore et al 1990).
3. Associated anomalies such as renal dysgenesis, peripheral lymphoedema, and ocular and aural defects.
4. There is an increased incidence of diabetes and autoimmune thyroid disease.

Anaesthetic problems

1. Intubation difficulties may occur as a result of the short neck and fused cervical vertebrae.
2. The distance between the vocal cords and carina may be short, with 15 or fewer tracheal rings (Wells et al 1989). A patient developed left lung collapse following accidental one-lung anaesthesia during laparoscopy (Divekar et al 1983). Subsequent X-rays showed that the bifurcation of the trachea was in an abnormally high position, at the level of the sternoclavicular joint.
3. Problems of renal disease.

Management

1. Assessment of abnormalities, particularly those of the cardiovascular system.
2. Potential intubation difficulties must be anticipated and the risk of inadvertent one-lung anaesthesia borne in mind.

BIBLIOGRAPHY
Divekar V M, Kothari M D, Kamdar B M 1983 Anaesthesia in Turner's syndrome. Canadian Anaesthetists' Society Journal 30: 417–418
Moore J W, Kirby W C, Rogers W M et al 1990 Partial anomalous pulmonary venous drainage associated with 45,X Turner's syndrome. Pediatrics 86: 273–276
Wells A L, Wells T R, Landing B H et al 1989. Short trachea, a hazard in tracheal intubation of neonates and infants: syndromal association. Anesthesiology 71: 367–373

VARICELLA

A common infectious disease of childhood caused by the DNA varicella zoster virus. In adults the disease may run a more severe course than in children, and anaesthetists may be involved in the treatment of patients with varicella pneumonia and other complications. Herpes zoster may follow, possibly as a result of reactivation of the virus within the spinal sensory ganglia.

Preoperative abnormalities

1. The incubation period is about 15–18 days. In children the rash starts immediately, whereas in adults there is a prodromal illness. Lesions begin in the mouth, hard palate, fauces and uvula. Those on the trunk spread from the back to the front, then onto the face and limbs. Hollows and protected parts may be particularly affected. There is cropping of the rash, in contrast to smallpox in which lesions tend to be of the same age. Thus in chickenpox macule, papule, vesicle, pustule and scab may be seen at any one time.
2. Complications, which particularly affect adults, include encephalitis, pneumonia, sepsis, hepatitis (Patti et al 1990) and thrombocytopenia.
3. Varicella pneumonia is more common in adults (almost exclusively affecting those who are smokers), in the immunologically compromised, and during pregnancy. It carries a significant morbidity and mortality. Cough and breathlessness usually starts 2–5 days after the rash appears, but occasionally before. CXR initially shows diffuse fine nodular shadowing, followed by an increase in nodular size, finally progressing to patchy consolidation. Patients may deteriorate rapidly, and the onset of hypoxia which is unresponsive to treatment is associated with a poor prognosis. Hyponatraemia is a common finding (Davidson et al 1988).

Anaesthetic problems

1. Anaesthetists are predominantly involved in the management of varicella pneumonia in patients who develop progressive hypoxaemia which is refractory to treatment (Clark et al 1991). Varicella pneumonia tends to be more common, and more severe, in pregnancy (Esmonde et al 1989).
2. It has been suggested that, if IPPV is required, there is an increased risk of laryngeal oedema following prolonged tracheal intubation. Laryngeal oedema has been reported after extubation in three adults (Boyd & Grounds 1991). In two, difficulties in reintubation resulted in cardiac arrest.

Management

1. Antiviral agents. There have been no really satisfactory studies to define the place of acyclovir in the management of varicella. There is some evidence that oral acyclovir 4 g/day reduces the severity of the illness in adults, provided that it is given within 24 hours of the rash appearing (Feder 1990). A retrospective study of varicella pneumonia in previously healthy adults suggested that i.v. acyclovir given within 36 hours of hospital admission was associated with a reduction in fever and tachypnoea and an improvement in

oxygenation (Haake et al 1990). A study of 21 cases of varicella pneumonia in pregnancy suggests that i.v. acyclovir reduces maternal morbidity and mortality and that it is safe for the developing fetus in the second and third trimesters (Smego & Asperilla 1991).

2. Treatment of hypoxia with oxygen, initially by mask. Assisted nasal breathing with inspiratory pressure support of 35 cmH$_2$O was used by Jankowski and Petros (1991) to improve oxygenation in a 44-year-old woman. However, this technique requires patient cooperation, and in cases of severe hypoxaemia, IPPV and PEEP
will usually be required. In one pregnant patient, the use of ECMO was reported to be life-saving (Clark et al 1991).

3. If view of the possibility of laryngeal oedema, it is important to inspect the larynx before extubation. If, in the presence of laryngeal oedema, the tracheal tube needs to be changed, the use of a bougie will be of assistance. It has been suggested that tracheal intubation be avoided, if possible. If not, tracheostomy should be considered at an earlier stage than normal, but at least 7 days after the last lesion has appeared.

BIBLIOGRAPHY

Boyd O F, Grounds R M 1991 Life threatening laryngeal oedema after prolonged intubation for chickenpox pneumonia. British Medical Journal 302: 516–517
Clark G P M, Dobson P M, Thickett A et al 1991 Chickenpox pneumonia, its complications and management. Anaesthesia 46: 376–380
Davidson R N, Lynn W, Savage P et al 1988 Chickenpox pneumonia: experience with antiviral treatment. Thorax 43: 627–630
Esmonde T F Herdman G, Anderson G 1989 Chickenpox pneumonia: an association with pregnancy Thorax 44: 812–815
Feder H M Jr 1990 Treatment of adult chickenpox with oral acyclovir. Archives of Internal Medicine 150: 2061–2065
Haake D A, Zakowski P C, Haake D L et al 1990 Early treatment with acyclovir for varicella pneumonia in otherwise healthy adults: retrospective controlled study and review. Review of Infectious Diseases 12: 788–798
Jankowski S, Petros A J 1991 Chickenpox pneumonia: NAB before IPPV? Anaesthesia 46: 993–994
Patti M E, Selvaggi K J, Kroboth F J 1990 Varicella hepatitis in the immunocompromised adult: a case report and review of the literature. American Journal of Medicine 88: 77–80
Smego R A, Asperilla M O 1991 Use of acyclovir for varicella pneumonia during pregnancy. Obstetrics and Gynecology 78: 1112–1116

VIPOMA
(WDHA SYNDROME)

One of the APUDomas (Amine Precursor Uptake and Decarboxylation), which secretes vasoactive intestinal polypeptide (VIP), but may also produce other hormones. Tumours in adults are most commonly of pancreatic endocrine origin, whereas in children they are usually ganglioneuroblastomas arising from the sympathetic chain. VIP may also be one of a number of hormones that can be secreted by bronchial carcinomas and paraganglionomas. Intravenous administration of VIP produces hypotension secondary to vasodilatation, hyperglycaemia, diarrhoea, inhibition of gastric acid output, and respiratory stimulation. About 50% of patients have metastatic spread at the time of diagnosis (Krejs 1987). Although surgery is the first-line treatment, the introduction of somatostatin analogues has resulted in dramatic improvement of symptoms (Philippe 1992), and in some cases long-term remission has been reported.

Preoperative abnormalities

1. The syndrome, as it was originally described, consisted of **W**atery **D**iarrhoea, **H**ypokalaemia and **A**chlorhydria or hypochlorhydria (WDHA syndrome). This is accompanied by weight loss and dehydration, and a history of abdominal colic and cutaneous flushing.
2. The picture may be complicated by the effects of additional hormones (see APUDomas).
3. Biochemical changes include hypokalaemia, acidosis, hypercalcaemia, increased blood urea, diabetic glucose tolerance, increased plasma VIP, and increased plasma pancreatic polypeptide levels.
4. Tumour location may be by CT scan and arteriography.

Anaesthetic problems

1. Gross fluid and electrolyte imbalance can be a major problem, since losses of up to 8 l/day may occur (Bouloux 1987). One patient, whose serum potassium level was only 1.3 mmol/l, presented with a quadriparesis. This resolved completely after potassium infusion (Taylor et al 1977).
2. Secretion of VIP during handling of the tumour may produce profound hypotension. The patient mentioned above had an adrenal ganglioneuroblastoma which secreted both VIP and noradrenaline. Prior to removal of the tumour, these had mutually antagonistic effects. However, following its removal there was severe hypotension, probably due to the more prolonged action of VIP.
3. There may be associated hypercalcaemia (Venkatesh et al 1989).

Management

1. Correction of fluid electrolyte imbalance before surgical removal.
2. Treatment with a somatostatin analogue by subcutaneous injection or infusion (octreotide 50–150 µg 8-hourly). Octreotide treatment has been associated with complete relief of diarrhoea, return of serum potassium levels to normal, and a decrease in plasma levels of VIP. Diarrhoea is reduced within 12–24 hours from 20 to 2 l/day,

and eleotrolyte imbalance resolves within 48 hours (Wynick & Bloom 1991). However, there is no evidence that somatostatin arrests the progression of the tumour (Brunani et al 1991).

3. Correction of hypercalcaemia, if present.

BIBLIOGRAPHY

Bouloux P-M 1987 Multiple endocrine neoplasia. Surgery 1: 1180–1185
Brunani A, Crespi C, De Martin M et al 1991 Four year treatment with a long acting somatostatin analogue in a patient with Verner-Morrison syndrome. Journal of Endocrinological Investigation 14: 685–689
Krejs G J 1987 VIPoma syndrome. American Journal of Medicine 82 (suppl 5B): 37–48.
Philippe J 1992 APUDomas: acute complications and their medical management. Bailliere's Clinical Endocrinology and Metabolism 6(1): 217–228
Taylor A R, Chulajata D, Jones D H et al 1977 Adrenal turnour secreting vasoactive intestinal peptide and noradrenaline. Anaesthesia 32: 1012–1016
Venkatesh S, Vassilopoulou-Sellin R, Samaan N A 1989 Somatostatin analogue: use in the treatment of VIPoma with hypercalcemia. American Journal of Medicine 87: 356–357
Wynick D, Bloom S R 1991 Clinical review 23. The use of long-acting somatostatin analog octreotide in the treatment of gut neuroendocrine tumours. Journal of Clinical Endocrinology and Metabolism 73: 1–3

VON GIERKE'S DISEASE

An autosomal recessive inherited glycogen storage disease (Cori type Ia) in which there is an absence, or reduction in levels, of glucose-6-phosphatase. Glycogen is a polymer made up of straight and branching chains of glucose monomer units. Blood glucose is normally maintained by breakdown of glycogen. Glucose-6-phosphatase is present in the liver, kidney, gut, and platelets. It is the enzyme involved in the final step in the conversion of glycogen to free glucose. An absence, or a reduction in levels, of the enzyme results in severe hypoglycaemia, multiple metabolic abnormalities, and accumulation of glycogen within the liver and kidney. Patients require a regular intake of glucose 2-3-hourly and limitation of fructose and lactose. Some patients have been helped by a portacaval shunt (Casson 1975), which improves most aspects of the disease apart from fasting hypoglycaemia, and by liver transplant.

Preoperative abnormalities

1. Presents in infancy with gross hepatomegaly, which results from accumulation of glycogen and fat in the liver. An increased incidence of cirrhosis and hepatocellular carcinoma has been reported (Conti & Kemeny 1992).
2. The kidneys are also enlarged, and renal disease (chronic proteinuria, renal stones, nephrocalcinosis) and renal failure are common (Chen et al 1988).

3. Severe hypoglycaemia occurs, which does not respond to glucagon, fructose or adrenaline. This may lead to fits and failure to thrive. In spite of this, patients tend to be obese, secondary to deposition of subcutaneous fat.
4. A chronic lactic acidosis results from free conversion of pyruvate to lactate, and increased pyruvate levels.
5. Hypertriglyceridaemia and high levels of free fatty acids occur as a result of increased synthesis, and stimulation of their release from fat.
6. Hyperuricaemia and gout, and gouty nephropathy.
7. Platelet dysfunction, secondary to biochemical derangements, may produce coagulation problems. These are reversed when treatment is instituted. Neutrophil dysfunction may also occur.
8. Diagnosis can be confirmed by liver biopsy, and histochemistry
9. Management includes measures such as continuous intragastric, nasogastric or parenteral feeding and portacaval shunt, all of which improve metabolic control and ameliorate the signs and symptoms of the disease.

Anaesthetic problems

1. Starvation produces severe hypoglycaemia and lactic acidosis. In a review of 12 patients, one 17-year-old boy developed a pH of 7.08 during surgery after 7 hours of starvation (Cox 1968). Death occurred in another child, who had a cardiac arrest at the end of a tonsillectomy, but no details were given.
2. The present, successful, continuous metabolic management of these children reduces the tolerance to low blood glucose levels, which normally occurs in the untreated child.
3. There may be epistaxis, bruising and coagulation problems secondary to platelet dysfunction, although strict metabolic control reverses this.
4. Muscle development is poor and may result in postoperative respiratory insufficiency.
5. Although there is a delay in sexual development and reproductive capacity is low, pregnancy has been reported (Johnson et al 1990, Chen et al 1984).

Management

1. To prevent an acidosis occurring at the beginning of surgery, a dextrose infusion should be given during the period of preoperative starvation. In one case, intragastric feeding was maintained until 3 hours preoperatively, and replaced by an infusion of glucose to give 0.4 g/kg per hour (Bevan 1980).
2. If major surgery, such as a portacaval shunt or liver transplant, is contemplated, preoperative parenteral nutrition is advisable (Casson 1975). Liver size is decreased and platelet function improved.

3. Plasma glucose and acid base status should be monitored regularly throughout the perioperative period (Bevan 1980). Acidaemia can occur without ketonuria, therefore testing for urinary ketones alone may be an unreliable predictor of acidosis. For the reasons stated above, hypoglycaemia should not be allowed to occur.

4. Lactate-containing solutions are absolutely contraindicated. Fructose should not be given because it induces hyperuricaemia.

5. Platelet function can be assessed by performing a bleeding time. If this is signicantly prolonged, regional anaesthesia is inadvisable.

6. Neuromuscular monitoring.

7. Careful postoperative observation is required to detect respiratory insufficiency.

8. The management of pregnancy and labour involving the use of 3-hourly cornstarch feeds has been described (Chen et al 1984). As much as 325 g cornstarch may be needed to meet the requirements of both mother and fetus. Protein loss secondary to severe pre-eclampsia necessitated the use of parenteral nutrition in one patient (Johnson et at 1990).

BIBLIOGRAPHY

Bevan J C 1980 Anaesthesia in Von Gierke's disease. Current approach to management. Anaesthesia 35: 699–702

Casson H 1975 Anaesthesia for portacaval bypass in patients with metabolic diseases. British Journal of Anaesthesia 47: 969–975

Chen Y T, Cornblath M, Sidbury J B 1984 Cornstarch therapy in type I glycogen-storage disease. New England Journal of Medicine 310: 171–175

Chen Y T, Coleman R A, Scheinman J I et al 1988 Renal disease in type I glycogen storage disease. New England Journal of Medicine 318: 7–11

Conti J A, Kemeny N 1992 Type Ia glycogenolysis associated with hepatocellular carcinoma. Cancer 69: 1320–1322

Cox J M 1968 Anesthesia and glycogen storage disease. Anesthesiology 29: 1221–1225

Johnson M P, Compton A, Drugan A et al 1990 Metabolic control of von Gierke disease (glycogen storage disease type IA) in pregnancy: maintenance of euglycemia with cornstarch. Obstetrics and Gynecology 75: 507–510

VON HIPPEL-LINDAU DISEASE

A rare autosomal dominant familial neuroectodermal disorder, usually presenting in young adults with one or more of a variety of manifestations. Amongst the most serious of these are cerebellar, medullary, or spinal haemangioblastomas, retinal angiomatosis, renal cell carcinoma and phaeochromocytoma (Horton et al 1976). A high incidence of pancreatic lesions has recently been found (Neumann et al 1991). Genetic studies suggest familial clustering of the features (Neumann & Wiestler 1991).

Preoperative abnormalities

1. Features usually present separately and, unless there is a known family history, the diagnosis of von Hippel-Lindau may only be

made in retrospect. Tumours may recur, or new tumours appear. A 14-year-old boy initially presented with a phaeochromocytoma and subsequently developed a cerebral angioblastoma, retinal angiomatosis and a second phaeochromocytoma (personal observation).

2. Other associated conditions include pancreatic cysts, islet cell tumours, angiomas of the liver and kidneys, renal cysts, epididymal cystadenoma and polycythaemia. About 25% of patients with CNS haemangioblastomas subsequently turn out to have von Hippel–Lindau disease.

Anaesthetic problems

1. Surgery for one manifestation of the disease may be complicated by the presence of an undiagnosed phaeochromocytoma (Potier et al 1989).
2. Those of the management of a phaeochromocytoma, if present.
3. Spinal anaesthesia may be hazardous in the presence of an undiagnosed cerebral or spinal tumour.
4. The safe management of the pregnant patient with a previously resected cerebral tumour has been reported (Matthews & Halshaw 1986).

Management

1. Careful assessment should be made for lesions other than the one for which anaesthesia is required, and in particular for any symptoms and signs of cerebral or cerebellar tumours. Patients with CNS haemangioblastomas have a 23% incidence of von.Hippel–Lindau disease.
2. Twenty-four-hour urinary screening for catecholamines.
3. Preparation for phaeochromocytoma surgery (see Phaeochromocytoma).

BIBLIOGRAPHY
Horton W A, Wong V, Eldridge R 1976 von Hippel–Lindau disease. Archives of Internal Medicine 136: 769–777
Matthews A J, Halshaw J 1986 Epidural anaesthesia in von Hippel–Lindau disease. Anaesthesia 41: 853–855
Neumann H P, Wiestler O D 1991 Clustering of features of von Hippel–Lindau syndrome: evidence for a complex genetic locus. Lancet 337: 1052–1054
Neumann H P Dinkel E, Brambs H et al 1991 Pancreatic lesions in the von Hippel–Lindau syndrome. Gastroenterology 101: 465–471
Potier F, Brasdfer D, Castier P et al 1989 Le pheochromocytome dans le maladie de

von Hippel Lindau. A propos d'un cas revelation per-operatoire. Bulletin des Societes d'Ophtalmologie de France 89: 251–252 (Eng abstr).

VON RECKLINGHAUSEN'S DISEASE
(SEE NEUROFIBROMATOSIS)

VON WILLEBRAND'S DISEASE

A group of autosomal dominant, inherited haemorrhagic diseases associated with reduced, abnormal or absent von Willebrand factor (vWF:Ag). In plasma, vWF:Ag forms a complex with Factor VIII (VIII/vWF:Ag), although the two proteins are controlled by genes on different chromosomes. During coagulation, the complexes are dissociated.

Since the formation of a complex with vWF:Ag protects Factor VIII from premature destruction, Factor VIII clotting activity levels are also reduced in most cases of von Willebrand's disease (vWD). However, levels usually remain above 5% and on occasions may even be normal.

vWF:Ag has been demonstrated to be present in endothelial cells, platelets, and megakaryocytes, and is involved in the link between platelets and damaged endothelium. Von Willebrand's disease is therefore associated with defects in platelet adhesiveness and aggregation, and a prolonged bleeding time. Von Willebrand factor is also found in plasma and intact subendothelium. Electrophoretic techniques have allowed laboratory classification of three major types, and further subtypes, of von Willebrand's disease (Cameron & Kobrinsky 1990).

1. Type I is the commonest form and is responsible for about 90% of cases; all vWF:Ag multimers are decreased quantitatively, and the haemophilic part (VIII:C) may also be decreased. The PT and PTT are usually normal; the bleeding time may be prolonged but can be normal despite a history of bleeding. In addition, results may vary on different occasions; for example, pregnancy and oestrogens may result in an increase in vWF:Ag and the menopause may be associated with excessive menstrual bleeding.
2. Type IIa (9%) in which vWF:Ag multimers are absent from plasma, and platelets and VIII:C levels may be normal or reduced.
3. Type IIb (1%) in which vWF:Ag multimers are reduced in the plasma but increased on the platelet surface. There is decreased platelet survival and a degree of thrombocytopenia.
4. Type IIc variants.
5. Type III, an autosomal recessive form, is the severest type, in which no vWF:Ag or VIII:C is detectable. The PTT will always be abnormal in this form.

The different types of the disease vary in their clinical severity, the mode of inheritance, laboratory abnormality and in their response to different therapies. Mild disease is common and may occur in up to 3% of the population.

Preoperative abnormalities

1. Clinically, the bleeding in vWD differs from that seen in haemophilia. Bruising occurs easily, and bleeding tends to be mucosal in type, from the nose, mouth, gastrointestinal tract, lungs, and uterus. Immediate bleeding tends to follow trauma and surgery in vWD, whereas in haemophilia it is usually delayed. In the homozygous form, cutaneous and deep tissue bleeding may also occur.

2. The bleeding time is usually prolonged, and platelet aggregation and adhesion reduced. Factor VIII clotting activity may be reduced or normal, and therefore the partial thromboplastin time may or may not be abnormal. There are a number of laboratory tests for vWF:Ag activity, which remain in the province of the haematologist. The Ristocetin cofactor activity is the most reliable in clinical terms.

Anaesthetic problems

1. Bleeding after trauma or surgery may occur, the degree being dependent upon the severity of the disease. Although bleeding is not usually as severe as in haemophilia, major anaesthetic problems may arise from time to time. The anaesthetic management of haemoptysis and haemothorax in vWD has been described (Bowes 1969).

2. Pregnancy and delivery may be complicated. Vaginal delivery may cause trauma and haemorrhage in infants of severely affected mothers, and in these patients Caesarean section is required. In such cases, blood loss at Caesarean section may be considerable.

3. Desmopressin may cause water retention. Two patients have been described in which the use of desmopressin in labour was associated with water retention. In one patient hyponatraemic fits occurred (Chediak et al 1986).

4. Menorrhagia may increase in menopausal women with vWD, because of the decrease in oestrogen levels. Oestrogens generally increase vWF:Ag levels in the commonest type of vWD, therefore care should be taken to exclude a history of other bleeding in women requiring hysterectomy.

Management

1. Careful clinical and haematological assessment of the type and severity of the disease is required. Advice must be obtained from a

haematologist as to the appropriate therapy to cover the proposed surgery. In the less severe form of the disease, a clinical and laboratory improvement is associated with both pregnancy and the administration of oestrogens or desmopressin (DDAVP). These have the advantage of avoiding the use of blood products.

2. Blood samples for coagulation studies should be taken with care. Stasis, or damage to blood by difficult aspiration, may produce unreliable results with some tests.
3. Salicylates may worsen the defect and their use should be avoided.
4. When treatment is required, either desmopressin 0.3 μ/kg, or both desmopressin and cryoprecipitate may be used, depending on the severity and type of vWD (Mannucci et al 1981). Cryoprecipitate contains large multimers and will increase the levels of Factor VIII:C and correct the bleeding time. Platelets alone do not correct the bleeding time, but may be required in addition to cryoprecipitate when blood loss occurs during surgery or trauma and results in thrombocytopenia. Desmopressin is probably unsuitable in type II disease because it may exacerbate the thrombocytopenia by increasing platelet/vWF:Ag binding. The use of a new pasteurized Factor VIII preparation (Humate-P) for treatment of a patient with type IIc vWD undergoing coronary artery bypass surgery has been described (Slaughter et al 1993).
5. In pregnant patients, haematological advice should be sought early on so that coagulation factors can be monitored through pregnancy. Opinion is divided as to whether regional anaesthesia should be performed. In normal pregnancy, Factor VIII levels increase, and it has been suggested that regional anaesthesia is feasible in patients with mild vWD, provided that the activated partial thromboplastin time and the bleeding time are close to normal. Caesarean section under extradural anaesthesia has been reported in a patient with vWD who fulfilled these criteria (Milaskiewicz et al 1990). As pregnancy progressed, the patient's bleeding time had decreased from 15 minutes to 6 minutes, and the Factor VIII:C level had increased from 42 to 108%. However, once the patient is delivered, the coagulation factors return to the prepregnant state, therefore early removal of the extradural catheter is probably advisable.
6. The clinical course of six pregnancies in patients with vWD has been described (Chediak et al 1986). Caesarean section will be required unless the defect is mild, because the trauma of delivery may cause haemorrhage in a susceptible infant. If both desmopressin and oxytocin are required, only small volumes of saline 0.9% should be used as the diluent, and the plasma sodium levels should be estimated regularly during treatment. Fluid retention may require treatment with frusemide 0.25–0.5 mg/kg.

BIBLIOGRAPHY

Bowes J B 1969 Anaesthetic management of haemothorax and haemoptysis due to von Willebrand's disease. British Journal of Anaesthesia 41: 894–897

Cameron C B, Kobrinsky N 1990 Perioperative management of patients with von Willebrand's disease. Canadian Journal of Anaesthesia 37: 341–347

Chediak J R, Alban G M, Maxey B 1986 von Willebrand's disease and pregnancy: management during delivery and outcome of offspring. American Journal of Obstetrics and Gynecology 155: 618–624

Conti M, Mari D, Conti E et al 1986 Pregnancy in women with different types of von Willebrand disease. Obstetrics and Gynecology 68: 282–285

Mannucci P M, Canciani M T, Rota L et al 1981 Response of factor VIII/von Willebrand factor to DDAVP in healthy subjects and patients with haemophilia and von Willebrand's disease. British Journal of Haematology 47: 283–293

Milaskiewicz R M, Holdcroft A, Letsky E 1990 Epidural anaesthesia and von Willebrand's disease. Anaesthesia 45: 462–464

Slaughter T F, Mody E A, Newland Oldham H et al 1993 Management of a patient with type IIC von Willebrand's disease during coronary artery bypass surgery. Anesthesiology 78: 195–197

WEGENER'S GRANULOMATOSIS

A systemic granulomatous vasculitis of the 20–40 years age group, in which granulomas of the upper and lower respiratory tract are associated with a focal necrotizing glomerulonephritis. and a widespread vasculitis involving other organs. The clinical features overlap with microscopic polyarteritis, and the antineutrophil cytoplasmic antibody is positive in both. A survey of 85 cases showed that all patients had either upper or lower respiratory tract involvement, and 85% had documented renal disease (Fauci et al 1983). Without treatment the prognosis is poor, and up to 90% of deaths are associated with renal failure. Treatment with cyclophosphamide and corticosteroids has improved the prognosis. In early cases, some response to sulphamethoxazole has been shown (Valeriano-Marcet & Spiera 1991). A limited form of the disease may occur in which there are mucosal lesions, and patients may require anaesthesia for oral or ENT procedures or for biopsy of airway lesions, before the diagnosis has been made.

Preoperative abnormalities

1. Upper airway problems include nasal discharge, crusting, bleeding and ulceration, sometimes progressing to septal perforation and nasal collapse. Infection or ulceration may occur in the sinuses, palate, and pharynx. Granulomas, ulceration and stenosis may involve the larynx.

2. More than 90% of patients have pulmonary involvement. Symptoms include cough, haemoptysis, chest pain, and breathlessness. CXR shows changing pulmonary opacities, which are often multiple and bilateral. Some of these cavitate and simulate lung carcinoma. In one series, fibreoptic bronchoscopy was found to be abnormal in

55% patients, the main lesions being inflammation, haemorrhage and ulceration (Cordier et al 1990). Partial bronchial stenosis was less common and occurred in 17.5%.

3. Renal disease may present with haematuria, proteinuria or red cell casts. Untreated, patients progress to kidney failure.

4. Ophthalmic and aural complications were reported in 58% and 61% of cases, respectively.

5. Other systems which may be involved in a diffuse vasculitis include the skin (45%), nervous (22%) and cardiovascular systems (12%). Cardiac complications include pericarditis, myopathy, valvular heart and coronary disease.

6. General symptoms include joint pains, malaise and fever.

7. Patients may be taking cyclophosphamide and steroids.

8. There may be anaemia, raised ESR, hypergammaglobulinaemia and leucocytosis (unless cyclophosphamide has caused a leucopenia), eosinophilia and thrombocytosis. The test for antineutrophil cytoplasmic antibody is usually positive in systemic disease but not necessarily so in the local form.

9. Plasmapheresis may have a place for those in renal failure.

Anaesthetic problems

1. Patients may present insidiously with ear, nose or throat problems some time before the diagnosis has been made (D'Cruz et al 1989). Granulomas of the upper airway may cause bleeding, or result in obstruction (Cohen et al 1978, Lake 1978). Subglottic stenosis, tracheal granulomas and tracheo-oesophageal fistula have all been described. Subglottic stenosis is usually circumferential, most frequently affects females, and usually requires permanent tracheostomy (Arauz & Fonseca 1982, McDonald et al 1982). Recurrent subglottic stenosis may occur (Hoare et al 1989). Rarely, proximal bronchial stenosis has been reported which in this case responded to cyclophosphamide and cotrimoxazole (Hirsch et al 1992).

2. Nasal intubation may dislodge tissue or cause bleeding.

3. Oral lesions have been reported, which may ulcerate and resemble malignancies (Allen et al 1991).

4. Renal failure is common.

5. A peripheral arteritis may result in digital ischaemia. In such cases, arterial cannulation is hazardous.

6. Pulmonary lesions may lead to consolidation, cavitation, bleeding, and arterial hypoxaemia.

7. Cardiac lesions can cause heart failure, conduction defects or coronary insufficiency, although this is rare.

8. Treatment for the disease may cause immunosuppression. Cyclophosphamide most commonly causes leucopenia, hair loss and

haemorrhagic cystitis (Fauci et al 1983). Plasma cholinesterase activity may be reduced.

Management

1. A careful assessment of the systems which may be affected by the disease must be undertaken. If there are signs that the airway is involved then indirect laryngoscopy and airway tomography may be indicated.
2. Investigations required may include Hb, WBC, platelet count, ESR, CXR, arterial blood gases, and tests of renal and liver function.
3. Corticosteroid supplements may be needed.
4. If airway obstruction is diagnosed, examination or intubation under local anaesthesia, or occasionally tracheostomy, may be necessary (D'Cruz et al 1989). Otherwise, examination of the palate, pharynx and larynx for lesions should be carried out during laryngoscopy.
5. The management of renal failure (see Renal failure).
6. If the patient has both airway lesions and renal failure, then local anaesthesia should be considered. However, any neurological lesions secondary to the disease should be documented accurately prior to anaesthesia.

BIBLIOGRAPHY

Allen C M, Camisa C, Salewski C et al 1991 Wegener's granulomatosis: report of three cases with oral lesions. Journal of Oral and Maxillofacial Surgery 49: 294–298
Arauz J C, Fonseca R 1982 Wegener's granulomatosis appearing initially in the trachea. Annals of Otology, Rhinology and Laryngology 91: 593–594
Cohen S R, Landing B H, King K K et al 1978 Wegener's granulomatosis causing laryngeal and tracheobronchial obstruction in an adolescent girl. Annals of Otology, Rhinology and Laryngology 87: (S52): 15–19
Cordier J F, Valeyre D, Guillevin L et al 1990 Pulmonary Wegener's granulomatosis. A clinical and imaging study of 77 cases. Chest 97: 906–912
D'Cruz D P, Baguley E, Asherson R A et al 1989 Ear, nose and throat symptoms in subacute Wegener's granulomatosis. British Medical Journal 299: 419–422
Fauci A S, Haynes B F, Katz P et al 1983 Wegener's granulomatosis: prospective clinical and therapeutic experiences. Annals of Internal Medicine 98: 76–85
Hirsch M M, Houssiau F A, Collard P et al 1992 A rare case of bronchial stenosis in Wegener's granulomatosis. Dramatic response to intravenous cyclophosphamide and oral cotrimoxazole. Journal of Rheumatology 19: 821–824
Hoare T J, Jayne D, Rhys Evans P et al 1989 Wegener's granulomatosis, subglottic stenosis and antineutrophil cytoplasm antibodies. Journal of Laryngology and Otology 103: 1187–1191
Lake C L 1978 Anesthesia and Wegener's granulomatosis: case report and review of the literature. Anesthesia and Analgesia 57: 353–359
McDonald T J, Neel H B, DeRemee A A 1982 Wegener's granulomatosis of the subglottis and the upper portion of the trachea. Annals of Otology, Rhinology and Laryngology 91: 588–592
Valeriano-Marcet J, Spiera H 1991 Treatment of Wegener's granulomatosis with sulfamethoxazole-trimethoprim. Archives of Internal Medicine 151: 1649–1652

WERDNIG-HOFFMANN DISEASE

One of a group of inherited diseases, the spinal muscular atrophies, in which there is neuronal degeneration and loss of neurones in the anterior horn cells. Werdnig-Hoffmann (type I or infantile spinal muscular atrophy or floppy infant syndrome) is the most severe. It is an autosomal recessive disease with an incidence of 1 in 10 000. Usually its onset is at birth or in the early week of life, and death occurs by the age of 3 years. Genetic mapping has recently shown the gene to be located on chromosome 5q (Editorial 1990).

Preoperative abnormalities

1. A floppy infant, with muscle weakness and wasting which begins in the back, and pelvic and shoulder girdles, and depressed tendon reflexes. There is tongue fasciculation and loss of sucking ability.
2. Intercostal and accessory muscles may be involved, resulting in increasing respiratory difficulty. Since the diaphragm is spared until late in the disease, lower rib indrawing may occur on inspiration. Respiratory failure, usually in association with pneumonia, is responsible for the early death.
3. Diagnosis is made on muscle biopsy, and this is the most common reason for anaesthesia.

Anaesthetic problems

1. Increasing muscle weakness and respiratory compromise, particularly in the later stages of the disease.
2. The possibility that suxamethonium may precipitate hyperkalaemia or rhabdomyolysis should be considered.

Management

1. Non-depolarizing neuromuscular blockers and respiratory depressants should be avoided because of the risks of hypoventilation and respiratory failure.
2. The use of ketamine for diagnostic muscle biopsy has been described (Ramachandra et al 1990). Thirty two children from 3 months to 12 years were given diazepam 0.2 mg/kg i.m. as premedication followed by either ketamine 2 mg/kg i.v. or ketamine 10 mg/kg i.m. as an anaesthetic.
3. For longer procedures, controlled ventilation and postoperative respiratory support may be required.

BIBLIOGRAPHY
Editorial 1990 Spinal muscle atrophies. Lancet 336: 280–281
Ramachandra P S, Anisya V, Gourie-Devi M 1990 Ketamine monoanaesthesia for diagnostic muscle biopsy in neuromuscular disorders in infancy and childhood: floppy infant syndrome. Canadian Journal of Anaesthesia 37: 474–476

WILLIAMS SYNDROME

An autosomal dominant condition in which cardiac abnormalities, in particular supravalvular aortic stenosis, are associated with an elfin face, mental retardation and hypercalcaemia. Myocardial ischaemia may occur and the cardiovascular elements of the disease are progressive (Greenberg 1989).

Preoperative abnormalities

1. A characteristic 'elfin' face with mandibular and dental hypoplasia, mental and physical retardation, and hypotonia.
2. Cardiovascular anomalies include supravalvular aortic stenosis or narrowing (Hallidie-Smith & Karas 1988), supravalvular and valvular pulmonary stenosis, a bicuspid aortic valve and carotid artery stenoses. In one echocardiographic and Doppler study, a high incidence of mitral or tricuspid valve prolapse was also found (Brand et al 1989).
3. Coronary artery stenosis and myocardial ischaemia has been reported in these children, possibly secondary to abnormal haemodynamics around the coronary ostia and limited diastolic coronary filling (Terhune et al 1985, Conway et al 1990). There is an increased risk of sudden death.
4. Systemic hypertension and a wide range of peripheral vascular anomalies may be present.
5. Idiopathic hypercalcaemia.
6. A spectrum of renal abnormalities, such as renal artery stenosis, nephrocalcinosis, urethral stenosis, reflux, kidney anomalies and systemic hypertension, have been described (Ingelfinger & Newburger 1991).
7. Bowel and joint problems.
8. Reports of adults with Williams syndrome are rare, but the small number of studies have shown progressive multisystem problems (Morris et al 1990). In particular, the vascular lesions may become more severe.

Anaesthetic problems

1. Intubation difficulties may occur because of mandibular hypoplasia. In adults, progressive joint limitation may exacerbate this.
2. Masseter muscle spasm after halothane and suxamethonium has been reported (Patel & Harrison 1991). However, this might have been a normal response to suxamethonium given in standard (Leary & Ellis 1990) or low dosages (Matthews & Vernon 1991) particularly since halothane had been given before the suxamethonium (Carroll 1987).
3. Cardiovascular disease is a prominent feature and may add to the risks of anaesthesia. In addition to the congenital cardiac lesions and left ventricular hypertrophy, myocardial insufficiency has been reported. A 16-month-old child with supravalvular aortic stenosis was admitted with episodes of cyanosis, which were associated with

ECG changes suggestive of subendocardial ischaemia (Terhune et al 1985). She was given morphine, but inadvertently in an overdose of 8 mg. The error was immediately recognized, naloxone 1 mg was given and a tracheal tube inserted. Ninety minutes later the child had a cardiac arrest and resuscitation failed. At postmortem, 80% occlusion of the lumen of the left anterior descending coronary artery was found, together with an area of recent myocardial infarction. Although the death was attributed to the child's cardiac state, rather than the morphine, the problems sometimes associated with the use of naloxone in cardiac disease cannot be ignored. The risk of sudden death during or after cardiac catheterization is well known to paediatric cardiologists, and a further three deaths, also associated with myocardial ischaemia, were reported in 1990 (Conway et al 1990). Two of the deaths took place immediately after cardiac catheterization, and the third at 72 hours. There was little detail apart from that of the postmortem reports and no mention of any anaesthetic having been given.

Management

1. Cardiovascular assessment is particularly important in view of the range of anomalies described. Management of the patient must be based on this knowledge. The reports of myocardial ischaemia and sudden deaths associated with cardiac catheterization means that these children should be treated with particular caution throughout the whole perioperative period. It has been suggested that in a patient suspected of having Williams syndrome, blood pressure should be measured at least once in all four limbs. When supravalvular aortic stenosis is present, the systolic and mean blood pressures may be higher in the right arm than in the other three extremities.
2. Management of difficult intubation, if applicable.
3. The problems of anaesthesia for surgical correction of supravalvular aortic stenosis under deep hypothermia, in a child who additionally had left carotid artery stenosis, have been described (Larson & Warner 1990).

BIBLIOGRAPHY
Brand A, Keren A, Reifen R M et al 1989 Echocardiographic and Doppler findings in the Williams syndrome. American Journal of Cardiology 63: 633–635
Carroll J B 1987 Increased incidence of masseter spasm in children with strabismus anaesthetised with halothane and succinyl choline. Anesthesiology 67: 559–561
Conway E E Jr, Noonnan J, Marion R W et al 1990 Myocardial infarction leading to sudden death in the Williams syndrome: report of three cases. Journal of Pediatrics 117: 593–595
Greenberg F 1989 Williams syndrome. Pediatrics 84: 922–923
Hallidie-Smith K A, Karas S 1988 Cardiac anomalies in Williams-Beuren syndrome. Archives of Disease in Childhood 63: 809–813
Ingelfinger J R, Newburger J W 1991 Spectrum of renal anomalies in patients with

Williams syndrome. Journal of Pediatrics 119: 771–773

Larson J S, Warner M A 1989 Williams syndrome: an uncommon cause of
supravalvular aortic stenosis in a child. Journal of Cardiothoracic Anesthesia 3:
337–340

Leary N P, Ellis F R 1990 Masseteric muscle spasm as a normal response to
suxamethonium. British Journal of Anaesthesia 64: 488–492

Matthews A J, Vernon J M 1991 Masseter spasm in Williams syndrome. Anaesthesia
46: 706

Morris C A, Leonard C O, Dilts C et al 1990 Adults with Williams syndrome.
American Journal of Medical Genetics Supplement 6: 102–107

Patel J, Harrison M J 1991 Williams syndrome: masseter spasm during anaesthesia.
Anaesthesia 46: 115–116

Terhune P E, Buchino J J, Rees A H 1985 Myocardial infarction associated with
supravalvular aortic stenosis. Journal of Pediatrics 106: 251–254

WOLFF-PARKINSON-WHITE SYNDROME

A congenital pre-excitation syndrome in which an accessory pathway
occurs between the atrial and ventricular myocardium (the bundle of
Kent). This permits the initiation of excitation and contraction of the
ventricles before the normal atrial impulse has crossed the AV node to
the bundle of His (Wellens et al 1987). The different excitation recovery
times of the two pathways allow repeated circulation of impulses
between the atria and ventricles. Subjects are thus liable to develop
episodes of supraventricular tachycardia, and sometimes rapid atrial
fibrillation. The myocardium is usually normal, but prolonged periods of
tachycardia may cause hypotension, and occasionally heart failure.

It may occur in up to 0.3% of the general population, and the
incidence can be even higher in close relatives of affected individuals.

In symptomatic patients who are refractory to treatment, surgical
division of the relevant accessory pathway may be required (Bennett
1988). This may be particularly appropriate to avoid long-term drug
therapy in the young patient (Hood et al 1991). However, it is probably
unnecessary to subject asymptomatic individuals, who are incidentally
found to have the WPW pattern on ECG, to electrophysiological studies
(Fisch 1990).

Preoperative abnormalities

1. The P–R interval is short, usually <0.12 seconds. This is best seen
   in lead V1.
2. The QRS interval is broader than normal (>0.12 seconds, best seen
   in leads II, V5 and V6), and the initial QRS deflection is slow rising
   and slurred, and known as the delta wave. Early depolarization
   occurs via the accessory pathway, but further spread is slow, as it
   does not involve specialized conducting tissue. It therefore merges
   into the normal QRS complex. In some cases the ECG may be
   entirely normal.
3. WPW was originally classified into two types; type A, in which the
   ventricular complex was predominantly positive in V1, and type B

in which it was predominantly negative. It is now known to be more complex than this since the pathway may be in any segment of the myocardium (Prystowsky et al 1984).

4. The clinical history is of episodes of 'palpitations' which are precipitated by exercise, stress, or excitement. During an attack the patient may complain of faintness, chest pain, breathlessness, or polyuria. If the arrhythmia persists, cardiac failure may occur.
5. The ECG during attacks may show an AV re-entrant tachycardia (120–140 b.p.m.), atrial fibrillation, or atrial flutter. Ventricular tachycardia, flutter, or fibrillation have been reported. Death occasionally occurs (Brechenmacher et al 1977). During the re-entrant tachycardia there will be narrow, regular ventricular complexes. If the P wave can be seen, it will occur midway between ventricular complexes. Atrial fibrillation will, in general, be faster than normal; most of the impulses will show delta waves, although some will not.

Anaesthetic problems

1. Since pre-excitation may be intermittent, WPW may present during anaesthesia, despite the patient having had a normal preoperative ECG (Nishikawa et al 1993). One case was unmasked by the development of glycine absorption syndrome during prostatectomy (Lubarsky & Wilkinson 1989).
2. Tachyatrhythmias may be precipitated by anxiety, surgical stimulation, induction of anaesthesia, intubation or hypotension (van der Starre 1978, Jacobson et al 1985).
3. During an attack, hypotension and a significant decrease in cardiac output may occur. Recurrent episodes of SVT were reported in a patient in late pregnancy. Failure to respond to drug therapy on one occasion, and the occurrence of hypotension and fetal distress from practolol therapy on the second, necessitated the use of direct current cardioversion on both occasions (Klepper 1981).
4. Anaesthesia for surgical ablation of the accessory pathway has two main requirements; the technique used must prevent sympathetic stimulation, to avoid tachyarrhythmias, yet must not materially alter conduction in the normal or accessory pathways, as this might hinder identification of the accessory pathway. Halothane, enflurane and isoflurane all depress conduction in normal and accessory pathways and may be unsuitable in these particular circumstances (Sharpe et al 1990, Dobkowski et al 1990).

Management

1. If the patient is already receiving antiarrhythmics, these should be maintained.
2. Sympathetic stimulants, such as atropine and pancuronium, should be avoided.

3. There is no agreement about the optimal agents for anaesthesia. However, on general principles, drugs producing tachycardia, or techniques of light anaesthesia resulting in sympathetic stimulation, should be avoided. Neuroleptic anaesthesia with droperidol and fentanyl has been recommended (van der Starre 1978). However, another report based on 13 cases, nine of which were for His or Kent bundle surgery, recommended inhalational anaesthesia (Sadowski & Moyers 1979). Three of these 13 patients developed tachycardias. Two of the three patients had morphine and pancuronium, and the third had halothane and d-tubocurarine. Of the 10 who had no arrhythmias, all but one had inhalation agents, and most received curare rather than pancuronium. It is possible that the episodes of tachycardia were triggered by a combination of pancuronium and light anaesthesia.

Anaesthesia has been described in a premature neonate for pyloric stenosis, using thiopentone, vecuronium, and isoflurane (Richmond & Conroy 1988).

Relatively little work has been done on the effect of anaesthetic drugs on the electrical pathways in patients with WPW. In one electrophysiological study on patients about to undergo surgical section of the accessory pathway, droperidol, in doses of 0.2–0.6 mg/kg, was found to increase the antegrade and retrograde effective refractory period of the action potential (Gomez-Arnau et al 1983). The effects of alfentanil-midazolam anaesthesia were studied in eight patients during accessory pathway ablation (Dobkowski et al 1991, Sharpe et al 1992). No effect was found on conduction in either the normal or the accessory pathway and there were no tachyarrhythmias. The authors concluded that this was a suitable technique for surgical ablation. Anaesthesia was induced with alfentanil 50 µg/kg, midazolam 0.15 mg/kg and vecuronium 20 mg, and maintained with a continuous infusion of alfentanil 2 µg/kg per min and intermittent midazolam 1–2 mg every 15 minutes.

4. If SVT occurs, vagal stimulation by carotid sinus massage, a Valsalva manoeuvre, or squatting, can be tried. To be effective, these need to be instituted as soon as possible after the beginning of the tachycarcia (Wellens et al 1987). If they fail, then drug or other methods of treatment will be needed. Individual patients may respond differently to different drugs. In addition, if atrial fibrillation is present, it can be made worse by verapamil and digoxin. Treatment can be aimed at abolishing the trigger mechanism, or preventing initiation or continuation of re-entry.

   a. For AV re-entrant tachycardias (Wellens et al 1987):

   i. verapamil 5–10 mg over 1 minute (but should not be used if the patient is receiving beta blockers or if atrial fibrillation or flutter with pre-excitation is present).

   ii. Other drugs which prolong the refractory period of either the aberrant pathway, or the AV node, can be tried. Adenosine 3 mg, given rapidly over 2 seconds, using cardiac monitoring if necessary, followed by 6 mg after 1–2 minutes, and then by 12 mg after a further 1–2 minutes. Others include flecainide, disopyramide, diltiazem, beta adrenoceptor blockers, procainamide, or amiodarone.

iii. Drugs producing reflex bradycardia may occasionally be successful. Phenylephrine 200 μg, and a subsequent phenylephrine infusion, finally terminated a refractory tachycardia in a patient having squint surgery, when other drugs had failed (Jacobson et al 1985).

b. For atrial fibrillation. Disopyramide, amiodarone and flecainide impair conduction in the bundle of Kent.

c. Direct current cardioversion should be considered early in atrial fibrillation, particularly if there is haemodynamic compromise. It can also be used if tachycardias fail to respond to drug treatment. Recurrent attacks of SVT which produced marked maternal hypotension in a patient in late pregnancy required cardioversion (Klepper 1981).

d. Atrial pacing may be used as a last resort.

e. Surgical transection may be considered for patients with recurrent arrhythmias or intolerance to drug therapy (Bennett 1988).

BIBLIOGRAPHY
Bennett J G 1988 Surgery for cardiac arrhythmias. British Medical Journal 296: 1687–1688
Brechenmacher R, Coumel P H, Fauchier J-P et al 1977 Intractable paroxysmal tachycardia which proved fatal in type A Wolff–Parkinson–White syndrome. Circulation 43: 408–417
Dobkowski W B, Murkin J M, Sharpe M D et al 1990 The effect of isoflurane (1 MAC) on the normal AV conduction system and accessory pathways. Anesthesia and Analgesia 70: S86
Dobkowski W B, Murkin J M, Sharpe M D et al 1991 The effect of combined alfentanil and midazolam anaesthesia on the normal A-V conduction system and accessory pathways in patients with Wolff–Parkinson–White syndrome. Canadian Journal of Anaesthesia 38: A168
Fisch C 1990 Clinical electrophysiological studies and the Wolff–Parkinson–White pattern. Circulation 82: 1872–1873
Gomez-Arnau J, Marquez-Montes J, Avello F 1983 Fentanyl and droperidol effects on the refractoriness of the accessory pathway in the Wolff–Parkinson–White syndrome. Anesthesiology 58: 307–313
Hood M A, Smith W M, Robinason M C et al 1991 Operations for Wolf–Parkinson–White syndrome. Journal of Thoracic and Cardiovascular Surgery 101: 998–1003
Jacobson L, Turnquist K, Masley S 1985 Wolff–Parkinson–White syndrome. Anaesthesia 40: 657–660
Lubarsky D, Wilkinson K 1989 Anesthesia unmasking benign Wolff–Parkinson–White syndrome. Anesthesia and Analgesia 68: 172–174
Kepper I 1981 Cardioversion in late pregnancy. Anaesthesia 36: 611–616
Nishikawa K, Mizoguchi M, Yukioka H et al 1993 Concealed Wolff–Parkinson–White syndrome detected during spinal anaesthesia. Anaesthesia (in press)
Prystowsky E N, Miles W M, Heger J J et al 1984 Pre-excitation syndromes: mechanisms and management. Medical Clinics of North America 68: 831–894
Richmond M N, Conroy P T 1988 Anesthetic management of neonate born prematurely with Wolff–Parkinson–White. Anesthesia and Analgesia 67: 477–478

Sadowski A R, Moyers J R 1979 Anesthetic management of the Wolff–Parkinson–
White syndrome. Anesthesiology 51: 553–556

Sharpe M D, Murkin J M, Dobkowski W B et al 1990 Halothane depresses conduction
of normal and accessory pathways during surgery for Wolff–Parkinson–White
syndrome. Anesthesia and Analgesia 70: S365

Sharpe M D, Dobkowski W B, Murkin J M et al 1992 Alfentanil-midazolam
anaesthesia has no electrophysiological effects upon the normal conduction system
or accessory pathways in patients with Wolff–Parkinson–White syndrome.
Canadian Journal of Anaesthesia 39: 816–821

van der Starre P J A 1978 Wolff–Parkinson–White syndrome during anaesthesia.
Anesthesiology 48: 369–372

Wellens H J J, Brugada P, Penn O C 1987 The management of the preexcitation
syndromes. Journal of the American Medical Association 257: 2325–2333

ZENKER'S DIVERTICULUM

An outpouching of pharyngeal mucosa in the posterior wall of the
hypopharynx at its junction with the oesophagus through Killian's
dehiscence. This is an area of weakness which lies between the
cricopharyngeus and the inferior pharyngeal constrictor muscles. There
may be a functional component to the condition, in that neuromuscular
dysfunction particularly in the relaxation of cricopharyngeus, has been
found.

Preoperative abnormalities

1. The main complaints are of food sticking in the throat and
   dysphagia bouts of coughing, swelling in the neck, and
   regurgitation.
2. Aspiration pneumonitis occurs in about 25% of patients and results
   in bronchitis or recurrent pneumonia (Aggerholm & Illum 1990).
3. Weight loss and poor nutrition.
4. It has been suggested that reflux oesophagitis and hiatus hernia
   occur more frequently than in the normal population, but this has
   been disputed (Gage-White 1988).
5. Treatment may be by diverticulectomy or by endoscopic dilatation.

Anaesthetic problems

1. Problems of aspiration and leakage around the tracheal tube.
2. The use of oral medication may be ineffective, because the tablets
   lodge within the pouch and absorption may be delayed.
3. Postoperative complications are most often associated with
   inhalation of food or debris from the pouch.

Management

1. The pouch should be emptied preoperatively.
2. Induction with a head-up tilt has been recommended.

3. There is agreement about the method of induction. Awake fibreoptic intubation has been recommended by some authors, and a smooth general anaesthetic induction by others (Thiagarajah et al 1990, Cope & Spargo 1990). Cricoid pressure may be contraindicated.
4. After surgery for the diverticulum, postoperative feeding for a week with a nasogastric tube is required.
5. Treatment with antibiotics after pouch surgery reduces the number of local infective complications, and possibly the incidence of pouch recurrence.

BIBLIOGRAPHY

Aggerholm K, lllum P 1990 Surgical treatment of Zenker's diverticulum. Journal of Laryngology and Otology 104: 312–314
Cope R, Spargo P 1990 Anesthesia for Zenker's diverticulum. Anesthesia and Analgesia 71: 312
Gage-White L 1988 Incidence of Zenker's diverticulum with hiatus hernia. Laryngoscope 98: 527–530
Thiagarajah S, Lean E, Keh M 1990 Anesthetic implications of Zenker's diverticulum. Anesthesia and Analgesia 70: 109–111

2

Emergency Conditions Arising During Anaesthesia or in the Immediate Perioperative Period

ADDISONIAN CRISIS OR ACUTE ADRENOCORTICAL INSUFFICIENCY
(see also SECTION 1)

An extremely rare cause of perioperative cardiovascular collapse. It may result from primary adrenocortical disease, in which case all three zones of the adrenal cortex will be affected, or be secondary, which manifests itself as pure glucocorticoid deficiency associated with atrophy of the zona fasciculata.

Although rare, it must not be overlooked. An unrecognized and untreated Addisonian crisis can be fatal. The preoperative diagnosis is difficult to make in patients with mild clinical disease, and yet it is these patients whose adrenal cortex may be incapable of responding to the stresses of anaesthesia and surgery. In patients with adenocarcinoma, adrenal metastases are not uncommon (Ihde et al 1990), but clinically apparent disease occurs only after a 90% loss of adrenocortical tissue.

Presentation

1. Acute cardiovascular collapse can occur under a wide variety of circumstances. (Occasionally, patients may be normotensive if they were hypertensive before the crisis.)

    a. Cardiac arrest during appendicectomy in a 15-year-old girl responded to cardiac massage, saline and bicarbonate (Salam & Davies 1974). She was subsequently found to have a normal resting blood cortisol, but no response to adrenal stimulation.

    b. An acute Addisonian crisis associated with a serum sodium of 106 mmol/l was deliberately provoked by a patient who stopped his own steroid therapy and then cut his neck and wrists (Smith & Byrne 1981).

    c. Severe perioperative hypotension, despite the administration of fluids and inotropic agents, occurred in a young man with an acute abdominal emergency (Hertzberg & Schulman 1985). An improvement in his condition only took place when steroids were given. His postoperative complications included myocardial infarction and pericarditis. A subsequent adrenal stimulation test indicated Addison's disease.

    d. Patients with adrenocortical insufficiency may be subfertile. Cardiovascular collapse occurred in a young woman undergoing infertility investigations under general anaesthesia (personal observation). Sudden death occurred a week later, in a period of steroid withdrawal, during adrenocortical investigations.

    e. A patient with severe diarrhoea and vomiting presented with hypotension, tachycardia and fever (Frederick et al 1991). Despite rehydration and inotropic support on ITU, he developed acute respiratory distress with hypoxia and died 10 hours later. It was subsequently discovered that his brother had primary Addison's disease and that the patient's own plasma cortisol level before death was $2 \mu g/100$ ml (Normal $6–25 \mu g/100$ ml).

f. Should pregnancy occur, which is rare because these patients are subfertile, then a crisis may present during pregnancy (Seaward et al 1989).

g. Adrenocortical insufficiency has been reported after the removal of apparently nonfunctioning adrenal adenomas (Huiras et al 1989). Although there were no stigmata of adrenal hyperactivity, it was postulated that there was sufficient secretion from the adenoma to produce basal cortisol levels, whilst suppressing the other gland.

h. Two patients with high-output circulatory failure and negative blood cultures were found to have primary adrenal insufficiency (Dorin & Kearns 1988).

i. In patients with cancer, adrenocortical insufficiency is particularly difficult to diagnose, since anorexia, nausea, orthostatic hypotension and confusion may be attributed to the disease itself (Kung et al 1990).

2. Other symptoms and signs include abdominal pain, vomiting, diarrhoea, orthostatic hypotension, syncope, confusion, stupor, and mucosal hyperpigmentation.

3. If Addison's disease is present, other endocrine abnormalities (hypothyroidism or panhypopituitarism) should be sought (Frederick et al 1991).

4. There may be a history of steroid therapy within the previous 12 months. Adrenocortical atrophy is detectable 5 days after the onset of glucocorticoid therapy with the equivalent of prednisone 20–30 mg/day. Hypothalamic-pituitary axis suppression may occur, and a return to completely normal homeostasis may take up to 1 year (Axelrod 1976).

Management

1. Hydrocortisone hemisuccinate i.v. 200 mg, followed by an infusion of hydrocortisone 400 mg in either dextrose 5% or saline 0.9%, to be given over 24 hours.

2. Saline 0.9% i.v., 1 litre rapidly initially, then more slowly.

3. Dextrose 10% i.v. to correct hypoglycaemia.

4. Subsequently, the presumptive diagnosis must be confirmed or refuted with plasma cortisol estimations and adrenal stimulation tests. Before this, the hydrocortisone should be changed to dexamethasone, which does not register in plasma cortisol assays.

BIBLIOGRAPHY
Axelrod L 1976 Glucocorticoid therapy. Medicine 55: 39–65.
Dorin R I, Kearns P J 1988 High output circulatory failure in acute adrenal insufficiency. Critical Care Medicine 16: 296–297.

Section 2

Addisonian Crisis or Acute Adrenocortical Insufficiency

Frederick R, Brown C, Renusch J et al 1991 Addisonian crisis: emergency presentation of primary adrenal insufficiency (clinical conference). Annals of Emergency Medicine 20: 802–806

Hertzberg L B, Schulman M S 1985 Acute adrenal insufficiency in a patient with appendicitis during anesthesia. Anesthesiology 62: 517–519

Huiras C M, Pehling G B, Caplan R H 1989 Adrenal insufficiency after operative removal of apparently nonfunctioning adrenal adenoma. Journal of the American Medical Association 261: 894–989

Ihde J K, Turnbull A D, Bajorunas D R 1990 Adrenal insufficiency in the cancer patient: implications for the surgeon. British Journal of Surgery 77: 1335–1337

Kung A W C, Pun K K, Lam K et al 1990 Addisonian crisis as presenting feature in malignancies. Cancer 65: 177–179

Salam A A, Davies D M 1974 Acute adrenal insufficiency during surgery. British Journal of Anaesthesia 46: 619–622

Seaward P G, Guidozzi F, Sonnendecker E W 1989 Addisonian crisis in pregnancy. Case report. British Journal of Obstetrics and Gynaecology 96: 1348–1350

Smith M G, Byrne A J 1981 An Addisonian crisis complicating anaesthesia. Anaesthesia 56: 681–684

AIR EMBOLISM

When a patient is in an upright position, air inadvertently entering the venous system will normally be carried to the right side of the heart, where it localizes initially at the junction of the right atrium and the superior vena cava. Some air may remain in the upper part of the right atrium, whilst the rest is carried through the tricuspid valve and into the pulmonary artery. There is experimental evidence to suggest that venous air emboli are eliminated primarily in the pulmonary arterioles (Presson et al 1989) and that this elimination depends on diffusion of gas across the arteriolar walls into the alveolar spaces. Larger amounts cause pulmonary outflow obstruction and a reduction in cardiac output. Air embolism can occur in any situation in which there is an open vein and a subatmospheric pressure.

Recent concern has focused on the subject of 'paradoxical' air embolism (Clayton et al 1985). At postmortem, 20–35% of all patients have a 'probe patent' foramen ovale, and transoesophageal echocardiographic studies showed passage of contrast across the interatrial septum in 22% of 50 patients (Konstadt et al 1991). In a patient with a patent foramen ovale, if the RAP were to exceed the LAP, venous air could theoretically enter the systemic circulation. It has been suggested that, if the incidence of air embolism in the sitting position is 30–40%, and that of patent foramen ovale is 20–35%, 1 in 10 patients operated on in this position could have conditions that predispose to the entry of air into the systemic circulation (Gronert et al 1979). This 'paradoxical' air embolism might account for a number of cases of air embolism in which Doppler changes occurred without ET_{CO_2} changes, when ST segment or QRS changes suggested entry of air into the coronary arteries, or where there were postoperative clinical signs of cerebral air embolism. The possibility of a transpulmonary route for access of venous air to the systemic circulation has also been postulated.

Haemodynamic studies have shown that in the sitting position, the interatrial pressure gradient can transiently be reversed (Perkins-Pearson et al 1982), particularly during sustained application of positive end-expiratory pressure (Jaffe et al 1992) or sudden release of positive airway pressure. However, work on preoperative identification of flow-patent foramen ovale is still in its early stages, interpretation is difficult and sometimes results are conflicting (Rafferty 1992).

Systemic air embolism, although a rare event, has been reported following blunt and penetrating injuries, induction of artificial pneumothorax, and laser surgery to bronchial carcinoma. There are pathognomonic antemortem signs, but the diagnosis may easily be missed at postmortem.

Presentation

1. Type of surgery
   The reported incidence of air embolism depends on the monitoring techniques employed. The Doppler method is particularly sensitive and capable of detecting extremely small emboli.
   a. Neurosurgery in the sitting position. Using Doppler detection, an incidence of up to 58% has been reported in patients having posterior fossa or cervical disc surgery in the sitting position.
   b. Craniectomy. Using new echocardiographic techniques, 66% of infants undergoing craniectomy in the supine position were shown to have evidence of venous air embolism (Harris et al 1987).
   c. Head and neck surgery. Emboli can also occur when large veins are opened in head and neck operations, if there is a head-up tilt.
   d. Hip surgery. In hip arthroplasty, Doppler evidence of air embolism has been reported in 30% of patients immediately following the insertion of the femoral cement. There was an accompanying decrease in blood pressure in only 4% (Michel 1980).
   e. Caesarean section. Air may also enter the uterine sinuses in up to 40% of Caesarean deliveries. However, massive emboli are rare, and most likely to occur in the hypovolaemic patient with placenta praevia, or placental abruption (Younker et al 1986, Fong et al 1990).
   f. Central venous catheter insertion or removal. The increasing use of CVP lines has been associated with a number of incidents of accidental introduction of air (Seidelin et al 1987). Disconnection of a three-way tap in a patient receiving chemotherapy at home resulted in a non-fatal paradoxical embolism (Jensen & Hansen 1989). Air embolism has also been reported after removal of central venous catheters (Turnage & Harper 1991), presumably

secondary to air entrainment through the track formed by the device.

g. Lumbar disc surgery. Three patients undergoing lumbar laminectomy in the prone position developed sudden air embolism (Albin et al 1991). This is a rare occurrence, but in each case a frame was used to retain the patient in a 'four-poster' position. In this posture, the pressure in the inferior vena cava is low and there is a considerable gravitational gradient between the right side of the heart and the operation site.

h. Transurethral resection of prostate. Fatal massive air embolism has been reported following TURP (Vacanti & Lodhia 1991). At the end of surgery, there was no drainage of urine from the Foley catheter, so repeated attempts to unblock it were made with a 60-ml syringe containing fluid and air. The patient collapsed after he was moved from the lithotomy position, and at postmortem air was found throughout the venous side of the circulation. The delay before collapse was presumably because the air was held in the femoral veins until the patient was moved.

i. Extradural injection. A suspected air embolism has been described during insertion of a Tuohy needle in the C7/C1 space for injection of extradural steroids in a seated patient (Jackson & Rauck 1991).

j. Laparoscopic cholecystectomy. A sudden decrease in end-tidal CO_2 with oxygen desaturation, which occurred just after accidental penetration of the liver by the sapphire tip of the neodymium:yttrium-aluminium-garnet laser, was the first sign of air embolism during laparoscopic cholecystectomy (Greville et al 1991). The surgeons were unaware that the laser was cooled with air flowing at 0.5 l/min from ports proximal to the tip, and this air must have entered the hepatic venous system in the 15 seconds of inadvertent penetration.

k. Transcervical resection of endometrium. Similar accidents resulted in two deaths during laser endometrial ablation using artificial sapphire tips with gaseous cooling systems (Baggish & Daniell 1989).

l. Laser application to a bronchial tumour. A massive, fatal, systemic air embolism, a rare event, resulted from a fistula produced between the right main bronchus and a branch of the pulmonary vein during Nd:YAG laser application to an obstructing bronchial carcinoma (Peachey et al 1988). The emergence of bright red froth from the arterial cannula, palpation of crepitus in the brachial, femoral and carotid arteries, and observation of air in the retinal vessels on ophthalmoscopy, confirmed the diagnosis.

m. During gastrointestinal endoscopy when, air accidentally delivered via the gastroscope entered a large hepatic vein (Loudon & Tidmore 1988).

n. After insertion of peritoneovenous shunt (Ahmat et al 1989).

o. Cardiac arrest in three patients during dental implant surgery performed by the same surgeon was found to be secondary to inadvertent injection into the facial and pterygoid venous plexuses of a mixture of air and water passing through a hollow drill (Davies & Campbell 1990).

2. Factors affecting clinical signs

The effects of air embolism depend on the rate of entry and quantity of air, the differences between the venous and atmospheric pressures, and the percentage of nitrous oxide being administered. Animal research indicates that of 0.5 ml/kg per min can produce symptoms. The entry of large boluses of air has been associated with the insertion of central venous lines, especially when the head-down position was not used, and if the CVP was low. Experiments have shown that with a pressure difference of 5 cm H_2O, much as 100 ml air/second can be drawn through a 2-mm needle. The concomitant administration of nitrous oxide effectively increases the volume of air drawn into the bloodstream. A concentration of 50% N_2O produces an effective increase of 200%, and 75% N_2O one of 400%.

3. Source or timing of entry

a. In neurosurgical procedures, air enters most frequently via veins held open by the neck muscles, or those in the dura, venous sinuses or bone.

b. During spinal fusion for scoliosis, two fatal cases were reported during instrumentation (McCarthy et al 1990).

c. In hip surgery, emboli can occur when cement is inserted into the femoral shaft.

d. Of 79 cases of air embolism associated with central venous lines, the majority involved technical problems (Seidelin et al 1987). One-third happened during catheter insertion, and death occurred in 32% of the cases reported.

e. During Caesarean section, there is evidence of entry of gas bubbles in 37-50% patients, sometimes associated with chest pain and dyspnoea, in the period between uterine incision and delivery (Malinow et al 1987, Matthews & Greer 1990); 71% were reported during uterine repair (Fong et al 1990). However, few emboli are haemodynamically detrimental, except during hypovolaemic states.

4. Clinical signs of venous air embolism

These may include a hissing sound from the wound, hypotension, arrhythmias, cyanosis, or changes in respiratory pattern in a spontaneously breathing patient. However, with adequate monitoring, subclinical air entry should be detected before many of these signs occur.

5. Clinical signs of systemic air embolism
   Circulatory collapse may occur, followed by pupillary dilatation. Although a brief preceding period of hypertension has been reported, this may be missed unless direct arterial monitoring is being undertaken. Other signs include marbling of the skin, air bleeding from arteries, bubbles of air in the retinal vessels, and pallor of part of the tongue. Although the mill wheel murmur is reported to be absent, it may be heard if large amounts of gas pass through the left ventricle from a pulmonary vein (Peachey et al 1988). Systemic air embolism may be missed at postmortem if the diagnosis is not suspected, because air disappears within a few hours of death.

Diagnosis

1. A precordial Doppler produces the earliest signs of air embolism, but is very sensitive to very small amounts of air. The use of an oesphageal Doppler has been described. The diagnosis may be confirmed by aspiration through a right heart catheter, which should have been placed high in the right atrium.

2. A decrease in ET_{CO_2} occurs before clinical signs, but will not necessarily change as quickly, or as much, if a paradoxical air embolus has also occurred.

3. Later signs of significant emboli include a 'mill wheel' murmur, arrhythmias, hypotension, a decrease in oxygen saturation, and increases in CVP or in PAWP.

4. The occurrence of paradoxical air embolism is difficult to prove, unless a neurosurgeon observes air in small cerebral arteries. However, its possibility may be suggested by the ECG changes of ST elevation or depression, or cardiac arrest. Monitored changes of cerebral function have been attributed to cerebral emboli. Localization of air in the cardiac chambers using two-dimensional transoesophageal echocardiography has been reported, but at present is primarily of research interest (Cucchiara et al 1984).

Management

1. **a.** In neurosurgery
   Identify the site of access and prevent further entry. Cover or flood the wound. Compress the neck to show open veins. Deal surgically with the open vein or apply bone wax, if appropriate. Although aspiration of air from a right heart catheter may have a diagnostic role, its therapeutic value is doubtful.
   b. Central venous lines
   To prevent air embolism during insertion of a central venous line,

it is important to have the patient in a head-down position. Occlusion of the catheter after insertion, and use of a three-way tap when disconnecting infusion sets, will reduce the risks. Catheter removal should be undertaken in the supine position and the site should be covered with an occlusive dressing. It has been suggested that patients remain supine for 1 hour afterwards (Turnage & Harper 1991).

c. Total hip replacement

It has been suggested that insertion of cement into the femoral shaft using a cement gun is less likely to produce air embolism than when the cement is inserted by hand (Evans et al 1989).

2. If the entry of a large amount of air occurs, cardiopulmonary resuscitation may be required. Place the patient in a head-down position to reduce pulmonary outflow obstruction.

3. It has been suggested that the morbidity and mortality is such that the sitting position should no longer be used for neurosurgical procedures. However, an analysis of 554 cases showed that with careful patient selection, monitoring, and anaesthetic and surgical skills, this can be minimized (Matjasko et al 1985). Increasing work is being done on the recognition of the flow-patent foramen ovale by transoesophageal echocardiographic techniques (Rafferty 1992), although techniques for identification are at an early stage and dependent on the skill of the operator. If a right-to-left shunt is demonstrated, the sitting position should not be used. Since reversal of pressure gradients can be caused by the sudden release of positive airway pressure, then positive end-expiratory airway pressures should be avoided in the seated patient.

4. An inflatable neck tourniquet, which could be used to identify venous bleeding points during the incision through muscle and bone, has been described (Sale 1984).

BIBLIOGRAPHY

Ahmat K P, Riley R H, Sims C et al 1989 Fatal air embolism following anesthesia for insertion of a peritoneovenous shunt. Anesthesiology 70: 702–704

Albin M S, Ritter R R, Pruett C E et al 1991 Venous air embolism during lumbar laminectomy in the prone position: report of three cases. Anesthesia and Analgesia 73: 346–349

Baggish M S, Daniell J F 1989 Death caused by air embolism associated with neodymium:yttrium-aluminium-garnet laser surgery and artificial sapphire tips American Journal of Obstetrics and Gynecology 161: 877–880

Black S, Cucchiara R F, Nishimura R A et al 1989 parameters affecting occurrence of paradoxical air embolus. Anesthesiology 71: 235–241

Clayton D G, Evans P, Williams C et al 1985 Paradoxical air embolism during neurosurgery. Anaesthesia 40: 981–989

Cucchiara R F, Nugent M, Seward J B et al 1984 Air embolism in upright neurosurgical patients: detection and localisation by two-dimensional transoesophageal echocardiography. Anesthesiology 60: 353–355

Davies J M, Campbell L A 1990 Fatal air embolism during dental implant surgery: a report of three cases. Canadian Journal of Anaesthesia 37: 112–121

Evans R D, Palazzo M G A, Ackers J W L 1989 Air embolism during total hip replacement: comparison of two surgical techniques. British Journal of Anaesthesia 62: 243–247

Fong J, Gadalla F, Pierri M K et al 1990 Are Doppler-detected venous emboli during Caesarean section air emboli? Anesthesia and Analgesia 71: 254–257

Greville A C, Clements E A F, Erwin D C et al 1991 Pulmonary air embolism during laparoscopic laser cholecystectomy. Anaesthesia 46: 113–114

Gronert G A, Messick J M Jr, Cucchiara R F et al 1979 Paradoxical air embolism from a patent foramen ovale. Anesthesiology 50: 548–549

Harris M M, Yemen T A, Davidson A et al 1987 Venous air embolism during craniectomy in supine infants. Anesthesiology 67: 816–819

Jackson K E, Rauck R L 1991 Suspected venous air embolism during epidural anesthesia. Anesthesiology 74: 190–191

Jaffe R A, Pinto F J, Schnittger I et al 1992 Aspects of mechanical ventilation affecting interatrial shunt flow during general anesthesia. Anesthesia and Analgesia 75: 484–488

Jensen A G, Hansen P A 1989 Non-fatal paradoxical air embolism. British Journal of Anaesthesia 63: 244

Konstadt S N, Louie E K, Black S et al 1991 Intraoperative detection of patent foramen ovale by transesophageal echocardiography. Anesthesiology 74: 212–216

Loudon J O, Tidmore T L 1988 Fatal air embolism after gastrointestinal endoscopy. Anesthesiology 69: 622–623

McCarthy R E, Lonstein J E, Mertz J D et al 1990 Air embolism in spinal surgery. Journal of Spinal Disorders 3: 1–5

Malinow A M, Naulty J S, Hunt C O et al 1987 Precordial ultrasonic monitoring during Cesarean delivery. Anesthesiology 66: 816–819

Matjasko J, Petrozza P, Cohen M et al 1985 Anesthesia and surgery in the seated position: analysis of 554 cases. Neurosurgery 17: 695–702

Matthews N C, Greer G 1990 Embolism during Caesarean section. Anaesthesia 45: 964–965

Michel R 1980 Air embolism in hip surgery. Anaesthesia 35: 858–862

Peachey T, Eason J, Moxham J et al 1988 Systemic air embolism during laser bronchoscopy. Anaesthesia 43: 872–875

Perkins-Pearson N, Marshall W, Bedford R 1982 Atrial pressures in the seated position. Anesthesiology 57: 493–497

Presson R G, Kirk K R, Haselby K A et al 1989 The fate of air emboli in the pulmonary circulation of the dog. Anesthesia and Analgesia 68: S227

Rafferty T D 1992 Intraoperative transesophageal saline-contrast imaging of flow-patent foramen ovale. Anesthesia and Analgesia 75: 475–480

Sale J P 1984 Prevention of air embolism during sitting neurosurgery. Anaesthesia 39: 795–799

Seidelin P H, Stolarek I H, Thompson A M 1987 Central venous catheterisation and fatal air embolism. British Journal of Hospital Medicine 38: 438–439

Turnage W S, Harper J V 1991 Venous air embolism occurring after removal of a central venous catheter. Anesthesia and Analgesia 72: 559–560

Vacanti C A, Lodhia K L 1991 Fatal massive air embolism during transurethral resection of the prostate. Anesthesiology 74: 186–187

Younker D, Rodriguez V, Kavanagh J 1986 Massive air embolism during Cesarean section. Anesthesiology 65: 77–79.

AMNIOTIC FLUID EMBOLISM

Entry of amniotic fluid into the maternal circulation is a rare cause of collapse or sudden haemorrhage during labour. However, it has also been described in association with Caesarean section, therapeutic abortion, amniocentesis, or immediately postpartum. The amniotic fluid, which contains electrolytes, nitrogenous compounds, lipids, prostaglandins, and fetal elements such as squames, hairs, vernix and meconium, enters the maternal venous plexuses via a tear in the amniotic membranes. The diagnosis is made primarily on the clinical triad of hypoxaemia, hypotension and coagulation defects.

Earlier papers suggested that pulmonary hypertension was the principal haemodynamic feature of the condition and that treatment should be with pulmonary vasodilators. More recently, invasive haemodynamic monitoring has been undertaken in several patients in the acute stage of the disease. An initial period of pulmonary hypertension, hypoxaemia and increased right heart pressures is succeeded by left ventricular failure secondary to impaired left ventricular function (Clark et al 1988, Clark 1991, Vanmaele et al 1990). The haemodynamic findings would thus vary according to the stage at which monitoring was first undertaken. This would account for the high incidence (70%) of pulmonary oedema seen on the CXR of survivors, and the variety of features described in the few patients in whom invasive monitoring has been undertaken. These features include pulmonary hypertension (Shah et al 1986), left heart failure (Girard et al 1986, Vanmaele et al 1990), and left and right heart failure (Moore et al 1982).

There is increasing evidence that the pathophysiology involves a two-stage response to the release of vasoactive metabolites of arachidonic acid (prostaglandins and leukotrienes) which directly or indirectly damage the myocardium and lead to left ventricular failure. In addition, circulating amniotic fluid has thromboplastic activity, and the entry of a significant amount is usually associated with disseminated intravascular coagulation. Abnormal fibrinolysis may occur as well. Immunoassays and functional assays suggest that coagulation changes are caused by tissue factors contained in amniotic fluid (Lockwood et al 1991).

In the past, the mortality was said to be in excess of 80% and the diagnosis was often made at postmortem. The condition is largely nonpreventable, but with better understanding of the pathophysiology, and an increasing use of intensive care facilities for haemodynamic monitoring, some improvement in mortality rate might be expected in the future.

Presentation

1. A review of 272 cases (Morgan 1979) showed that 90% occurred during labour, and that 88% were in multiparous patients. Presenting symptoms were respiratory distress with cyanosis (51%), cardiovascular collapse (27%), convulsions (10%), or haemorrhage (12%). Associated features can include coagulation abnormalities, coma and pulmonary oedema (Lumley et al 1979, Mainprize & Maltby 1986). Bronchospasm is rare.
2. The onset is often dramatic.
3. One fatal case presented with an asymptomatic decrease in oxygen saturation, as a measured by pulse oximetry, during Caesarean section under extradural anaesthesia (Quance 1988).

Diagnosis

1. Initially, this is made on clinical grounds. The primary concern is that of resuscitation of the collapsed patient; 25% will be dead within the first hour. Of those who survive for more than an hour, the incidence of DIC is 40% (Morgan 1979).
2. The diagnosis may be confirmed if fetal squames are seen on sputum examination, or by the finding of amniotic fluid and anucleate squames in a blood sample taken from a CVP line or a pulmonary artery catheter (Shah et al 1986).

Treatment

1. Cardiovascular collapse, or even cardiac arrest, may be the initial event. Cardiopulmonary resuscitation is instituted and, if the fetus is still in utero, the Cardiff wedge (Oates et al 1988) should be used to prevent aortocaval compression (see Section 3, Resuscitation during pregnancy). Hypoxaemia is treated with high-flow oxygen and, if necessary, IPPV and PEEP.
2. Hypotension requires careful management on an ITU, such as is provided for any patient with cardiogenic shock. In the situation in which the obstetric unit is geographically isolated from such facilities, a decision must be made on the optimum time for transfer. Clark (1991) suggests initial treatment with fluids followed by circulatory support with an inotropic agent such as dopamine, and careful monitoring with a pulmonary artery catheter is advised. Once the blood pressure improves, fluid restriction may be required to prevent or treat pulmonary oedema.
3. Replacement of blood volume may be needed if there is significant haemorrhage. Treatment of any bleeding diathesis will require repeated clotting screens and specialist haematological advice. In general, packed red cells are followed by fresh frozen plasma and the tests repeated. There is not sufficient evidence to support the use of heparin, which has sometimes been recommended.
4. Cardiopulmonary bypass and pulmonary artery thrombectomy was carried out in one patient who developed shock 1 hour after Caesarean section (Exposito et al 1990). A pulmonary perfusion scan showed a massive embolus to the left lung, and friable thrombus was removed which contained a high concentration of fetal squames.

BIBLIOGRAPHY
Clark S L 1991 Amniotic fluid embolism. Critical Care Clinics 7: 877–882
Clark S L, Cotton D B, Gonik B et al 1988 Central hemodynamic alterations in, amniotic fluid embolism. American Journal of Obstetrics and Gynecology 158: 1124–1126
Davies M G, Harrison J C 1992 Amniotic fluid embolism: maternal mortality revisited. British Journal of Hospital Medicine 47: 775–776

Esposito R A, Grossi E A, Coppa G et al 1990 Successful treatment of postpartum shock caused by amniotic fluid embolism with cardiopulmonary bypass and pulmonary artery thromboembolectomy. American Journal of Obstetrics and Gynecology 163: 572–574

Girard P, Mal H, Laine J-F et al 1986 Left heart failure in amniotic fluid embolism. Anesthesiology 64: 262–265

Lockwood C J, Bach R, Guha A et al 1991 Amniotic fluid contains tissue factor, a potent initiator of coagulation. American Journal of Obstetrics and Gynecology 165: 1335–1341

Lumley J, Owen R, Morgan M 1979 Amniotic fluid embolism. A report of three cases. Anaesthesia 34: 33–36

Mainprize T C, Maltby J R 1986 Amniotic fluid embolism: a report of four probable cases. Canadian Anaesthetists' Society Journal 33: 382–387

Morgan M 1979 Amniotic fluid embolism. Anaesthesia 34: 20–32

Moore P G, James O F, Saltos N 1982 Severe amniotic fluid embolism: case report with haemodynamic findings. Anaesthesia and Intensive Care 10: 40–44

Oates S, Williams G L, Rees G A D 1988 Resuscitation in late pregnancy. British Medical Journal 297: 404–405

Quance D 1988 Amniotic fluid embolism: detection by pulse oximetry. Anesthesiology 68: 951–952

Shah K, Karlman R, Heller J 1986 Ventricular tachycardia and hypotension with amniotic fluid embolism during Cesarean section. Anesthesia and Analgesia 65: 533–535

Vanmaele L, Noppen M, Vincken W et al 1990 Transient left heart failure in amniotic fluid embolism. Intensive Care Medicine 16: 269–271

Section 2

Anaphylactoid
Reactions to
Intravenous Agents

ANAPHYLACTOID REACTIONS TO INTRAVENOUS AGENTS

A general term for a drug-related clinical event which either threatens life or disrupts the course of an operation. It is a multisystem response to a drug, or drug combination, to which the patient may or may not have been previously exposed. The term anaphylactoid does not explain the mechanism. Usually, the type of reaction may only be elucidated subsequently, by evaluation of history, immunology and, if appropriate, skin testing. Unfortunately more than one drug may have been given immediately before the reaction. The collection of blood samples for immunological studies should start as soon as possible after the event. Understanding the mechanism of the reaction is important for the subsequent management of the patient.

There appears to be an increase in the number of these reactions (Stoelting 1983). Reactions occur more frequently in women than in men. An analysis of 154 serious cases in France showed that 70% occurred in women (Laxenaire et al 1985).

1. Drugs producing reactions
    a. Induction agents
       Thiopentone causes more reactions than either methohexitone or etomidate. Etomidate is considered to be 'immunologically safe' (Watkins 1983), and a low incidence of anaphylactoid reactions has been reported. There have now been a number of reports of reactions to propofol (Laxenaire et al 1992, de Leon-Casasola et al 1992).

b. Neuromuscular blocking agents

Produce a surprising number of anaphylactoid responses and may be involved in up to 50% of reactions occurring during anaesthesia. In decreasing order of frequency, those reported to have been involved in anaphylactoid reactions are: suxamethonium, alcuronium, atracurium, tubocurarine, pancuronium, vecuronium, and gallamine (Watkins 1985). At the time of Watkins' study, pancuronium was in very common use, yet rarely involved. Subsequently, the use of either vecuronium or atracurium (despite the incidence of local histamine release) has been suggested as being relatively safe in patients with allergy or atopy.

Controversy exists about the potential for cross-reactivity between muscle relaxants, based on common quaternary or tertiary ammonium ions (Baldo 1986, Watkins 1987). Confusion may also occur with intradermal testing because neuromuscular blockers can cause skin histamine release, even at dilutions of 1:1000 or 1:10 000 (Watkins & Nimmo 1985).

c. Plasma expanders

Anaphylactoid reactions to colloid volume substitutes have been studied (Ring & Mesmer 1977) and were shown to occur most commonly in the dextrans. A study of 50 dextran-induced reactions identified a metabolic acidosis as having occurred in all the severe reactions, and also frequently in the less severe ones (Ljungstrom & Renck 1987). A technique of hapten administration (dextran 1) prior to the use of dextran has been reported to have dramatically reduced the number of serious reactions in Sweden (Ljungstrom et al 1988). However, serious reactions have occurred despite immunoprophylaxis, including one which was thought to have resulted in fetal brain damage. In view of this, the use of dextrans before Caesarean section has been questioned (Berg et al 1991). A severe reaction to hydroxyethyl starch has been reported, although this is rare (Cullen & Singer 1990).

d. X-ray contrast media

Adverse systemic reactions to contrast media occur in 5% of patients (Goldberg 1984). The majority of those who receive intravenous contrast media have an increased serum osmolality, a decreased haematocrit, and a subsequent osmotic diuresis. In addition, some patients will develop an actual anaphylactoid response, usually within 2 minutes of the injection. There may be nausea and vomiting, cardiovascular collapse, upper airway obstruction, bronchospasm, and hypoxaemia.

The newer contrast media are likely to be much safer.

e. Local anaesthetic agents

The differentiation between anaphylactoid and toxic reactions is difficult. However, the incidence of true allergy is probably very low (Incaudo et al 1978).

f. Antibiotics

Penicillin produces a high incidence of anaphylactic reactions, a proportion of which are fatal. IgE is frequently involved (Sogn 1984). Up to 8% of patients allergic to penicillin also react to cephalosporins. It has been suggested that all intraoperative antibiotics, particularly those of the penicillin type, should be given slowly, diluted into 50–250 ml of fluid (Levy 1986). Requests that they be given at induction of anaesthesia should be resisted. If a reaction occurs, there may be considerable difficulty in identifying the drug responsible.

g. Latex anaphylaxis

This is increasingly being reported. Extracted from the sap of Hevea brasiliensis, latex is used in the manufacture of rubber gloves, balloons, catheters, and elastic adhesives. Reactions, which have included rash, wheezing, urticaria, and hypotension, are of delayed onset, the earliest time being 40 minutes from induction of anaesthesia (Gold et al 1991) but they may occur much later because elution of the protein from the rubber gloves is required (Hirshman 1992).

2. Types of reactions

This is a controversial area. Some immunologists believe that non-specific anaphylactoid reactions are more common than immune-mediated ones, and that skin testing is only of value when clinical and laboratory evidence strongly favours immune involvement (Watkins & Nimmo 1985). This view is not shared by other workers (Fisher 1984). In general, the immune-mediated response tends to be more severe, and is more likely to result in death.

a. Type I hypersensitivity response

A true anaphylactic or allergic response which depends upon previous exposure to the drug. On the first occasion, lymphocytes produce specific IgE antibodies which become attached to the membrane of mast cells and basophils. A second exposure results in cross-linkages between these primed cells, changes in the cell membrane, and mast cell and basophil degranulation. Mediators such as histamine and leukotriene C are released from mast cells, causing some or all of the pharmacological effects associated with anaphylactic reactions. Complement is not involved. IgE involvement is most common, IgG may be concerned and C4 is consumed. Disappearance of basophils is said to be highly indicative of a type I reaction (Watkins 1987). This type of reaction may occur after multiple exposures to thiopentone and, although uncommon, can be fatal.

b. Complement-mediated reaction

This classical reaction can occur on initial exposure to the drug. Activation of Cl–C9, the complement cascade, occurs and C4 and C3 are consumed. C3a and C5a (anaphylatoxins) are mast cell degranulators. Once again, chemical mediators are released.

c. Alternate complement pathway

Activation of this results in direct conversion of C3, C3a once again being released. A previous exposure is not necessary. Reactions to cremophor-containing drugs were frequently of this type.

d. Non-immune anaphylactoid responses

These are common and it may be difficult to identify the drug responsible. Chemical mediators are released as a result of a direct or an indirect effect on mast cells and basophils. The diagnosis is generally one of exclusion. No IgE changes occur, and complement C3 and C4 are not consumed. It has been suggested that this reaction may occur on exposure to a particular group of drugs, such as muscle relaxants, when they share common molecular characteristics (Baldo 1986).

There may be predisposing factors, such as chronic atopy, complement abnormalities, or a history of regular exposure to the drug concerned. The greater the amount of drug and the more rapid its administration, the more severe the reaction is likely to be.

e. Miscellaneous

In some cases, a similar response may be due to drug interactions or drug overdose. Rarely, it is secondary to an unexpected pathology, such as a hormone-secreting tumour.

Presentation

Life-threatening effects include cardiovascular collapse (90%), bronchospasm (30%), angio-oedema (25%), and pulmonary oedema (49%) (Fisher 1992).

1. Cutaneous effects

   These include flushing and urticaria and may cause significant fluid depletion. The development of a 1-mm layer of subcutaneous fluid over the whole body is approximately equivalent to a loss of 1.5 litres of extracellular volume.

2. Cardiovascular effects

   Feature most commonly and vary in severity from moderate hypotension to cardiovascular collapse. Hypotension is secondary to release of histamine (and other vasoactive peptides), which causes widespread capillary vasodilatation and increased capillary permeability. Changes in heart rate or rhythm accompany the hypotension. ECG changes were analyzed in 186 cases (Fisher 1986). A supraventricular tachycardia developed in 153 (82%) and this was accompanied by ST elevation in a further eight patients. The remaining arrhythmias included asystole, rapid AF, and ventricular fibrillation. Arrhythmias other than SVT tended to be associated with pre-existing cardiac disease. This was so in 24 out of 26 patients with heart disease, whereas 151 out of the 160 patients without cardiac disease had SVT alone. The four episodes of VF came from both groups, and were usually associated with the administration of adrenaline in the presence of halothane.

3. Bronchospasm
   Was noted to have occurred in 39% of cases studied in France (Laxenaire et al 1985). It is serious and can be responsible for deaths, secondary to cerebral hypoxia.
4. Glottic oedema
   May occur occasionally.
5. Gastrointestinal effects
   Immediately after recovery from the reaction, the patient may complain of abdominal pain, diarrhoea or vomiting. This may be secondary to hyperperistalsis and oedema of the gut.
6. Miscellaneous
   Other effects include AV conduction defects, leucopenia, and coagulation disorders. Widespread fibrin deposition and haemorrhage found at postmortem examination suggested disseminated intravascular coagulation in a patient who had died on induction of anaesthesia with thiopentone and suxamethonium (Wright et al 1989). The formation of colloid aggregates was thought to be the cause.

Management

1. Resuscitation
   a. Stop administration of the suspected drug and turn off all inhalational agents. There is no place for these in the treatment of anaphylactoid bronchoconstriction.
   b. Administer 100% oxygen and maintain the airway.
   c. Give adrenaline i.v., 50–100 μg (0.5–1 ml of 1:10 000 solution) for cardiovascular collapse. Repeat as required; 5–8 μg/kg may be needed.

   Adrenaline is the drug of first choice in anaphylactoid reactions and should be given early. The route of administration has been the subject of debate; there is evidence that any route (i.v., i.m., s.c., or via the airway) is better than none (Fisher 1992). In view of its brevity of action, in severe reactions an adrenaline infusion may be required subsequently. Additional to its cardiovascular effects, adrenaline inhibits further degranulation of mast cells and basophils, by increasing levels of intracellular AMP. In six out of seven fatal reactions, adrenaline had been given late in the treatment (Fisher 1986). For patients who are receiving beta adrenoceptor antagonists, the hypotension does not respond well to adrenaline (Laxenaire et al 1985), and isoprenaline may have to be given in higher than normal doses. Its effects require close monitoring, and caution is essential if halothane has been in use, since VF may be precipitated.

d. Give crystalloid or colloid i.v. 10 ml/kg rapidly to expand the vascular volume. Following analysis of treatment given to 203 cases, it was concluded that colloid was preferable (Fisher 1986). Whilst colloid is important for the replacement of intravascular losses, it should not be relied upon solely. It cannot be given sufficiently fast to counteract hypotension in severe cases, and does not have the additional benefits of adrenaline in stopping the progress of the reaction, and treating oedema and bronchospasm.

e. Manage the airway. In the presence of severe laryngeal oedema and failure of tracheal intubation, tracheostomy or cricothyroidotomy may be required.

f. Measure pH and arterial blood gases. Significant acidosis may occur and require treatment with sodium bicarbonate (Ljungstrom & Renck 1987).

2. Second line treatment
   a. Antihistamines
   Chlorpheniramine i.v. 10–20 mg can be given slowly over 1 minute. Antihistamines occupy cellular H_1-receptor sites and are competitive inhibitors of histamine binding. However, they only partially reverse anaphylactoid responses, because chemicals other than histamine are involved. Also, it may not be possible to achieve complete block of certain histamine receptor sites.

   b. Aminophylline
   A dose of 250–500 mg (5 mg/kg) given slowly over 20 minutes may be required if bronchospasm persists. Aminophylline prevents degradation of 3,5-cyclic AMP, and reduces the release of histamine and arachidonic acid metabolites. Its effect on respiratory function is not solely that of bronchodilatation

   c. Corticosteroids
   There is little place for corticosteroids in the immediate treatment, since their onset of action at a cellular level may take several hours. However, they may be used when the reaction does not quickly resolve and hypotension persists.

3. Investigations
   a. Immediate
      i. As soon as possible, blood samples should be taken for subsequent assessment of the mechanisms of the reaction.
      ii. Additional advice can be obtained from specialist centres.
      iii. Take two sets of venous blood samples in two EDTA tubes

as soon as possible after the start of the reaction. (EDTA stabilizes plasma complement proteins). Further duplicated samples should be taken at 3 hours, 6 hours, 12 hours and 24 hours.

iv. The first set should go to the local haematology department for Hb, WCC (total and differential), platelet count and haematocrit.

v. Plasma should be separated from the second set. This should be stored at – 20° to – 25°C until ready for dispatch (without ice) by first class post to an Immunology Laboratory, as soon as the 24-hour collection is complete. Alternatively, some hospitals may have their own facilities for performing complement and immunoglobulin levels.

vi. Detailed documentation should accompany the samples. This will include a full record of the incident, the agents and batch numbers, details of previous administration of these substances, and relevant history, such as allergies and atopy.

vii. Other similar, but more complex protocols exist, arising from recommendations by a joint European workshop in Nancy (Laxenaire et al 1983).

viii. Plasma histamine levels are increased but they are difficult to measure. Histamine has a short half-life and studies suggest that plasma levels should be measured 10 minutes to 1 hour after the reaction and samples should not be haemolyzed (Laroche et al 1991).

ix. Measurement of plasma tryptase concentrations has been reported (Laroche et al 1991). Plasma tryptase, a protease in mast cell granules, has a longer half life (approximately 2 hours) than histamine. Thus, increases may be documented 1–2 hours after the reaction, but in any case not more than 6 hours (Laroche et al 1991).

If these samples have been taken correctly, it should be possible to resolve the mechanism of the reaction. Should the results of immunological testing indicate an immune reaction (by changes in IgE and disappearance of basophils), then skin testing is appropriate.

b. Subsequent
   i. Skin testing with drugs at low dilutions 6 weeks after the initial reaction. A regimen for intradermal testing has been described, with recommendations on drug dilutions (Fisher 1984). This should preferably be undertaken by someone experienced in the technique. However, controversy exists over the indications for skin testing and its reliability if used indiscriminately. There is debate as to whether cross-reactivity, based on common quaternary or tertiary ammonium ions, occurs between muscle relaxants. Detection of serum IgE

antibodies which reacted with more than one relaxant has been reported (Baldo & Fisher 1983).

ii. The basophil degranulation test, or measurement of basophil histamine release (Withington et al 1987).

iii. RAST test. This radioallergosorbent test involves the use of commercially prepared antigen to detect drug-specific IgE antibodies. At present, the usefulness of this test is limited, both by the availability of preparations, and by the occurrence of false-positive and false-negative results. The suxamethonium test proved to be reliable, and the thiopentone test may be so (Assem 1990).

4. Communication of information

   a. Report the reaction to the Committee on Safety of Medicines via the Yellow Card system.

   b. Inform the patient of the results of investigations. Issue a warning card or suggest a Medic Alert bracelet.

   c. Document the results clearly in the patient's notes.

   d. Inform the patient's general practitioner.

5. Management of subsequent anaesthetics

   a. If the reaction is shown to be immune-mediated and the drug is identified by skin testing, then this drug should not be used again. In an immune-mediated reaction, there is no place for the use of i.v. test doses, since even minute amounts of a drug may prove fatal. Follow-up of patients after previous anaphylactic reactions showed that there was evidence of persistence of antibodies in the majority of patients (Fisher & Baldo 1992).

   b. If the reaction is non-specific, then future anaesthetics should be conducted using drugs considered to be relatively safe, whilst avoiding those known to produce reactions more readily. Currently, drugs with the fewest reports of serious problems are fentanyl, etomidate, vecuronium, and pancuronium. If closely repeated anaesthetics are required in the same patient, consideration should be given to varying the techniques and drugs used. All drugs should be given slowly.

   c. Pretreatment with H_1 and H_2 antagonists has been recommended by some authors. However, since other mediators are also involved, this does not guarantee freedom from a response.

6. Establishing a diagnosis following a fatal reaction. Since death from anaphylaxis is associated with only non-specific postmortem changes, there may be medicolegal pressures to establish a diagnosis. The use of sera, taken before or after death, has been described (Fisher et al 1991). Radioimmunoassay for drug-specific IgE antibodies was performed on blood taken for preoperative laboratory tests in two cases, and resulted in revision of the preliminary postmortem diagnosis to one of anaphylaxis.

BIBLIOGRAPHY

Assem E S K 1990 Anaphylactic anaesthetic reactions. The value of paper radioallergosorbent tests for IgE antibodies to muscle relaxants and thiopentone. Anaesthesia 45: 1032–1038

Baldo B, Fisher M McD 1983 Detection of serum IgE antibodies that react with alcuronium and tubocurarine after life-threatening reactions to muscle relaxants. Anaesthesia and Intensive Care 11: 194–197

Baldo B A 1986 Cross-reactions of neuromuscular blocking drugs and anaphylactoid reactions. Anaesthesia 41: 550–551

Berg E M, Fasting S, Sellevold O F M 1991 Serious complications with dextran-70 despite hapten prophylaxis. Is it best avoided prior to delivery? Anaesthesia 46: 1033–1035

Clarke R S J, Dundee J W, Garrett R T et al 1975 Adverse reactions to intravenous anaesthetics. A survey of 100 reports. British Journal of Anaesthesia 47: 575–585

Cullen M J, Singer M 1990 Severe anaphylactoid reaction to hydroxyethyl starch. Anaesthesia 45: 1041–1042

Fisher M M 1984 Intradermal testing after anaphylactoid reactions to anaesthetic drugs. Practical aspects of performance and interpretation. Anaesthesia and Intensive Care 12: 115–120

Fisher M McD 1986 Clinical observations on the pathophysiology and treatment of anaphylactic cardiovascular collapse. Anaesthesia and Intensive Care 14: 17–21

Fisher M McD, Baldo B A, Silbert B S 1991 Anaphylaxis during anesthesia: use of radioimmunoassay to determine etiology and drugs responsible in fatal cases. Anesthesiology 75: 1112–1115

Fisher M M, Baldo B A 1992 Persistence of allergy to anaesthetic drugs. Anaesthesia and Intensive Care 20: 143–146

Fisher M 1992 Treating anaphylaxis with sympathomimetic drugs. In severe anaphylaxis adrenaline by any route is better than none. British Medical Journal 305: 1107–1108

Gold M, Swartz J S, Braude B M et al 1991 Intraoperative anaphylaxis: an association with latex sensitivity. Journal of Allergy and Clinical Immunology 87: 662–666

Goldberg M 1984 Systemic reactions to intravascular contrast media. Anesthesiology 60: 46–56

Hirshman C A 1992 Latex anaphylaxis. Anesthesiology 77: 223–225

Incaudo G, Schatz M, Patterson R et al 1978 Administration of local anesthetics to patients with a history of prior adverse reaction. Journal of Allergy and Clinical Immunology 61: 339–345

Laroche D, Vergnaud M-C, Sillard B et al 1991 Biochemical markers of anaphylactoid reactions to drugs. Anesthesiology 75: 945–949

Laxenaire M-C, Moneret-Vautrin D A, Watkins J 1983 Diagnosis of the causes of anaphylactoid anaesthetic reactions. A report of the recommendations of the joint Anaesthetic and Immuno-allergological Workshop, Nancy, France: 19 March 1982. Anaesthesia 38: 147–148

Laxenaire M-C, Moneret-Vautrin D A, Vervloet D 1985 The French experience of anaphylactoid reactions. International Anesthesiology Clinics 23: 145–160

Laxenaire M-C, Mata-Bermejo E, Moneret-Vautrin D A et al 1992 Life-threatening anaphylactoid reactions to propofol (Diprivan). Anesthesiology 77: 275–280

de Leon-Casasola O A, Weiss A, Lema M J 1992 Anaphylaxis due to propofol. Anesthesiology 77: 384–386

Leynadier F, Pecquet C, Dry J 1989 Anaphylaxis to latex during surgery. Anaesthesia 44: 547–550

Levy J H 1986 Anaphylactic reactions in Anesthesia and Intensive Care. Butterworths, London

Ljungstrom K-G, Renck H 1987 Metabolic acidosis in dextran–induced anaphylactic rections. Acta Anaesthesiologica Scandinavica 31: 157–160

Ljungstrom K G, Renck H, Hedin H, Richter W, Wilholm B E 1988 Hapten inhibition and dextran anaphylaxis. Anaesthesia 43: 729–732

Nimmo W S 1990 Anaphylactic reactions associated with anaesthesia. Report of a working party. Association of Anaesthetists of Great Britain and Ireland, London

Ring J, Messmer K 1977 Incidence and severity of anaphylactoid reactions to colloid volume substitutes. Lancet i: 466–469

Sogn D D 1984 Penicillin allergy. Journal of Allergy and Clinical Immunology 74: 589–593

Stoelting R K 1983 Allergic reactions during anesthesia. Anesthesia and Analgesia 62: 341–356

Watkins J, Thornton J A, Clarke R S J 1979 Adverse reactions to i.v. agents. British Journal of Anaesthesia 51: 469

Watkins J 1983 Etomidate: an 'immunologically safe' anaesthetic agent. Anaesthesia 38 (suppl): 34–38

Watkins J 1985 Adverse anaesthetic reactions. An update from a proposed national reporting and advisory service. Anaesthesia 40: 797–800

Watkins J, Nimmo W S 1985 'Allergic' drug reactions during anaesthesia. Anaesthesia 40: 813–814

Watkins J 1987 Investigation of allergic and hypersensitivity reactions to anaesthetic agents. British Journal of Anaesthesia 59: 104–111

Weiss M E, Adkinson N F, Hirshman C A 1989 Evaluation of allergic drug reactions in the perioperative period. Anesthesiology 71: 483–486

Withington D E, Leung K B P, Bromley L et al 1987 Basophil histamine release. Anaesthesia 42: 850–854

Wright P J, Shortland J R, Stevens J D et al 1989 Fatal haemopathological consequences of general anaesthesia. British Journal of Anaesthesia 62: 104–107

ANGIONEUROTIC OEDEMA

A general term applied to the development of acute oedema in the subcutaneous or submucous tissues. Anaesthetic assistance may be sought during an attack, when oedema of the lips, tongue or larynx may cause respiratory problems. Angio-oedema may be secondary to release of histamine, or a number of other vasoactive substances such as the bradykinins, prostaglandins or leukotrienes. The development of oedema may be:

1. Part of a general anaphylactoid or anaphylactic reaction to a drug, bite, sting, or the ingestion of a substance (see this section: Anaphylactoid reactions).

2. A manifestation of hereditary angioneurotic oedema, a familial condition caused by a deficiency of C1 esterase inhibitor (see Section 1: Hereditary angioneurotic oedema).

3. A result of an acquired form of C1 esterase inhibitor deficiency which usually occurs in association with a B-lymphocyte malignancy (see Section 1: C1 esterase inhibitor deficiency).

4. A known side-effect of a drug. Recently, there have been a number of cases reported of angio-oedema, usually involving the tongue, floor of the mouth, epiglottis, and aryepiglottic folds, secondary to treatment with ACE inhibitors (Gannon & Eby 1990, Rodgers et al 1991). The onset can be early or delayed and may be associated with elevated serum bradykinin levels. In a profile of cases, 22% were considered to be life-threatening (Slater et al 1988) and fatalities have occurred. At present, it is impossible to predict which patients are likely to develop it.

Presentation

1. There may be a history of a predisposing factor. This can be ingestion of food or a drug, an infection, bite or sting, a family history of angioneurotic oedema, or a B-lymphocytic malignancy.
2. Oedema of subcutaneous tissue may occur on its own, or be accompanied by hypotension.
3. Angio-oedema of the tongue occurred 15 minutes after tracheal tube removal in a patient receiving ACE inhibitors (Kharasch 1992).

Management

1. If the angio-oedema is part of an anaphylactic or anaphylactoid reaction, see appropriate section.
   a. Give adrenaline i.v. or i.m., 0.1–0.5 mg, depending on the severity.
   b. If the condition is severe and involves the glottis, an airway should be established, either by intubation, cricothyroidotomy or tracheostomy.
   c. Second-line treatment includes i.v. fluids, chlorpheniramine i.v. 10–20 mg, and steroids.
2. Hereditary angio-oedema, or acquired C1 esterase inhibitor deficiency. These do not respond to adrenaline or antihistamines, but to replacement of the deficient inhibitor by either:
   a. An infusion of fresh frozen plasma. There is a risk that the additional presence of C2 and C4 may initially cause a deterioration, but this objection appears to be largely theoretical.
   b. Purified C1 esterase inhibitor can be obtained from Immuno Ltd, (Rye Lane, Dunton Green, Sevenoaks, Kent TN14 5HB. UK. Tel: 0732 458101).

BIBLIOGRAPHY

Gannon T H, Eby T L 1990 Angioedema from angiotensin converting inhibitors: a cause of upper airway obstruction. Laryngoscope 100: 1156–1160

Kharasch E D 1992 Angiotensin-converting enzyme inhibitor-induced angioedema associated with endotracheal intubation. Anesthesia and Analgesia 74: 602–604

Rodgers G K, Galos R S, Johnson J T 1991 Hereditary angioedema: case report and review of management. Otolaryngology, Head and Neck Surgery. 104: 394–398

Slater E E, Merrill D D, Guess H A et al 1988 Clinical profile of angioedema associated with angiotensin-converting-enzyme inhibitor. Journal of the American Medical Association 260: 967–970

AORTOCAVAL FISTULA

Rare, but most commonly the result of rupture of an atheromatous abdominal aortic aneurysm. Other causes are trauma (vehicular or gunshot) or following surgery for lumbar discectomy. Occasionally, the aneurysm may be syphilitic, or associated with a connective tissue disorder such as Marfan's or Ehlers-Danlos syndrome.

Aortocaval fistulae may present pre-, intra- or postoperatively. A significant portion of the cardiac output may flow into the inferior vena cava; this steal phenomenon reduces arterial pressure and flow to the coronary circulation. In these circumstances, vasopressors are ineffective and will simply increase the shunt of blood through the fistula.

If the aortocaval fistula is associated with an aneurysm, the signs and symptoms will depend upon the presence or absence of external rupture of the aneurysm, and whether or not there is compression of the inferior vena cava by the aneurysm (Phipps 1988). If compression exists, the increased venous pressure is directed distally; if it does not, the pressure is transmitted in both directions. The diagnosis is easily missed and even if it is made, the condition carries a mortality of up to 50%.

Presentation

1. Abdominal signs and symptoms. Lower abdominal or back pain radiating into the testes or legs. There is a pulsatile, tender mass, an abdominal bruit and thrill.
2. Cardiac signs. Inappropriate jugular venous distension and a hyperdynamic circulation, despite hypotension and shock. High output cardiac failure, hepatomegaly, and signs of myocardial insufficiency or decompensation.
3. Systemic signs. Shock and poor perfusion if the aortic aneurysm is ruptured. Anuria, increased blood urea, and renal failure may ensue.
4. Venous signs in the lower part of the body with truncal dusky cyanosis. Limb discolouration and oedema, haematuria, rectal bleeding, or priapism.
5. Paradoxical embolism from mural thrombus (Hecker & Lynch 1983).
6. Unexpected presentation during aortic aneurysm surgery (Bodenham 1990), sometimes with massive venous haemorrhage after cross clamping of the aorta.
7. Signs of blood loss during or after lumbar disc surgery.
8. In an analysis of seven cases without aortic rupture, the median Hb level was within normal limits but the PCV was low. This is because no blood has actually been lost from the vascular compartment. An absolute lymphocytopenia was also found, probably associated with cardiac failure (Burke & Jamieson 1983).
9. If invasive monitoring is undertaken, there is a high mixed venous oxygen saturation and a discrepancy between right and left heart pressures.

Diagnosis

Diagnosis can be made in a variety of ways. It may be demonstrated on CT scan, DVI, MRI, or an aortogram. A femoral catheter can be passed into the IVC to show increased pressure, oxygen content, or oxygen saturation. Fibreoptic oximetry was used to confirm the diagnosis in a patient following resection of an unruptured aneurysm (Khan et al 1992). An oximetric flotation catheter was passed up the femoral vein. A damped arterial waveform was identified, which was maximal at 15 cm, and increasing oxygen saturations were recorded as the fistula was approached.

Management

1. Attempts at resuscitation are fruitless and will simply overload the circulation. Surgery must be undertaken expeditiously. Preliminary control of the fistula with a balloon catheter has been reported, but this may risk venous damage or thrombosis (Ingoldby et al 1990).
2. Agents should be used which minimize changes in arterial pressure. Vasopressor drugs which will increase the shunt should be avoided. Although vasodilators may reduce blood flow through fistulae, they may worsen the haemodynamics.

BIBLIOGRAPHY

Bodenham A 1990 Anaesthetic hazards of aortocaval fistula. British Journal of Anaesthesia 65: 723–725
Burke A M, Jamieson G G 1983 Aorto-caval fistula associated with ruptured aortic aneurysm. British Journal of Surgery 70: 431–433
Editorial 1991 Aortocaval fistula. Lancet 338: 415–416
Ingoldby C J, Case W G, Primrose J N 1990 Aortocaval fistulas and the use of transvenous balloon tamponade. Annals of the Royal College of Surgeons of England 72: 335–338
Hecker B R, Lynch C 1983 Intraoperative diagnosis and treatment of massive pulmonary embolism complicating surgery of the abdominal aorta. British Journal of Anaesthesia 55: 689–691
Khan K J, Tsnag G M K, Fielding J W L et al 1992 Fibreoptic oximetry in the diagnosis of aortocaval fistula. A case study and review of the literature. Anaesthesia 47: 237–239
Phipps R F 1988 Spontaneous aortocaval fistulas. British Journal of Hospital Medicine 39: 306–307

ARRHYTHMIAS

The diagnosis and treatment of certain cardiac arrhythmias can on occasions be complex and may require cardiological expertise. At present, the Vaughan Williams classification of arrhythmias is being re-examined, and attempts are being made to classify arrhythmias and their therapy on the basis of molecular mechanisms, and identification of the parameters which are most vulnerable to treatment (Rosen & Schwartz 1991). Reference to this article is recommended for those who wish to understand why antiarrhythmics with such different electrophysiological effects may have similar clinical actions.

However, during anaesthesia a cardiologist may not be available immediately, therefore the anaesthetist needs a basic working knowledge of the common abnormalities and their likely causes. There is often a correctable surgical or anaesthetic precipitating factor, so the need for complex antiarrhythmic therapy in theatre is unusual, and potentially dangerous.

If the use of an antiarrhythmic is contemplated, careful thought should be given to possible interactions. In the presence of anaesthetic agents, or preoperative drug therapy, the i.v. administration of potent cardiac drugs can precipitate serious side-effects. The anaesthetist must be aware of these and be prepared to treat complications should they arise. However, on occasions, the urgent treatment of a life-threatening arrhythmia may be essential.

In general, if rhythm disturbances appear for the first time in the perioperative period, the initial search should be for a precipitating cause, associated with either the surgery or the anaesthesia.

Predisposing factors

1. General problems. Hypoxia, hypercarbia, metabolic and electrolyte abnormalities, light anaesthesia, or manoeuvres which stimulate the output of endogenous catecholamines.
2. Drug causes. Accidental overdose with local anaesthetics, absorption of adrenaline during surgical infiltration or pre-existing medication with drugs such as digoxin.
3. Pre-existing cardiac disease. Ischaemic heart disease, congenital heart disease, cardiomyopathy, WPW, mitral valve prolapse or the prolonged QT syndromes.
4. Rare causes. Diagnosed thyrotoxicosis, phaeochromocytoma, carcinoid syndrome, 'athlete's heart', malignant hyperthermia, and drug or solvent abuse.

Presentation

1. Atrial fibrillation
    Fast chaotic atrial activity, irregular fibrillation waves of 350–600/min best seen in V1. An irregular ventricular response of 100–200/min and varying AV conduction. Only if AF is associated with AV block is the ventricular rate regular. Causes include ischaemic, hypertensive and rheumatic heart disease, thyrotoxicosis, sick sinus syndrome, alcohol abuse, and atrial septal defect. Transient AF may occur during an acute toxic illness. Patients are at risk from systemic embolism.
2. Atrial flutter
    Regular atrial rate of 250–350/min with saw-toothed flutter waves, which are best seen in leads II, III, AVF and V1. There may be a 2:1 or 3:1 AV block. The ventricular rate is also regular, varying from 125–350/min. Causes are similar to those of AF.
3. Atrial tachycardia with AV block
    P waves are visible but often inverted in leads II, III and AVF. The

atrial rate is regular at 120–250/min, with a fixed or varying degree of AV block. Ventricular activity is usually normal, but occasionally bundle branch block occurs. Most often associated with digitalis toxicity, but can be due to ischaemic heart disease, cardiomyopathy or sick sinus syndrome.

4. Paroxysmal supraventricular tachycardia (AV nodal re-entrant tachycardia)
Ventricular rate regular at 130–250/min. No normal P waves seen, but inverted ones follow the QRS complex. Normal ventricular activity, sometimes with BBB. Often occurs in the absence of cardiac disease, but can be associated with WPW or Ebstein's anomaly. An abrupt onset of palpitations may cause hypotension, syncope, chest pain, polyuria and, if it persists, occasionally heart failure occurs.

5. Atrial ectopic beats
A premature, abnormal-shaped or sometimes inverted, P wave, best shown in V1. The QRS is usually normal and there is no compensatory pause after the ectopic. The next beat occurs exactly one sinus cycle after the ectopic, thus resetting the cycle. Atrial ectopics are frequently benign, but if they occur with heart disease, they may presage AF.

6. Ventricular ectopic beats
A widened bizarre-shaped QRS, without a preceding ectopic P wave. There is a short interval between a normal beat and the ectopic, followed by a compensatory pause before the next normal beat. If the ectopic falls early onto the T wave of the previous contraction (R on T), then ventricular tachycardia or fibrillation may be precipitated. Causes include ischaemic heart disease, cardiomyopathies, digoxin toxicity, and valvular disease. However, the cause may not be obvious.

7. Ventricular fibrillation
An incoordinated contraction of ventricular myocardial fibres associated with loss of consciousness and an absence of cardiac output.

8. Ventricular tachycardia (see also Torsade de pointes)
A rapid ventricular rhythm of 120–20/min, lasting for at least three or more beats, with abnormal-shaped complexes. Evidence of separate atrial activity occurring at a slower rate, with P-waves dissociated from ventricular complexes, helps to distinguish it from supraventricular tachycardia. If in doubt, the distance between any visible P waves may be shown to be mathematically related. R waves occur only in V1 and the QRS width is >140 ms.

Problems

1. The presenting arrhythmia may cause hypotension and a reduction in cardiac output. Ventricular fibrillation and occasionally ventricular tachycardia, cause circulatory arrest.

2. Myocardial ischaemia may be provoked.
3. If there is pre-existing left-sided heart disease, there may be cardiac decompensation and pulmonary oedema.
4. The arrhythmia may precipitate a more serious or fatal one, such as ventricular tachycardia or ventricular fibrillation.

Management (see also Prys-Roberts 1993)

1. Atrial fibrillation
   Digoxin slows the ventricular response rate to atrial activity.
   Verapamil will slow the ventricular rate. In AF of acute onset, direct current cardioversion will result in sinus rhythm. Amiodarone can also be used, but only after expert advice.
2. Atrial flutter
   Verapamil and digoxin may not control the ventricular rate.
   Cardioversion may be successful in reverting flutter to sinus rhythm.
   Atrial pacing can be tried.
3. Atrial tachycardia with AV block
   Stop digoxin, correct any hypokalaemia and give lignocaine i.v. 1 mg/kg. Should this fail, direct current cardioversion or rapid atrial pacing may be tried. If the patient is not already taking digoxin, treatment with this may control the ventricular rate.
4. Paroxysmal supraventricular tachycardia
   Carotid sinus massage or a Valsalva manoeuvre to increase vagal tone (for details see Autonomic dysfunction, Section 1). Pressure should be exerted by two fingers over the carotid artery at the level of the thyroid cartilage. Verapamil i.v. 5–10 mg is usually successful, but should not be given if the patient is taking beta blockers. Alternatively, adenosine by rapid i.v. injection of 3 mg over 2 seconds, if necessary followed by 6 mg after 1–2 minutes, then by 12 mg after a further 1–2 minutes. Digoxin, propranolol, quinidine, procainamide, disopyramide and DC cardioversion can also be used. (for treatment of Wolff-Parkinson–White syndrome, see Section 1).
5. Atrial ectopic beats
   No treatment is usually necessary, unless they are very frequent, or are associated with cardiac disease. In such a case digoxin may help.
6. Ventricular ectopic beats
   In general, no treatment is needed, unless the ectopic beats are frequent, or of the early R on T type. A lignocaine infusion or a beta bocker may then be needed.
7. Ventricular fibrillation
   A single precordial blow can be tried, otherwise defibrillation is required. If the heart is resistant to defibrillation then prior treatment with bretylium tosylate i.v. 400 mg may raise the fibrillation threshold.
8. Ventricular tachycardia (see also Torsade de pointes)
   The urgency and method of treatment depends upon the degree of

haemodynamic impairment. In the presence of shock, direct current cardioversion is required. When there is no significant hypotension, or for brief episodes of tachycardia, drug treatment can be used. Lignocaine is the first choice. If this fails, disopyramide, flecainide, amiodarone or mexiletine can be used.

BIBLIOGRAPHY
Prys-Roberts C 1993 Strange bedfellows: amiodarone, adenosine, and dopamine. Current Opinion in Anaesthesiology 6: 187–196
Rosen M R, Schwartz P J 1991 The 'Sicilian Gambit'. A new approach to the classification of antiarrhythmics drugs based on their actions on arrhythmogenic mechanisms. Task Force of the Working Group on Arrhythmias of the European Society of Cardiology. European Heart Journal 12: 1112–1131

BRONCHOSPASM
(see also Section 1, ASTHMA)

In a large study of anaesthesia, an incidence of bronchospasm of 0.17% was reported. It was usually triggered in susceptible patients by mechanical stimuli (Olsson 1987). Other causes include anaphylactoid reactions, inhalation of gastric contents, and rarely, certain hormone-secreting tumours. Recent emphasis has been placed on the inflammatory element of the disease, and preoperative treatment must be directed towards the control of this, in addition to the prevention of bronchospasm (Guidelines 1990).

Presentation

1. Predisposing factors to intraoperative bronchospasm include asthma, obstructive airways disease, respiratory infection, and tracheal intubation. It is most likely to occur during airway manipulation in a patient who has previously exhibited a capacity for airway constriction.
2. Bronchospasm may be one manifestation of an anaphylactoid reaction. Other signs such as flushing, urticaria, hypotension and tachycardia should be sought.
3. It may be due to silent aspiration of gastric contents. This may have been associated with intubation difficulties.
4. In rare hormone-secreting tumours, such as carcinoids, flushing and hypotension may additionally occur.

Management

1. Bronchospasm is frequently associated with intubation or airway manipulation in a patient with a history of bronchitis, asthma, or wheezing. Its incidence can be significantly reduced by preoperative preparation, with a combination of inhaled bronchodilators and anti-inflammatory agents with or without oral corticosteroids, the use of

i.v. lignocaine 1–1.5 mg/kg before induction, and avoidance of tracheal intubation during light anaesthesia (Kingston Hirshman 1984). If bronchospasm occurs in spite of these measures, an attempt should be made to deepen the anaesthetic, using an inhalational agent and oxygen. Halothane, enflurane and isoflurane are all effective at reversing antigen-induced bronchospasm. However, halothane sensitizes the heart to the effects of exogenous and endogenous catecholamines. In addition, it interacts with aminophylline to produce arrhythmias. Isoflurane, therefore, is probably the best choice.

2. A bronchodilator, such as a salbutamol infusion 5–20 μg/min or aminophylline 5 mg/kg over 10–15 minutes can be given.
3. If the clinical situation suggests an anaphylactoid reaction, or the bronchospasm is severe enough, then adrenaline 1–10 ml of 1:10 000 i.v. is the treatment of choice (see also Anaphylactoid reactions)
4. If there is evidence of gastric inhalation, appropriate treatment should be instituted (see Mendelson's syndrome).

BIBLIOGRAPHY

Cottm S, Eason J 1991 The intensive care management of acute asthma. In: Kaufman L (ed) Anaesthesia Review 8. Churchill Livingstone, Edinburgh

Guildelines for the management of asthma in adults 1990, Statement by the British Thoracic Society, Research Unit of the Royal College of Physicians, King's Fund Centre, National Asthma Campaign. I – Chronic persistent asthma in adults. British Medical Journal 301: 651–653. II – Acute severe asthma in adults. British Medical Journal 301: 797–800

Hirshman C A 1991 Perioperative management of the asthmatic patient. Canadian Journal of Anaesthesia 38: R26–32

Hirshman C A, Bergman N A 1990 Factors influencing intrapulmonary airway calibre during anaesthesia. British Journal of Anaesthesia 65: 30–42

Kingston H G G, Hirshman C A 1984 Perioperative management of the patient with asthma. Anesthesia and Analgesia 63: 844–855

Olsson G L 1987 Bronchospasm during anaesthesia. A computer-aided incidence study of 136 929 patients. Acta Anaesthesiologica Scandinavica 31: 244–252

CARCINOID SYNDROME
(see also Section 1)

Less than 25% of patients with carcinoid tumours have the carcinoid syndrome. The majority of those with the syndrome have liver metastases. Exceptions are the tumours whose venous drainage bypasses the liver. Flushing and hypertension have occurred during anaesthesia in the absence of metastases (Jones & Knight 1982), and these were attributed to release of hormones resulting from manipulation of the tumour itself. Preoperative features include flushing, diarrhoea, wheezing and valvular lesions of the heart. The patient may present unexpectedly, during anaesthesia or investigative procedures, with cardiovascular or respiratory complications from secretion of vasoactive chemical mediators such as serotonin, bradykinins, tachykinins, prostaglandins, or histamine.

Presentation

1. Release of hormones from carcinoid tissue may occur as a result of certain stimuli during anaesthesia, surgery, or investigative procedures. These include tracheal intubation, biopsy, tumour handling, hypotension, and catecholamine release.

2. Serotonin is known to cause hyperkinetic states of hypertension, tachycardia, and certain sorts of flushing. Bradykinins and tachykinins may produce hypotension, increased capillary permeability, oedema, flushing and bronchospasm. The tachykinins possibly play a rôle in fibrosis of the cardiac valves. Other vasoactive peptides such as histamine and prostaglandins may be involved, but their part in the syndrome has not as yet been elucidated.
3. Serious reactions during anaesthesia have included severe hypertension which responded to ketanserin (Casthely et al 1986) and to ketanserin and octreotide (Hughes & Hodkinson 1989), cardiovascular collapse which responded to a somatostatin analogue (Marsh et al 1987), severe bronchospasm (Miller et al 1980), and facial oedema (Lippmann & Cleveland 1973).
4. General anaesthesia is not always a requirement; a fatal acute crisis has occurred immediately after fine-needle liver biopsy of liver metastases (Bissonnette et al 1990) and a non-fatal one after bronchial biopsy (Sukamaran et al 1982), both of which procedures were performed under local anaesthesia.

Management

1. Somatostatin analogues, which inhibit the release of active mediators from carcinoid tumours, now form the basis of therapy for acute carcinoid crises, as well as being used in the preoperative management of patients with known carcinoid syndrome. The authors of several case reports have suggested that in the situation of an acute crisis it has been lifesaving. Octreotide (in doses of 25–100 μg i.v. diluted 1:1 with 0.9% saline) was used for intraoperative treatment during excision of metastatic carcinoid tumours (Roy et al 1987), and in one case in which cardiovascular collapse occurred the beneficial effect was dramatic (Marsh et al 1987).
2. A number of different antiserotoninergic drugs have been used in attempts to treat complications arising during anaesthesia. These include: methotrimeprazine i.v. 2.5 mg (Mason & Steane 1976), cyproheptadine i.v. 1 mg (Solares et al 1987), and ketanserin i.v. 10 mg over 3 minutes and an infusion of 3 mg/h (Fischler et al 1983, Casthely et al 1986). The choice is often governed by availability of the drug.

3. Antibradykinin drugs include aprotinin (infusion of 200 000 kiu in 250 ml saline) and corticosteroids. However, there have been variable reports of their effectiveness in treating complications, and with the advent of somatostatin analogues they probably have little rôle in the management of acute carcinoid crisis.

4. The rôle of histamine is uncertain. Flushing was successfully blocked in a patient with a gastric carcinoid using a combination of H1 and H2 antagonists (Roberts et al 1979).

5. It should be remembered that acute events during surgery are not always the result of tumour hormone secretion. Intractable hypotension without flushing or bronchospasm occurred following cardiopulmonary bypass in a patient undergoing valve replacement. This was thought to be of cardiac origin, and the cautious use of adrenaline resulted in an improvement in the patient's condition (Hamid & Harris 1992). Cardiovascular collapse after propofol and suxamethonium occurred in a patient who had an atypical carcinoid tumour (Bachelor & Conacher 1992) and the authors discussed the problems in differentiating a carcinoid crisis from an anaphylactoid reaction.

BIBLIOGRAPHY

Bachelor A M, Conacher I D 1992 Anaphylactoid or carcinoid? British Journal of Anaesthesia 69: 325–327

Bissonnette R T, Gibney R G, Berry B R et al 1990 Fatal carcinoid crisis after percutaneous fine-needle biopsy of hepatic metastasis: case report and review of the literature. Radiology 174: 751–752

Casthely P A, Jablons M, Griepp R B et al 1986 Ketanserin in the preoperative and intraoperative management of a patient with carcinoid tumour undergoing tricuspid valve replacement. Anesthesia and Analgesia 65: 809–811

Fischler M, Dentan M, Westerman M N et al 1983 Prophylactic use of ketanserin in a patient with carcinoid syndrome. British Journal of Anaesthesia 55: 920

Hamid S K, Harris D N F 1992 Hypotension following valve replacement surgery in carcinoid heart disease. Anaesthesia 47: 490–492

Hughes E W, Hodkinson B P 1989 Carcinoid syndrome: the combined use of ketanserin and octreotide in the management of an acute crisis during anaesthesia. Anaesthesia and Intensive Care 17: 367–370

Jones R M, Knight D 1982 Severe hypertension and flushing in a patient with a non-metastatic carcinoid tumour. Anaesthesia 37: 57–59

Lippmann M, Cleveland R J 1973 Anesthetic management of a carcinoid patient undergoing tricuspid valve replacement. Anesthesia and Analgesia 52: 768–771

Marsh H M, Martin J K, Kvols L K et al 1987 Carcinoid crisis during anesthesia: successful treatment with a somatostatin analogue. Anesthesiology 66: 89–91

Mason R A, Steane P A 1976 Carcinoid syndrome: its relevance to the anaesthetist. Anaesthesia 31: 228–242

Miller R, Boulukos P A, Warner R R P 1980 Failure of halothane and ketamine to alleviate carcinoid syndrome-induced bronchospasm during anesthesia. Anesthesia and Analgesia 59: 621–623

Roberts L J II, Marney S R Jr, Oates J A 1979 Blockade of the flush associated with metastatic gastric carcinoid by combined histamine H1 and H2 receptor antagonists. New England Journal of Medicine 300: 236–238

Roy R C, Carter R F, Wright P D 1987 Somatostatin, anaesthesia, and the carcinoid syndrome. Anaesthesia 42: 627–632

Solares G, Blanco E, Pulgar S et al 1987 Carcinoid syndrome and intravenous cyproheptadine. Anaesthesia 42: 989–992

Sukumaran M, Wilkinson Z S, Christianson L 1982 Acute carcinoid syndrome: a complication of flexible fibreoptic bronchoscopy. Annals of Thoracic Surgery 34: 702–705

CARDIAC TAMPONADE

Can occur when a pericardial effusion, or a collection of blood within the pericardial cavity, restricts cardiac filling during diastole, by the effect of external pressure. At the point at which the pericardium becomes no longer distensible, small volume increases result in a rapid increase in intrapericardial pressure. There is a fixed decreased diastolic volume of both ventricles. Induction of anaesthesia may cause cardiovascular collapse, although in the case of aortic dissection, problems are more likely to occur after relief of tamponade. Tamponade secondary to aortic dissection is frequently fatal and requires special management if the patient is to survive (Norman & Mycyk 1989).

Presentation

1. Causes include:
   a. Malignancy, which may present as a large mediastinal mass on CXR (Keon 1981) .
   b. Recent cardiac surgery (Skacel et al 1991).
   c. Blunt or sharp chest trauma, especially in the presence of sternal tenderness, chest bruising, or wedge fractures of the thoracic or upper lumbar vertebrae (Cyna et al 1990).
   d. Closed cardiac massage.
   e. Intracardiac injection.
   f. CVP or pacemaker insertion.
   g. Anticoagulant therapy.
   h. Aortic dissection (Bond et al 1987, Norman & Mycyk 1989)
   i. Systemic disease such as rheumatoid arthritis (Bellamy et al 1990).
2. In the presence of one of the predisposing factors, raised venous pressure, rapid low volume pulse, hypotension, and reflex peripheral arterial and venous vasoconstriction, may arouse suspicions of tamponade, particularly if respiratory distress is accentuated in the supine position or there is a history of 'fainting' attacks.
3. Pulsus paradoxis. Normally on inspiration there is a slight decrease in systolic pressure. In cardiac tamponade this decrease is accentuated, usually to >10 mmHg, and sometimes even to >20 mmHg. Pulsus paradoxus is easily detected by palpation, but may be detected by an auscultation method (Lake 1983). Using a sphygmomanometer, the cuff pressure should first be reduced until the sound is intermittent, then deflation continued until all beats are heard. The difference between the two pressures is then measured.

4. Tamponade presented as cardiovascular collapse on induction of anaesthesia in two children with mediastinal masses (Keon 1981, Halpern et al 1983). At postmortem, both were found to have lymphomas enveloping the heart and infiltrating the pericardium.

5. Cardiac tamponade may complicate aortic dissection (Bond et al 1987), in which case median sternotomy may relieve the tamponade. However, under these circumstances exsanguination may occur because of the sudden increase in arterial pressure in a patient under light anaesthesia (Norman & Mycyk 1989).

Diagnosis

1. Initially, the diagnosis must be thought of either on the history or on clinical examination.

2. If the fluid collection is >250 ml, the CXR may show an enlarged globular cardiac outline, the border of which may be straight or even convex. The right cardiophrenic angle is less than 90°. The lung fields are clear. Reduced cardiac pulsation may be detected on fluoroscopy. Echocardiography is the most reliable method of diagnosis (Horgan 1987).

3. In the case of aortic dissection, the diagnosis may also be made during angiography.

Management

1. Monitor direct arterial and central venous pressures.

2. Minimize factors which worsen the haemodynamic situation. These include:

   a. An increase in intrathoracic pressure. If artificial ventilation is already being undertaken, for example after cardiac surgery, then PEEP should be avoided since it further reduces cardiac output, especially at slow rates of ventilation (Mattila et al 1984).

   b. A low intravascular volume. Maintain the blood volume with i.v. fluids, according to the haemodynamic responses.

   c. A decreased myocardial contractility. Dopamine may have a favourable effect on haemodynamics, even in the presence of severe tamponade (Mattila et al 1984).

3. Relief of tamponade, except in patients with aortic dissection. If possible, needle pericardiocentesis, with or without catheter insertion, should be performed under local anaesthesia, with ECG and radiological screening and facilities for emergency thoracotomy. The subxiphoid approach can be used, in which the needle enters the angle between the xiphisternum and the left costal margin and is aimed towards the left shoulder. An alternative apical approach can be made through the fifth intercostal space on the left side (Lake 1983). In either case, a soft catheter should be introduced using a Seldinger wire technique, to avoid perforating the

myocardium as the fluid or blood is aspirated. Safety may be increased by use of a sterile ECG lead attached to the needle.

4. Sudden drainage of a chronic cardiac tamponade may cause acute haemodynamic changes and pulmonary oedema (Vandyke et al 1983, Downey et al 1991). This gradually resolves over 24 hours. In one patient a volume of 500 ml of pericardial fluid had been removed. Full haemodynamic monitoring was being undertaken and in both there was a sudden increase in pulmonary artery pressure after periocardiocentesis. In cardiac tamponade it is the right, rather than the left, ventricle that is compressed. After release of the tamponade there is sudden overload of the left ventricle while the PVR is still high. Acute dilatation of the thinner walled right ventricle and temporary mismatch between the outputs of the two ventricles were thought to have been responsible for the pulmonary oedema in these cases.

5. In the case of aortic dissection, the management may have to be modified. Norman and Mycyk (1989) described two patients: the first, who was managed conventionally, exsanguinated when sudden relief of tamponade restored cardiac output; in the second patient, who survived, femoro-femoral bypass was instituted before sternotomy, and propranolol and vasodilators were given to control systemic arterial pressure.

BIBLIOGRAPHY
Bellamy M C, Natarajan V, Lenz R J 1990 An unusual presentation of cardiac tamponade. Anaesthesia 45: 135–136
Bond D M, Milne B, Pym J et al 1987 Cardiac tamponade following anaesthetic induction for repair of ascending aorta dissection. Canadian Journal of Anaesthesia 34: 291–293
Cobbe S M 1980 Pericardial effusions. British Journal of Hospital Medicine 23: 250–255
Cyna A M, Rodgers R C, McFarlane H 1990 Hypotension due to unexpected cardiac tamponade. Anaesthesia 45: 140–142
Downey R J, Bessler M, Weissman C 1991 Acute pulmonary oedema following pericardiocentesis for chronic cardiac tamponade secondary to trauma. Critical Care Medicine 19: 1323–1325
Halpern S, Chatten J, Meadows A T et al 1983 Anterior mediastinal masses: anesthesia hazards and other problems. Journal of Pediatrics 102: 407–410
Horgan J H 1987 Cardiac tamponade. British Medical Journal 295: 563
Keon T P 1981 Death on induction of anesthesia for cervical node biopsy. Anesthesiology 55: 471–472
Lake C L 1983 Anesthesia and pericardial disease. Anesthesia and Analgesia 62: 431–443
Mattila I, Takkunen O, Mattila P et al 1984 Cardiac tamponade and different modes of ventilation. Acta Anaesthesiologica Scandinavica 28: 236–240
Norman P H, Mycyk T 1989 Dissection of ascending thoracic aorta complicated by cardiac tamponade. Canadian Journal of Anaesthesia 36: 470–472
Skacel M, Harrison G A, Verdi I S 1991 A case of isolated right atrial compression following cardiac surgery. Anaesthesia and Intensive Care 19: 114–115
Vandyke W H, Cure J, Chakko C S et al 1983 Pulmonary edema after

Section 2

Cardiac Tamponade

pericardiocentesis for cardiac tamponade. New England Journal of Medicine 309: 595–596

CENTRAL ANTICHLOLINERGIC SYNDROME

A term given to a syndrome of blockade of central cholinergic neurotransmission, probably involving muscarinic receptors, which produces a clinical picture similar to that of atropine intoxication. May be caused by any drug with anticholinergic actions, and sometimes following normal doses. It may occur after acute intoxication with drugs in association with sedation on the ITU or during acute withdrawal states.

The conscious level is usually impaired, or the patient may exhibit unpredictable behaviour. The syndrome has been described following a wide variety of drugs including atropine, hyoscine, benzodiazepines, phenothiazines, butyrophenones, cimetidine, opiates, tricyclic antidepressants and datura stramonium, and patients vary in their sensitivity to the anticholinergic effects. This is a difficult condition to diagnose with absolute certainty, since nothing is measurable. However, an improvement in conscious level after small doses of physostigmine, a cholinesterase inhibitor that crosses the blood-brain barrier and increases brain acetylcholine levels, is suggestive of the diagnosis.

Presentation

1. Restlessness, stupor, amnesia, hallucinations, respiratory depression or seizures. In the perioperative period, after premedication with morphine 10 mg and hyoscine 0.4 mg, a young man developed hyperthermia (39.3°C increasing to 42°C), tachycardia and confusion, which resolved immediately after administration of physostigmine 3 mg (Torline 1992). A young woman given glycopyrrolate 0.2 mg became hot and dry, and developed headache, tachycardia and widely dilated pupils; this responded to physostigmine 1 mg (Grum & Osborne 1991). This, however, is a surprising reaction, since glycopyrrolate has limited passage across the blood-brain barrier, and it was subsequently suggested that ranitidine might have potentiated the effects of glycopyrrolate (Wingard 1991). In one patient, dramatic extrapyramidal symptoms after anaesthesia responded to physostigmine; in this case fentanyl was thought to have been responsible, but naloxone had failed to reverse the symptoms (Dehring et al 1991).

2. After overdoses involving psychoactive drugs which have anticholinergic effects.

3. On the ITU after prolonged sedation.

Differential diagnosis

Disturbances of glucose and electrolytes, endocrine disorders (myxoedema and thyrotoxicosis), hypoxia and hypercarbia, neuropsychiatric disorders, stroke, neuroleptic malignant syndrome, and drug dependence.

Management

1. Increase the levels of acetylcholine in the brain by the use of a drug such as physostigmine, a cholinesterase inhibitor which crosses the blood-brain barrier, and which possesses minimal muscarinic effects. A small dose of physostigmine (increments of 0.5 mg) can be used as a diagnostic test and for treatment of the more serious symptoms (arrhythmias, seizures, autonomic side-effects or delirium) of drug overdose. In the case of overdoses, it should not be used simply to arouse the patient. Physostigmine has a relatively brief duration of action; most is eliminated within 2 hours, therefore repeated doses may be required.
2. Ensure oxygenation and respiratory adequacy. If in doubt, tracheal intubation should be performed and IPPV instituted.

BIBLIOGRAPHY
Dehring D J, Gupta B, Peruzzi W T 1991 Postoperative opisthotonos and torticollis after fentanyl, enflurane and nitrous oxide. Canadian Journal of Anaesthesia 38: 919–925
Grum D F, Osborne L R 1991 Central anticholinergic syndrome following glycopyrrolate. Anesthesiology 74: 191–193
SchneckH J, Rupreht J 1989 Central anticholinergic syndrome in anesthesia and intensive care. Acta Anaesthesiologica Belgica 40: 219–228
Torline R L 1992 Extreme hyperpyrexia associated with central anticholinergic syndrome. Anesthesiology 76: 470–471
Wingard D W 1991 Glycopyrrolate and the central anticholinergic syndrome. Anesthesiology 75: 1125–1126

DISSEMINATED INTRAVASCULAR COAGULATION
(DIC)

A general term for a derangement of the coagulation process, in which activation of the clotting system results in consumption of platelets and clotting factors, and subsequent overactivation of the fibrinolytic system (Preston 1982). Clinically evident DIC, which presents with bleeding, usually only occurs in critically ill patients.

The occurrence of DIC signals an underlying disease. Therefore the mortality in patients with severe DIC, reported to be as high as 6–85%, is usually a function of the precipitating condition, rather than the DIC itself.

The original stimulus may be tissue damage, toxin production or a drug reaction. Initially there may only be local fibrin deposition at the

Section 2

Disseminated
Intravascular
Coagulation (DIC)

sites of endothelial damage, or thromboplastin or phospholipid release. This can produce mild abnormalities in laboratory tests, without overt clinical problems. On rare occasions, and if the underlying cause is not removed, a pathological state of widespread fibrin deposition can develop, with consumption of clotting factors and secondary fibrinolysis. A wide variety of disease processes can be responsible for the initiating stimulus of a severe DIC, and treatment should be directed towards the correction of this in the first instance. Some doubt has been cast on the rôle and extent of microvascular thrombosis and organ infarction in the condition (Mant & King 1979). In their series of 47 patients with severe DIC the mortality was 85%. At autopsy, microvascular thrombosis and organ infarction was found to be uncommon. DIC was a contributing factor in only a quarter of the deaths, and was considered to be a preterminal event.

Presentation

1. Predisposing factors include Gram-negative septicaemia, malignancy, trauma, surgery, burns, amniotic fluid embolism, pregnancy-induced hypertension, placental abruption, transfusion reactions, intrauterine death, fat embolism, malignant hyperthermia, late midtrimester abortion (White et al 1983), drug interactions (Tackley & Tregaskis 1987), and bilateral cemented hip arthroplasty (Pugh 1991). Five adverse reactions to vascular grafts were associated with hypotension, erythema and DIC; in two, activation of the complement and kinin systems were demonstrated (Roizen et al 1989). Contact activation of plasma by the prosthetic graft was suspected. The three patients whose grafts were replaced survived, whereas the two in whom they were not, died. Evidence of DIC was found at postmortem following a fatal drug reaction (Wright et al 1989).

2. The clinical picture is that of widespread oozing from a variety of previously damaged sites, such as wounds, puncture sites, or incisions. More clinically serious bleeding may occur from the gastrointestinal tract, the lungs, or the uteroplacental bed.

3. The patient is often shocked and acidotic, and proceeds to develop hypoxaemia and respiratory distress.

4. Coagulation tests basically show evidence of consumption of coagulation factors and platelets, and increased fibrinolysis. The findings are therefore of prolonged one-stage prothrombin time, and partial thromboplastin time, and thrombin clotting time, and usually a thrombocytopenia. There is a reduced fibrinogen level and increased fibrin degradation products.

Management

1. Early involvement of a haematologist is essential.

2. The diagnosis and treatment, if possible, of the underlying cause, such as infection, retained placenta, etc.
3. The treatment of other abnormalities such as hypoxaemia, acidosis, electrolyte imbalance, and renal failure.
4. Correction of clinically significant abnormalities of haemostasis, as a temporizing measure, with the hope that the initial pathological process might be arrested. On a haematologist's advice, the following may be required:
    a. Fresh frozen plasma.
    b. Cryoprecipitate, especially if hypofibrinogenaemia is present.
    c. Platelet concentrates.
    Coagulation tests should be repeated to assess the progress of the condition and its treatment.
5. There is considerable dispute about the advisability of using heparin. In a detailed study of 47 patients, heparin was rarely found to be beneficial, and was often suspected to be the cause of severe bleeding (Mant & King 1979). Again, haematological advice is essential.

BIBLIOGRAPHY

McIntyre A J 1992 Blood transfusion and haemostatic management in the perioperative period. Canadian Journal of Anaesthesia 39: R101–107

Mant M J, King E G 1979 Severe, acute disseminated intravascular coagulation. American Journal of Medicine 67: 557–563

Preston F E 1982 Disseminated intravascular coagulation. British Journal of Hospital Medicine 28: 129–137

Pugh S C 1991 Disseminated intravascular coagulation complicating bilateral cemented total hip arthroplasty. Anaesthesia and Intensive Care 19: 106–108

Roizen M F, Rodgers G M, Valone F H et al 1989 Anaphylactoid reactions to vascular graft material presenting with vasodilatation and subsequent disseminated intravascular coagulation. Anesthesiology 71: 331–338

Tackley R M, Tregaskis B 1987 Fatal disseminated coagulation following a monoamine oxidase inhibitor/tricyclic interaction. Anaesthesia 42: 760–763

White P F, Coe V, Dworsky W A et al 1983 Disseminated intravascular coagulation following midtrimester abortions. Anesthesiology 58: 99–101

Wright P J, Shortland J R, Stevens J D et al 1989 Fatal haemopathological consequences of general anaesthesia. British Journal of Anaesthesia 62: 104–107

Section 2

Higher Oxides of
Nitrogen Poisoning

GLYCINE ABSORPTION
(SEE TURP SYNDROME)

HIGHER OXIDES OF NITROGEN POISONING

In 1967, an incident occurred in which a batch of nitrous oxide, contaminated with impurities, was used for anaesthesia in the south west of England (Clutton-Brock 1967). Three cases of poisoning occurred, and two of the patients died. The impurities included nitric oxide, nitrogen dioxide and carbon monoxide. A clinical picture of respiratory damage, similar to that produced by a severe acid aspiration syndrome, and circulatory failure, was produced.

Presentation

1. Intense cyanosis occurs from a combination of methaemoglobinaemia, which reduces the oxygen-carrying capacity of the blood, and arterial desaturation due to pulmonary oedema.
2. The onset of tachypnoea, tachycardia and respiratory distress.
3. Hypotension and circulatory failure. Nitrates and nitrites relax smooth muscle, causing vasodilatation.
4. Respiratory and metabolic acidosis. Nitrogen dioxide dissolves in body fluids to produce nitrous and nitric acids. Lactic acidosis also occurs due to tissue hypoxia.

Diagnosis

Crude testing: moistened starch iodide paper is placed in a large syringe, into which 15 ml of the suspect nitrous oxide and 5 ml oxygen is drawn. If contamination of >300 p.p.m. is present, then the starch iodide paper will turn blue within 10 minutes.

Management

1. Give 100% oxygen. IPPV and PEEP may be required.
2. Insert a radial artery cannula and take serial samples for blood gases, acid base status and oxygen content. Estimate the haemoglobin and methaemoglobin levels.
3. Attempt to convert the methaemoglobin using methylene blue 1–2 mg/kg. This should be titrated against blood levels of methaemoglobin, as excess methylene blue can in itself cause methaemoglobinaemia, as well as a haemolytic anaemia.
4. Hypotension should be treated with a vasopressor, such as methoxamine or noradrenaline, both of which have specific peripheral smooth muscle effects. Other cadiovascular support may be required.
5. Antibiotics, parenteral steroids and bronchodilators have been suggested for the pneumonitis (Prys-Roberts 1967).
6. In a severe case, specific treatment with dimercaprol has been recommended (Prys-Roberts 1967).

BIBLIOGRAPHY
Clutton-Brock J 1967 Two cases of poisoning by contamination of nitrous oxide with higher oxides of nitrogen. British Journal of Anaesthesia 39: 388–392
Prys-Roberts C 1967 Principles of treatment of poisoning by higher oxides of nitrogen. British Journal of Anaesthesia 39: 432–439

LOCAL ANAESTHETIC TOXICITY

Local anaesthetic toxicity may occur if the maximum safe dose is exceeded, or if transient high blood levels are achieved by accidental intravenous injection, or rapid absorption from an inflamed or vascular area. However, maximum safe doses are extremely difficult to define, since they depend upon a large number of factors including the concentration of the local anaesthetic and the site of administration (Scott 1986). When continuous infusion techniques are employed, additional factors, in particular those which affect the rate of absorption and drug metabolism and excretion, become important.

In adults, in the field of extradural analgesia, there has been increasing use of local anaesthetics combined with opiates. This decreases the amount of local anaesthetic required, which in turn reduces sympathetic vasodilatation, muscular paralysis, and the risk of systemic local anaesthetic toxicity. However, in the US in particular, techniques of continuous caudal or lumbar extradural analgesia in children using local anaesthetic alone, have become more popular. Sometimes these are continued for several days and there have been reports of seizures, and in some cases cardiotoxicity, occurring without warning (Berde 1992).

Now that bupivacaine is no longer recommended for intravenous regional anaesthesia, the safety of this technique seems to have increased. However, the lessons learned from the deaths which occurred in accident and emergency units, when the technique was used by non-anaesthetic staff, must not be forgotten (Heath 1982). In unfamiliar hands, accidental deflation of an automatic tourniquet can occur before the local anaesthetic has become fixed. Inappropriately high doses of the drug may be given. Standard resuscitation procedures in casualty may be inadequate.

Problems with bupivacaine, either injected accidentally into a vessel or given in doses at the upper limit of safety, continue to be reported. The acceptance that the two longer-acting local anaesthetics, bupivacaine and etidocaine, possess cardiotoxic properties (Albright 1979, Reiz & Nath 1986), and have a narrower margin between the CNS and cardiac effects, has led to a search for less toxic agents. Early studies on ropivacaine have been encouraging.

Presentation

1. Contributory factors include administration of a local anaesthetic in doses exceeding the toxic levels, the sudden release of a normal dose into the circulation, or the injection of small amounts into an artery supplying the brain. The arterial concentration, and in particular the proportion of blood going to the brain, is important in acute toxicity. Toxicity is therefore likely to be most serious in a hypovolaemic or shocked patient (Scott 1986). The threshold for CNS toxicity with lignocaine is a blood level of 5 μg/ml, which is close to the therapeutic dose for treatment of ventricular

extrasystoles. In the case of bupivacaine, reports of convulsions have occurred at blood concentrations ranging from 2–10 μg/ml (Berde 1992).

a. Interscalene block. Accidental injection into the vertebral artery during interscalene brachial plexus block resulted in transient, reversible 'locked-in' syndrome (Durrani & Winnie 1991), probably as a result of a direct toxic effect of mepivacaine and tetracaine on the brainstem. Unconsciousness, apnoea and hypotension occurred after interscalene injection of 20 ml 0.75% bupivacaine and adrenaline (Tuominen et al 1991); this was also attributed to accidental entry into the vertebral artery.

b. The presence of inhalation anaesthetics may prevent convulsions. Accidental i.v. injection of lignocaine 20 mg/kg instead of 2 mg/kg into an anaesthetized patient before tracheal intubation resulted in cardiovascular collapse and tachyarrhythmias. Convulsions only appeared 10 minutes later, after discontinuance of anaesthesia (Yukioka et al 1990). These had presumably been suppressed by anaesthesia.

c. Stellate ganglion block (Wulf et al 1991). In a study of plasma bupivacaine concentrations after stellate ganglion block, three out of 11 exceeded the threshold for CNS toxicity of 2 μg/ml. Maximum values were reached in 5 minutes. Intra-arterial injection may still occur even with negative aspiration tests.

d. Continuous intrapleural block with bupivacaine resulted in convulsions in a child 21 hours after the start (Agarwal et al 1992). The blood bupivacaine level was 5.6 μg/ml.

e. A continuous lumbar extradural technique in a child was associated with convulsions at 56 hours and a blood bupivacaine level of 5.4 μg/ml (Agarwal et al 1992).

f. Three cases of bupivacaine toxicity with continuous caudal anaesthesia have been reported (McCloskey et al 1992). A neonate developed bradycardia, hypotension and ventricular tachycardia, then seizures 2 hours later; an 8-year-old child had convulsions at 25 hours, and a 4-year-old had convulsions at 34 hours. The blood bupivacaine levels taken at the time of the events were 5.6 μg/ml, 6.6 μg/ml and 10.2 μg/ml respectively. In none of the children had warning signs of toxicity been detected.

2. Symptoms of toxicity include lightheadedness, circumoral tingling, numbness of the tongue, a metallic taste, tinnitus, visual disturbances, anxiety, and restlessness. Convulsions and apnoea may follow.

3. The combination of apnoea and convulsions leads to hypoxia, and respiratory and metabolic (in particular lactic) acidosis. With drugs such as lignocaine, it had been accepted that a wide margin existed between CNS and cardiovascular toxicity. However, the situation

with bupivacaine is different, in that following convulsions, hypotension, serious ventricular arrhythmias, or cardiac arrest have been reported. Resuscitation had proved to be particularly difficult or impossible (Albright 1979, Prentiss 1979). Successful resuscitation has however been reported on occasions (Davis & de Jong 1982, Mallampati et al 1984). In late pregnancy, the associated problems of aortocaval occlusion and supine resuscitation cannot be ignored.

4. In the cases of bupivacaine and etidocaine, the margin between CNS and cardiac toxicity is narrower than that with lignocaine. The cardiac effects of bupivacaine, of which depression of cardiac function is the main one, do not appear to be attributable solely to hypoxaemia and acidosis, and may in part be related to differences in myocardial uptake of the drug (Morishima et al 1985). An inhibition of energy metabolism has been suggested as one explanation for bupivacaine-induced cardiotoxicity (Eledjam et al 1989). Acute toxicity studies in fit volunteers suggested that ropivacaine caused less CNS symptoms and was at least 25% less toxic than bupivacaine (Scott et al 1989). Animal experiments also suggest that it is less cardiotoxic than bupivacaine (Reiz et al 1989).

5. All the clinical and experimental evidence indicates that pregnant patients are particularly vulnerable to bupivacaine toxicity (Morishima et al 1983). In addition, the combination of severe lactic acidosis and hypoxaemia during convulsions increases the resuscitation difficulties. However, severe ventricular arrhythmias occurred with bupivacaine in pregnant sheep, even when the acidosis was rapidly corrected (Marx 1984). A pregnancy-associated increase in availability of free bupivacaine, which does not occur with mepivacaine, has been suggested to account for the differences (Santos et al 1989). Recent studies with ropivacaine seem to indicate that ovine pregnancy, at least, is not associated with a gestation-related increase in the availability of free drug (Santos et al 1991).

6. Toxic doses of prilocaine (exceeding 600–900 mg or 8 mg/kg) are associated with methaemoglobinaemia. Probably due to a metabolite, orthotoluidine (Duncan & Kobrinsky 1983, Bardoczky et al 1990). After the administration of prilocaine, peak blood levels of methaemoglobin occur at 60–90 minutes, but may sometimes be delayed for 6 hours. Unexpectedly low oxygen saturation readings are recorded using a pulse oximeter, in the presence of a normal Pao_2 on a blood gas sample. The effect of methaemoglobin on the oximeter reading however is complex (Ralston et al 1991). For technical reasons, the presence of MetHb will bias the saturation reading towards 85%, so that either over- or underestimation may occur. Very high MetHb levels will therefore mask profound desaturation (Rieder et al 1989). A brachial plexus block with 35 ml 1.5% prilocaine resulted in a pulse oximetry reading of 88% despite a Pao_2 of 48.6 kPa (Bardoczky et al 1990). There have been several

reports of toxicity in infants and children given EMLA cream, a eutectic mixture of prilocaine and lignocaine (Duncan & Kobrinsky 1983, Jakobsen & Nilsson 1985, Frayling et al 1990).

7. Physical injury may sometimes result from local anaesthetic toxicity. Convulsions caused posterior dislocation of the shoulder in two cases, after bupivacaine injection during sacral and extradural anaesthesia respectively (Pagden et al 1986).

Prophylaxis

1. A benzodiazepine premedication may suppress some of the manifestations of local anaesthetic toxicity. In pigs however, although convulsions were suppressed, the threshold for cardiovascular toxicity was unaltered (Bernards et al 1989).

2. Do not exceed the maximum safe dose for the particular local anaesthetic being used. When continuous infusions are used for prolonged periods, this requires particular care. It has been suggested that doses for prolonged caudal or lumbar extradural analgesia should not exceed 0.2–0.4 mg/kg per h in infants and 0.2–0.75 mg/kg per h in children, and that caudal analgesia should be limited to 48 hours (Berde 1992).

3. With extradural anaesthesia, there is no foolproof method of ensuring that intravascular or subarachnoid injection has not occurred.

4. All injections should be given slowly and the dose should be fractionated. Where a large volume of local anaesthetic is required, a rate not exceeding 1 ml/s and the use of a 10-ml rather than a 30-ml syringe has been recommended (Moore & Bonica 1985).

5. Aspiration for blood and CSF should always be performed. However, a negative test does not ensure safe placement of the extradural catheter.

6. The use of a test dose is controversial. It has been suggested that for a single test dose of local anaesthetic to be of value in signalling the possibility of an i.v. or subarachnoid injection, it must contain a dose of local anaesthetic sufficient to rapidly produce evidence of spinal anaesthesia, plus 0.015 mg adrenaline. Thus, a systemic tachycardia will give warning of an accidental intravascular injection (Moore & Batra 1981). This means the use of 3 ml of local anaesthetic containing 1:200 000 adrenaline. However, there are doubts about the safety of using adrenaline in obstetric patients. It was found to decrease uterine blood flow in up to 50% of pregnant ewes, sometimes with signs of fetal distress (Hood et al 1986). The heart rate in the pregnant patient is so variable that its reliability has also been called into question (Leighton et al 1987). In addition, the use of adrenaline does not guarantee identity of inadvertent subarachnoid or i.v. injection (Blomberg et al 1991). The test dose will not consistently identify misplaced catheters. Failures to identify

subdural placement have been reported. Extensive sensory neural blockade followed injection of 13 ml lignocaine 1.5% into a catheter thought to be positioned extradurally (Crosby & Halpern 1989). Response to the test dose had not led to suspicions of misplacement.

7. The patient's mental state should be continuously assessed throughout the injection, usually by engaging her in active conversation. Each subsequent dose of local anaesthetic should be considered as if it were a test dose. Pulse oximetry should be used if the patient is sedated.
8. The immediate availability of resuscitation equipment and experienced personnel.

Management
The method by which the convulsions are controlled is arguable and depends partly upon the experience of the attendant.

1. Oxygenation and control of convulsions
   a. Suxamethonium will immediately control convulsions, and allow oxygen to be given by bag and mask ventilation, before tracheal intubation. During local anaesthetic-induced convulsions, severe hypoxaemia, hypercarbia and lactic acidosis occur simultaneously. Lactic acid production stops immediately after administration of suxamethonium. Rapid intubation is permitted, no myocardial depression occurs, and its effects wear off rapidly (Moore & Bonica 1985).
   b. Thiopentone 150–200 mg has been promoted as preferable to suxamethonium, on the grounds that the latter is unsafe unless given by someone capable of managing a paralyzed patient, and may result in an awake, intubated patient (Scott 1986).
   c. Diazepam 2–5 mg has also been recommended. However, it takes several minutes to become effective, during which time the convulsions continue and acidosis progresses. It is a long-acting drug, and has respiratory-depressant properties.
   d. Midazolam 2.5–5 mg.
2. Cardiac resuscitation
   May be required with a massive local anaesthetic overdose or if bupivacaine has been used. ECG monitoring may show bradycardia, asystole, ventricular tachycardia, or ventricular fibrillation.
   a. Cardiac massage must be sustained and effective, since bupivacaine remains longer in the myocardium than lignocaine.
   b. Hypoxaemia and acidosis must be corrected rapidly.
   c. If ventricular fibrillation occurs, defibrillation may not be successful on the first occasion.
   d. Ventricular tachycardia is treated. The ventricular tachycardia threshold has been tested during bupivacaine toxicity in dogs (Kasten & Martin 1985). Bretylium increased the ventricular tachycardia threshold, whereas lignocaine either was ineffective

or further decreased it. It was noted that bupivacaine prolonged the Q–T interval and produced a ventricular tachycardia similar to that of a torsade de pointes atypical VT. Bretylium tosylate 5–10 mg/kg (diluted to 10 mg/ml with 5% dextrose or 0.9% saline) can be given slowly over 8–10 minutes, with ECG observation.

e. Hypotension may need to be treated with inotropes or vasopressors.

f. Cardiopulmonary bypass was successful in treating bupivacaine-induced cardiac arrest (Long et al 1989).

BIBLIOGRAPHY

Agarwal R, Gutlove D P, Lockhart C H 1992 Seizures occurring in pediatric patients receiving continuous infusion of bupivacaine. Anesthesia and Analgesia 75: 284–286

Albright G A 1979 Cardiac arrest following regional anesthesia with etidocaine or bupivacaine. Anesthesiology 51: 285–287

Bardoczky G I, Wathieu M, D'Hollander A 1990 Prilocaine-induced methemoglobinemia evidenced by pulse oximetry. Acta Anaesthesiologica Scandinavica 34: 162–164

Berde C B 1992 Convulsions associated with pediatric regional anesthesia. Anesthesia and Analgesia 75: 164–166

Bernards C M, Carpenter R L, Rupp S M et al 1989 Effect of midazolam and diazepam premedication on central nervous system toxicity and cardiovascular toxicity of bupivacaine in pigs. Anesthesiology 70: 318–323

Blomberg R G, Löfström J B 1991 The test dose in regional anaesthesia. Acta Anaesthesiologica Scandinavica 35: 465–468

Crosby E T, Halpern S 1989 Failure of a lidocaine test dose to identify subdural placement of an epidural catheter. Canadian Journal of Anaesthesia 36: 445–447

Dawling S, Flanagan R J, Widdop B 1989 Fatal lignocaine poisoning: report of two cases and review of the literature. Human Toxicology 8: 389–392

Davis N L, de Jong R H 1982 Successful resuscitation following massive bupivacaine overdose. Anesthesia and Analgesia 61: 62–64

Duncan P, Kobrinsky N 1983 Prilocaine-induced methemoglobinemia in a newborn infant. Anesthesiology 59: 75–76

Durrani Z, Winnie A P 1991 Brainstem toxicity with reversible locked-in syndrome after intrascalene brachial plexus block. Anesthesia and Analgesia 72: 249–252

Eledjam J J, de la Coussaye J E Brugada J et al 1989 In vitro study on bupivacaine-induced depression of myocardial contractility. Anesthesia and Analgesia 69: 732–735

Frayling I M, Addison G M, Chattergee K, et al 1990 Methaemoglobinaemia in children treated with prilocaine-lignocaine cream. British Medical Journal 301: 153–154

Heath M 1982 Deaths after intravenous regional anaesthesia. British Medical Journal 285: 913–914

Hood D D, Dewan D M, James F M 1986 Maternal and fetal effects of epinephrine in gravid ewes. Anesthesiology 64: 610–613

Jakobson B, Nilsson A 1985 Methaemoglobinaemia associated with a prilocaine-lidocaine cream and trimethoprim-sulphamethazole. Acta Anaesthesiologica Scandinavica 29: 453–455

Kasten G W, Martin S T 1985 Bupivacaine cardiovascular toxicity. Comparison of treatment with bretylium and lignocaine. Anesthesia and Analgesia 64: 911–916.

Leighton B, Norris M, Sosis M et al 1987 Limitations of ephedrine as a marker of intravascular injection in laboring women. Anesthesiology 66: 688–691

Long W B, Rosenblum S, Grady I P 1989 Successful resuscitation of bupivacaine-induced cardiac arrest using cardiopulmonary bypass. Anesthesia and Analgesia 69: 403–406

McCloskey J J, Haun S E, Deshpande J K 1992 Bupivacaine toxicity secondary to continuous caudal epidural infusion in children. Anesthesia and Analgesia 75: 287–290

Mallampati S R, Liu P L, Knap R M 1984 Convulsions and ventricular tachycardia from bupivacaine with epinephrine: successful resuscitation. Anaesthesia and Analgesia 63: 856–859

Marx G F 1984 Cardiotoxicity of local anesthetics – the plot thickens. Anesthesiology 60: 3–5

Moore D C, Batra M S 1981 The components of an effective test dose prior to epidural block. Anesthesiology 55: 693–696

Moore D C, Bonica J J 1985 Convulsions and ventricular tachycardia from bupivacaine with epinephrine: successful resuscitation – congratulations. Anesthesia and Analgesia 64: 844–845

Moore D C, Crawford R D, Scurlock J E 1980 Severe hypoxia and acidosis following local anesthetic-induced convulsions. Anesthesiology 53: 259–260

Morishima H O, Pedersen H, Finster M et al 1983 Is bupivacaine more cardiotoxic than lignocaine? Anesthesiology 59S: A409

Morishima H O, Pedersen H, Finster M et al 1985 Bupivacaine toxicity in pregnant and non-pregnant ewes. Anesthesiology 63: 134–139

Pagden D, Halaburt A S, Wirpszor R et al 1986 Posterior dislocation of the shoulder complicating regional anesthesia. Anesthesia and Analgesia 65: 1063–1065

Prentiss J E 1979 Cardiac arrest following regional anesthesia with etidocaine or bupivacaine. Anesthesioloy 51: 285–287

Ralston A C, Webb R K, Runciman W B 1991 Potential errors in pulse oximetry. III. Effects of interference, dyes, dyshaemoglobins and other pigments. Anaesthesia 46: 291–295

Reider H U, Frei F J, Zbinden A M, Thomson D A 1989 Pulse oximetry in methaemolobinaemia. Anaesthesia 44: 326–327

Reiz S, Nath S 1986 Cardiotoxicity of local anaesthetic agents. British Journal of Anaesthesia 58: 736–746

Reiz S, Haggmark S, Johansson G et al 1989 Cardiotoxicity of ropivacaine – a new amide local anaesthetic agent. Acta Anaesthesiologica Scandinavica 33: 93–98

Santos A C, Pedersen H, Harmon T W et al 1989 Does pregnancy alter the systemic toxicity of local anesthetic? Anesthesiology 70: 991–995

Santos A C, Arthur G R, Pedersen H et al 1991 Systemic toxicity of ropivacaine during ovine pregnancy. Anesthesiology 75: 137–141

Scott D B 1986 Toxic effects of local anaesthetic agents on the central nervous system. British Journal of Anaesthesia 58: 732–735

Scott D B, Lee A, Fagan D et al 1989 Acute toxicity of ropivacaine compared with that of bupivacaine. Anesthesia and Analgesia 69: 563–569

Tuominen M K, Pere P, Rosenber P H 1991 Unintentional arterial catheterization and bupivacaine toxicity associated with continuous interscalene brachial plexus block. Anesthesiology 75: 356–358

Yukioka H, Hayashi I M, Fujimori M 1990 Lidocaine toxicity during general anesthesia. Anesthesia and Analgesia 71: 200–212

Wulf H, Maier C, Schele H-A et al 1991 Plasma concentrations of bupivacaine after stellate ganglion blockade. Anesthesia and Analgesia 72: 546–548

Section 2

Malignant
Hyperthermia

MALIGNANT HYPERTHERMIA
(see also Section 1)

Nowadays, a fulminant malignant hyperthermia (MH) crisis – the commonest form of presentation in the early days – will be unusual. The widespread use of monitoring means that signs are likely to be detected at an earlier stage. However, many of these signs are non-specific, so that the problem arises as to how seriously they should be taken, particularly since a decreasing percentage of the patients referred to the Leeds Unit for investigation subsequently turn out to be MHS (Ellis et al 1990).

The anaesthetist must be aware, therefore, of the spectrum of signs associated with MH. Should the possibility of MH be entertained during surgery, certain observations and investigations must be undertaken at the time of the event. There is nothing worse for a family, (or for subsequent anaesthetists), to be told that an individual could possibly be MH susceptible, when no effort was made at the time to seek evidence of muscle involvement.

Presentation

1. The clinical signs and symptoms of MH can be broadly divided into two;
   a. Signs of metabolic stimulation.
   b. Signs of abnormal muscle activity.
      However, it should be remembered that there are conditions other than MH that can cause either or both, of these signs. A combination of metabolic and muscle signs under anaesthesia may occur with Duchenne or Becker muscular dystrophy, spinal muscle atrophy, myotonia congenita, McArdle's disease, and carnitine palmitoyl transferase deficiency.
2. Signs of metabolic stimulation
   a. Hypercarbia. Tachypnoea occurs in a spontaneously breathing patient, whilst in the paralyzed patient there is an apparently increased requirement for neuromuscular blockers. Both states initially result from stimulation of respiration by an increasing alveolar CO_2. If a capnograph is being used, an increase in ET_{CO_2} in a patient receiving IPPV may be the earliest sign of MH (Thomas et al 1987).
   b. Metabolic acidosis. In early reports of fulminating cases, an arterial pH of less than 7.0 was not uncommon. Severe acidosis may have been responsible for the cases in which sudden death occurred unexpectedly in the operating theatre.
   c. Arrhythmias.
   d. Increase in core temperature; this is a late sign.
   e. Hypoxaemia. In the later stages of an MH crisis, cyanosis occurs secondary to the combination of a massive increase in oxygen consumption, and ventilation perfusion defects.
3. Signs of abnormal muscle activity
   a. Failure of the jaw to relax after suxamethonium. An increase in tone in the masseter muscle is a normal response to suxamethonium and in some patients the tension developed may be very marked (Leary & Ellis 1990, Saddler et al 1990). However, it may also be an early sign of MH. Susceptibility to MH was found in about half of a series of 77 patients who developed masseter muscle rigidity (MMR) (Rosenberg & Fletcher

1986). In view of this, it was suggested that any patient who developed MMR after suxamethonium should be assumed to be MH susceptible and anaesthesia terminated. However, a 1% incidence of MMR was found in children receiving halothane and suxamethonium (Carroll 1987) and it soon became apparent that MMR, although occurring frequently in MH, was not exclusive to it (see masseter muscle rigidity).

b. Rigidity of certain, but not necessarily all, groups of muscles. Although a non-rigid group has been described, it is not yet known whether this is a different biochemical process, or an earlier stage of the same process. A contracture of the muscle actually takes place and, if the process is not aborted, oedema of the muscle and subsequently ischaemia can develop.

c. Hyperkalaemia, with or without cardiac arrest; potassium may be released in large quantities, usually after the use of suxamethonium. However, once again, this complication is not exclusive to MH, and can occur with other muscle diseases, particularly the muscular dystrophies. In addition, hyperkalaemia may occur even when suxamethonium has not been given. Hyperkalaemia and cardiac arrest has been reported after inhalation anaesthesia alone in both Duchenne (Chalkiadis & Branch 1990) and Becker muscular dystrophies (Bush & Dubovitz 1991).

d. Myoglobin and potassium may be released in large quantities, sometimes resulting in massive myoglobinuria and renal failure. Myoglobin may be detected in the blood and urine almost immediately, but its transient appearance means that its presence is frequently missed.

e. A greatly elevated serum CK level; this may be in excess of 100 000 iu/l. Unlike myoglobin, which can be detected almost immediately and is transient in its appearance, the serum CK takes several hours to increase. Often, the maximum blood concentration will not be seen until the following day, and levels will remain elevated for several days after this.

4. Later complications:
   a. Disseminated intravascular coagulation may occur in advanced cases, possibly secondary to thromboplastin release.
   b. Cerebral and pulmonary oedema may develop.

Management

1. Nowadays, the increased quality of monitoring means that the fulminant case is rarely seen. However, it also means that there is an increase in the number of aborted or doubtful cases. Since the early signs of MH are non-specific, it is the responsibility of the anaesthetist, should MH be suspected, to gain as much information as possible at the time of the event.

2. What should be done if intraoperative signs occur which are not specific to MH, and are not life-threatening, but raise the suspicion of MH? Under these circumstances, Ellis et al (1990) recommended that attention is paid to the following features:
   a. Good record keeping of the time sequence of clinical events:
      i. MMR (duration and degree).
      ii. Presence or absence of generalized rigidity.
      iii. Arrhythmias.
      iv. Tachypnoea with signs of CO_2 production.
      v. Cyanosis.
      vi. Increase in core temperature.
   b. Laboratory tests:
      i. Arterial blood gases.
      ii. Serum potassium.
      iii. Initial, 12- and 24-hour serum CK levels. Serial CK levels taken under these circumstances are very important. Whilst a random CK level is normally of little diagnostic help in MH, if an anaesthetic has been given which is associated with evidence of hypermetabolism, the serum CK may be of considerable value. If the CK is very high, it is likely that the event that occurred was of significance. It may not necessarily be MH, but could be associated with one or another of a variety of myopathies, as mentioned above.
      iv. Evidence of myoglobinuria.
3. If a tentative intraoperative diagnosis of MH is made, the treatment required will depend upon the severity of the reaction at the time of diagnosis. The patient's susceptibility, the promptness of the diagnosis and hence the dose of the triggering agent received, are important factors (Gronert 1980). With a short exposure and a rapid diagnosis the syndrome will be aborted by the first measure in (4.) alone.
4. Treatment of established MH
   a. Stop the use of all MH trigger agents. Terminate surgery if possible, or change to a non-triggering anaesthetic. Observe ECG and capnograph. Estimate blood gases.
   b. Delegate one person to prepare dantrolene sodium, 1 mg/kg.
   c. Record core temperature, pulse rate and blood pressure every 5 minutes.
   d. Hypercarbia should be treated with hyperventilation.
   e. Treat acidosis with sodium bicarbonate 2–4 mmol/kg and oxygenation maintained.
   f. Send venous samples for electrolytes, calcium and CK.
   g. Give dantrolene sodium i.v. 1 mg/kg and repeat, up to 10 mg/kg.
   h. If the syndrome is severe, treat symptomatically. Institute cooling and treat hyperkalaemia if necessary.

i. Save the first urine sample for myoglobin estimation. Measure urine output. If there is obvious myoglobinuria, give i.v. fluids, with mannitol or frusemide to reduce the possibility of renal failure.

j. The use of steroids is debatable. They may be indicated in the severe case, particularly if there is cerebral oedema.

k. Repeat the serum CK at 24 hours.

l. Treat DIC if necessary.

m. The half-life of dantrolene is only 5 hours, therefore if retriggering occurs in the first 24 hours it may need to be repeated.

BIBLIOGRAPHY

Bush A, Dubowitz V 1991 Fatal rhabdomyolysis complicating general anaesthesia in a child with Becker muscular dystrophy. Neuromuscular Disorders 1: 204–210

Carroll J B 1987 Increased incidence of masseter spasm in children with strabismus anaesthetised with halothane and succinyl choline. Anesthesiology 67: 559–561

Chalkiadis G A, Branch K G 1990 Cardiac arrest after isoflurane anaesthesia in a patient with Duchenne's muscular dystrophy. Anaesthesia 45: 22–25

Ellis F R, Halsall P J 1984 Suxamethonium spasm. British Journal Anaesthesia 56: 381–384

Ellis F R, Halsall P J, Christian A S 1990 Clinical presentation of suspected malignant hyperthermia during anaesthesia in 402 probands. Anaesthesia 45: 838–841

Gronert G A 1980 Malignant hyperthermia. Anesthesiology 53: 395–423

Leary N P, Ellis F R 1990 Masseteric muscle spasm as a normal response to suxamethonium. British Journal of Anaesthesia 64: 488–492

Rosenberg H, Fletcher J E 1986 Masseter muscle rigidity and malignant hyperthermia susceptibility. Anaesthesia and Analgesia 65: 161–164

Saddler J M, Bevan J C, Plumley M H et al 1990 Jaw muscle tension after succinylcholine in children undergoing strabismus surgery. Canadian Journal of Anaesthesia 37: 21–25

Thomas D W, Dev V J, Whitehead M J 1987 Malignant hyperpyrexia and isoflurane. British Journal of Anaesthesia 59: 1196–1198

Section 2

Masseter Muscle
Rigidity (MMR)

MASSETER MUSCLE RIGIDITY
(MMR)

Masseter muscle rigidity is a clinical diagnosis; it has been defined as jaw tightness to a degree which interferes with tracheal intubation and occurs despite usually adequate doses of suxamethonium (Saddler et al 1990). Since MMR occurs in 50% patients who are MHS, it was assumed to be an exclusive sign presaging an MH crisis. However, it is now known that an increase in masseter muscle tone may be a normal response to suxamethonium.

In a study of 50 healthy patients, the majority showed myotonia which lasted for less than 100 seconds. (Leary & Ellis 1990). In about 40%, the maximum tone was greater than 500 g, and in 1% it was greater than 1 kg. On occasions, the rigidity can last several minutes, and may be such that the jaw can barely be opened. Intubation may temporarily be impossible, although ventilation on a mask is usually feasible. A similar situation was found in studies on eight patients having squint surgery (Saddler et al 1990). At the same time, an increase in tension, but to a lesser degree, was found in the adductor pollicis muscles. This hypertonus is more likely to occur in young patients, particularly if a volatile agent has been given before the suxamethonium. Most cases have a minor degree of rhabdomyolysis, as evidenced by an increase in serum CK level. The masseter spasm may be associated with ventricular arrhythmias and myoglobinuria.

Thus, although MMR is certainly one sign of MH, and features in a high proportion of patients subsequently found to be MHS, transient MMR commonly occurs in normal patients and is pronounced in about 1% of the population. As a result, the significance of MMR, and its subsequent management if it occurs, has been a controversial subject.

Previously it was assumed that, since a proportion of cases would be associated with MH, anaesthesia should be stopped, or the drugs used should be changed to non-triggering agents. The masseter muscle is known to contain a unique form of myosin. This may explain the localization of the spasm to the jaw muscles (Fletcher 1987).

The controversies

1. MMR as normal response to suxamethonium
   Two studies claim that masseter spasm occurs in as many as 1% of children after a halothane induction folowed by suxamethonium administration (Schwartz et al 1984, Carroll 1987). Littleford et al (1991), in a study of 42 000 anaesthetics over a 10-year period, found that it occurred in 0.3% of inhalational anaesthetics in which suxamethonium was given. They found no morbidity or mortality in 57 children who developed isolated MMR, and suggested that anaesthesia could continue in the presence of this sign. However, this is controversial. The discrepancy between these figures, and the 50% incidence of MHS with MMR, is difficult to explain. A difference in definition of MMR may contribute (Rosenberg 1987). MMR is a situation in which the jaw can hardly be opened, even with considerable effort by the anaesthetist. This situation, which is rare, must be differentiated from a mere increase in muscle tone, which is common among children (van der Spek et al 1987) and passes off fairly rapidly. In addition, those referred to a centre for screening are likely to have been a selected group of patients who had additional signs of MH.

2. MMR associated with malignant hyperthermia
   The exact percentage of patients with MMR found subsequently to be MHS varies with the studies reported. One claimed an incidence of 100% in 15 patients (Schwartz et al 1984). However, the diagnosis of MH was made on the basis of a sarcoplasmic reticulum calcium uptake test. This has not been accepted as diagnostic by a number of workers in the field, and an incidence as high as this has therefore been disputed (Ellis & Halsall 1986).

Using caffeine and halothane contracture tests, other workers have found the incidence to be between 40% and 60%. Nearly 50% of 77 patients who had developed MMR after suxamethonium were found to be MHS using these tests (Rosenberg & Fletcher 1986). Another study reported four out of six boys with isolated MMR to be MHS (Flewellen & Nelson 1984).

Muscle rigidity, not necessarily of the masseter alone, is a common feature in MH episodes. It appeared in about 80% of MHS patients studied by Britt and Kalow (1970). In 31 out of 75 patients, MH episodes with muscle rigidity occurred after the use of suxamethonium. In another study of 147 patients found to be MHS after referral for investigation (Ellis & Halsall 1984), 65% had responded to suxamethonium with muscle spasm. In 5% of these MHS patients, the suxamethonium spasm was the only sign of MHS.

3. MMR not associated with malignant hyperthermia but with other muscle disorders.

Further investigations of the group of patients with MMR who were shown not to be susceptible to malignant hyperthermia, revealed a small number who had some other myopathy. These included Duchenne and Becker muscle dystrophies and myotonia congenita. The remainder must be assumed to have had an abnormal reaction to suxamethonium.

Presentation

1. Administration of suxamethonium is associated with a degree of rigidity of the jaw muscles such that the patient's mouth can hardly be opened. It may last anywhere between 90 seconds and several minutes. Sometimes it results in intubation difficulty.
2. Peripheral muscles are usually flaccid, and there is no response to nerve stimulation.
3. The episode may be accompanied by tachycardia or ventricular arrhythmias.
4. Pyrexia can develop subsequently or the patient may be apyrexial.
5. Myoglobinuria may occur and the serum CK level may be increased within the first 24 hours after anaesthesia.
6. Muscle pains, stiffness, and occasionally weakness may last for several days.
7. A small number of patients may proceed to MH, although this may not be immediately clinically obvious.

Management

1. If a patient develops increased masseter muscle tone after suxamethonium, it should be remembered that in the majority of cases this is a normal reaction. However, rarely, it is an early sign of

MH and this should be borne in mind. At present there is no way of distinguishing the types of MMR, except that the 'normal' myotonia usually returns to baseline after 60–90 seconds (Leary & Ellis 1990) and the patient's lungs can be ventilated with oxygen by mask during this time. Anaesthetists should be wary if the rigidity is particularly severe or prolonged.

2. At the time of writing, the profession is divided as to whether or not surgery should be continued if masseter spasm occurs, and a vigorous correspondence on the matter continues (Rosenberg & Shutack 1991, van der Spek 1991). If the surgery is elective, postponement has been advised on the grounds that, even in the absence of an overt MH episode, significant rhabdomyolysis may occur (Rosenberg 1987). Other authors have suggested that surgery should be continued with close metabolic and acid base monitoring, and only stopped if there is an abnormal metabolic response (Gronert 1988) and other signs of muscular involvement. Undoubtedly, an experienced anaesthetist should be consulted.

3. In all cases, heart rate, core temperature, end-tidal CO_2, blood gas tensions, and serum potassium level must be measured. At the same time blood should be taken for serum CK and the urine examined for myoglobin.

4. If there is no evidence of hypermetabolism, it is safe to continue surgery.

5. If there is evidence of hypermetabolism, if the MMR is very severe and prolonged, or if the patient has generalized rigidity, MH should be suspected and elective surgery stopped. If surgery is urgent, a non-triggering technique MH (N_2O/narcotic analgesic/non-depolarizing relaxant) should be used, and CO_2 temperature and biochemistry closely monitored. If necessary, dantrolene 2.5 mg/kg may be administered.

6. Postoperative serum CK levels should always be measured. In all patients with MMR, the serum CK is likely to be elevated to some degree. However, in one study, levels above 20 000 u occurred only in patients found to be MHS, or in patients with muscle dystrophy (Rosenberg & Fletcher 1986). The peak serum CK level does not usually occur until the following day.

7. If there is frank myoglobinuria, intravenous fluids and an osmotic diuretic should be given. Renal function requires monitoring. Myoglobin is present in the blood and urine almost immediately, and its appearance may be missed.

8. If any patient shows evidence of both hypermetabolism and muscle signs they should subsequently be referred for investigation of possible MH. If there is doubt, discussion with an investigating unit is suggested. Ellis et al (1990) have outlined the important information required to elucidate the diagnosis of an event during

anaesthesia suspected of being MH. This requires good record keeping of the clinical events, including:

a. Duration and degree of MMR.

b. Generalized rigidity.

c. Arrhythmias.

d. Tachypnoea and/or signs of increased CO_2 production.

e. Cyanosis

f. Increase in core temperature.

g. Arterial blood gases.

h. Serum potassium.

i. Initial, 12- and 24-hour serum CK level.

j. Evidence of myoglobinuria.

9. The results of investigations should be clearly conveyed to the patients and recorded in the notes.

Section 2

**Masseter Muscle
Rigidity (MMR)**

BIBLIOGRAPHY

Britt B A, Kalow W 1970 Malignant hyperthermia: a statistical review. Canadian Anaesthetists' Society Journal 17: 293–315

Carroll J B 1987 Increased incidence of masseter spasm in children with strabismus anesthetised with halothane and succinyl choline. Anesthesiology 67: 559–561

Christian A S, Ellis F R, Halsall P J 1989 Is there a relationship between masseteric muscle spasm and malignant hyperpyrexia? British Journal of Anaesthesia 62: 540–544

Ellis F R, Halsall P J 1984 Suxamethonium spasm. A differential diagnostic conundrum. British Journal of Anaesthesia 56: 381–384

Ellis F R, Halsall P J 1986 Improper diagnostic test may account for high incidence of malignant hyperthermia associated with masseter spasm. Anesthesiology 64: 291

Ellis F R, Halsall P J, Christian A S 1990 Clinical presentation of suspected malignant hyperthermia during anaesthesia in 402 probands. Anaesthesia 45: 838–841

Fletcher R 1987 4th International Hyperpyrexia Workshop. Report of a meeting. Anaesthesia 42: 206

Flewellen E H, Nelson T E 1982 Masseter spasm induced by succinylcholine in children: contracture testing for malignant hyperthermia: report of 6 cases. Canadian Anaesthetists' Society Journal 29: 42–49

Flewellen E H, Nelson T E 1984 Halothane-succinylcholine induced masseter spasm: indicative of malignant hyperthermia susceptibility? Anesthesia and Analgesia 63: 693–697

Gronert G A 1988 Management of patients in whom trismus occurs following succinylcholine. Anesthesiology 68: 653–654

Leary N P, Ellis F R 1990 Masseteric muscle spasm as a normal response to suxamethonium. British Journal of Anaesthesia 64: 488–492

Littleford J A, Patel L R, Bose D et al 1991 Masseter muscle spasm in children: implications of continuing the triggering anesthetic. Anesthesia and Analgesia 72: 151–160

Rosenberg H 1987 Trismus is not trivial. Anesthesioloy 67: 453–455

Rosenberg H 1988 Clinical presentation of malignant hyperthermia. British Journal of Anaesthesia 60: 268–273

Rosenberg H, Fletcher J E 1986 Masseter muscle rigidity and malignant hyperthermia susceptibility. Anesthesia and Analgesia 65: 161–164

Rosenberg H, Shutack J G 1991 Masseter muscle spasm in children. Anesthesia and Analgesia 73: 361–363

Saddler J M, Bevan J C, Plumley M H et al 1990 Jaw muscle tension after succinylcholine in children undergoing strabismus surgery. Canadian Journal of Anaesthesia 37: 21–25

Schwartz L, Rockoff M A, Koka B V 1984 Masseter spasm and anesthesia: incidence and implications. Anesthesiology 61: 772–775 van der Spek A F L, Fang W B, Ashton-Miller J A et al 1987 The effect of suxamethonium on mouth opening. Anesthesiologgy 67: 459–465

MENDELSON'S SYNDROME, ACID ASPIRATION SYNDROME

A syndrome that follows pulmonary aspiration of acid gastric contents. Gastric fluid, particularly that with a pH of 2.5 or less, causes chemical damage to the alveolar epithelium and the capillary endothelium. As a result of permeability changes, fluid and protein leak from the capillaries into the alveoli and interstitial spaces, causing pulmonary oedema and hypoxaemia. This leakage is enhanced by increases in pulmonary artery pressure. It is particularly, but not exclusively, associated with obstetric anaesthesia, and is more likely to occur in patients in whom intubation difficulties have been encountered, in gross obesity, hiatus hernia, and gastroduodenal obstruction.

A recent retrospective study has suggested that, if patients who have had clinical evidence of perioperative aspiration do not develop symptoms (cough or wheeze), or hypoxaemia on room air or CXR abnormalities, within 2 hours, serious sequelae are unlikely to occur (Warner et al 1993). In fact, clinically important pulmonary aspiration is extremely uncommon and the morbidity from it is low. In a study of more than 200 000 anaesthetics, the risk of aspiration was found to be related to ASA status and the nature of the surgery. Thus, risks were greatest in ASA 4 and 5 patients undergoing emergency procedures.

Although there have been suggestions that treatment with H2-receptor antagonists before elective surgery should be routine, at present there is no evidence to justify use in patients other than those at high risk (Editorial 1989).

Presentation

1. Regurgitation and aspiration may be obvious at induction, or it may pass unnoticed, particularly if there are problems during intubation. Under the latter circumstances, signs may be delayed for several hours. The syndrome has been reported to follow the aspiration of as little as 25 ml of acid. However, recent work in primates has suggested that the critical volume required to produce severe pneumonitis may be 50 ml (0.8 ml/kg), double that previously thought (Raidoo et al 1990), thus reducing the percentage of patients at risk.

2. Unexplained bronchospasm may occur during the anaesthetic. In the absence of a history of asthma, pulmonary aspiration should be suspected.

3. Postoperatively, tachycardia, tachypnoea, cyanosis, and respiratory difficulty may develop.

4. CXR may be normal initially, but can progress from patchy pulmonary infiltration, most commonly in the basal or perihilar regions, to signs of gross pulmonary oedema.
5. If significant inhalation has occurred, serial blood gases will show a deterioration in oxygenation. A decreasing Pao_2 and a metabolic acidosis will occur.

Management

1. Prophylaxis is the best form of management. The use of H_2-receptor antagonists and 0.3 mol/l sodium citrate given before surgery in cases considered to be at risk will reduce the pH of the gastric contents, should aspiration take place. An increase in gastric pH will occur 30–120 minutes after oral ranitidine.
2. The patient should be placed in a head-down position and the pharynx or tracheal tube aspirated. There is little place for bronchoscopy unless solid pieces of food have been inhaled.
3. If inhalation has occurred or is suspected, treatment should be aggressive. The tracheal tube should be kept in situ and IPPV and PEEP instituted. The aim of treatment is to provide respiratory support until pulmonary function returns to normal. A policy of waiting for deterioration may prove to be disastrous.
4. The advisability of using high-dose steroids remains controversial. One view is that there is little evidence to support their use, and that if infection occurs there may also be interference with tissue immunity. High-dose steroids were of no benefit in treating pneumonitis induced in rabbits (Wynne et al 1979). On the contrary, a clinical impression has been gained that, in man, their use for a 72-hour period may limit the extent of damage (Zorab 1984).
5. If the inhaled material is obviously contaminated, then antibiotics can be given. Otherwise they should be reserved for the presence of proven infection, and the appropriate antibiotic used to which the organism is sensitive.
6. Bronchodilators may be given for bronchospasm. A salbutamol infusion 5–20 μg/min can be given, or aminophylline i.v. 5 mg/kg over 10–15 minutes, can be followed by an infusion of 0.5 mg/kg per hour.
7. Occasionally, dopamine 5–20 μg/kg per min may be required for inotropic support.

BIBLIOGRAPHY
Coombs D W 1983 Editorial. Aspiration pneumonia prophylaxis. Anesthesia and Analgesia 62: 1055–1058
Jacobs B R, Swift C A, Dubow H D et al 1991 Time required for oral ranitidine to decrease gastric fluid acidity. Anesthesia and Analgesia 73: 787–789
Editorial 1989 Routine H2 receptor antagonists before elective surgery? Lancet 1: 1363–1364
Raidoo D M, Rocke D A, Brock-Utne J G et al 1990 Critical volume for pulmonary

acid aspiration: reappraisal in a primate model. British Journal of Anaesthesia 65: 248–250

Tordoff S G, Sweeney B P 1990 Acid aspiration prophylaxis in 288 obstetric departments in the United Kingdom. Anaesthesia 45: 776–780

Warner M A, Warner M E, Weber J G 1993 Clinical significance of pulmonary aspiration in the perioperative period. Anesthesioloy 78: 56–62

Wynne J W, Reynolds J C, Hood I et al 1979 Steroid therapy for pneumonitis in rabbits by aspiration of foodstuffs. Anesthesiology 51: 11–19

Zorab J S M 1984 Pulmonary aspiration. British Medical Journal 288: 1631–1632

METHAEMOGLOBINAEMIA

Methaemoglobin is produced when iron in the haem group of the haemoglobin molecule is oxidized from the ferrous to the ferric form. Methaemoglobin is continuously formed during red cell metabolism, but it is then converted back to reduced Hb. Under normal circumstances, its concentration never exceeds 1%. However, sometimes the capacity of the enzyme system is exceeded. Methaemoglobinaemia is a clinical condition in which more than 1% of the blood has been oxidized to the ferric form. It can arise from:

1. Congenital methaemoglobinaemia due to NADH-diaphorase deficiency. The inheritance is autosomal recessive.
2. Toxic methaemoglobinaemia, which occurs when various drugs or toxic substances oxidize haemoglobin, e.g. aniline and nitrobenzene.
3. Haemoglobin M disease, a form of haemoglobinopathy.

Cyanosis is seen when the level of methaemoglobin exceeds 1.5 g/dl. In congenital methaemoglobinaemia, the level of methaemoglobin varies between 8% and 40%. In general, 20% of methaemoglobin is required before symptoms occur. Higher levels can be tolerated without symptoms in the congenital condition, as compared with the acute toxic form.

Presentation

1. The patient looks cyanosed, his actual appearance often being described as a 'slatey grey'. Arterial blood takes on an unusual chocolate-brown colour. About 1.5 g/dl of methaemoglobin causes cyanosis, compared with the 5 g/dl required for reduced Hb. The diagnosis may also be suspected when unexpectedly low oxygen saturation readings are recorded using a pulse oximeter, in the presence of a normal Pao_2 on a blood gas sample. The effect of methaemoglobin on the oximeter reading however is complex (Ralston et al 1991). For technical reasons, the presence of MetHb will bias the saturation reading towards 85%, so that either over- or underestimation may occur (Bardoczky et al 1990). Very high MetHb levels can therefore mask profound desaturation (Rieder et al

1989). Carboxyhaemoglobin, and dyes such as methylene blue, have also caused spurious oximeter readings (Eisenkraft 1988).

2. Methaemoglobinaemia has been reported to have been caused in normal subjects by a variety of substances:

   a. Ingestion of aniline or nitrobenzene compounds (Harrison 1977).
   b. Prilocaine in doses exceeding 600–900 mg (or 8 mg/kg), due to a metabolite, orthotoluidine (Duncan & Kobrinsky 1983, Bardoczky et al 1990). Methaemoglobinaemia peaks at 60–90 minutes after administration of prilocaine, but may sometimes be delayed for 6 hours.
   c. Benzocaine in toxic doses (O'Donohue et al 1980). Infants and children are more susceptible to benzocaine because fetal Hb is more easily oxidized, and they have lower levels of NADH-methaemoglobin reductase, catalase and glutathione peroxidase (Severinghaus et al 1991).
   d. Methylene blue, in doses of >7 mg/kg, due to oxidation of haemoglobin.
   e. Treatment with antimalarials.
   f. Antileprosy drugs (Mayo et al 1987).
   g. A combination of 'EMLA' cream (prilocaine and lignocaine) and a sulphonamide in a baby (Jakobsen & Nilsson 1985).

3. Techniques
   a. 'Three-in-one block' (Bellamy et al 1992).
   b. Brachial plexus block (Bardoczky et al 1990, Marks & Desgrand 1991).
   c. During methylene blue infusion for parathyroid location.

Anaesthetic or resuscitative problems

1. The oxygen carrying capacity is reduced, and the oxygen dissociation curve is shifted to the left.
   a. 20% methaemoglobin is required before symptoms occur.
   b. 20–50% produces tachycardia, giddiness, headache and dyspnoea.
   c. 60–70% or more may be associated with vascular collapse, coma and death.
2. Unexplained cyanosis may occur. Cyanosis during appendicectomy in a child, was subsequently found to be due to dapsone 200 mg, administered to him by his father (Mayo et al 1987).
   Although methylene blue, 1–2 mg/kg is used in the treatment of methaemoglobinaemia, higher doses may in fact oxidize haemoglobin to methaemoglobin. Thus, a rapid infusion of methylene blue can itself produce transient cyanosis. An infusion of methylene blue 5 mg/kg is frequently used to assist in identification of the parathyroid glands during parathyroid surgery. Studies of the resulting methaemoglobin levels have shown a peak of 7.1% (Whitwam et al 1979) in one, and a range

from 4.5–17.4% (Lamont et al 1986) in another. The first authors thought that such levels might be dangerous in a patient with haemoglobin M disease, or where there was an abnormality of the hexose monophosphate pathway. The second paper concluded that with normal doses problems were unlikely.

Management

1. Ascorbic acid 300–600 mg daily can be used for chronic methaemoglobinaemia.
2. If acute symptomatic methaemoglobinaemia occurs, methylene blue, 1–2 mg/kg should be given. This stimulates the relevant reducing enzymes. Excess methylene blue (>7 mg/kg) can itself cause methaemoglobinaemia.
3. In cases of severe poisoning, exchange transfusion may be required (Harrison 1977).

BIBLIOGRAPHY

Anderson S T, Hajduczek J, Barker S J 1988 Benzocaine-induced methemoglobinemia in adults: accuracy of pulse oximetry with methemoglobinemia. Anesthesia and Analgesia 67: 1099–1101

Bardoczky G I, Wathieu M, D'Hollander A 1990 Prilocaine-induced methemoglobinemia evidenced by pulse oximetry. Acta Anaesthesiologica Scandinavica 34: 162–164

Barker S J, Tremper K K, Hyatt J 1989 Effects of methemoglobinemia on pulse oximetry and mixed venous oximetry. Anesthesiology 70: 112–117

Bellamy M C, Hopkins P M, Halsall P J et al 1992 A study into the incidence of methaemoglobinaemia after 'three-in-one' block with prilocaine. Anaesthesia 47: 1084–1085

Duncan P, Kobrinsky N 1983 Prilocaine-induced methemoglobinemia in a newborn infant. Anesthesiology 59: 75–76

Eisenkraft J B 1988 Pulse oximeter desaturation due to methemoglobinemia. Anesthesiology 68: 279–280

Harrison M R 1977 Toxic methaemoglobinaemia. Anaesthesia 32: 270–272

Jakobson B, Nilsson A 1985 Methaemoglobinaemia. associated with a prilocaine-lidocaine cream and trimethoprim-sulphamethazole. Acta Anaesthesiologica Scandinavica 29: 453–455

Lamont A S M, Roberts M S, Holdsworth D G 1986 et al Relationship between methaemoglobin production and methylene blue plasma concentrations under general anaesthesia. Anaesthesia and Intensive Care 14: 360–364

Marks L F, Desgrand D 1991 Prilocaine associated methaemoglobinaemia and the pulse oximeter Anaesthesia 46: 703

Mayo W, Leighton K, Robertson B et al 1987 Intraoperative cyanosis: a case of dapsone-induced methaemoglobinaemia. Canadian Journal of Anaesthesia 34: 79–82

O'Donohue W J, Moss L M, Angelillo V A 1980 Acute methemoglobinemia induced by topical benzocaine and lidocaine. Archives of Internal Medicine 140: 1508–1509

Ralston A C, Webb R K, Runciman W B 1991 Potential errors in pulse oximetry. III: Effects of interference, dyes, dyshaemoglobins and other pigments. Anaesthesia 46: 291–295

Rieder H U, Frei F J, Zbinden A M et al 1989 Pulse oximetry in methaemoglobinaemia. Anaesthesia 44: 326–327

Severinghaus J W, Xu F-D, Spellman M J 1991 Benzocaine and methemolobinemia: recommended actions. Anesthesioloy 74: 385–386
Whitwam J G, Taylor A R, White J M 1979 Potential hazard of methylene blue. Anaesthesia 34: 181–182

PHAEOCHROMOCYTOMA

Patients with unsuspected phaeochromocytoma may undergo anaesthesia for surgical, investigative, or obstetric procedures. The danger of this situation is underlined by the results of a study of 54 patients in whom tumours were shown at autopsy. These had been clinically unsuspected prior to the event leading to death, or were only diagnosed postmortem (Sutton et al 1981). One-third of these patients had died suddenly during, or immediately after, minor operations for unrelated conditions. Death was associated with either hypotensive or hypertensive crises.

Severe complications may occur with remarkable rapidity. If disaster is to be averted, the anaesthetist must be aware of the possibility of the diagnosis, the detailed pharmacology of the condition, and the correct method of treatment. Tachycardia treated blindly with beta adrenoceptor antagonists may result in extreme hypertension. Patients are at risk from cerebral haemorrhage, encephalopathy, pulmonary oedema, myocardial infarction, ventricular fibrillation, or renal failure. Phaeochromocytoma during pregnancy carries a particularly bad prognosis. A maternal mortality of 48%, and a fetal mortality of 55% has been reported in the past (Mitchell et al 1987), although the maternal mortality in pregnancy for 1980–1987 was said to be 17% (Harper et al 1989). Crises may also occur after drugs, chemotherapy and tumour embolization.

The most frequent preoperative clinical features are episodes of headache, pallor, palpitations, and sweating. Patients may have an unusually labile blood pressure and a pressor response to the induction of anaesthesia.

Presentation

1. Severe hypertension or severe hypotension during the perioperative period (Sutton et al 1981, Wooster & Mitchell 1981, Bittar 1979, 1982, Jones & Hill 1981). However, the classical signs are not always present and sometimes the signs are masked by other pathology. Several cases have been reported following cardiopulmonary bypass (Brown & Caplan 1986, Fenje et al 1989).
2. Tachyarrhythmias. A patient with an abdominal mass, high-output left ventricular failure, and hypertension underwent laparotomy. Severe cardiovascular instability was treated with practolol and phentolamine. Massive blood loss was reduced by means of sodium

nitroprusside. Direct arterial and pulmonary artery pressure monitoring assisted cardiovascular control. Subsequent histology confirmed a phaeochromocytoma (Darby & Prys-Roberts 1976).

3. Acute pulmonary oedema has been described in several cases. A 43-year-old man with a history of attacks of sweating and palpitations was admitted to ITU with pulmonary oedema and shock (Blom et al 1987). He was treated with IPPV and cardiovascular monitoring. Biochemistry indicated a predominantly adrenaline-secreting phaeochromocytoma.

4. Myocardial depression, cardiogenic shock, and segmental ST changes after massive catecholamine release in two patients with metastatic phaeochromocytoma have been described (Quezado et al 1992). In both, high levels of all three catecholamines were found, and as levels decreased haemodynamic function improved. In one, the episode had been precipitated by an injection of metoclopramide, whilst the second occurred 24 hours after embolization of the right superior gluteal artery. Both had large tumours.

5. Phaeochromocytomas presenting in pregnancy are associated with a high mortality. The condition may be forgotten, or misdiagnosed as pregnancy-induced hypertension (PIH). One patient actually presented with a convulsion and the diagnosis was only made at autopsy (Harper et al 1989). Intra- or postoperative tachycardia, hypotension, pulmonary oedema, and death are the commonest modes of presentation (Sardesai et al 1990). Tachycardia and gross pulmonary oedema occurred on extubation at the end of a Caesarean section in a patient with pregnancy-induced hypertension (personal communication). Death occurred 3 days later, and the diagnosis was only made at autopsy.

6. An acute abdominal emergency. Haemorrhagic necrosis of the tumour mimicked an acute abdominal emergency in two cases (Jones & Durning 1985). One patient developed pulmonary oedema after induction, and surgery was abandoned. The second developed a tachycardia of 180/min and an unrecordable arterial pressure during surgery. Both died postoperatively.

7. Bilateral dilated, nonreactive pupils, accompanied by only moderate cardiovascular changes were the only signs of a phaeochromocytoma in a patient undergoing nephrectomy for renal cell carcinoma (Larson & Herman 1992). The possibility of phaeochromocytoma was suspected (and later confirmed), therefore appropriate management was instituted.

8. Presentation may mimic malignant hyperthermia (Crowley et al 1988). Hypertension, tachycardia, pyrexia, acidosis, hypoxaemia, and cardiac arrest occurred perioperatively in a patient undergoing cholecystectomy. The patient survived and subsequently underwent surgical removal of the tumour (Allen & Rosenberg 1990).

9. Rarely, phaeochromocytoma presents as a crisis with multiple system organ failure, hyperthermia, encephalopathy and hyper- or hypotension (Newell et al 1988).

Management

1. Incidental surgery in a patient with an undiagnosed phaeochromocytoma carries a high mortality. The patient's best chance of survival lies in the early recognition of the condition, cessation of the proceedings, and admission to an ITU for haemodynamic monitoring (Smith et al 1978).
2. Phentolamine, phenoxybenzamine and sodium nitroprusside have all been used to control hypertension. The use of magnesium sulphate in a pregnant patient has been reported (James et al 1988). Magnesium is known to inhibit catecholamine release from the adrenal medulla, to decrease the sensitivity of the alpha adrenergic receptors to catecholamines, and to cause vasodilatation. A bolus of magnesium sulphate i.v. 4 g over 15 minutes was used, followed by an infusion of 1.5 g/h.
3. If hypotension occurs, phenylephrine or dopamine have been suggested as the most appropriate agents to use (Roizen et al 1982). Aggressive ITU support, invasive monitoring, and treatment with alpha and beta adrenoceptor antagonists for cardiogenic shock, are required.
4. Beta blockers should only be used to treat a tachycardia after alpha blockers have been given.

BIBLIOGRAPHY

Allen G C, Rosenberg H 1990 Phaeochromocytoma presenting as acute malignant hyperthermia – a diagnostic challenge. Canadian Journal of Anaesthesia 37: 593–595

Bittar D A 1979 Innovar-induced hypertensive crises in patients with pheochromocytoma. Anesthesiology 50: 366–369

Bittar D A 1982 Unsuspected phaeochromocytoma. Canadian Anaesthetists' Society Journal 29: 183–184

Blom H J, Karsdop V, Birnie R et al 1987 Phaeochromocytoma as cause of pulmonary oedema. Anaesthesia 42: 646–650

Brown P, Caplan R A 1986 Recognition of an unsuspected phaeochromocytoma during elective coronary artery bypass surgery. Canadian Anaesthetists' Society Journal 33: 785–789

Crowley K J, Cunningham A J, Conroy B et al 1988 Phaeochromocytoma – a presentation mimicking malignant hyperthermia. Anaesthesia 43: 1031–1032

Darby E, Prys-Roberts C 1976 Unusual presentation of phaeochromocytoma. Management of anaesthesia and cardiovascular monitoring. Anaesthesia 31: 913–916

Fenje N, Lee L W, Jamieson W R E et al 1989 Phaeochromocytoma and mitral valve replacement. Canadian Journal of Anaesthesia 36: 198–199

Greaves D J, Barrow P M 1989 Emergency resection of phaeochromocytoma presenting with hyperamylasaemia and pulmonary oedema. Anaesthesia 44: 841–842

Harper M A, Murnaghan G A, Kennedy L et al 1989 Phaeochromocytoma in pregnancy. Five cases and a review of the literature. British Journal of Obstetrics and Gynaecology 96: 594–606

5   James M F M, Huddle K R L, Owen A D et al 1988 Use of magnesium sulphate in the anaesthetic management of phaeochromocytoma in pregnancy. Canadian Journal of Anaesthesia 35: 178–182

Jones D J, Durning P 1985 Phaeochromocytoma presenting as an acute abdomen: report of two cases. British Medical Journal 291: 1267–1269

Jones R M, Hill A B 1981 Severe hypertension associated with pancuronium in a patient with a phaeochromocytoma. Canadian Anaesthetists' Society Journal 28: 394–396

Larson M D, Herman W C 1992 Bilateral dilated nonreactive pupils during surgery in a patient with undiagnosed pheochromocytoma. Anesthesiology 77: 200–202

Mitchell S Z, Freilich J D, Brant D et al 1987 Anesthetic management of pheochromocytoma resection during pregnancy. Anesthesia and Analgesia 66: 478–480

Newell K A, Prinz R A, Pickleman J et al 1988 Pheochromocytoma multisystem crisis. Archives of Surgery 123: 956–959

Quezado Z N, Keiser H R, Parker M M 1992 Reversible myocardial depression after massive catecholamine release from pheochromocytoma. Critical Care Medicine. 20: 549–551

Roizen M F, Horrigan R W, Koike M et al 1982 A prospective randomised trial of 4 anesthetic techniques for resection of pheochromocytoma. Anesthesioloy 57: A43

Sardesai S H, Mourant A J, Sivathandon Y et al 1990 Phaeochromocytoma and catecholamine-induced cardiomyopathy presenting as heart failure. British Heart Journal 63: 234–237

Smith D S, Aukberg S M, Levit J D 1978 Induction of anesthesia in a patient with undiagnosed pheochromocytoma. Anesthesiology 49: 368–369

Sutton M St J, Sheps S G, Lie J T 1981 Prevalence of clinically unsuspected pheochromocytoma. Mayo Clinic Proceedings 56: 354–360

Wooster L, Mitchell R I 1981 Unsuspected phaeochromocytoma presenting during surgery. Canadian Anaesthetists' Society Journal 28: 471–474

PITUITARY APOPLEXY

A complication of a previously undiagnosed pituitary adenoma caused by its sudden enlargement, usually as a result of spontaneous haemorrhage into the adenoma, or tumour infarction. Pituitary adenomas may be susceptible to infarction because of compromised blood supply from abnormal tumour vessels. Symptoms may be related to compression of the optic chiasma and other structures around the sella, or associated with hormonal disturbances. A number of precipitating factors have been identified, of which anaesthesia and surgery are two.

Presentation

1. Headache, visual disturbances, ophthalmoplegias, and impaired conscious level. May present with meningism and blood in the CSF and be difficult to distinguish from subarachnoid haemorrhage. The majority of perioperative cases have occurred after coronary artery bypass surgery (Shapiro 1990); however, pituitary apoplexy has been reported after cholecystectomy under combined general and extradural anaesthesia (Yahagi et al 1992). The day after surgery, the patient developed diplopia and cranial nerve palsies involving the fifth and sixth cranial nerves.

2. Endocrine disturbances, usually mild, either due to the adenoma or secondary to pituitary or hypothalamic damage. Multiple pituitary hormone deficiencies may occur.
3. Diagnosis by CT scan or MRI.
4. The differential diagnosis includes subarachnoid haemorrhage, brain abscess, and cavernous sinus thrombosis.

Management

1. Suspicion of pituitary apoplexy should be aroused if a patient develops unusual symptoms and signs in the perioperative period which are referable to the cranial nerves.
2. A neurological opinion should be sought; CT scan or MRI will confirm the diagnosis.
3. May need early diagnosis and urgent surgical decompression.
4. Check endocrine function; disturbances may be mild. Treat any hypopituitarism.

BIBLIOGRAPHY
Cardoso E R, Peterson E W 1984 Pituitary apoplexy: a review. Neurosurgery 14: 363–373
Editorial 1986 Pituitary tumours and the empty sella syndrome. Lancet ii: 1371–1372
Lewin I G, Mohan J, Norrnan P F et al Pituitary apoplexy. British Medical Journal 297: 1526–1527
Shapiro L M 1990 Pituitary apoplexy following coronary artery bypass surgery. Journal of Surgical Oncology 44: 66–68
Yahagi N, Nishikwa A, Matsui S et al 1992 Pituitary apoplexy following cholecystectomy. Anaethesia 47: 234–236

PNEUMOTHORAX

May cause compression and collapse of lung tissue, resulting in atelectasis and intrapulmonary shunting. During anaesthesia a pneumothorax may increase in size, either due to the diffusion of nitrous oxide, or secondary to positive pressure ventilation. Conversion to a tension pneumothorax will cause compression of mediastinal structures. In the absence of treatment this can result in cardiovascular collapse and death. Bilateral pneumothorax may occasionally occur during anaesthesia.

Presentation

1. Factors predisposing to the development of a pneumothorax include:
   a. Chronic bronchitis and emphysema.
   b. Congenital lung cysts. An increase in tension within the cyst, due to rapid diffusion of nitrous oxide, may cause it to rupture.
   c. Fractured ribs. With or without surgical emphysema.

d. IPPV. Particularly with high inspiratory pressures. This has occurred secondary to pulmonary barotrauma as a result of ventilator dysfunction (Hilton & Clement 1983). Bilateral pneumothoraces can occur following tracheal intubation and IPPV without other predisposing factors (Biswas et al 1989).

e. Jet ventilation techniques. Unilateral pneumothorax occurred as a result of the catheter being placed in the left main bronchus (Chang et al 1980). High alveolar pressures may be achieved with laryngeal obstruction of only brief duration.

f. Cystic fibrosis. Pneumothorax is a common complication of cystic fibrosis in adults. It tends to be recurrent, and may be difficult to treat (Penketh et al 1982, Robinson & Branthwaite 1984).

g. In neonates. May occur in association with tracheo-oesophageal fistula, diaphragmatic hernia (Diaz 1987), and during prolonged ventilation for RDS.

h. Surgical procedures. Including nephrectomy, cervical sympathectomy and rib resection.

i. Local anaesthetic procedures such as supraclavicular and interscalene brachial plexus block, stellate ganglion or intercostal blocks.

j. Subclavian venous cannulation. Fatalities have been reported due to bilateral pneumothorax during attempted subclavian venous cannulation (Schapira & Stern 1967).

k. In association with laparoscopy. Bilateral pneumothoraces which required urgent treatment (Doctor & Hussain 1973), and a transient pneumothorax which spontaneously resolved and was probably due to nitrous oxide (Batra et al 1983, have been reported in association with laparoscopy.

l. Tracheal intubation. Subcutaneous emphysema and pneumothorax resulted from accidental oesophageal intubation and perforation (Johnson & Hood 1986).

2. Clinical signs
If the patient's lungs are being ventilated, there will be a decreased compliance, difficulty in ventilation, hyper-resonance on percussion, and diminished movement of one side of the chest. If unrelieved, it may progress to signs of mediastinal shift, cyanosis, tachycardia, and hypotension. Further progression may lead to cardiovascular collapse and death.

3. Desaturation recorded by pulse oximetry led to the diagnosis in one patient after insertion of a double-lumen tube (Laishley & Aps 1991).

Diagnosis

1. Clinical. Decreased chest movement on one side, with absent breath sounds, hyper-resonance, tracheal shift, a decrease in oxygen saturation, and eventual frank cyanosis.
2. If time and the clinical situation permit, confirmation is by CXR.

Management

1. Stop nitrous oxide administration.
2. Immediately insert a chest drain. In an emergency, when the patient is receiving IPPV, a 12-gauge needle can be inserted into the second intercostal space in order to relieve the tension. An Argyle-type catheter and introducer can then be inserted at leisure into the second intercostal interspace anteriorly, in the mid-clavicular line, and connected to an underwater seal drain.

   Alternatively, the fifth interspace can be used, in the anterior axillary line, posterior to pectoralis major.
3. If anaesthesia is required in the presence of a pneumothorax, nitrous oxide should not be used and spontaneous respiration should be maintained. The use of a computer-controlled propofol infusion has been described (Crofts & Hutchison 1991).

BIBLIOGRAPHY

Batra M S, Driscoll J J, Coburn W A 1983 Evanescent N_2O pneumothorax after laparoscopy. Anesthesia and Analgesia 62: 1121–1123
Biswas C, Jana N, Maitra S 1989 Bilateral pneumothorax-following tracheal intubation. British Journal of Anaesthesia 62: 338–339
Chang J-L, Bleyaert A, Bedger R 1980 Unilateral pneumothorax following jet ventilation during general anesthesia. Anesthesiology 53: 244–246
Crofts S L, Hutchison G L 1991 General anaesthesia and undrained preumothorax. The use of a computer-controlled propofol infusion. Anaesthesia 6: 192–194
Diaz J 1987 Tension pneumoperitoneum-pneumothorax during repair of congenital diaphragmatic hernia. Anesthesia and Analgesia 66: 577–580
Doctor N H, Hussain Z 1973 Bilateral pneumothorax associated with laparoscopy. Anaesthesia 28: 75–81
Hilton P J, Clement J A 1983 Surgical emphysema resulting from ventilator malfunction. Anaesthesia 38: 342–345
Johnson K G, Hood D D 1986 Esophageal perforation associated with endotracheal intubation. Anesthesiology 64: 281–283
Laishley R S, Aps C 1991 Tension pneumothorax and pulse oximetry British Journal of Anaesthesia 66: 250–252
Penketh A, Knight R K, Hodson M E, et al 1982 Management of pneumothorax in adults with cystic fibrosis. Thorax 37: 850–853
Robinson D A, Branthwaite M A 1984 Pleural surgery in patients with cystic fibrosis. A review of anaesthetic management. Anaesthesia 39: 655–659
Schapira M, Stern W Z 1967 Hazards of subclavian vein cannulation for central venous monitoring. Journal of the American Medical Association 201: 327–329

PULMONARY OEDEMA
(SEE SECTION 1)

SUBDURAL BLOCK (ACCIDENTAL)

The subdural space is a potential space between the arachnoid mater and the dura mater which contains minimal amounts of serous lubricating fluid. It extends from S2 into the cranial cavity and runs for a short distance along the spinal and cranial nerves. Autopsy studies have confirmed that it is possible to open up the subdural space with saline, using both a Tuohy needle and an extradural catheter (Blomberg 1987). During myelography, an incidence of subdural injection as high as 13% has been reported, occasionally with extensive spread of contrast medium the whole length of the subdural space. The extensive spread is presumably because the space has a limited capacity and the injected fluid cannot escape. Accidental subdural injection may account for the 'massive epidurals' previously described (Boys & Norman 1975).

The incidence of penetration of this space during extradural blocks is difficult to estimate, but it may be 0.05–1.125%. In a study of 2182 patients receiving extradural analgesia, 0.82% patients met the criteria for subdural block (Lubenow et al 1988). The signs and symptoms produced can vary widely, although the chief features are those of a more extensive block than would normally be expected for the dose of local anaesthetic given, but in the presence of a negative aspiration test. The presentation presumably depends upon the site of the catheter, the precise distribution of the local anaesthetic, its volume and concentration, and the force with which the solution has been injected. Several papers have included X-rays or CT scans showing the distribution of contrast injected through the misplaced catheter. Since there is potentially more capacity posteriorly and laterally in the subdural space, a sensory block is more likely to occur. However, the subsequent positioning of the patient may influence the symptoms and signs (McMenemin et al 1992). Clinical signs of mixed blocks may occur, and CT scans have shown evidence of spread within both the extradural and subdural spaces. Motor blockade seems to be associated with the use of larger volumes or more concentrated solutions.

Reynolds and Speedy (1991) suggest that there are nine possible sequences when a catheter is passed through a needle which has penetrated the dura. They believe that this may account not only for the typical delayed onset and the profound and extensive conduction blockade, but also for a series of other unexplained features. Radio-opaque dye introduced into 100 catheters thought to be in the extradural space showed that 17 were just outside the spinal canal or only partly in the space (Mehta & Salmon 1985).

Presentation

1. Extensive segmental spread of local anaesthetic following an extradural block in the presence of a negative aspiration test. Slow progressive ascent of signs may occur from 15 minutes for up to 1.5 hours. There is less of a reduction in systemic blood pressure than would be expected with spinal anaesthesia, and the hypotension is easy to control. The sensory block extends high, but sacral sensation is retained (Morgan 1990). Occasionally a motor block occurs (Soni & Holland 1981), but this is relatively unusual. Progressive respiratory depression may occur. There is usually complete recovery within 2 hours.

2. The volume of local anaesthetic in the subdural space may lead to compression of the dural contents (Reynolds & Speedy 1991, McMenemin et al 1992). This second paper reported a patient in whom frontal headache occurred on injection of local anaesthetic, and this was followed by the development of atypical signs. A subsequent CT scan with contrast showed the catheter lying anteriorly within the spinal canal, and a long posterior fluid level, clearly influenced by gravity, with pooling at the most dependent level. An axial scan at T7 showed anterior displacement of the spinal cord within the subarachnoid space by the contrast. The authors considered that such displacement could potentially produce direct spinal cord damage, or indirect damage from ischaemia secondary to pressure on a vessel. They suggested that subdural injection might account for the occasional reports of permanent nerve damage following extradural analgesia.

3. A predominantly unilateral block occurs in some patients (Brindle-Smith et al 1984). Total unilateral (left-sided) analgesia occurred in one patient, and injection of 2 ml of a contrast material showed it ascending within the left lateral subdural space, with minimal spread to the right side, or caudal to the site of entry of the catheter (Manchanda et al 1983).

4. Although the aspiration test is usually negative, if the bevel of the needle straddles the subdural and subarachnoid spaces CSF may be obtained (Stevens & Stanton-Hicks 1985)

5. The incidence of subdural block may be increased by dural tears (caused by a preceding lumbar puncture, a spinal anaesthetic, or dural puncture), rotation of the needle, or intermittent advancement of the needle using loss of resistance to air.

6. Often there has been a failure to use a test dose, or to fractionate the local anaesthetic (Collier 1992), although one paper showed that test doses of local anaesthetic do not consistently identify misplaced catheters (Crosby & Halpern 1989).

7. Injection of morphine 2–3 mg has been reported in three gravid patients in whom subdural placement of the catheter was

subsequently confirmed radiologically (Chadwick et al 1992). Although there were atypical signs during the development of the block, anaesthesia for Caesarean section and postoperative opiate analgesia were successful in each case. In no patient did signs of opiate respiratory depression occur.

8. Occasionally, if the local anaesthetic reaches the cranial nerves, pupillary dilatation, trigeminal nerve block, and respiratory depression occurs.

9. Migration of the catheter into the subdural space can occur following successful extradural blockade (Abouleish & Goldstein 1986).

Diagnosis

1. Accidental subdural placement should be suspected if abnormal symptoms and signs follow extradural analgesia, particularly if a more extensive block than expected is obtained.

2. Injection of contrast medium into the catheter will show a characteristic 'string of beads' dorsally and laterally around the nerve roots, with a 'rail-road track' appearance on the anteroposterior view.

3. A range of findings on CT scan have been shown (Dake et al 1986, McMenemin et al 1992).

Management

1. Inadvertent subdural block is difficult to detect; however, it may be avoided by the application of constant pressure to the plunger of a saline-filled syringe, so that the dura is pushed away.

2. Appropriately trained staff, who can recognize the signs of abnormal placement of an extradural catheter and treat the resulting complications, must be present at all times.

3. Symptomatic treatment for hypotension or respiratory depression. Oxygen, tracheal intubation, and IPPV may sometimes be required (Abouleish & Goldstein 1986).

4. Alternative forms of analgesia must be given, although satisfactory anaesthesia may be produced (Chadwick et al 1992).

5. Perform an X-ray to confirm misplacement, then remove the catheter.

BIBLIOGRAPHY

Abouleish E, Goldstein M 1986 Migration of an extradural catheter into the subdural space. A case report. British Journal of Anaesthesia 58: 1194–1197

Blomberg R G 1987 The lumbar subdural extra-arachnoid space of humans; an anatomical study using spinaloscopy in autopsy cases. Anesthesia and Analgesia 66: 177–180

Boys J E, Norman P F 1975 Accidental subdural analgesia. British Journal of Anaesthesia 47: 1111–1126

Brindle-Smith G, Barton F L, Watt J H 1984 Extensive spread of local anaesthetic solution following subdural insertion of an epidural catheter during labour. Anaesthesia 39: 355–358

Chadwick H S, Bernards C M, Kovarik D W et al 1992 Subdural injection of morphine for analgesia for Cesarean section: a report of three cases. Anesthesiology 77: 590–594

Collier C B 1992 Accidental subdural block: four more cases and radiographic review. Anaesthesia and Intensive Care 20: 215–232

Crosby E T, Halpern S 1989 Failure of a lidocaine test dose to identify subdural placement of an epidural catheter. Canadian Journal of Anaesthesia 36: 445–447

Dake M D, Dillon W P, Dowart R H 1986 CT of extraarachnoid metrizamide installation. American Journal of Roentgenology 147: 583–586

Lee A, Dodd K W 1986 Accidental subdural catheterisation. Anaesthesia 41: 847–849

Lubenow T, Keh-Wong E, Kristof K et al 1988 Inadvertent subdural injection: a complication of an epidural block. Anesthesia and Analgesia 67: 175–179

Manchanda V N, Murad S H N, Shilyansky G et al 1983 Unusual clinical course of accidental subdural local anesthetic injection. Anesthesia and Analgesia 62: 1124–1126

McMenemin I M, Sissons G R J, Brownridge P 1992 Accidental subdural catheterization: radiological evidence of a possible mechanism for spinal cord damage. British Journal of Anaesthesia 69: 417–419

Mehta M, Salmon N 1985 Exadural block. Confirmation of the injecion site by X-ray monitoring. Anaesthesia 40: 1009–1012

Morgan B 1990 Unexpectedly extensive conduction blocks in obstetric analgesia. Anaesthesia 45: 148–152

Paech M J 1988 A most unusual subdural block. Anaesthesia and Intensive Care 16: 488–490

Reynolds F, Speedy H M 1991 The subdural space: the third place to go astray. Anaesthesia 45: 120–123

Soni N, Holland R 1981 An extensive lumbar epidural block. Anaesthesia and Intensive Care 9: 150–153

Stevens R A, Stanton-Hicks M A 1985 Subdural injection of local anesthetic: a complication of epidural anesthesia. Anesthesiology 63: 323–326

SUXAMETHONIUM APNOEA
(see also Section 1: PLASMA CHOLINESTERASE ABNORMALITIES)

Prolonged apnoea and neuromuscular blockade may occur following the administration of suxamethonium, either from the presence of a genetic variant of plasma cholinesterase, or as a result of low levels of the normal enzyme.

Presentation

1. Spontaneous respiration fails to return after suxamethonium has been given in a normal clinical dosage.
2. The patient may have a known family history of plasma cholinesterase abnormalities.
3. A low level of the normal enzyme may result from a number of pathological causes. These include severe liver disease, tetanus, malnutrition, renal failure, malignant disease, Huntington's chorea, and collagen disorders.
4. Iatrogenic causes include radiotherapy, renal dialysis, plasmapheresis, cardiac bypass, cytotoxic drugs, ecothiopate eye

drops, oral contraceptives, propanidid, neostigmine, chlorpromazine, pancuronium, and exposure to organophosphorus compounds (Whittaker 1980).

Diagnosis

Confirm complete neuromuscular blockade with a peripheral nerve stimulator. During the return of neuromuscular function there will be signs of a phase II block, with fade in response to train-of-four stimulation.

Management

1. Continue IPPV until adequate respiration is re-established. Maintain light anaesthesia to reduce distress.
2. After full recovery, a detailed anaesthetic, family, and drug history should be taken from the patient.
3. A clotted blood sample should be taken for plasma cholinesterase activity, and dibucaine and fluoride numbers. This may be sent to the Cholinesterase Research Unit, Royal Postgraduate Medical School, Hammersmith Hospital, London W12 OHS (Whittaker & Britten 1987).
4. The results should be given to the patient, and a warning card issued, if applicable. The investigation of other close relatives may be suggested.

BIBLIOGRAPHY
Whittaker M 1980 Plasma cholinesterase variants and the anaesthetist. Anaesthesia 35: 174–197
Whittaker M, Britten J J 1987 Phenotyping of individuals sensitive to suxamethonium. British Journal of Anaesthesia 59: 1052–1055

THYROTOXIC CRISIS OR STORM

The abrupt onset of symptoms of a severe hypermetabolic state, associated with the output of thyroxine, in a patient with pre-existing thyroid disease. This is a clinical, not a biochemical, diagnosis and biochemically it is difficult to distinguish between the two. However, serum free T4 concentrations are significantly higher in a thyroid crisis compared with thyrotoxicosis. It may occur in a patient with occult thyroid disease, in whom a crisis can be precipitated by an acute medical, traumatic, or surgical event. It may also occur in a treated thyrotoxic patient following thyroidectomy, either if there is inadequate preoperative control (Jamison & Done 1979), or if antithyroid therapy has been discontinued too early in the postoperative period. Thyrotoxicosis may be difficult to diagnose during pregnancy, and a thyroid crisis may be precipitated by delivery or Caesarean section (Halpern 1989, Clark et al 1985).

Although the onset of the crisis is most likely to occur in the postoperative period, intraoperative problems have also been described. A thyroid crisis can also be concealed by the use of beta adrenoceptor blockers (Jones & Solomon 1981). Beta blockers only affect the peripheral effects on beta adrenoceptors, not the output of thyroid hormone, or the biochemical tests.

Section 2

Thyrotoxic Crisis or Storm

Presentation

1. Intraoperative tachycardia or atrial fibrillation (Robson 1985, Bennett & Wainwright 1989), ventricular tachycardia, and cardiac arrest (Peters et al 1981).
2. A hypermetabolic state which may resemble malignant hyperthermia (Murray 1978, Peters et al 1981, Stevens 1983, Bennett & Wainwright 1989). Respiratory and metabolic acidosis occurs, with increased oxygen consumption.
3. Intraoperative pulmonary oedema has been descibed. This may present as cyanosis, tachycardia, and respiratory distress. It is secondary to a combination of increased cardiac output, tachycardia or atrial fibrillation, mild hypertension, increased red cell mass, and increased blood volume. An undiagnosed thyrotoxic patient with a fractured hip developed pulmonary oedema, pyrexia, and tachycardia during surgery (Stevens 1983). This state was diagnosed and treated as malignant hyperthermia, and the true diagnosis was only discovered during postoperative investigations.
4. Depression of myocardial function. A dilated cardiomyopathy complicated by a septic abortion (Hankins et al 1984) and ventricular dysfunction during Caesarean section (Clark et al 1985) have been described. In pregnant patients with untreated disease, thyroid crisis is most likely to occur during labour, surgery, or infection, or with pregnancy-induced hypertension. Heart failure is common. The stillbirth rate is high.
5. The sudden onset of confusion or mania in the perioperative period; alternatively, patients may occasionally present to the emergency department in coma (Gilbert et al 1992).
6. Postoperatively it can present with hyperpyrexia, tachycardia, agitation, nausea, vomiting, abdominal pain, diarrhoea, jaundice, hepatomegaly, dehydration, and infection.
7. A thyrotoxic crisis may also occur in an adequately prepared toxic patient in whom therapy is stopped too soon postoperatively, or when the thyrotoxicosis is being treated with propranolol alone (Eriksson et al 1977).

Management

1. Antithyroid drugs
   a. Carbimazole 60–120 mg or propylthiouracil 600–1200 mg, given orally or if necessary, by nasogastric tube. This usually starts to act within 1 hour of administration.
   b. Potassium or sodium iodide acts immediately to inhibit further release of thyroid hormone; this should not be given until 1 hour after the antithyroid drug (Smallridge 1992).
2. Beta adrenoceptor antagonists. Propranolol orally 20–80 mg 6-hourly, or i.v. 1–5 mg 6-hourly. In the short term, an esmolol infusion may be used (Thorne & Bedford 1989, Vijayakumar et al 1989).
3. Active cooling to reduce metabolic demands.
4. IPPV and muscle paralysis if necessary.
5. Steroids. Hydrocortisone i.v. 100 mg 6-hourly.
6. In the presence of atrial fibrillation digoxin may be required, in which case beta blockers should be given with caution.
7. Fluid i.v. (including dextrose) to replace insensible losses and vitamins. In the elderly, haemodynamic monitoring may be required.
8. Sources of infection should be sought, and some authors recommend the empirical use of antibiotics.
9. Dantrolene has been used to treat a child with thyroid storm who failed to respond to conventional treatment (Christensen & Nissen 1987). Although dantrolene successfully controlled the hypermetabolic state, the patient subsequently died from respiratory and renal failure. Dantrolene was also used in a young man who developed a hypermetabolic state on induction of anaesthesia and who subsequently proved to have thyrotoxicosis (Bennett & Wainwright 1989).

BIBLIOGRAPHY
Bennett M H, Wainwright A P 1989 Acute thyroid crisis on induction of anaesthesia. Anaesthesia 44: 28–30
Christensen P A, Nissen L R 1987 Treatment of thyroid storm in a child with dantrolene. British Journal of Anaesthesia 59: 522–526
Clark S L, Phelan J P, Montoro M et al 1985 Transient ventricular dysfunction associated with cesarean section in a patient with hyperthyroidism. American Journal of Obstetrics and Gynecology 151: 384–386
Erikkson M, Rubenfeld S, Garber A J et al 1977 Propranolol does not prevent thyroid storm. New England Journal of Medicine 296: 263–264
Gilbert R E, Thomas G W, Hope R N 1992 Coma and thyroid dysfunction. Anaesthesia and Intensive Care 20: 86–87
Halpern S H 1989 Anaesthesia for Caesarean section in patients with uncontrolled hyperthyroidism. Canadian Journal of Anaesthesia 36: 454–459
Hankins G D V, Lowe T W, Cunningham F G 1984 Dilated cardiomyopathy and thyrotoxicosis complicated by septic abortion. American Journal of Obstetrics and Gynecology 149: 85–86
Jamison M H, Done H J 1979 Postoperative thyrotoxic crisis in a patient prepared for thyroidectomy with propranolol. British Journal of Clinical Practice 32: 82–83

Jones D K, Solomon S 1981 Thyrotoxic crisis masked by treatment with beta blockers. British Medical Journal 283: 659
Murray J F 1978 Hyperpyrexia of uncertain origin. British Journal Anaesthesia 50: 387–388
Peters K R, Nance P, Wingard D W 1981 Malignant hyperthyroidism or malignant hyperthermia? Anesthesia and Analgesia 60: 613–615
Robson N J 1985 Emergency surgery complicated by thyrotoxicosis and thyroid periodic paralysis. Anaesthesia 40: 27–31
Smallridge R C 1992 Metabolic and anatomic thyroid emergencies: a review. Critical Care Medicine 20: 276–291
Stevens J J 1983 A case of thyrotoxic crisis that mimicked malignant hyperthermia. Anesthesiology 59: 263
Thorne A C, Bedford R F 1989 Esmolol for perioperative management of thyrotoxic goiter. Anesthesiology 71: 291–294
Vijayakumar H R, Thomas W O, Ferrara J J 1989 Perioperative management of severe thyrotoxicosis with esmolol. Anaesthesia 44: 406–408

TORSADE DE POINTES
(See also Section 1)

An atypical paroxysmal ventricular tachycardia associated with delayed repolarization of the ventricles. It is frequently drug induced, but may also occur with metabolic abnormalities.

Presentation

1. The patient may complain of episodes of palpitations, faintness, or fatigue. Sudden death may occur.
2. ECG shows paroxysms of an atypical ventricular tachycardia in which the QRS complexes vary in form and amplitude, and the axis of the complexes twists around the baseline. During periods of ordinary sinus rhythm there is a prolonged Q-Tc of >0.44 seconds or an uncorrected Q-T interval of >0.5 seconds. Immediately before the onset of the event there is a characteristic 'long-short' sequence (Raehl et al 1985) in which a premature ectopic is followed by a long pause, then a second premature ectopic initiates the torsade de pointes.
3. Predisposing factors
   a. Any disease that causes prolongation of the Q–T interval, such as the Romano–Ward, Jervell, and Lange-Nielsen syndromes or familial ventricular tachycardia.
   b. Metabolic abnormalities. Including hypokalaemia (Alexander & Potgieter 1983), hypomagnesaemia and hypocalcaemia. It has been suggested that hypomagnesaemia should be considered in any patient vith a combination of gastrointestinal losses and torsade de pointes (Ramee et al 1985). Torsade de pointes occurred following massive blood transfusion and hypomagnesaemia (Kulkarni et al 1992).
   c. Drug induced. A number of drugs, some of which prolong myocardial repolarization, have been reported to precipitate

torsade de pointes. These include amiodarone, disopyramide, lidoflazine, prenylamine, procainamide, propranolol, quinidine, sotalol, amitriptyline, imipramine, maprotiline, thioridazine, trifluoperazine, vasopressin, and diuretics (Raehl et al 1985).
 d. Following surgery which involved a block dissection of the right side of the neck (Otteni et al 1983).

Diagnosis

Torsade de pointes can be differentiated from polymorphous ventricular tachycardia by the long Q–Tc and the 'long-short' initiating sequence.

Management

1. Stop any potentially causative drug.
2. Avoid the use of class I antiarrhythmics, or any of those already mentioned.
3. Correct potential metabolic causes such as hypokalaemia, hypocalcaemia or hypomagnesaemia.
4. Defibrillation, if VF occurs.
5. Atrial or ventricular pacing may be required until the Q–Tc is normal. The duration of pacing required will depend upon the half-life of the precipitating drug.
6. Treatment can either be directed towards shortening the action potential duration with beta agonists or vagolytic agents, or suppressing early after-depolarization (Rosen & Schwartz 1991).
7. Thus, isoprenaline may increase the heart rate and therefore shorten the Q–T interval. A dose of 1–2 µg/min has been recommended. However, this is a potentially dangerous treatment and should be used with caution. Contraindications to its use include myocardial ischaemia and hypertensive heart disease (Raehl et al 1985).
8. Early after-depolarization can be suppressed with calcium channel blockers, magnesium sulphate (Ramee et al 1985, Martinez 1987) or beta adrenoceptor blockers.
9. Occasionally, bretylium (Raehl et al 1985) and lignocaine have been reported to be effective.

BIBLIOGRAPHY

Alexander M G, Potgieter P D 1983 Atypical ventricular tachycardia (torsade de pointes). Anaesthesia 38: 269–274
Kulkarni P, Bhattacharya S, Petros A J 1992 Torsade de pointes and long QT syndrome following major blood transfusion. Anaesthesia 47: 125–127
Martinez R 1987 Torsade de pointes: atypical rhythm, atypical treatment. Annals of Emergency Medicine 16: 878–884
Otteni J C, Pottecher R T, Bronner G et al 1983 Prolongation of the Q–T interval and sudden cardiac arrest following right radical neck dissection. Anesthesiology 59: 358–361
Raehl C L, Patel A K, LeRoy M 1985 Drug-induced torsade de pointes. Clinical Pharmacy 4: 675–-690
Ramee S R, White C J, Svinarich J T, et al 1985 Torsade de pointes and magnesium deficiency. American Heart Journal l09: 164–167

Rosen M R, Schwartz D J 1991 The 'Sicilian Gambit'. A new approach to the classification of antiarrythmic drugs based on their actions on arrhythmogenic mechanisms. Taskforce of the Working Group on arrhythmias of the European Society of Cardiology. European Heart Journal 12: 1112–1131

TOTAL SPINAL ANAESTHESIA

A syndrome of central neurological blockade. It occurs when a volume of local anaesthetic solution intended for extradural anaesthesia enters the subarachnoid space and ascends to the cervical region. This results in cardiovascular collapse, phrenic nerve paralysis and unconsciousness. Deaths have occasionally been reported.

Accidental total spinal analgesia may occur in association with the original extradural, or subsequently following a top-up dose, due to accidental puncture of the dura by the catheter.

Presentation

1. The circumstances.
   a. After a known dural tap. Three cases of total spinal anaesthesia have been reported after extradural injections of local anaesthetic were given into the interspace adjacent to an inadvertent dural perforation (Hodgkinson 1981). All three incidents occurred when the patient was in active labour. It was postulated that frequent uterine contractions can result in some of the local anaesthetic solution being forced through a puncture hole into the subarachnoid space.
   b. After extradural top-ups. High spinal anaesthesia after top-ups of extradural catheters has been reported (Philip & Brown 1976). This is unlikely to result from catheter migration, but may occur when part of the catheter lies within the extradural space and part within the subarachnoid. With a slow injection, the solution will emerge from the proximal holes, and with a rapid one from the more distal (Morgan 1990). Cardiovascular collapse usually takes place immediately after the extradural injection, although delays of up to 45 minutes have been reported (Woerth et al 1977). There is severe hypotension because of widespread blockade of the sympathetic outflow. Occasionally cardiac arrest occurs.
2. Rapidly increasing paralysis involves the respiratory muscles, resulting in apnoea and hypoxaemia (Philip & Brown 1976).
3. The pupils become dilated and consciousness is lost.
4. Apnoea may vary from 20 minutes to 6 hours, and unconsciousness from 25 minutes to 4 hours, while full recovery of sensation may take up to 9 hours (Gillies & Morgan 1973). The lengths of time vary with the agent, the dose and the volume of local anaesthetic given. Bupivacaine lasts longer than lignocaine.

Management

1. Precautions should be taken to prevent the occurrence of total spinal anaesthesia. A test dose of local anaesthetic through the extradural catheter is recommended. The injection of 3 ml of the local anaesthetic containing adrenaline 1:200 000, followed by an adequate pause to assess the effects, has been suggested (Moore & Batra 1980). The use of this during labour is controversial (see Local anaesthetic toxicity). It has been recommended that if dural puncture occurs during active labour when a Caesarean section is required, then further attempts should not be made. Either a spinal or a general anaesthetic should be employed as an alternative (Hodgkinson 1981). Others claim never to have seen this complication, and challenge the advice (Crawford 1983).

2. The assumption cannot be made that once a successful extradural is established, a total spinal anaesthesia cannot occur. Thus if a top-up is performed, facilities for resuscitation should still be available. It has been suggested that those mothers with previous dural punctures should only have top-ups performed by anaesthetists (Morgan 1990).

3. If an accidental total spinal does occur, a non-pregnant patient should be turned supine, tilted head-down and the legs elevated to encourage venous return. The pregnant patient should be tilted in the lateral position to prevent aortocaval compression (Rees & Willis 1988).

4. The lungs should be inflated with oxygen.

5. A pressor agent such as ephedrine i.v. in 5–10-mg increments up to 30 mg is recommended. Adrenaline 0.1–0.5 mg may occasionally be required, but should preferably be avoided in patients in labour.

6. Intravenous fluids should be infused rapidly.

7. A tracheal tube can then be inserted. IPPV may have to be continued for up to 2 hours, depending upon the local anaesthetic and the volume used.

BIBLIOGRAPHY

Crawford J S 1983 Collapse after epidural injection following inadvertent dural perforation. Anesthesiology 59: 78–79

Gillies I D S, Morgan M 1973 Accidental total spinal analgesia. Anaesthesia 28: 441–445

Hodgkinson R 1981 Total spinal block after epidural injection into an interspace adjacent to an inadvertent dural perforation. Anesthesiology 55: 593–595

Moore D C, Batra M S 1981 The components of an effective test dose prior to epidural block. Anesthesiology 55: 693–696

Morgan B 1990 Unexpectedly extensive conduction blocks in obstetric analgesia. Anaesthesia 45: 148–152

Philip J H, Brown W U 1976 Total spinal late in the course of an obstetric bupivacaine epidural block. Anesthesiology 44: 340–341

Rees G A D, Willis B A 1988 Resuscitation in late pregnancy. Anaesthesia 43: 347–349

Woerth S D, Bullard J R, Alpert C C 1977 Total spinal anesthesia. A late complication of epidural anesthesia. Anesthesiology 47: 380–381

TURP SYNDROME

A syndrome which may occur during transurethral resection of the prostate, in which large quantities of glycine 1.5% irrigating fluid are absorbed into the circulation through open veins in the prostatic bed, although some is also absorbed extravascularly into the periprostatic and retroperitoneal spaces. Glycine 1.5% is a non-electrolytic, slightly hypotonic solution (2.1% would be isotonic), which on absorption is mainly confined to the extracellular fluid (ECF). Plasma sodium levels are decreased by more than that which would be caused by an equivalent volume of water alone.

In general, the amount absorbed depends upon the number and size of prostatic venous sinuses opened, the hydrostatic pressure of the irrigating fluid and the length of exposure (although this has been disputed, since development of the syndrome has been reported after quite brief resection times). Absorption studies suggest an average rate of 20 ml/min, but as much as 87 ml/min has been reported (Alexander et al 1986). Risk factors for the development of a severe syndrome may include a large prostate, profuse bleeding from open prostatic veins, pre-existing hyponatraemia and excessive resection times. Several deaths from the syndrome have been reported (Aasheim 1973, Osborn et al 1980, Rhymer et al 1985). In patients undergoing regional anaesthesia it has been found that the smallest volume absorbed which gives rise to symptoms is 1000 ml, and more severe symptoms occur when it exceeds 2000 ml (Hahn 1989, 1990).

In some centres, isotonic dextrose was used as the irrigating fluid. In a study of 22 patients, dextrose was found to give a significantly greater decrease in plasma sodium than glycine, and some patients developed severe hyperglycaemia (Allen et al 1981).

A decrease in body temperature usually accompanies significant absorption of glycine, and surgery is associated with increased systemic vascular resistance, decreased stroke volume, and decreased cardiac output (Evans et al 1992). Haemodynamic stresses have been suggested to contribute to the higher long-term mortality found following TURP compared with open prostatectomy (Roos et al 1989, Editorial 1991).

Presentation

1. The patient is usually undergoing a TURP, and glycine 1.5% is being used as an irrigating fluid. It has also been described during percutaneous ultrasonic lithotripsy (Sinclair et al 1985) and endoscopic intrauterine surgery (Van Boven et al 1989).
2. The time of onset is variable. In one case, a convulsion occurred during spinal anaesthesia after only 15 minutes of resection

(Hurlbert & Wingard 1979). There were no warning signs despite the plasma sodium having decreased to 104 mmol/l. Absorption of glycine may continue beyond the resection time into the postoperative period.

3. Initially there is an increase in systolic blood pressure and a widening of pulse pressure. This is followed by bradycardia, hypotension, and occasionally cardiac arrest (Charlton 1980). Other ECG abnormalities, including nodal rhythm and U waves, have been reported. Blood loss may mask the initial hypertensive phase.

4. The syndrome is likely to present earlier in a conscious patient undergoing spinal anaesthesia than in one having a general anaesthetic. Facial warmth, visual disturbances, restlessness, confusion, headache, nausea, and retching may herald its onset. Convulsions have been reported. During general anaesthesia, detection may be delayed, particularly if the initial hypertensive phase is masked by blood loss.

5. Pulmonary oedema may occur (Aasheim 1973, Allen et al 1981). The patient can present with respiratory distress and cyanosis in the postoperative period (Rhymer et al 1985).

6. Cerebral oedema may result in mental confusion and fits. Several cases of visual disturbances (Ovassapian et al 1982) and transient blindness have been described (Russell 1990). These have been attributed to the effects of high glycine levels on the retinal synapses, although oedema of the occipital cortex has also been suggested as a cause. (Ovassapian et al 1982). Delayed awakening from anaesthesia has been reported (Roesch et al 1983).

7. Profound hyponatraemia can occur, plasma sodium levels of 102–105 mmol/l often being reported. In one fatal case, the plasma sodium, after more than 5 hours' resection, was 83 mmol/l. The sodium level does not necessarily correlate with the amount of fluid absorbed since the presence of glycine enhances the hyponatraemia. In a study of 372 prostatectomies, 15% of patients had plasma sodium levels of less than 125 mmol/l. All had clinical evidence of hyponatraemia (Shearer & Standfield 1981). In contrast, other authors claimed to have seen patients with levels of 104 mmol/l, without clinical signs (Allen et al 1981).

8. Decreased serum osmolality usually occurs, but the degree is very variable.

9. The extent to which high levels of glycine and its metabolites contribute to the CNS effects of the syndrome is the subject of continuing discussion. Products of glycine metabolism include serine, ammonia, oxalate, and glycolate. Glycine (and to a lesser extent serine) is known to be an inhibitory neurotransmitter in the brain, spinal cord and retina, with a similar action to GABA on chloride channels.

Although early reports indicated that ammonia accumulation was not a problem, in one case delayed recovery from anaesthesia was associated with a blood ammonia level of 500 μmol/l (Roesch et al 1983). It was suggested that some patients may be more susceptible to ammonia production and toxicity than others.

Twenty-four-hour urinary oxalate and glycolate levels were studied in three patients, who were selected from a total of 34 patients, on the basis of hyponatraemia the morning after surgery (Fitzpatrick et al 1981). Urinary levels of oxalate and glycolate were high in all three patients, and oxalate continued to be excreted for up to 2 weeks.

Diagnosis

1. Plasma sodium. Values as low as 83 mmol/l have been reported.
2. Plasma osmolality may be reduced.
3. Hb and haematocrit levels are decreased.
4. The use of irrigating fluid tagged with 1% or 2% ethanol. Absorption in litres has been calculated to be equal to 3.6 EB-ethanol (max) divided by the ethanol concentration in % in the irrigating fluid (Hulten et al 1991).
5. Plasma glycine levels are high (N = 176–332 μmol/l). The results of glycine level estimations may take several days to become available, and are therefore not of immediate use. Levels as high as 8000 μmol/l have been reported.
6. Blood ammonia levels may be increased (N = 11–35 μmol/l). In the patient with delayed recovery from anaesthesia, the blood ammonia was 500 μmol/l.
7. When isotonic dextrose was used as the irrigating fluid, one patient developed a blood glucose of 61.8 mmol/l (Allen et al 1981).
8. Urinary oxalate (N = 0.1–0.5 mmol/24 h) and glycolate levels (N = 0.10–0.35 mmol/24 h) may be elevated.

Management

1. Prophylaxis and anticipation
   a. Prostatic resection time should, in general, be limited to 1–1.5 hours. However, one case of convulsions and a sodium of 104 mmol/l developed after only 15 minutes (Hurlbert & Wingard 1979).
   b. Irrigating pressure should be kept to about 60–70 cm H_2O, and certainly should never be allowed to exceed 100 cmH_2O.
   c. Sodium-free i.v. solutions should not be used during prostatic resection.
   d. Postoperatively, the bladder irrigation fluid should be changed from glycine to saline.
2. Early detection of absorption of glycine and prompt cessation of surgery if the amount suspected approaches 2000 ml. Methods of

detecting this include the use of an ethanol 'marker' in the glycine. Hahn (1990) reported the use of glycine 1.5% containing ethanol 1% in 100 consecutive patients having TURP under extradural anaesthesia, and subsequently the technique was found to be applicable to anaesthetized patients (Hulten et al 1991). An alcohol meter (Alcolmeter S-D2, Lions Laboratories Ltd, Barry, Wales) was used each 10 minutes (or each 5 minutes if absorption was detected), and irrigant absorption was calculated according to a formula determined in a previous study (Hahn 1989), where EBV is the expired breath volume:

Absorption of glycine   3.6 EBV-ethanol (max) divided by the ethanol
     in litres = concentration in % in the irrigating fluid.

The use of 1% alcohol allowed the absorption of 100–150 ml/10 minute period to be detected, and if 2% alcohol was used, as little as 50 ml/10 minute period could be detected.

3. Treatment of hyponatraemia

This is controversial. Recommendations range from no treatment at all, to saline 0.9%, hypertonic saline, mannitol, loop diuretics and peritoneal dialysis. Those who have reservations about the use of active therapy observed that some patients with a sodium of 104 mmol/l were asymptomatic, and that spontaneous correction of hyponatraemia normally occurred within 12–24 hours. In addition, rapid correction of hyponatraemia is potentially dangerous because of osmotic gradients which may occur between the brain and vascular compartments. These may result in cerebral damage (Arieff 1986, Sterns et al 1986, Sterns 1992). However, a number of deaths associated with the TURP syndrome have been reported, and in the elderly patient, cardiac arrhythmias, convulsions, and pulmonary and cerebral oedema are dangerous complications.

a. Each case must be dealt with individually with a knowledge of the patient's clinical state, his cardiovascular and respiratory status, and the biochemical results.

b. If active therapeutic correction of the hyponatraemia is required, it should be carried out with extreme caution. Saline 0.9% is usually sufficient, perhaps with the addition of a loop diuretic. However, a loop diuretic is less effective in dilutional hyponatraemia, and has the disadvantage of causing the loss of sodium in addition to water. If the serum osmolality is very low, hypertonic saline may be required. However, a plasma sodium correction rate of not more than 6–8 mmol/l/day has been suggested (Sterns 1992).

c. Prophylactic IPPV and ITU monitoring are essential, at least until the plasma sodium and hypervolaemia are corrected, if the hyponatraemia is severe. This will prevent hypoxaemia, minimize the effects of cerebral oedema or convulsions, and allow detection and treatment of cardiac arrhythmias.

4. Calcium and inotropic agents may be required. The routine use of calcium gluconate 10% 10 ml, has been recommended, and particularly when cardiovascular collapse has occurred.
5. Coagulation studies should be performed if there is persistent bleeding and hyponatraemia. Dilutional abnormalities are the most frequent, although DIC may also occur. Defects should be treated appropriately.
6. Should blindness occur, ophthalmological advice should be sought; however, in those cases reported, sight has always been restored within 12–24 hours.
7. Urinary volumes should be maintained postoperatively, to prevent the deposition of calcium oxalate in the urinary tract.

BIBLIOGRAPHY

Aasheim G M 1973 Hyponatraemia during transurethral surgery. Canadian Anaesthetists' Society Journal 20: 274–280

Alexander J P, Polland A, Gillespie I A 1986 Glycine and transurethral resection. Anaesthesia 41: 1189–1195

Allen P R, Hughes R G, Goldie D J et al 1981 Fluid absorption during transurethral resection. British Medical Journal 282: 740

Anathana A, Rayan G 1991 The TURP syndrome. Canadian Journal of Anaesthesia 38: 543–544

Arieff A I 1986 Hyponatremia, convulsions, respiratory arrest and permanent brain damage after elective surgery in healthy women. New England Journal of Medicine 314: 1529–1535

Charlton A J 1980 Cardiac arrest during transurethral prostatectomy after absorption of 1.5% glycine. Anaesthesia 35: 804–806

Crowley K, Clarkson K, Hannon V et al 1990 Diuretics after transurethral prostatectomy: a double-blind controlled trial comparing frusemide and mannitol. British Journal of Anaesthesia 65: 337–341

Editorial 1991 Monitoring TURP. Lancet 338: 606–607

Evans J W H, Singer M, Chapple C R et al 1992 Haemodynamic evidence for cardiac stress during transurethral resection of the prostate. British Medical Journal 304: 666–671

Fitzpatrick J M, Kasidas G P, Rose G A 1981 Hyperoxaluria following glycine irrigation for transurethral prostatectomy. British Journal of Urology 53: 250–252

Hahn R G 1989 Early detection of the TUR syndrome by marking the irrigating fluid with 1% ethanol. Acta Anaesthesiologica scandinavica 33: 146–151

Hahn R G 1990 Prevention of TURP syndrome by detection of trace ethanol in the expired breath. Anaesthesia 45: 577–581

Hahn R G 1991 The transurethral resection syndrome. Acta Anaesthesiologica Scandinavica 35: 557–567

Hatch P D 1987 Surgical and anaesthetic considerations in transurethral resection of the prostate. Anaesthesia and Intensive Care 15: 203–211

Hulten J, Sarma V J, Hjertberg H et al 1991 Monitoring of irrigating fluid absorption during transurethral prostatectomy. A study in anaesthetised patients using a 1% ethanol solution. Anaesthesia 46: 349–353

Hurlbert B J, Wingard D W 1979 Water intoxication after 15 minutes of transurethral resection of the prostate. Anesthesiology 50: 355–356

Osborn D E, Rao P N, Greene M J et al 1980 Fluid absorption during transurethral resection. British Medical Journal 281: 1549–1550

Ovassapian A, Joshi C W, Brunner E A 1982 Visual disturbances: an unusual symptom of transurethral prostate resection reaction. Anesthesiology 57: 332–334

Rhymer J C, Bell T J, Perry K C et al 1985 Hyponatraemia following transurethral resection of the prostate. British Journal of Urology 57: 450–452

Roesch R P, Stoelting R K, Lingeman J E et al 1983 Ammonia toxicity resulting from glycine absorption during a transurethral resection of the prostate. Anesthesiology 58: 577–579

Roos N P, Wennberg J E, Malenka D J et al 1989 Mortality and reoperation after open and transurethral resection of prostate for benign prostatic hyperplasia. New England Journal of Medicine 320: 1120–1124

Russell D 1990 Painless loss of vision after transurethral resection of the prostate. Anaesthesia 45: 218–221

Shearer R J, Standfield N J 1981 Fluid absorption during transurethal resection. British Medical Journal 282: 740

Sinclair J F, Hutchison A, Baraza R et al 1985 Absorption of 1.5% glycine after percutaneous ultrasonic lithotripsy for renal stone disease. British Medical Journal 291: 691–692

Stalberg H P, Hahn R G, Jones A W 1992 Ethanol monitoring of transurethral resection of the prostate during inhaled anesthesia. Anesthesia and Analgesia 75: 983–988

Sterns R H, Riggs J E, Schochet S S Jr 1986 Osmotic demyelination syndrome following correction of hyponatremia. New England Journal of Medicine 1535–1542

Sterns R H 1992 Severe hyponatraemia: the case for conservative management. Critical Care Medicine 20: 534–539

Van Boven M J, Singelyn F, Donnez J et al 1989 Dilutional hyponatremia associated with intrauterine endoscopic laser surgery. Anesthesiology 71: 449–450

Wang J M, Creel D J, Wong K C 1989 TURP, serum glycine levels and ocular evoked potential. Anesthesiology 70: 36–41.

Miscellaneous Problems

AUTOMATIC IMPLANTABLE CARDIOVERTER-DEFIBRILLATOR (AICD)

A device used in the treatment of patients with recurrent tachyarrhythmias which are unresponsive to medical treatment. The automatic implantable cardioverter-defibrillator (AICD) senses VT or VF and responds with countershocks to the heart. Although there are significant complications from this procedure and its subsequent aftercare, survival in this high risk group of patients is said to be improved (Borbola et al 1988). However, no controlled clinical trials have been performed and doubts about its benefits have been expressed (Fogoros 1991).

Unlike pacemaker implantation, which can be performed under local anaesthesia, AICD implantation requires a general anaesthetic because of the need to expose the apex of the heart. Increasing numbers of devices are being inserted and anaesthesia is usually required on at least two occasions. Consequently there is an increasing chance of a patient with an implanted AICD needing incidental surgery.

Description

The device is implanted subcutaneously into the thorax or abdomen. The cardiac connections consist of two unipolar screw-in sensing leads in the anterobasal part of the left ventricular septum and two epicardial patch electrodes (about 5 × 6 cm) which are sewn in place. One is usually sited posterolaterally over the left ventricle, the other anteriorly over the right ventricle. The screw-in leads sense electrical activity, and the charger delivers a countershock via the two patch electrodes.

The AICD can be programmed to detect tachycardias in certain ranges. If and when the predetermined criteria are fulfilled, the device charges and delivers a shock to the heart and will recharge at a higher level, giving, if necessary, up to five countershocks of 30 joules each. The device can be deactivated by a programmer or a magnet.

From time to time, pulse generators and electrodes will need replacement.

Indications for insertion
Recurrent ventricular tachyarrhythmias in patients who are not controlled by drugs or who do not tolerate them.

Anaesthetic problems

1. The patient may need two anaesthetics, the first for insertion, the second about three months later to test device function. However, this is not always necessary (Lee 1992). These patients are high-risk candidates for surgery and the average operative mortality is 3.5%, although ranges of 0–8% have been reported.

2. Testing of the device. Repeated intraoperative induction of VF may be required to test thresholds, during which time haemodynamics may be compromised (Carr & Whiteley 1991). Testing with the patient awake is also necessary, so that he can experience the sensation of a shock (Crozier & Ward 1988). However, if reversion to sinus rhythm fails, an anaesthetist will be required urgently so that external defibrillation can be applied. Each time a test is performed there is a risk that normal rhythm will not be restored (Horrow & Pharo 1991).

3. The presence of the AICD patches may increase the energy requirements for external defibrillation to a level higher than usual with the paddles in the standard position. In one case, failure to convert an induced episode of VF was finally resolved by placing the internal paddles perpendicular to the plane of the epicardial patches and delivering two near-simultaneous (orthogonal) shocks, discharged 50 ms apart (Horrow & Pharo 1991).

4. Most patients are receiving antiarrhythmic therapy, usually amiodarone. This drug may increase the threshold for defibrillation. Possible amiodarone pulmonary toxicity was reported in two patients undergoing one-lung anaesthesia with high oxygen concentrations for AICD insertion (Herndon et al 1992).

5. Anaesthetic agents may alter cardiac conduction or the threshold for defibrillation.

6. The AICD can be triggered by any form of electromagnetic radiation, including electrocautery (Gaba et al 1985). In one patient, the countershock sequence that precipitated VT was initiated by the diathermy.

7. An AICD may discharge at any time. Staff handling such patients should wear gloves (Lee 1992).
8. Poor ventricular function is common and associated with an increased mortality at operation. Ventricular arrhythmias can occur at any time, with a resultant decrease in cardiac output.
9. Problems associated with specific procedures:
   a. Shock-wave lithotripsy (SWL). In patients undergoing SWL for fragmentation of calculi there is a danger of the piezoelectric crystal being shattered by the shock wave (Long & Venditti 1991, Horrow & Pharo 1991).
   b. ECT needs special precautions. If the patient is earthed, the ECT current may pass through the heart via the AICD and cause VF.
   c. Problems of using transcutaneous electrical nerve stimulation (TENS).
10. Complications of initial AICD insertion include wound infection, seroma of the pocket holding the device, pleural effusion, device failure, and inappropriate activation.

Section 3

Automatic
Implantable
Cadioverter-
Defibrillator (AICD)

Management

1. If incidental surgery is required in a patient with an AICD, the cardiology department should be informed in advance to allow the function and frequency of firing to be assessed. An expert must be present in theatre. An external defibrillator is also needed.
2. Surgical diathermy should be used with caution. If it is essential, bipolar electrodes should be used and the AICD put into the inactive mode. The indifferent electrode should be placed as far from the pulse generator and AICD leads as possible (Gaba et al 1985).
3. Anaesthesia for implantation of AICD. Intra-arterial monitoring is advisable as testing involves the induction of VF (Gaba et al 1985). This can be associated with adverse cardiopulmonary effects, which sometimes require treatment with inotropic agents (Hachenberg et al 1991). However, others have suggested that ET_{CO_2} monitoring may be sufficient to indicate decreases in cardiac output (Cashman et al 1992). Central venous access is needed both for the passage of pacing wires and for administration of vasoactive drugs.
4. During AICD implantation or testing, anaesthetic drugs should be given that interfere as little as possible with the procedure of threshold determination. It has been suggested that lignocaine be avoided and procaine used as an alternative local anaesthetic. The use of nitrous oxide, oxygen, an analgesic and only low doses of isoflurane, has been recommended.
5. Staff handling these patients should wear gloves because a shock can occur at any time (Lee 1992).
6. Anaesthesia for electroconvulsive therapy (ECT). The device needs disabling before ECT is applied. An external defibrillator and full

resuscitation equipment should be immediately available. Earthing the patient should be avoided, otherwise the current may pass through the heart and trigger VF.

7. Shock-wave lithotripsy. To investigate methods of protecting the device from the shock wave, an AICD generator was strapped to a patient who was undergoing SWL It was protected from the shockwave with a 2.5 cm thick styrofoam board and was subsequently examined for damage. None was found (Long & Venditti 1991). When SWL is being undertaken, the AICD should be deactivated with a magnet by the cardiologist, and it should be protected from the effects of the shock-wave.

8. Transcutaneous pacing. Investigations have shown that emergency non-invasive transcutaneous pacing is possible in patients with AICD patches despite the fact that there is insulation of the epicardial patch electrodes (Kemnitz et al 1992). No difference in thresholds was found when compared with patients without the patches who were undergoing routine coronary artery bypass surgery.

9. Access to extracorporeal circulation facilities may be life-saving if there is refractory VF (Horrow & Pharo 1991).

BIBLIOGRAPHY

Borbola J, Denes P, Ezri M D et al 1988 The automatic implantable cardioverter-defibrillator. Archives of Internal Medicine 148: 70–76

Carr C M E, Whiteley S M 1991 The automatic implantable cardioverter-defibrillator Implications for anaesthetists. Anaesthesia 46: 737–740

Cashman J N, Garcia-Rodriguez C, Lamond C 1992 Anaesthesia for transvenous insertion of an automatic implantable converter-defibrillator. Anaesthesia 47: 720–721

Crozier I G, Ward D E 1988 Automatic implantable cardioverter-defibrillator. British Journal of Hospital Medicine 40: 136–139

Fogoros R N 1991 The implantable defibrillator backlash. American Journal of Cardiology 67: 1424–1427

Gaba D M, Wynder J, Fish K J 1985 Anesthesia and the automatic implantable cardioverter defibrillator. Anesthesiology 62: 786–792

Hachenberg T, Hammel D, Mollhoff I et al 1991 Cardiopulmonary effects of internal cardioverter defibrillator implantation. Acta Anaesthesiologica Scandinavica 35: 626–630

Herndon J C, Cook A O, Ramsay M A E et al 1992 Postoperative unilateral pulmonary edema: possible amiodarone toxicity. Anesthesiology 76: 308–311

Horrow J C, Pharo G 1991 Successful defibrillation with near-simultaneous orthogonal discharges. Anesthesiology 75: 362–364

Kemnitz J, Winter J, Vester E G et al 1992 Transcutaneous cardiac pacing in patients with automatic implantable cardioverter defibrillators. Anesthesiology 77: 258–262

Lee E M 1992 More on automatic cardioverter-defibrillators. Anaesthesia 47: 637–638

Long A L, Venditti F J 1991 Lithotripsy in a patient with an automatic implantable cardioverter defibrillator. Anesthesiology 74: 937–938

SURGERY IN JEHOVAH'S WITNESSES

Problems

1. Ethical, moral and practical issues (see also Layon et al 1990, Benson 1989).

   a. Limitations placed on the physician and their effects
   Jehovah's Witnesses will not accept the transfusion of blood or blood products, on religious grounds. If an adult is accepted for elective surgery, the surgeon and anaesthetist must also accept the limitations placed on their practice of medicine by the patient's wishes. In the case of an emergency, or in the case of essential treatment if the practitioner is the only suitably qualified person available, there may be no choice but to undertake treatment. In general, however, it is the anaesthetist who has to administer blood, and, as the likely resuscitator in the event of life-threatening haemorrhage, has to face the impact of these restrictions on his normal practice. The devastating effect of watching a patient exsanguinate and being unable to administer blood cannot be underestimated. Another problem is that the original agreement to surgery was usually made between the surgeon and patient. The anaesthetist, who may only be involved at a late stage, is an outsider to this agreement and may not be party to its exact terms. Not only must he know whether or not the patient understands the full implications of his decision but, almost more importantly, whether the surgeon does as well.

   b. The type of surgery
   Blood transfusion is now undertaken in fewer operations. In addition, substantial blood loss is unlikely for many types of surgery. As a result, the fact that a Jehovah's Witness has signed a form to say that he refuses blood transfusion often has little impact on the anaesthetist's relationship with his patient. If, on the other hand, substantial blood loss is anticipated, there is likelyto have been extensive discussion. Thus, all parties in the agreement will have accepted the remote possibility of the patient's death. Practical preparation of the patient, for example by haemodilution techniques, is also likely to have taken place. The worst scenario is when completely unexpected bleeding occurs in a situation in which transfusion would be most unusual.

2. In the UK, legal issues have been decided by case, not statute, law.

   a. The child in an emergency situation
   Courts have been consistent in their support of children, or a viable fetus, against parental objection. When a child's life is in danger, transfusion is allowed despite religious objections by the parents. Technically, application can be made for the child to

become a ward of court. However, in an emergency this is not necessary, provided a second physician has seen the patient and agreed that blood is essential (See Management b.).

b. The adult for elective surgery

If a fully informed adult has refused blood transfusion and subsequently dies, the physician is legally protected. Unless the physician believes that the patient did not understand the implications, the undertaking not to give blood should not be reversed.

c. Adults and third party problems

Certain situations may modify the legal judgments in the case of adults. These involve the protection of innocent third parties, such as a mature fetus or a child, and may take precedence over an individual's expression of religious freedom. Adults have rights to refuse (for details see Benson 1989).

d. Unconscious or incompetent adult

The situation may be different in the case of an emergency, or with an unconscious patient, when the physician becomes an 'involuntary host'. However, a Canadian doctor was found guilty of battery when he transfused an unconscious patient who was in possession of an undated card indicating that she would not accept blood transfusion (Brahams 1989).

e. Problems with administration of treatment which may result in an increased risk of bleeding

A patient with a myocardial infarction, randomized in a clinical trial to receive streptokinase subsequently died from haemorrhagic complications (Sugarman et al 1991).

3. On certain issues there is a lack of clarity. The use of albumin, immune globulins and haemophiliac preparations appears to be a matter of individual discretion (Dixon & Smalley 1981). In addition, the decision whether or not to accept autologous blood transfusions is an individual one. Patients will often accept if they are satisfied that there is continuity between the blood and their own circulation.

4. Mortality was found to be dependent on the blood loss at surgery not the preoperative Hb (Spence et al 1990).

5. Haematological problems:
   a. Circulating volume.
   b. Oxygen carriage.
   c. Platelets and coagulation.
   d. Oncotic pressure.
   e. Immune status.

6. Reactions to plasma expanders have been reported. Transfusion of hydroxyethyl starch 2.66 g/kg in a child (which represented 60% of his blood volume) undergoing scoliosis correction resulted in a severe coagulopathy which did not revert to normal until 72 hours

later (Lockwood et al 1988). Defects included prolonged PT and APTT, and decreased levels of Factor X, Factor VII, Factor VIII and vWF. In clinical studies, up to 1.4 g/kg had been used with only minor laboratory abnormalities.

7. The problems of managing a post-spinal headache.

Management

1. Preliminary discussions
   a. For an elective procedure, a physician may decide not to accept the limitations placed on his treatment, but to refer the patient to a colleague, or to another hospital specializing in the treatment of Jehovah's Witnesses.
   b. For a child who needs transfusion, support in writing from a colleague should be obtained first. If time allows, and in his presence, the reason for treatment and the risks if blood is not given are discussed with the parents. In the event of refusal by the parents, a record is made in the case notes. Both physicians should sign this record. An application to a magistrate for custody of the child is not usually necessary (Medical Defence Union 1989). If there is particular concern, the practitioner may contact a defence union for advice.
   c. If in adults a decision is made to proceed, there should be a proper assessment of risk factors. Both patient and surgeon must understand the consequences of refusal (Editorial 1992). It has been suggested that an adult should also be interviewed alone at some point, without the presence of relatives or a minister.
   d. The anaesthetist must be involved at an early stage, so that he can discuss the options for treatment with the patient or his family. It is important to establish exactly what the individual is willing to accept (Dixon & Smalley 1981). In particular, the patient's views on albumin, haemophiliac factors, and autologous intraoperative transfusion must be absolutely clarified.
   e. Proper informed consent in the presence of a witness and if wished, a relative or adviser. A full explanation of the benefits of surgery, and the hazards if he refuses blood transfusion, must be undertaken. Consent or refusal should be witnessed and signed by a relative.
   f. If a patient is accepted for elective surgery, the physician must accept the individual's decision.

2. Preoperative preparation
   a. In advance of surgery, if autologus blood is accepted, it can be withdrawn and stored. For elective surgery, the patient's Hb and Hct may be improved by restoration of iron stores, nutritional support and, if acceptable to the patient, treatment with erythropoietin. There have been several reports of its use in anaemic patients requiring major elective surgery (Connor &

Olsson 1992, Atabek et al 1992). Seven weeks treatments with
r-HuEPO, 100 units/kg 2–3 times a week given to an adolescent
for scoliosis surgery improved the Hct from 39.5–47% and
increased the Hb by 2 g/dl (Rothstein et al 1990). Erythropoietin
was also used in a Jehovah's Witness with a Hb of 3.2 g/dl
following multiple trauma, to expedite weaning from mechanical
ventilation (Kraus & Lipman 1992). Hypertension and
thrombocythaemia may occur as side-effects of treatment.

b. Limit blood withdrawal after admission, by performing only
essential investigations, by the use of paediatric sample tubes,
and in the case of ITU patients by returning the flush from
arterial lines.

3. Methods of minimizing blood loss

a. Techniques that minimize surgical blood loss should be
employed. These include a meticulous surgical technique with
extensive use of diathermy, ligation of vessels before transection,
the use of sharp dissection, and dissection along anatomical
tissue planes (Spence et al 1990).

b. If blood losses of greater than 500 ml are anticipated, monitor the
CVP and replace losses with colloid as they occur.

c. Induced hypotension to 50–55 mmHg may be considered if a
blood loss of greater than 20% of the blood volume is
anticipated. Careful technique in 100 Jehovah's Witnesses undergoing total hip arthroplasty, 89 of whom had hypotensive
anaesthesia, showed a 43% reduction in blood loss when
compared with a control group of patients who were not
Jehovah's Witnesses and who had surgery under normotensive
anaesthesia (Nelson & Bowen 1986).

d. Haemodilution techniques with a glucose crystalloid prime were
used for cardiopulmonary bypass in surgery for congenital heart
disease in 110 children of Jehovah's Witnesses. Only one death
was attributed to blood loss (Henling et al 1985).

e. Acute hypervolaemic haemodilution at the start of surgery has
been used to achieve a moderate (20–25%) or low (<20%
haematocrit, so that any blood lost involved a reduced loss of
blood cells. Haemodilution to a Hct of 0.20 was induced in an
anaemic patient who required emergency surgery after full
invasive monitoring was established (Trouwborst et al 1990).
Dextran 40, 500 ml and Ringer's lactate 500 ml were infused on
two occasions over a period of 40 minutes and measurements
repeated each 15 min. During surgery, blood loss was replaced
by equal volumes of gelatin and Ringer's lactate, given as urine
volume plus 500 ml/h.

4. Methods of treating blood loss
   a. Use of plasma expanders or crystalloid to replace blood loss as it occurs.
   b. Blood substitutes. Fluosol (perfluorocarbon emulsion) may increase dissolved oxygen in the first 12 hours (Atabek et al 1992), but is probably of little use otherwise.

5. Use of patient's own blood in a continuous system
   a. Autotransfusion of blood collected just before surgery (Schaller et al 1983). Blood was removed and replaced with three times the volume of a balanced electrolyte solution. After most of the surgical blood loss had stopped, the blood was returned and frusemide given. Preoperative collection of whole anticoagulated blood, storage in a blood cell processor, and simultaneous reinfusion of saline and the collected blood at rates in relation to surgical requirements has also been reported (Lichtiger et al 1982). The processes, as described, are acceptable to many patients because the extracorporeal blood is always in continuity with the patient's circulation.
   b. Return of blood by intraoperative use of a cell saver and autotransfusion. In this case, a continuous circuit is made from the patient to the cell saver device and back to the patient. A dedicated line is 'piggybacked' from the autotransfusion device to the patient and kept open with a saline infusion via a three-way tap until enough blood is collected to transfuse. The three-way tap is then turned to re-establised flow. Again, this technique is acceptable to most Jehovah's Witnesses because the blood never leaves a continuous circuit with the body. In all haemodilution techniques there is the question of whether crystalloid or colloid should be used for dilution. A mixture may be appropriate.
6. Reducing oxygen requirements or maximizing oxygenation
   a. Oxygenation and IPPV.
   b. Hypothermia to reduce oxygen consumption, with simultaneous haemodilution. A patient with a Hct of 4%, was treated with hypothermia, isovolaemic haemodilution, muscular paralysis, IPPV and sedation for 4 hours whilst awaiting a court decision concerning transfusion (Lichtenstein et al 1988).
7. The prophylactic use of DDAVP, 0.3 μg/kg i.v. over 20 minutes has been suggested (Stone & DiFazio 1988). DDAVP may also correct vWF: Ag and platelet abnormalities after large infusions of colloids.
8. A blood patch was performed in a patient with a postspinal headache, using manometer tubing, a three way tap and a syringe, so that no continuity of blood was lost (Tyers 1988).

BIBLIOGRAPHY
Atabek U, Spence R K, Pello M et al 1992 Pancreaticoduodenectomy without homologous blood transfusion in an anemic Jehovah's Witness. Archives of Surgery 127: 349–351

Blajchman M A 1991 Transfusion-related issues in Jehovah's Witness patients. Transfusion Medicine Review 5: 243–246

Benson K T 1989 The Jehovah's Witness patient: considerations for the anesthesiologist. Anesthesia and Analgesia 69: 647–656

Brahams D 1989 Jehovah's Witness transfused without consent: a Canadian case. Lancet 2: 1407–1408

Connor J P, Olsson C A 1992 The use of recombinant human erythropoietin in a Jehovah's Witness requiring major reconstructive surgery. Journal of Urology 147: 131–132

Dixon J L, Smalley M G 1981 Jehovah's witnesses. The surgical/etnical challenge. Journal of the American Medical Association 246: 2471–2472

Editorial 1992 When a patient says no. Lancet 340: 345

Henderson A M, Maryniak J K, Simpson J C 1986 Cardiac surgery in Jehovah's Witnesses. A review of 36 cases. Anaesthesia 41: 748–753

Henling C E, Carmichael M J, Keats A S et al 1985 Cardiac operation for congenital heart disease in children of Jehovah's Witnesses. Journal of Thoracic and Cardiovascular Surgery 89: 914–920

Kraus P, Lipman J 1992 Erythropoietin in a patient following multiple trauma. Anaesthesia 47: 962–964

Layon A J, D'Amico R, Caton D et al 1990 And the patient chose: medical ethics and the case of the Jehovah's Witness. Anaesthesiology 73: 1258–1262

Lichtenstein A. Eckhart W F, Swanson K J et al 1988 Unplanned intraoperative and postoperative hemodilution: oxygen transport and consumption during severe anemia. Anesthesiology 69: 119–122

Lichtiger B, Dupuis J F, Seski J 1982 Hemotherapy during surgery for Jehovah's Witnesses: a new method. Anaesthesia and Analgesia 61: 618–619

Lockwood D N, Bullen C, Machin S J 1988 A severe coagulopathy following volume replacement with hydroxyethyl starch. Anaesthesia 43: 391–393

Medical Defence Union 1989 Consent to Treatment. Medical Defence Union, London

Nelson C L, Bowen W S 1986 Total hip arthroplasty in Jehovah's Witnesses without blood transfusion. Journal of Bone and Joint Surgery 68: 350–353

Ott D A, Cooley D A 1977 Cardiovascular surgery in Jehovah's Witnesses. Report of 542 operations without blood transfusion. Journal of the American Medical Association 238: 1256–1258

Panchal H I, Ramwell J, Lawler P G 1989 Severe coagulopathy in Jehovah's witness Anaesthesia 44: 71–72

Rothstein P, Roye D, Verdisco L et al 1990 Preperative use of erythropoietin in an adolescent Jehovah's witness. Anesthesiology 73: 568–570

Schaller R T, Sehaller J, Morgan A et al 1983 Hemodilution anesthesia: a valuable aid to major cancer surgery in children. American Journal of Surgery 146: 79–84

Spence R K, Carson J A, Poses R et al 1990 Elective surgery without transfusion: influence of preoperative hemoglobin level and blood loss on mortality. American Journal of Surgery 159: 320–324

Stone D J, DiFazio C A 1988 DDAVP to reduce blood loss in Jehovah's Witnesses. Anesthesiology 69: 1028

Sugarman J, Churchill L R, Moore J K et al 1991 Medical, ethical and legal issues regarding thrombolytic therapy in the Jehovah's Witness. American Journal of Cardiology 68: 1525–1529

Trouwborst A, Hagenouw R R P M, Jeekel J et al 1990 Hypervolaemic haemodilution in an anaemic Jehovah's witness. British Journal of Anaesthesia 64: 646–648

Tyers M 1988 Blood patch in a Jehovah's witness. Anaesthesia and Intensive Care 16: 127–128

Wong D H W, Jenkins L C 1989 Surgery in Jehovah's Witnesses. Canadian Journal of Anaesthesia 36: 578–585

MANAGEMENT OF PATIENTS WITH CERVICAL SPINE INJURY

The non-neurosurgical anaesthetist may be involved in the transport or emergency management of patients with potential or actual cervical spine injury. It is therefore important that the general principles and problems are understood, since poor management at this stage may result in neurological deterioration. Over the last few years there has been lively debate in the anaesthetic and trauma literature about the optimum method of achieving airway control in the patient with cervical spine injury. The resolution of this debate is not assisted by the difficulties of performing prospective, controlled clinical trials.

Section 3

Management of
Patients with Cervical
Spine Injury

The cervical spine can be considered to be composed of three major supporting columns: an anterior, middle and posterior column. Disruption of ligaments and bone in any two of these will result in cervical instability and a risk of spinal cord damage (Crosby & Lui 1990). Initial management is directed towards the early diagnosis of neck injuries, and the prevention of any extension of existing neurological damage which might occur during transport or emergency airway control.

Problems

1. Neurological
   Vertebral fractures, dislocations, or subluxations may result in damage to the spinal cord and loss of neuronal conduction, with flaccid paralysis and loss of reflexes below the level of injury. The possibility exists of further neurological deterioration during treatment. Factors likely to be associated with this are:
   a. Severity of the original injury.
   b. Damage during transport.
   c. Failure to make an early diagnosis. Cervical X-rays may have been misread or misinterpreted, or even not performed.
   d. Overdistraction of the neck by either manual or mechanical in-line traction.
   e. Movement during cricoid pressure.
   f. Movement during tracheal intubation.
2. Airway problems
   Avoidance of hypoxaemia and hypercapnoea may mean that tracheal intubation is required. There is a risk that primary airway management, or intubation for emergency surgery, may be associated with neurological deterioration secondary to subluxation or distraction of the vertebrae. As a result, the profession is divided about the safest method of intubation. There are individual proponents of conventional orotracheal, blind nasotracheal, and awake fibreoptic intubation.
3. Cardiovascular
   a. At the time of the initial injury there is intense sympathetic activity with hypertension, bradycardia and arrhythmias.
   b. Spinal shock occurs within minutes and can last from hours to weeks. This is a state of hypotension with decreased systemic

vascular resistance and increased venous capacitance associated with venous pooling.

c. For lesions above T5 level, severe bradycardia and hypotension with or without cardiac dysfunction occur, because of interruption to the sympathetic outflow to the heart. The absence of tachycardia means that signs of hypovolaemia from blood loss may be missed, although the tachycardia in response to hypoxaemia or hypercarbia may still be present.

d. The subsequent return of reflex activity below the level of the lesion may be associated with autonomic hyper-reflexia.

4. Respiratory

a. Lesions above the innervation of the diaphragm (C4/C5) cause complete diaphragmatic paralysis and death often takes place before hospital admission.

b. Lesions below C6 are variable, and dependent upon the degree of involvement of intercostal or abdominal muscles. There is a decrease in all respiratory volumes, with hypoventilation and hypercapnoea, an inability to cough, atelectasis, and pneumonia. Occasionally, neurogenic pulmonary oedema may occur.

5. Gastrointestinal
Paralytic ileus may develop.

6. Body temperature
Thermal regulation may be disturbed and the patient becomes poikilothermic.

7. Neuromuscular changes
Denervation sensitivity starts at about 48 hours, after which suxamethonium should be avoided.

8. Blood sugar
Pre-existing hyperglycaemia has been shown to intensify subsequent ischaemic injury to the spinal cord in experimental animals, possibly secondary to lactic acidosis (Drummond & Moore 1989).

9. Anaesthesia
Anaesthesia may be required for:
a. Decompression.
b. Reduction and stabilization.
c. Incidental surgery.

Management

The key to management is the care of the patient in the early stages, when neurological deterioration is likely to occur. Suspicion of cervical trauma, and immobilization of the neck until it can be excluded, is crucial. The improvements in morbidity and mortality over the last 20 years have been attributed to better care at the site of the injury and during transport (Crosby 1992). The advent of Advanced Trauma Life Support courses from America has improved awareness and management, but the absence of the anaesthetist as a member of the team has decreased its relevance to the situation in the UK (Bennett et al 1992, Wood & Lawler 1992).

1. Clinical assessment (Meschino et al 1992)
   a. Sunnybrook cord injury scale
      Grade 1   Complete motor loss; complete sensory loss.
      Grade 2   Complete motor loss; incomplete sensory loss.
      Grade 3   Incomplete motor useless; complete sensory loss.
      Grade 4   Incomplete motor useless; incomplete sensory loss.
      Grade 5   Incomplete motor useless; normal sensory.
      Grade 6   Incomplete motor useful; complete sensory loss.
      Grade 7   Incomplete motor useful; incomplete sensory loss.
      Grade 8   Incomplete motor useful; normal sensory.
      Grade 9   Normal motor; incomplete sensory loss.
      Grade 10 Normal motor; normal sensory.
2. Radiological assessment by:
   a. Odontoid views.
   b. AP and lateral cervical views.
   c. Occasionally may require CT scan.
3. Immobilization of neck either by mechanical or manual means.
4. Careful transport.
5. Airway management may be required for:
   a. Surgery.
   b. Airway protection.
   c. Respiratory problems.
   d. Tracheobronchial toilet.
6. Alternative methods of managing the airway have included:
   a. Orotracheal intubation under general anaesthesia.
   b. Nasotracheal intubation under general anaesthesia.
   c. Fibreoptic intubation either awake or asleep, either via the oral or the nasal route.
   d. Laryngeal mask airway.
   e. Bullard laryngoscope.
   f. Retrograde intubation.
   g. Cricothyroidotomy.
7. Anaesthesia in a patient with a cervical spine injury. The main controversy surrounds the conduct of tracheal intubation. Previous fears that manipulation of the neck under general anaesthesia might be responsible for neurological deterioration are now being questioned. A retrospective review of 150 patients for elective stabilization of the neck did not show any differences between the group whose tracheas were intubated after general anaesthesia (55%) and those intubated awake (45%) (Suderman et al 1991). Another comparison between 165 patients undergoing awake tracheal intubation within 2 months of injury and 298 who remained unintubated within that period did not reveal any

significant differences in neurological deterioration (Meschino et al 1992). These authors therefore concluded that awake intubation was a safe method of airway management in patients with cervical spine injury.

Retrospective reports such as these have inherent defects as scientific papers. The numbers involved are relatively small and for obvious reasons randomization cannot take place. However, in a review by the Cervical Spine Research Society of 5356 major cervical spinal procedures, the overall incidence of neurological complications was 1.04% and none were presumed to be related to intubation (Graham 1989).

One advantage of an awake technique is that following intubation the patient can be examined to ascertain that no new neurological deficit has developed. However, fibreoptic intubation is unsuitable for the unconscious or uncooperative patient. Experience of the operator should also be taken into account. A badly performed awake intubation may cause more movement of an unstable spine than a carefully performed one under general anaesthesia.

If general anaesthesia is undertaken, several authors have advised careful oral intubation with manual in-line axial traction, without extension of the neck (Doolan & O'Brien 1985) and with a second assistant applying cricoid pressure (Grande et al 1988). However, it has been pointed out that the exact definition of manual in-line traction is lacking (Wood & Lawler 1992). Any type of traction should be limited to 20–25 kg and applied gradually. The use of two sandbags and 3-inch forehead tape is also an effective method of stabilization and limitation of movement during tracheal intubation. It has been shown that the normal orotracheal position actually provides reasonable stability in the lower cervical spine (Horton et al 1989).

Although blind nasal intubation has been suggested, the technique requires flexion and extension of the neck, together with anterior neck pressure. Since these manoeuvres create substantial movement of the cervical vertebrae, it is a totally unsuitable method. In addition, nasal bleeding may be a problem and death has followed failure to intubate.

The consensus of opinion is that no clear evidence exists to show that awake fibreoptic intubation is better than conventional orotracheal intubation. It is probable that the actual method used is less important than the care with which it is performed (Crosby 1992). Decisions about management must be based on the individual patient and the experience of the operator in a particular technique.

8. Dextrose-containing solutions should be avoided and the blood sugar kept at less than 17 mmol/l with insulin.

BIBLIOGRAPHY
Bennett J R, Bodenham A R, Berridge J C 1992 Advanced trauma life support. A time for reappraisal. Anaesthesia 47: 798–800
Crosby E T, Lui A 1990 The adult spine: implications for airway management. Canadian Journal of Anaesthesia 37: 77–93
Crosby E T 1992 Tracheal intubation in the cervical-spine injured patient. Canadian Journal of Anaesthesia 39: 105–109
Doolan L A, O'Brien J F: 1985 Safe intubation in cervical spine injury. Anaesthesia and Intensive Care 13: 319–324
Drummond J C, Moore S S 1989 The influence of dextrose administration on neurologic outcome after temporary spinal cord ischemia in the rabbit. Anesthesiology 70: 64–70
Graham J J 1989 Complications of cervical spine surgery. A five year report on a survey of the membership of the Cervical Spine Research Society. Spine 14: 1046–1050
Grande C M, Barton C R, Stene J K 1988 Appropriate techniques for airway management of emergency patients with suspected spinal cord injury Anesthesia and Analgesia 67: 714–715
Hastings R H, Marks J D 1991 Airway management for trauma patients with potential cervical spine injury. Anesthesia and Analgesia 73: 471–482
Horton W A, Fahy L, Charters P 1989 Disposition of cervical vertebrae, atlanto-axial joint, hyoid and mandible during X-ray laryngoscopy. British Journal of Anaesthesia 63: 435–438
Lam A M 1991 Acute spinal cord injury: monitoring and anaesthetic implications. Canadian Journal of Anaesthesia 38: R60–R70
Meschino A, Devitt J H, Koch J-P et al 1992 The safety of awake tracheal intubation in cervical spine injury Canadian Journal of Anaesthesia 39: 114–117
Suderman V S, Crosby E T, Lui A 1991 Elective oral tracheal intubation in cervical spine-injured adults. Canadian Journal of Anaesthesia 38: 785–789
Wood P R, Lawler P G P 1992 Managing the airway in cervical spine injury. A review of the Advanced Trauma Life Support protocol. Anaesthesia 47: 792–797

Section 3

Management and Training for Awake Fibreoptic Intubation

MANAGEMENT AND TRAINING FOR AWAKE FIBREOPTIC INTUBATION

The problems of training in fibreoptic bronchoscopy and awake fibreoptic intubation are well known (Mason 1992). The following are guidelines used by the author for teaching, and are regularly updated. Training is undertaken using a graduated method. The novice is first instructed in the prediction of difficult intubation, the components of sedation, local anaesthesia, bronchoscopic visualization of the larynx, passage of the tracheal tube, reasons for failure, and indications and contraindications to awake intubation.

Instruction in the handling and manipulation of the bronchoscope is paramount, and the trainee must become familiar with these aspects first of all. After this, practice is undertaken on an airway training model. Only then is the trainee allocated to the diagnostic bronchoscopy list where he is instructed in sedation, local anaesthesia, and passage of the bronchoscope on a patient.

Awake fibreoptic intubation in a patient with intubation problems must only be undertaken under the supervision of an experienced person. Even for the experienced bronchoscopist, there are considerable advantages in the presence of a second anaesthetist. In addition, it is not simply a technical procedure and requires considerable judgement as well as technical skill. Awake fibreoptic bronchoscopy is not necessarily the answer to every airway problem and in some patients there may be contraindications to its use.

The fibreoptic bronchoscope

This is a delicate instrument consisting of insulated glass fibres bound into a flexible bundle. In addition, there is a light guide cable, a working channel which is used for suction, local anaesthetic or oxygen insufflation, and angulation wires to allow movement of the tip in an anterior-posterior plane. Actual specifications such as length, diameter and tip angulation can vary. Those designed for intubation tend to be longer (600 mm compared with 550 mm), of smaller diameter (4 mm or 2.5 mm compared with 6 mm) and possess lesser degrees of tip deflection and hence field of view (75° compared with 90–120°) than diagnostic bronchoscopes.

Indications

1. Previous difficult or failed intubation as a result of 'structural' abnormality, but with a normal airway, e.g. receding lower jaw, rigid neck, ankylosing spondylitis, trismus, etc.
2. Patients predicted, at the preoperative visit, as being potentially difficult to intubate. (A combination of a modified Mallampati test class III or IV – (no posterior pharyngeal wall seen behind the soft palate) plus a thyromental distance of less than 7 cm (Frerk 1991).
3. Risk of damage to teeth or dental work.

   Additional uses have been suggested, such as in patients at high risk from gastric aspiration and those with upper airway obstruction from epiglottitis and upper airway tumours. However, these indications are controversial and certainly not suitable conditions for the inexperienced bronchoscopist. It is quite possible for a patient to inhale whilst awake, even when the local anaesthetic is not applied until the bronchoscope is ready to be inserted through the vocal cords. It is also inadvisable to use the technique in critical upper airway obstruction, since it is possible to precipitate complete airway obstruction from laryngeal spasm, bleeding or dislodged tumour fragments. Under these circumstances, tracheostomy under local anaesthesia, or an inhalational induction with an ENT surgeon present, are safer techniques.

Other uses

1. Airway evaluation.
2. Checking or changing a tracheal tube.
3. Tracheobronchial toilet.

4. Placement of a double-lumen bronchial tube.
5. Placement or checking of a nasogastric tube.

Premedication

Patients who have experienced previous failed intubation are usually extremely apprehensive about the succeeding anaesthetic. It is imperative that their first experience of awake fibreoptic intubation is as atraumatic as possible. This anaesthetist therefore carries a considerable burden of responsibility. An unpleasant experience may lead to subsequent refusal to undergo an awake procedure. An inexperienced bronchoscopist should not therefore undertake this unsupervised. Unless there is some contraindication, an effective premedication should be given. In all patients a drying agent should be used since excess secretions prevent satisfactory mucosal anaesthesia.

Equipment

1. Fibreoptic bronchoscope, adapter, light source, suction, saline, swabs.
2. Midazolam 10 mg diluted to 1 mg/ml.
3. 10% lignocaine spray with nozzle.
4. Topical lignocaine 4%, 3 ml diluted up to 5 ml.
5. Cotton wool buds, galley pot.
6. ECG, oximeter, MC oxygen mask.
7. Green needle, mediswabs.

Monitoring

1. ECG.
2. Pulse oximeter.

Sedation

1. Dilute midazolam 10 mg up to 10 ml with saline.
2. Give 2–2.5 mg depending on age and fitness.

Local anaesthesia method I (patient sitting up at 45°)
This technique is suitable for diagnostic bronchoscopy and for the novice, because cricothyroid puncture probably gives the best local anaesthesia below the level of the vocal cords. When the operator is experienced, he may prefer method II, the 'spray as you go' technique.

1. Anaesthetize the tip of the tongue with a single spray of lignocaine 10%. Then grasp the tip with a swab and give 5–6 sprays of lignocaine to the back of tongue and pharynx using a long, plastic (or metal) nozzle, with its tip bent slightly downwards. Pause for 20 seconds and repeat, advancing the nozzle.

2. Dip two cotton wool buds in lignocaine 4% from galley pot and insert one into each nostril, along the floor of the nose. Select the more patent nostril of the two and insert a second swab. Leave in place.

3. Perform a cricothyroid puncture with the patient's head fully extended by the assistant. Feel the thyroid cartilage and the cricothyroid membrane below it. Place index and middle fingers vertically on either side of the membrane. Insert a 21–G needle mounted on a syringe containing lignocaine (4% topical lignocaine 3 ml diluted further with 2 ml saline) through the membrane and aspirate. If air is withdrawn, inject 1 ml solution and quickly withdraw the needle. Wait for 20 seconds and repeat, using 2 ml on the next occasion. The last 2 ml is reserved for use down the bronchoscope, if necessary.

4. Lie the patient flat, secure eye pads and remove the nasal swabs. Gently introduce a Mackintosh laryngoscope. Suck out any secretions and give 2–3 more sprays of lignocaine 10% directly onto the vocal cords.

5. If necessary, give additional midazolam 1–2.5 mg. Administer oxygen through the mouth via an MG mask.

Local anaesthetic method II
Instead of using cricothyroid puncture, use a 'spray as you go' technique down the side channel of the bronchoscope, having ensured that the suction is turned off.

Local anaesthetic method III
If there is some contraindication to cricothyroid puncture, lignocaine 4% can be given in advance, using a nebulizer. However, this takes about 20–30 minutes and its duration of action is quite short. Timing therefore has to be meticulous. In addition, the anaesthesia produced is much less reliable than in methods I and II.

Put 3 ml 4% topical lignocaine into the nebulizer and nebulize with oxygen until the nebulizer is empty (20–30 minutes).

Bronchoscopy technique

1. Remove the pillow and extend the neck. This opens up the airspace around the glottis.

2. Focus the bronchoscope on a printed document (if the diagnostic bronchoscope is being used, check that the brake is not applied).

3. Gently check the movement of the tip.

4. Lubricate the insertion cord and tip generously and hold the distal end of the bronchoscope in a swab. Ensure that there is no twist on the light source cable.

5. Insert the bronchoscope into the more patent nostril, standing back so that the bronchoscope is not bent. Negotiate the tip along the

floor of the nose below the inferior turbinate under direct vision, steering as you go. Do not push when the scope is up against mucosa otherwise bleeding will result. Follow the dark triangular slit of the nasal passage, rotating, flexing or extending the tip of the bronchoscope gently, but exerting fairly firm pressure. A definite 'give' is felt as you pass from the nose into the pharynx. This is probably the most uncomfortable part of the whole manoeuvre and the patient may wince or complain. However, I have not yet encountered any patient who could subsequently recall any part of the procedure. If the nasal passages are exceptionally tight, this approach may have to be abandoned in favour of the oral route, particularly if the bronchoscopy is being performed as part of a nasal intubation technique.

6. At this stage the bronchoscope is in the pharynx and the vocal cords may be seen in the distance. However, in some patients, particularly the obese, redundant mucosa may make visualization of recognizable structures difficult simply because of lack of airspace. Under such circumstances the scope is advanced gently under direct vision, until it is inserted about 12 cm. The area is re-inspected by gently flexing and extending the tip, then rotating it in both directions, followed by flexion and extension until an identifiable structure appears.

7. There is usually no doubt when the epiglottis and vocal cords come into view. However, if vague curves that resemble glottic structures are repeatedly seen, the scope is probably in one or other pyriform fossa, usually the right. Rotation of the scope to the left will finally allow identification of the epiglottis. The fibrescope is advanced underneath and through the vocal cords. This may be difficult if the epiglottis is overhanging. If necessary, ask the patient to take a deep breath which will maximally abduct the cords. Loss of vision before entering the cords is probably due to impaction of the scope on the front of the epiglottis. Withdrawal a short distance will restore the view. When insertion is successful, the tracheal rings and then the carina will be seen. Sometimes at this stage there is a 'red-out' and the scope cannot be advanced further. This is usually because it is impacted on the anterior tracheal wall, (in which case the light can be seen through the skin of the neck). The tip should be lowered a little before advancing the instrument.

Common difficulties

The most difficult part is to learn to handle and manipulate the bronchoscope. However, much can be learned by practice on an airway training model, long before the first patient is encountered. Try 20 insertions on the model down each nostril. It is more difficult to pass the bronchoscope on the model than it is on an actual patient because it tends to adhere to the rubber of the manikin. This occurs even when antistatic lubricant is used. Do not become disheartened, patients are much easier!

Remember that there are three components involved in fibreoptic bronchoscopy. The secret is continuously to remind yourself of these three components and at all times to steer the bronchoscope to maintain your target exactly in the centre of the field of view.

1. Flexion or extension, using the tip bending lever, to move the scope anteriorly or posteriorly.
2. Rotation of the scope, followed by flexion or extension, to move it laterally. If your target is off to the left, then rotate your hand to the left (anticlockwise) and vice versa. This is the most difficult manoeuvre for the trainee to learn and is the most important when dealing with a difficult intubation, when the vocal cords may not be in the midline. Rotation should be a wrist not a shoulder movement and should primarily involve rotation of the scope handle, but with assistance from the hand holding the tip, which should follow the movement simultaneously. Use the arrow on the eyepiece to check that you are actually rotating the instrument and also to assist with orientation. Thus, if the cords are situated at 10 o'clock, rotate the handle so that the arrow points towards your target and then move the control lever to flex or extend the tip appropriately.

    There is a tendency for a right-handed bias. Right-handed operators most commonly end up with the bronchoscope in the right pyriform fossa. This is because they tend to insert it with their right hand rotated with a slight bias to the right. Make a deliberate effort to straighten the wrist.
3. Forward movement. In an anxiety to achieve the other two movements, novices frequently forget to actually advance the bronchoscope. There is no point in searching for the glottis when the scope is only 5–10 cm beyond the nares. Under direct vision gently push it down to 12 cm, then look for landmarks.

Helpful tips

1. Topical local anaesthesia does not work well if there are a lot of secretions. A drying agent is therefore an important part of the technique.
2. The distance between the nares and the epiglottis in an adult is about 15 cm (check the distances of the markings on the bronchoscope first of all). Markings vary with the design of bronchoscope; they may be at 5-cm intervals from the tip, at 5-cm intervals from the 15-cm mark, or from the 20-cm mark. If you are much beyond 15 cm, the scope is likely to be in the oesophagus. If not, advance under direct vision to 12 cm and look again.
3. 'Red out'. The scope is abutting the mucosa or there is blood on the lens. First slightly withdraw the tip from the mucosa and vision

should be restored. If not, suck out any blood. Remember that to be able to see, you need an air space.

4. 'White out'. Caused by secretions. Suck out, but if the mucus is adherent, withdraw the scope and clean the end.
5. Whenever suction is performed, always advance and retract the tip a little as you do it, so that you are aspirating secretions rather than sucking up, and hence traumatizing, the mucosa.
6. If the vocal cords keep appearing and disappearing, the patient is usually talking, swallowing or coughing. A little more local anaesthetic may need to be applied to the vocal cords, but turn off the suction before injecting it via the working channel, and then inject some air to clear the dead space. Keep the syringe in place until the patient has stopped coughing, so that the anaesthetic is not coughed straight out.

Section 3

Management and Training for Awake Fibreoptic Intubation

Awake intubation

Decide on your route of intubation. Nasal is easier than oral. Choose a small tracheal tube (6.0 mm for women, 6.5 or 7.0 mm for men) so that you do not have the embarrassment of passing the scope into the trachea but failing to pass the tube through the nose. Mount the tube on the bronchoscope before starting and tape it in place. When the bronchoscope is above the carina, lubricate the tube well and pass it over the scope through the vocal cords. If there is difficulty in the passage through the glottis, rotate the tube anticlockwise through 90° and ask the patient to take a deep breath. When the tube is in the trachea, inflate the cuff, remove the bronchoscope and connect to a Bain system to check movement of the reservoir bag.

If you select the oral route, it is easier to pass the fibrescope through a Berman (or equivalent) airway which is designed specially for the purpose. This stops the patient biting the bronchoscope, prevents the tongue from interfering with insertion, and if the airway needs to be removed it can be split down the side. However, problems may be encountered with this technique if the glottis is not centrally placed, as may be the case in a patient with a difficult intubation.

Finally, before you embark on an awake intubation, check that you have all the drugs and equipment ready for induction of anaesthesia once the tube is securely in place.

At the end of surgery, do not remove the tracheal tube until you are certain that the patient is awake. The onset of laryngeal spasm at this stage in a patient with a difficult airway is a hazardous situation to manage. Nasotracheal intubation has particular advantages when it comes to tube removal; patients tolerate its presence for much longer than they would an orotracheal tube.

BIBLIOGRAPHY
Frerk C M 1991 Predicting difficult intubation. Anaesthesia 46: 1005–1008

Mason R A 1992 Learning fibreoptic intubation: fundamental problems. Anaesthesia 47: 729–731

Middleton R M, Shah A, Kirkpatrick M B 1991 Topical nasal anesthesia for flexible fiberoptic bronchoscopy – a comparison of four methods in normal subjects and in patients undergoing transnasal bronchoscopy. Chest 99: 1093–1096

Ovasapian A 1990 Fiberoptic airway endoscopy in anesthesia and critical care. Raen Press, New York

Section 3

Anaesthesia for
Laser surgery of the
Airway (Light
Amplification by
Stimulated Emission
of Radiation)

ANAESTHESIA FOR LASER SURGERY OF THE AIRWAY
(LIGHT AMPLIFICATION BY STIMULATED EMISSION OF RADIATION)

Anaesthesia for laser surgery of the airway may constitute a formidable challenge for the anaesthetist, both from the point of view of sharing the airway with the surgeon, and from the various potential hazards of fire and tracheal tube ignition from the laser beam. Increasing experience with the technique and the development of new techniques and tracheal tubes has improved the safety aspects, but the importance of adequate training of staff must be emphasized. Fewer complications were found to occur when surgeons had attended a course on the use of the laser (Ossoff 1989).

Problems

1. Fire hazards. Although they are rare events, airway fires and tracheal tube combustion have occasionally resulted in serious burns to a patient. Ignition of a foil-wrapped PVC tube resulted in extensive injury to lung parenchyma and the airway, necessitating tracheostomy and IPPV (Cozine et al 1981). The type of fire generated, and the resultant damage, will depend upon a number of factors. These include whether ignition originates from the outside or from the unprotected inside of the tube (Hirshman & Smith 1980), the nature of the material ignited, whether or not the gases support combustion, and the nature of any toxic products of the combustion. Fires from the outside will damage the tube, but if they burn through to the inside of the tube, then heat and toxic effects of the products of combustion may damage the lungs. The polyvinyl chloride tube is more easily ignited and penetrated by CO_2 lasers than red rubber tubes, and produces more toxic products of combustion, and a carboniferous debris (Patel & Hicks 1981). In laboratory trials of three types of tube, PVC tubes ignited during shuttered mode trials, and both Xomed Laser-Shield and Rusch red rubber tubes ignited during continuous mode trials (Ossoff 1989). It was recommended that PVC tubes should not be used, even wrapped, and that Xomed Laser-Shield and red rubber tubes should be wrapped if used for microlaryngeal laser surgery.

2. Gaseous combustion. Oxygen and nitrous oxide both support combustion. If the tracheal cuff bursts, it allows spread of fire onto the operative site. Helium 60% retards tube fires, and oxygen 30% in helium was found to be the safest anaesthetic gas mixture (Pashayan & Gravenstein 1985). Halothane 2% could be added without increasing the risks.

3. Ignition of cottonoids, if they are permitted to dry out.
4. Ignition of the surgical drapes by a misdirected beam.
5. Laser damage to eyes of patients or staff.
6. Laser damage to skin of patients or staff.
7. Hazards of misdirection of energy, by incorrect focusing or direction of the beam, perforation of tissues and beam reflection, perforation of a vessel, or a gas embolism.
8. The use of a Venturi or jet ventilation technique may be associated with barotrauma, particularly in the presence of obesity, a large obstructing upper airway lesion, or reduced pulmonary or thoracic compliance. Location of the orifice of the needle below the vocal cords increases the potential of trauma. Pneumothorax, pneumomediastinum and surgical emphysema have all been reported. A fire occurred during supraglottic jet ventilation when a misdirected laser beam ignited the surgeon's gloves and the burning vapours were entrained by the Venturi (Wegrzynowicz et al 1992). Both patient and surgeon sustained burns.
9. Potential of transfer of virus or bacterial particles from infected tissue in laser smoke plumes (Hallmo & Naess 1991).

Management and safety aspects

1. General safety, for protection of staff and patient
   a. Access to theatre limited and the doors closed.
   b. Warning notices placed on theatre doors.
   c. Protective goggles with side pieces for all staff.
   d. Patient's eyes taped shut and eye pads soaked in saline, or metal shields placed on top of the tape.
   e. Exposed skin and mucous membranes covered with saline soaked towels or sponges. Towels should be kept wet during the procedure. Teeth must be protected.
   f. Two suction apparatuses are required for the surgeon: one, which should have an in-line filter, for aspiration of smoke and steam from the laser; the second for aspirating blood and mucus.
   g. The microlaryngoscope should be of wide bore, with non-reflective surface.
   h. Avoidance of vaporization of tissue below the tip of the tube, to prevent indirect fires.
2. Administration of anaesthesia
   a. Tracheal tube techniques
      i. Externally protected tubes. Red rubber tubes are more resistant

Section 3

Anaesthesia for
Laser surgery of the
Airway (Light
Amplification by
Stimulated Emission
of Radiation)

Section 3

Anaesthesia for
Laser surgery of the
Airway (Light
Amplification by
Stimulated Emission
of Radiation)

to ignition than are polyvinyl chloride tubes, provided they are wrapped with reflective metal tape. To apply the metal foil, wipe the tube with an alcoholic solution, then spirally wrap it with the foil, allowing a 30% overlap, and beginning at the junction of the tube with the proximal part of the cuff. No bare areas should be left through which the tube might be ignited, and wrinkles which might abraid the trachea should be avoided (Rampil 1992). Silicone tubes are also less ignitable than PVC ones, but they produce white silica ash if they burn (Ossoff et al 1983) and should also be wrapped (Ossoff 1989).

ii. Special tubes. These include flexible stainless steel tubes, without cuffs (Oswal-Hunton; Hunton & Oswal 1985), silicone tubes with an outer coating of metallic oxide (Xomed Laser-Shield) and stainless steel spiral tubs with two distal cuffs to be filled with saline (Mallinkrodt Laser-Flex).

b. Protection of the cuff from perforation

i. Fill with saline, coloured with methylene blue. The saline acts as a heat sink and the methylene blue will indicate if the cuff has burst.

ii. Keep the cuff as distal as possible, so that it is not within the view of the operator.

iii. Protect cuff with saline-soaked cotton swabs.

iv. Count the swabs and keep them moist.

c. 'Tubeless' techniques

i. Use of 'jet' ventilation techniques. The advantages of dispensing with a tube must be balanced against the possibility of barotrauma to the lungs, the inhalation of debris, gastric distension, and regurgitation (O'Sullivan & Healy 1985). Expiration must not be obstructed even for a few seconds and the technique should be avoided in the obese, those with poor lung compliance, or where the laryngeal lesions are large and potentially obstructing. Adequate neuromuscular blockade is essential to prevent laryngeal spasm. For infants, the use of a metal-wrapped, triple-lumen, central venous catheter has been described. Ventilation was with an impulse ventilator (Model 303 Healthdyne) and airway pressure was monitored through the middle catheter lumen (Dhara & Butler 1992). Increase in pressure above a preset level will inhibit the ventilator.

ii. Apnoeic anaesthesia. Inhalational or intravenous induction and neuromuscular blockers is followed by insertion of a PVC tube; inhalation agents are added. When the operating laryngoscope is in place, the PVC tube is removed and the laser is applied, allowing up to 2 minutes of apnoea at a time

(Hawkins & Joseph 1990). The tube is replaced between each laser application. Pulse oximetry must be used.

d. Anaesthetic gases

i. Should be non-flammable.

ii. Limit oxygen concentration to 40% maximum.

iii. Avoid nitrous oxide if possible.

iv. Mixture of O_2 30% with helium is the safest.

e. Management of an airway fire

i. Remove the source of fire.

ii. Disconnect gases to stop enrichment of the fire.

iii. Extinguish flames with bucket of water. Flush operative area with sterile water or saline.

iv. Once the fire is extinguished, ventilate the lungs with a mask and oxygen, and continue the anaesthetic. Insert a new tube.

v. Laryngoscopy and bronchoscopy are performed to assess any damage. Look out for foreign bodies and if necessary wash the airways.

vi. Examine the more distal airways for damage.

vii. If damage is serious, consider tracheostomy.

viii. Inspect the face and mouth for damage.

ix. CXR for evidence of smoke inhalation injury, or hydrochloric acid damage if a PVC tube has ignited.

x. A short course of high-dose steroids has been recommended. Humidification, antibiotics, IPPV, and monitoring may be required, depending upon the extent of the injury (van der Spek et al 1988).

Section 3

Anaesthesia for
Laser surgery of the
Airway (Light
Amplification by
Stimulated Emission
of Radiation)

BIBLIOGRAPHY

Cozine K, Rosenbaum L M, Askanazi J et al 1981 Laser-induced endotracheal tube fire. Anesthesiology 55: 583–585

Dhara S S, Butler P J 1992 High frequency jet ventilation for microlaryngeal laser surgery. Anaesthesia 47: 421–424

Hallmo P, Naess O 1991 Laryngeal papillomatosis with human papillomavirus DNA contracted by a laser surgeon. European Archives of Otolarynology 248: 425–427

Hawkins D B, Jospeh M M 1990 Avoiding wrapped endotracheal tubes in laser laryngeal surgery: experiences with apneic anesthesia and metal Laser Flex endotracheal tubes. Laryngoscope 100: 1283–1287

Hirshman C A, Smith J 1980 Indirect ignition of the endotracheal tube during carbon dioxide laser surgery. Archives of Otolaryngology 106: 639–641

Hunton J, Oswal V H 1985 Metal tube anaesthesia for ear, nose and throat carbon dioxide laser surgery. Anaesthesia 40: 1210–1212

Johans T G, Reichert T J 1984 An insufflation device for anesthesia during subglottic carbon dioxide laser microsurgery in children. Anesthesia and Analgesia 63: 368–370

Ossoff R H, Eisenman T S, Duncavage J A et al 1983 Comparison of tracheal damage from laser-ignited endotracheal tube fire. Annals of Otology, Rhinology and Laryngology 92: 333–336

Ossoff R H 1989 Laser safety in otolaryngology, head and neck surgery: anesthetic and educational considerations for laryngeal surgery. Larynogscope 99 (suppl 48) 1–26

O'Sullivan T J, Healy G B 1985 Complications of Venturi jet ventilation during microlaryngeal surgery. Archives of Otolaryngology 111: 127–131

Paes M L 1987 General anaesthesia for carbon dioxide laser surgery within the airway. A review British Journal of Anaesthesia 59: 1610–1620

Pashayan A G, Gravenstein J S 1985 Helium retards endotracheal tube fires from carbon dioxide lasers. Anesthesiology 62: 274–277

Patel K F, Hicks J N 1981 Fire hazards associated with the use of carbon dioxide lasers. Anesthesia and Analgesia 60: 885–888

Rampil I J 1992 Anesthetic considerations for laser surgery. Anesthesia and Analgesia 74: 424–435

van der Spek A F L, Spargo P M, Norton M L 1988 The physics of lasers and implications for their use during airway surgery. British Journal of Anaesthesia 60: 709–729

Wegrzynowicz E S, Jensen N F, Pearson K S et al 1992 Airway fire during jet ventilation for laser excision of vocal cord papillomata. Anesthesiology 76: 468–469

PROBLEMS OF ANAESTHESIA FOR MAGNETIC RESONANCE IMAGING

The purpose of this section is not to provide a recipe to allow anaesthetists unfamiliar with magnetic resonance imaging to immediately administer anaesthesia within the MRI environment. Nor is it intended to enable precise planning of a new unit. The aim is to outline the general problems and to provide a checklist for consideration of these problems and a bibliography for more detailed reading. Many articles which, in the early days of MRI units, specified adaptations of equipment have rapidly become out of date. Units are now more likely to be built with anaesthesia in mind, and equipment is being designed specifically for use in a magnetic field, so that modifications are less necessary.

Advance planning of units

It is crucial that anaesthetists are involved in the early planning so that there is proper design to allow general anaesthesia and sedation. It is much easier to build radio frequency filters into the magnetic shielding and isolated, filtered alternating current power circuits at the beginning of the project. In addition, adequate space for anaesthesia and recovery should be provided for safety and to improve the throughput of cases. The cost of MRI-compatible anaesthetic and monitoring equipment should be included in the initial installation price. Anaesthesia should not be permitted to become a cheap afterthought lest serious problems for the service and patients result.

Introduction

Magnetic resonance imaging (MRI) is an investigative procedure used for examination of the brain and soft tissue, for stereotaxy and spectroscopy. It takes place within a magnetic field whose strength might vary from 0.15–2 tesla. A tesla (t) is a measure of magnetic field strength and is equal to 10 000 gauss. If anaesthesia is required, the problems can be broadly divided into two:

1. The effect of the magnetic field on the patient and equipment.
2. The effect of the equipment and the patient on the quality of the image produced.

These problems increase in proportion to the increasing strength of the magnet and the reduction in the size of the bore of the magnet in which the patient is placed. In addition, time is required to build up the magnetic field. The magnet should therefore only be switched off in an emergency.

Section 3

Problems of
Anaesthesia for
Magnetic Resonance
Imaging

Problems

1. Effect of environment on patient
   a. The surroundings are noisy and claustrophobic. Although the majority of adults can cope awake, most children and a few adults may require anaesthesia or sedation.
   b. Implants such as metal clips, middle-ear implants, or metal foreign bodies in the eye may cause problems. Aneurysmal clips may become detached or eyes may be damaged by movement of the metal. Implanted devices, particularly pacemakers or automatic implanted cardioverter-defibrillators may fail, be reprogrammed, or cause microshock.
   c. Injury to personnel from ferromagnetic missiles in the room, or metal objects carried by the patient or on staff.
   d. Burns to patients from the pulse oximeter (Bashein & Syrovy 1991).
2. Access to the patient for anaesthesia or for CPR.
3. Factors which may affect quality of image.
   a. Patient movement or change in patient position.
   b. Introduction of radiofrequency signals from electrical connections can distort the image.
   c. Monitors disturb the signal/noise ratio.
4. Effect of environment on monitoring or anaesthetic equipment. The problems encountered depends upon the strength of the magnetic field.
   a. Propulsion of ferromagnetic objects across the room by the magnet.
   b. Interference with, and distortion of, electron beams on monitors.
   c. Noise interferes with audible signals from monitoring equipment.
   d. Actual malfunctioning of monitoring equipment.
5. Problems of having suddenly to extinguish a magnetic field in an emergency; once the magnet has been turned off it needs several hours to build up the field again.

Management

1. Preparation of patient for MRI without anaesthesia, must include counselling and education.

2. If doubt exists about the patient's ability to keep still, or for exceptionally nervous patients, a decision must be made about whether sedation or anaesthesia would be the more appropriate. A sedated patient still needs monitoring and oxygenation.

3. Preoperative asessment for anaesthesia. In addition to routine assessment, the use of a checklist for prostheses and contraindications to MRI is advised (Menon et al 1992). A similar checklist, to be consulted before anaesthesia for MRI is undertaken, is also recommended (Menon et al 1992).

4. Adequate staffing. Ideally there should be two anaesthetists, in addition to a trained assistant.

5. Equipment may be positioned outside the magnetic field, using long extension leads. Alternatively, purpose built equipment can be used within the field. The development of radiofrequency shields and special MRI equipment means that detailed discussion of present adaptations and models is inappropriate, since it is likely to become out of date. However, the following equipment must be considered in the light of its use in a magnetic field:
   a. Anaesthetic machine: either bolt to wall or floor or construct using non-ferromagnetic parts and cylinders.
   b. Breathing systems; a long Mapleson D system may be appropriate.
   c. Ventilators with non-ferromagnetic components.
   d. Laryngoscopes with non-ferromagnetic batteries.

6. Monitoring
   a. Indirect BP and direct arterial monitoring will require the use of extra long cables.
   b. ECG: twist the cables and keep electrodes close together; keep the plane of the cable parallel to the magnetic field lines.
   c. Pulse oximeter: there now are several MRI compatible models on the market.
   d. Capnography.
   e. Gas analyzers.
   f. Thermometry.
   g. Oesophageal stethoscopes.

7. Miscellaneous equipment
   a. Blood warmers.
   b. Infusion pumps.

8. Induction of anaesthesia can take place within or outside the field. If it takes place outside, the patient must be transported on a non-ferromagnetic stretcher.

9. If cardiopulmonary resuscitation is required, the patient should first be removed from the bore of the magnet. Ferromagnetic items must be taken from members of the cardiac arrest team before they enter the magnetic field.

10. The use of a mobile trolley, which carries adapted monitoring, for transporting critically ill patients should be considered (Peden et al 1992).

BIBLIOGRAPHY

Bashein G, Syrovy G 1991 Burns associated with pulse oximetry during magnetic resonance imaging. Anesthesiology 75: 382–383

Boutros A, Pavlicek W 1987 Anesthesia for magnetic resonance imaging. Anesthesia and Analgesia 66: 367

Geiger R S, Cascorbi H F 1984 Anesthesia in an NMR scanner. Anesthesia and Analgesia 63: 622–623

Menon D K, Peden C J, Hall A S et al 1992 Magnetic resonance for the anesthetists. Part I: physical principles, applications, safety aspects. Anaesthesia 47: 240–255

Patteson S K, Chesney J T 1992 Anesthetic management for magnetic resonance imaging: problems and solutions. Anesthesia and Analgesia 74: 121–128

Peden C J, Menon D K, Hall A S et al 1992 Magnetic resonance for the anaesthetist. Part II: anaesthesia and monitoring in MR units. Anaesthesia 47: 508–517

Rao C C, Brandl R, Mashak J N 1988 Modification of Ohmeda (R) Excel anesthesia machine for use during magnetic resonance imaging. Anesthesiology 68: 640–641

Rao C C, Krishna G, Emhardt J 1990 Anesthesia machine for use during magnetic imaging. Anesthesiology 73: 1054–1055

Tobin J R, Spurrier E A, Wetzl R C 1992 Anaesthesia for critically ill children during magnetic resonance imaging. British Journal of Anaesthesia 69: 482–486

Section 3

Cardiopulmonary Resuscitation (CPR)

A. Cardiac Resuscitation in the Adult

CARDIOPULMONARY RESUSCITATION
(CPR)

A. CARDIAC RESUSCITATION IN THE ADULT (GUIDELINES ON CARDIOPULMONARY RESUSCITATION 1989, EUROPEAN RESUSCITATION COUNCIL GUIDELINES 1992. N.B. NEW GUIDELINES ARE ANTICIPATED IN 1994).

1. ECG shows ventricular fibrillation or pulseless VT precordial thump.
   a. Defibrillate with 200 joules.
   b. Defibrillate with 200 joules.
   c. Defibrillate with 360 joules.
   d. Tracheal intubation and i.v. access.
   e. Give adrenaline 1 mg i.v.
   f. 10 CPR sequences of 5:1.
   g. Defibrillate with 360 J.
   h. Repeat defibrillations 360 J × 2.
   i. Consider different paddle positions and/or a different defibrillator.
   j. Consider bretylium tosylate 400 mg.
   k. Consider sodium bicarbonate 50 mmol or according to blood gas results.
   Continue CPR for up to 2 minutes after each drug. Do not interrupt CPR for more than 10 seconds, except for defibrillation.

If an i.v. line cannot be established, consider giving double doses of adrenaline or atropine via a tracheal tube.

2. ECG shows apparent asystole (isoelectric ECG)

Precordial thump and exclude ventricular fibrillation. If VF, DC shock 200 J, 200 J, 360 J, as above.

If still asystole:

a. Start cardiopulmonary resuscitation.

b. Tracheal intubation and i.v. access.

c. Give adrenaline 1 mg i.v.

d. 10 CPR sequences of 5:1.

e. Atropine 3 mg once only

f. Consider pacing if P waves or any other electrical activity is present.

g. After 3 cycles consider adrenaline 5 mg i.v.

Continue CPR for up to 2 minutes after each manoeuvre. Do not interrupt CPR for more than 10 seconds except for defibrillation. If an i.v. line cannot be established, consider giving double doses of adrenaline or atropine via a tracheal tube.

3. Electromechanical dissociation (QRS complexes present but no palpable pulse)

Consider, and if necessary give, specific therapy for hypovolaemia, pneumothorax, cardiac tamponade, pulmonary embolism, drug overdose, hypothermia or electrolyte imbalance.

a. Tracheal intubation and i.v. access.

b. Adrenaline 1 mg i.v.

c. 10 CPR sequences of 5:1.

d. Consider pressor agents, calcium, bicarbonate, and adrenaline 5 mg i.v.

Continue CPR for up to 2 minutes after each drug. Do not interrupt CPR for more than 10 seconds except for defibrillation If an i.v. line cannot be established, consider giving double doses of adrenaline or atropine via a tracheal tube.

4. Post-resuscitation care

a. Check arterial blood gases, electrolytes CXR.

b. Observe, monitor and treat the patient in an intensive care area.

5. Routes of administration of resuscitation drugs

a. Intravenous. Drugs should preferably be given via a central vein to avoid thrombophlebitis in peripheral veins.

b. Intratracheal. Administration of drugs by this route is still controversial (Greenbaum 1987). It is suitable for adrenaline, atropine or naloxone, when each is diluted to 10 ml, but blood levels achieved may be unreliable (Quinton et al 1987) and the possibility of introducing foreign bodies exists. Bicarbonate and calcium are NOT suitable for intratracheal use.

6. Defibrillation technique

a. One paddle should be placed to the right of the upper sternum just below the clavicle, the other to the apex of the heart. Contact is achieved with electrode jelly, or impregnated pads. Use special paddles for children and infants (see Paediatric resuscitation).

b. Remove any trinitrate patches from chest wall.

c. Charge the defibrillator to 200 J.

d. All personnel must be warned to stand back and avoid any contact with the patient during defibrillation.

e. Discharge the shock, by pressing appropriate button(s) on paddles.

B. RESUSCITATION IN PREGNANCY

A number of factors contribute to problems encountered in the resuscitation of the pregnant patient, and modifications to the conventional treatment of cardiac arrest are needed. The differences in management are necessitated by the altered cardiovascular physiology in the pregnant patient, and by the presence of the fetus. Effective ECM must be combined with a lateral tilt to reduce aortocaval compression. Crucial decisions may have to be made on the possible therapeutic benefits and ethical considerations of immediate Caesearean section, and the question of initiating open cardiac massage at an early stage. The maturity of the fetus is also important. Prior to 24–26 weeks, primarily maternal considerations operate. After this, the question of fetal viability enters the equation.

1. Altered maternal cardiovascular physiology
   Changes include an increase in cardiac output, vascular volume and oxygen consumption. The volume distribution of blood flow is altered, such that about 25% goes to the uterus. in the later stages of pregnancy, a key factor contributing to resuscitation difficulties at cardiac arrest is aortocaval compression by the gravid uterus when the patient is supine. This may markedly decrease venous return, in addition to reducing arterial blood flow to the uterus and kidneys. The contribution of aortocaval compression to poor outcome was stressed in reports on bupivacaine toxicity (Marx 1982), and in the death of a patient with sickle cell trait, when insufficient lateral tilt was applied during Caesarean section (Anaesthetic Advisory Committee 1987).

2. Special considerations in CPR in late pregnancy
   a. Relief of aortocaval compression
   This is a crucial factor influencing outcome and can be achieved by:
   i. Maintenance of a lateral tilt
   This is essential, but it hampers effective cardiac massage. A head-down position, with a wedge under one buttock, and

manual displacement of the uterus by an assistant, have been suggested. A special resuscitation wedge for pregnant patients has also been described (Rees & Willis 1988). It is 100 cm long, inclined at an angle of 27°, and has a fixed side piece to retain the patient during external cardiac massage. In the absence of this, the use of a 'human wedge' has been described (Goodwin & Pearce 1992). One assistant kneels on the floor, sitting on his heels, such that his thighs form the wedge on which the back of the patient to be resuscitated is supported. The assistant uses one arm to stabilize the patient's shoulders and the other to stabilize the pelvis. The head should be supported by a pillow.

ii. Immediate Caesarean section

Maternal survival without neurological deficit has been accomplished by this method of relieving compression (Marx 1982). Even if fetal death has occurred, this may be an effective therapeutic manoeuvre (Lindsay & Hanson 1987). Successful outcome for both mother and child has been reported after 'postmortem' Caesarean section (DePace et al 1982). A paediatrician should therefore form part of the resuscitation team.

b. Open cardiac massage

Should be seriously considered if a satisfactory circulation has not been achieved after 15 minutes of closed cardiac massage (Lee et al 1986).

c. Drug therapy

May require modification in the pregnant patient. Both acidosis and the administration of adrenaline cause reductions in uterine blood flow. Treatment with bicarbonate at a stage earlier than usual has therefore been recommended. The use of adrenaline should be delayed if possible (Lee et al 1986).

C. PAEDIATRIC RESUSCITATION

1. Causes of cardiac arrest in infants and children:
   a. Hypoxia, secondary to ventilatory failure or upper respiratory tract obstruction.
   b. Secondary to hypovolaemia.
   c. A result of sudden infant death syndrome.
   d. Secondary to septicaemia.
   e. Associated with congenital heart disease.

2. Paediatric tracheal tube sizes

	Diameter (mm)	Length of oral tube (cm)
Premature	2.5–3.0	11
Newborn	3.5	12
1 yr	4.0	13
2 yr	4.5	14
4 yr	5.0	15
6 yr	5.5	17
8 yr	6.0	19
10 yr	6.5	20
12 yr	7.0	21
14 yr	7.5	22

Section 3

Cardiopulmonary Resuscitation (CPR)
C. Paediatric Resuscitation

3. Respiratory rate = 20–40 breaths/minute
4. Cardiac massage rate = >100/minute
5. Sternal depression 1–2 cm
6. Maximum airway pressure = 40 cmH$_2$O
7. Massage to breathing ratio = 5:1
8. DC shock = 5 joules/kg
9. Drugs for paediatric resuscitation
  a. Adrenaline
    0.2 ml/kg of a 1:10 000 dilution.
    Used for asystole, bradycardia, ventricular fibrillation. Injection should be via a central vein or via tracheal tube.
  b. Atropine
    0.2 ml/kg of 100 μg/ml solution.
    Used for bradycardia or AV block.
  c. Lignocaine
    0.2 ml/kg of a 10 mg/ml solution.
  d. Calcium chloride
    0.2 ml/kg of a 100 mg/ml solution.
    Used for asystole.
  e. Dextrose 50%
    2 ml/kg in ALL cases
  f. Dexamethasone
    1 mg in infants, 8 mg in adolescents.
  g. Dopamine 5–20 μg/kg per min.
  h. Isoprenaline
    0.1–0.5 μg/kg per min.
  i. Lignocaine
    0.5 mg/kg.
    Used for ventricular tachycardia.
  j. Mannitol
    0.5–1 g/kg infusion over 20 minutes.
    Used to improve urinary output.

k. Naloxone
0.01mg/kg i.v., i.m., or s.c.
Used for reversal of respiratory depression due to opiates.

10. Paediatric defibrillation
Only use special paediatric electrodes. They should be positioned so that the heart lies in between the two electrodes:
Positive electrode: left midclavicular line, at xiphoid level.
Negative electrode: right of sternum, second rib level.
a. Infants
Neonate to age 3 years
Paddles 4.5 cm diameter

Defibrillator charge for infants

1.5 kg	premature	3–6 J
3.5 kg	neonate	7–14 J
7 kg	6 months	14–28 J
10 kg	1 year	20–40 J
15 kg	3 years	30–60 J

b. Children
Aged 3–15 years
Paddles 8.0 cm diameter

Defibrillator charge for children

15 kg	3 years	45 J
20 kg	5 years	100 J
22 kg	7 years	110 J
30 kg	10 years	150 J
50 kg	15 years	200 J

D. NEONATAL RESUSCITATION

1. Apgar scoring for assessment at 1 minute and 5 minutes
   a. Appearance:
      0 = blue, pale
      1 = body pink, peripheries blue
      2 = pink all over
   b. Heart rate:
      0 = absent
      1 = <100/min
      2 = >100/min
   c. Reflex irritability on stimulation of the soles of the feet:.
      0 = no response
      1 = some movement
      2 = a cry

d. Muscle tone:

  0 = flaccid, limp

  1 = some flexion

  2 = good flexion

e. Respiratory effort:

  0 = absent

  1 = irregular respiration

  2 = strong cry

  Assessment on total scoring:

  0–3 severe depression

  4–6 moderate depression

  7–10 good state

2. Normal birth

   a. Aspirate mucus from the mouth.

   b. Dry the skin and reduce heat loss by covering body and head.

   c. Fit name bands and complete identification procedures.

3. Moderate depression of the neonate

   a. Give 100% oxygen.

   b. Stimulate the feet and dry the skin.

   c. If there is a bradycardia of <100/min or breathing is inadequate, perform IPPV with bag and mask until improvement occurs.

   d. If there is no improvement, perform laryngoscopy, intubate, and treat as for severe neonatal depression.

4. Severe depression of the neonate

   a. Ventilate with 100% oxygen using a bag and mask.

   b. Perform pharyngeal suction, laryngoscopy and endotracheal intubation.

   c. If there is a bradycardia of <100/min, start ECM at a rate of 120/min, with fingers behind the chest and thumbs over the lower third of the sternum.

   d. Drug therapy should be given via the umbilical artery or vein. A useful technique for the anaesthetist to achieve rapid catheterization of the umbilical artery has been described (Cole & Rolbin 1980). This must be performed within 15 minutes of birth, before the onset of arterial spasm. It can subsequently be used for blood sampling, drug and fluid administration, and aortic pressure monitoring.

   i. Sodium bicarbonate 1 mmol/kg, then according to the acid base state.

   ii. Dextrose 0.5–2 g/kg for hypoglycaemia.

   iii. Adrenaline: up to 0.05 mg/kg may be required for the acidotic neonate, and 0.01 mg/kg for the non-acidotic one.

   iv. Naloxone i.v. 0.01 mg/kg (or 0.02 mg/kg i.m.), but only if the mother has received opiate analgesia. Naloxone is short acting, so depression may recur after 30 minutes.

BIBLIOGRAPHY

Anaesthesia Advisory Committee to the Chief Coroner of Ontario 1987 Intraoperative death during Caesarean section in a patient with sickle cell trait. Canadian Journal of Anaesthesia 34: 67–70

Anonymous 1992 Guidelines for basic life support. A statement by the Basic Life Support Working Party of the European Resuscitation Council. Resuscitation 24: 103–110

Baskett P J F 1985 Towards better resuscitation. British Journal of Hospital Medicine 34: 345–350

Baskett P J F 1992 Advances in cardiopulmonary resuscitation. British Journal of Anaesthesia 69: 182–193

Bembridge M, Lyons G 1988 Myocardial infarction in the first trimester of pregnancy. Anaesthesia 43: 202–204

Bennett J R, Bodenham A R, Berridge J C 1992 Advanced trauma life support. A time for reappraisal. Anaesthesia 47: 798–800

Bray R J 1985 The management of cardiac arrest in infants and children. British Journal of Hospital Medicine 34: 72–81

Cole A F D, Rolbin S H 1980 A technique for rapid catheterisation of the umbilical artery. Anesthesiology 53: 254–255

DePace N L, Betesh J S, Kotler M N 1982 'Postmortem' Cesarean section with recovery of both mother and offspring. Journal of the American Medical Association 248: 971–973

Goodwin A P L, Pearce A J 1992 The human wedge a manoeuvre to relieve aortocaval compression during resuscitation in late pregnancy. Anaesthesia 47: 433–434

Greenbaum R 1987 Down the tube. Anaesthesia 42: 927–928

Guidelines for cardiopulmonary resuscitation. Basic life support. Revised recommendations of the Resuscitation Council (UK). Marsden A K 1989 British Medical Journal 299: 442–445

Guidelines for cardiopulmonary resuscitation. Advanced life support. Revised recommendations of the Resuscitation Council (UK). Chamberlain D A 1989 British Medical Journal 299: 446–448

Lee R V, Rodgers B D, White L M et al 1986 Cardiopulmonary resuscitation of pregnant women. American Journal of Medicine 81: 311–318

Lindsay S L, Hanson G C 1987 Cardiac arrest in near-term pregnancy. Anaesthesia 42: 1074–1077

Lissauer T 1980 Paediatric emergencies. Cardiorespiratory arrest. Hospital Update 6: 1067–1077

Marx G F 1982 Cardiopulmonary resuscitation of late-pregnant women. Anesthesiology 56: 156

Quinton D N, O'Byrne G, Aitkenhead A R 1987 Comparison of endotracheal and peripheral venous adrenaline in cardiac arrest. Lancet 1: 828–829

Rees G A D, Willis B A 1988 Resuscitation in late pregnancy. Anaesthesia 43: 347–349

Safar P, Bircher N G 1988 Cardiopulmonary cerebral resuscitation. W B Saunders, Philadelphia

Schleien C L, Berkowitz I D, Traystman R et al 1989 controversial issues in cardiopulmonary resuscitation. Anesthesiology 71: 133–149

CRITERIA FOR BRAIN DEATH

1. Certification

   Two doctors, clinically independent of each other, are required for certification; one a consultant, the other either a consultant or a senior registrar. Both should have expertise in brain death diagnosis. and neither should be a member of the transplant team. A formal checklist should be used

2. Preconditions
   a. 'Does the patient suffer from a condition that has led to irremediable brain damage?'
   b. 'What was the time of onset of unresponsive coma?'
   c. 'Have potentially reversible causes for the patient's condition been adequately excluded?' In particular:
      i. Depressant drugs.
      ii. Neuromuscular blocking drugs.
      iii. Hypothermia.
      iv. Metabolic or endocrine disturbances.
3. Tests for absence of brain stem function
   a. 'Do the pupils react to light?'
      Pupils should be fixed and dilated. Sudden changes in light intensity should not cause any response.
   b. 'Are there corneal reflexes?'
   c. 'Is there eye movement on caloric testing?'
      The slow injection of 20 ml ice-cold water in turn into each auditory canal, free of blood or wax, should not produce any eye movements.
   d. 'Are there motor responses in the cranial nerve distribution in response to stimulation of the face, limbs or trunk?'
      Somatic stimulation, such as firm supraorbital or eye pressure, should not produce any motor response.
   e. 'Is there a gag reflex?'
      If the test is practicable.
   f. 'Is there a cough reflex?'
      There should be no response to the passage of a suction catheter down the tracheal tube.
   g. 'Have the recommendations concerning testing for apnoea been followed?'
   h. 'Were any respiratory movements seen?'
   The test for apnoea is extremely important (Rudge 1988). A sufficiently high Pa_{CO_2} must be produced to cause respiratory stimulation, but not at the expense of hypoxia. It has been suggested that the initial Pa_{CO_2} should be 6 kPa, and that the period of apnoea must be sufficient to produce a further rise of 6.66 kPa, confirmed by blood gases estimation. Prior to the test, 100% oxygen should be given for 15 minutes. At the end of this time, the patient should be disconnected from the ventilator, and oxygen 6 l/min insufflated using a narrow catheter which is passed down the endotracheal tube. Observation of the patient for any signs of respiratory movement must continue for 10 minutes, after which the patient is reconnected to the ventilator.
4. Confirmatory testing
   Brain death can only be conclusively established when the criteria have been satisfied on two successive occasions. The interval

Section 3

Criteria for Brain Death

between testing will depend on the original condition. Patients with possible drug overdosage or hypothermia may require a longer period of observation. In the case of drug toxicity, blood levels of the relevant drug may be required.

MANAGEMENT OF THE BRAIN DEAD DONOR FOR ORGAN HARVEST

1. General criteria of suitability
   a. A diagnosis of brain stem death has been made.
   b. No damage has been sustained by the organ to be harvested.
   c. No sepsis or systemic infection is present.
   d. No malignancy, except in the case of a proven primary brain tumour.
   e. No prolonged period of hypotension.
   f. HIV negative, HBV negative, no slow virus disease.
   g. No i.v. drug abuse.
   h. Consent has not been refused by relatives, coroner or equivalent legal officer.
   i. No juvenile-onset diabetes mellitus.
2. Guidelines for suitability for specific organ harvest
   a. Kidney
      i. Age range: 2–70 years.
      ii. No hepatic or renal damage, no history of hypertension.
      iii. A good urinary output (>0.5 ml/kg per h).
      iv. HLA compatibility.
   b. Liver
      i. Age range: 4 months–65 years.
      ii. No clinical liver damage, no history of alcohol abuse.
      iii. Normal liver function tests.
      iv. Gall bladder must be present.
      v. Normal gross appearance of the liver.
   c. Pancreas
      i. Age range: 15–50 years.
      ii. Normal serum amylase.
      iii. No diabetes mellitus.
   d. Heart or heart/lung
      i. Age: Male <40 years.
         Female <45 years.
      ii. No heart disease, chronic lung disease, hypertension, or myocardial trauma. For lung transplant, only non-smokers are acceptable.
      iii. No prolonged cardiac arrest period, a stable cardiovascular system requiring minimal or no inotropic support.
      iv. No abnormality of the heart. The lungs should be normal on clinical examination.

v. ECG and CXR normal.

vi. A short ventilatory period of <24 hours, to reduce risk of infection.

vii. Size compatibility with the potential recipient.

3. Preliminary intensive care management

a. Discussion with relatives

The patient may have carried a signed donor consent card. If not, the relatives should be approached by an experienced, and preferably a senior, member of staff to obtain their views. Even if the patient has signed a donor card, discussion with the relatives is appropriate and their feelings must be considered. (For further discussion and medicolegal details, see DHSS 1983.) Donor confidentiality should be maintained unless the relatives indicate otherwise. All details of discussion should be recorded in the patient's case records.

b. Discussion with the coroner

The coroner, or equivalent officer, need only be approached if the case would normally be reported to him because of the circumstances leading to the patient's death. In such situations, the prodedures set out by the local coroner must be followed.

c. Discussion with the transplant team

Contact should be made early with the regional transplant coordinator or the transplant team, giving the details listed below. At this stage it must be clearly indicated whether or not consent from the relatives has already been obtained.

d. Profile of the donor

i. The transplant centre will require information on the medical history and cause of brain stem death, age, sex, and height and weight of patient.

ii. Blood should be taken for ABO grouping, HLA typing, and HIV and HBV status.

iii. The results of recent investigations, where appropriate for the organs being taken, will be needed. These may include electrolytes and urea, full blood count, liver function tests, serum amylase, a 12-lead ECG, a recent CXR, and blood gases.

e. Maintenance of physiological homeostasis of donor

i. Respiratory support

Continued respiratory support with either air and oxygen or nitrous oxide and oxygen. Should aim to maintain a Pa_{O_2} of 10 kPa and a Pa_{CO_2} of about 43 kPa. The reduction in CO_2 production by brain-dead patients may necessitate the addition of a dead space to the respiratory circuit. PEEP may be required to maintain oxygenation, especially in the case of heart/lung donors. Metabolic acidosis may need treatrnent, although a cause should be sought.

ii. Blood pressure

In order to maintain the systolic BP >90 mmHg, inotropic support, with a dopamine infusion of not more than 5 μg/kg per min, may be required. The lowest possible dose should be used to avoid the alpha adrenergic effects which occur at doses above 10 μg/kg per min. Drugs with alpha-1 adrenergic effects should not be used, as they may compromise vital organ blood flow. This could subsequently impair the function of the transplanted organ. Persistent hypertension can be treated with hydralazine.

iii. Vascular volume and fluid management

The CVP should be maintained at 5–10 cmH$_2$O with gelatin or PPF, or with blood, should there be a continuing blood loss, to keep the Hb >8 g/dl. If diabetes insipidus is present, desmopressin (DDAVP) i.v. or i.m., 0.5–2 μg 6– hourly is given. Desmopressin is preferable to vasopressin, since it has no vasoconstrictor effect, starts to act at about 30 minutes, and is longer acting with a duration of 12 hours. Correction of serum electrolytes may be required, particularly sodium and potassium. up to 20 mmol potassium may be needed each hour if there is hypokalaemia.

iv. Urinary output

Is monitored and a volume of >0.5 ml/kg per hour maintained. Urinary fluid and electrolyte losses from diabetes insipidus are replaced and the CVP kept in the desired range. If the urine output remains low, a diuretic may be required. Frusemide i.v. 1–2 mg/kg or a frusemide infusion of <4 mg/min, or a mannitol infusion of 0.5 mg/kg can be used. Alpha-1 adrenergic agonists are not given because of the accompanying decrease in organ perfusion.

v. Body temperature

Is maintained at 34–36°C to prevent arrhythmias or cardiac arrest. Brain stem death is usually accompanied by a gradual decrease in body temperature. A warming blanket, warm fluids, and humidification may be required.

vi. Prevention of infection

Infection must be prevented, so a strict aseptic technique is used for all procedures.

vii. Hormonal therapy

After brain death thyroid hormone levels are depleted and adrenocortical function is depressed. The administration of intravenous tri-iodothyronine prevents the metabolic effects of brain death (Novitsky et al 1988), while adrenal suppression can be corrected with hydrocortisone 100 mg, and hyperglycaemia treated with insulin to keep the serum glucose levels between 8 and 13 mmol/l (Odom 1990, Soifer

& Gelb 1989). Actrapid 0.5–2 units/h are usually sufficient unless the patient is diabetic.

4. Management of the organ donor in the operating theatre

   a. Maintenance of monitoring and physiological homeostasis should be continued. Plasma expanders or blood transfusion may be needed to replace blood loss which occurs during dissection. The average blood loss during multiple organ harvesting was found to be 4 units in adults and 2 units in children (Rosenthal et al 1983). In heart-lung donors, the use of 20% albumin has been recommended.

   Direct arterial monitoring is useful, even if inotropic support is not required. It provides access for rapid arterial blood sampling for blood gases during the procedure, should there be any doubt about the suitability of the lungs for harvest. Similarly, a CVP line will enable intraoperative blood samples to be obtained for subsequent immunological testing. For heart and heart-lung donors, left-sided arterial and right-sided venous lines are recommended, because the right subclavian artery and the brachiocephalic vein are divided early thus curtailing access from the respective vessels (Ghosh et al 1990).

   b. A neuromuscular blocker such as pancuronium is required for abdominal relaxation and to prevent spinal reflexes. There may be haemodynamic responses to surgery, which can be alarming to inexperienced staff but which do not invalidate the diagnosis of brain death (Wetzel et al 1985). Marked increases in systolic and diastolic pressures and heart rate, persisting for up to 25 minutes, can occur in response to skin incision and may require treatment with narcotic analgesics, isoflurane, or sodium nitroprusside.

   Occasionally, inhalational agents may be required to control these responses (Kang & Gelman 1987).

   c. The exact drug regimen will depend upon the organ(s) being harvested and the individual preferences of the transplant team. The following are commonly required:

   i. A broad-spectrum antibiotic, such as a cephalosporin, with or without gentamicin.

   ii. Phenoxybenzamine i.v. 1 mg/kg prior to removal of the kidneys. This prevents vasoconstriction.

   iii. Heparin 3 mg/kg i.v. is given, after mobilization of the viscera or in heart-lung donors after the heart and lungs have been inspected), but before the organs are excised.

   iv. Methylprednisolone may be needed in the case of heart/lung removal.

   v. Tri-iodothyronine.

   vi. Prostacyclin 10–20 ng/kg per min into the pulmonary artery.

5. In heart-lung harvest, the tracheal tube and all venous lines should be withdrawn before division of the trachea and SVC.

6. Cardiac perfusion and preservation are beyond the scope of this book, but further details may be obtained from the articles by Hakim et al 1988 and Ghosh et al 1990.

7. Factors adversely affecting organ survival

Prolonged hypotension, and the use of vasopressors, dopamine and vasopressin, were all found to be factors contributing to the occurrence of tubular necrosis, and hence a decrease in the chance of kidney survival.

BIBLIOGRAPHY

Conference of Medical Royal Colleges and their Faculties in the United Kingdom 1976 Diagnosis of brain death. British Medical Journal 2: 1187–1188

Department of Health and Social Security 1983 Cadaveric organs for transplantation. HMSO, London

Ghosh S, Bethune D W Hardy I et al 1990 Management of donors for heart and heart-lung transplantation Anaesthesia 45: 672–675

Graybar G B, Tarpey M 1987 Kidney transplantation. Anesthesia and Organ Transplantation. W B Saunders, Philadelphia

Grebenik C R, Hinds C J 1987 Management of the multiple organ donor. British Journal of Hospital Medicine 38: 62–65

Hakim M, Higenbottam T, Bethune D et al 1988 Selection and procurement of combined heart and lung grafts for transplantation. Journal of Thoracic and Cardiovascular Surgery 95: 474–479

Jennett B 1981 Brain death. British Journal of Anaesthesia 53: 1111–1119

Kang Y G, Gelman S 1987 Liver transplantation. Anesthesia and Organ Transplantation. W B Saunders, Philadelphia

Novitsky D, Cooper D K C, Human P A et al 1988 Triiodothyronine therapy for heart donor recipient. Journal of Heart Transplantation 7: 370–376

Odom N J 1990 Organ donation. I – Management of the multiorgan donor. British Medical Journal 300: 1571–1573

Robertson K M, Ryan Cook D 1990 Perioperative management of the multiorgan donor. Anesthesia and Analgesia 70: 546–556

Rolles K 1986 Management of the multiple organ donor. Hospital Update 12: 633–638

Rosenthal J T, Shaw B W Jr, Hardesty R L et al 1983 Principles of multiple organ procuremenf from cadaver donors. Annals of Surgery 1 98: 617–621

Rudge C J 1988 Organising organ donation. British Journal of Hospital Medicine 40: 127–130

Soifer B E, Gelb A W 1989 The multiple organ donor: identification and management. Annals of Internal Medicine 110: 814–823

Timmins A C, Hinds C J 1991 Management of the multiple-organ donor. Current Opinion in Anaesthesiology 4: 287–292

Wetzel R C, Setzer N, Stiff J L et al 1985 Hemodynamic responses in brain-dead organ donor patients. Anesthesia and Analgesia 64: 125–128

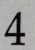

Rare and unusual syndromes

Rare or unusual conditions which as yet have few references in the literature, but which may have implications for the anaesthetist.

Asherman's syndrome

Intrauterine synechiae form after dilatation and curettage of a puerperal uterus and result in the cervix and part of the uterine cavity being obliterated. Infertility may result, but in the event of subsequent pregnancy, severe obstetric complications, in particular peripartum haemorrhage, may ensue. Emergency Caesarean hysterectomy may be required.

Smith C E, Weeks S K 1988 Anesthesia for Cesarean section in a patient with Asherman's syndrome. Anesthesiology 68: 615–618

Beckwith-Wiedemann syndrome

A syndrome of macroglossia, omphalocoele, visceromegaly, hemihypertrophy and neonatal hypoglycaemia secondary to islet cell hyperplasia. Adrenal hyperplasia and a variety of neural crest tumours can be present. If the hypoglycaemia is untreated, brain damage and seizures will occur. Most patients have congenital heart disease. Macroglossia can cause airway obstruction in the awake patient. Pulmonary hypertension may develop.

Management of an infant having subtotal pancreatectomy for severe hypoglycaemia is described (Gurkowski & Rasch 1989). Treatment of hypoglycaemia with dextrose, diazoxide, glucagon, and steroids may be required until the age of 4 years, when improvement occurs. If intubation difficulties are anticipated, attempts should be made to visualize the vocal cords under local anaesthesia. If they cannot be seen, awake intubation is required. Blood glucose monitoring for hypoglycaemia is required.

Gurkowski M A, Rasch D 1989 Anesthetic considerations for Beckwith-Wiedemann syndrome. Anesthesiology 70: 711–712

Churg-Strauss syndrome

A condition similar to polyarteritis nodosa in which there is eosinophilia and systemic vasculitis together with asthma, which may be intractable, and allergic rhinitis. Three distinct phases are described: an allergic phase which may be prolonged; an eosinophitic phase; and a more serious vasculitic phase (Lanham et al 1984). Diagnosis requires the presence of asthma, peak levels of eosinophils $>1.5 \times 10^9/1$, and vasculitis of two or more organs. Other features include arthralgia, skin rash, renal impairment, hypertension, and peripheral neuropathy secondary to ischaemia. CXR shows pulmonary infiltrates. Two patients had decreased serum cholinesterase activity (Taylor et al 1990). However, both were receiving immunosuppressive agents and had multiple organ imvolvement.

Lanham J G, Elkon K B, Pusey C D et al 1984 Systemic vasculitis with asthma and eosinophilia: a clinical approach to the Churg-Strauss syndrome. Medicine 63: 65–80
Taylor B L, Whittaker M, Van Heerden V et al 1990 Cholinesterase deficiency and the Churg-Strauss syndrome. Anaesthesia 45: 649–652

Crigler–Najjar syndrome

Unconjugated hyperbilirubinaemia resulting from a deficiency of bilirubin uridine diphosphate glucuronyl transferase. Encephalopathy (kernicterus) can result, particularly in type 1 disease. Phototherapy transforms bilirubin into forms which do not require conjugation for excretion, and this may be needed up until the time of surgery.

Drugs that are highly protein-bound should be avoided because they displace bilirubin and increase the amount going to the brain. Fasting and infection exacerbate hyperbilirubinaemia. Elective surgery should be postponed in the presence of infection. Cephalosporins should be avoided. Liver transplant in a child has been described (Prager et al 1992). The use of barbiturates, morphine, neuromuscular blocking, and inhalational agents are thought to be safe.

Prager M C, Johnson K L, Ascher N L et al 1992 Anesthetic care of patients with Crigler–Najjar syndrome. Anesthesia and Analgesia 74: 162–164

Dandy-Walker syndrome

Includes cerebellar hypoplasia, cystic dilatation of the fourth ventricle, obstructive hydrocephalus and ventricular dilatation, craniofacial abnormalities, and renal and skeletal anomalies (Asai et al 1989). There is a gradual increase in intracranial pressure until a shunt is required. Central ventilatory abnormalities with apnoeic spells may occur. Anaesthesia is required for CT scan, ventriculoperitoneal or cyst-peritoneal shunt, or resection of cyst membranes. Multiple anaesthetics were needed for treatment of hydrocephalus in a single individual (Ewart & Oh 1990).

Asai, A, Hoffman H J, Hendrick E B et al 1989 Dandy-Walker syndrome: experience at the Hospital for Sick Children, Toronto. Pediatric Neuroscience 15: 66–73
Ewart M C, Oh T E 1990 The Dandy-Walker syndrome. Relevance to anaesthesia and intensive care. Anaesthesia 45: 646–648

Edward's syndrome (trisomy 19)

A syndrome secondary to the chromosomal abnormality, trisomy 19. Cataracts, glaucoma and ptosis, mental retardation, and microcephaly can be present. Tracheal intubation may be difficult and the baby is prone to apnoeic attacks. Death usually occurs before the age of one year. A laryngeal mask airway was used for ear surgery in an infant with micrognathia (Bailey & Chung 1992).

Bailey C, Chung R 1992 Use of the laryngeal mask airway in a patient with Edward's syndrome. Anaesthesia 47: 713

EEC syndrome

A syndrome of anomalies in which Ectrodactyly, Ectodermal dysplasia, and Cleft lip/palate form the classical triad. Additionally, there is a high incidence of genitourinary abnormalities. The clinical course of eight operations has been described (Mizushima & Satoyoshi 1992). Malnutrition, skin fragility, thick tracheal secretions, and wide variations in body temperature proved to be particular problems.

Mizushima A, Satoyoshi M 1992 Anaesthetic problems in a child with ectrodactyly, ectodermal hypoplasia and cleft lip/palate. Anaesthesia 47: 137–140

Familial amyloid polyneuropathy (Portuguese type)

An autosomal dominant polyneuropathy secondary to amyloid accumulation in peripheral nerve fibres. It develops in early middle–age with sensory and motor features. Autonomic disturbances occur and degeneration of cardiac conduction tissue leads to cardiac arrhythmias. Severe hypotension occurred in a single patient after local anaesthesia, thiopentone, and hypnosis. Each was given in an attempt to perform dental extractions (Tavares & Maciel 1989). Subsequent anaesthesia with midazolam and isoflurane was uneventful. Severe bradycardias and heart block have occurred after induction of anaesthesia (Eriksson et al 1986).

Eriksson P, Boman K, Jacobbson B et al 1986 Cardiac arrhythmias in familial amyloid polyneuropathy during anaesthesia. Acta Anaesthesiologica Scandinavica 30: 317–320

Tavares J C, Maciel L 1989 Anaesthetic management of a patient with familial amyloid polyneuropathy of the Portuguese type. Canadian Journal of Anaesthesia 36: 209–211

Gerstmann-Straussler-Scheinker dtsease (see Creutzfeldt-Jakob disease, Section 1).

Gorlin's syndrome

Multiple basal cell naevi, jaw cysts, bifid ribs, scoliosis, cervical or thoracic vertebral fusion, meningiomata, ovarian cysts, and frontal and temporal bossing. Acute hypotension, bradycardia, and bronchospasm has been observed on induction of anaesthesia (Southwick & Schwartz 1979). In all three cases this was sufficiently severe for the surgery to be cancelled. Handling of a malignant ovarian tumour produced hypertension and tachycardia (Yoshizumi et al 1990). Subsequent immunohistochemistry showed the presence of prorenin/renin within the cells.

Southwick C J, Schwartz R A 1979 The basal cell nevus syndrome. Disasters occurring among a series of 36 patients. Cancer 44: 2294–2305
Yoshizumi J, Vaughan R S, Jasani B 1990 Pregnancy associated with Gorlin's syndrome. Anaesthesia 45: 1046–1048

Hallermann–Streiff syndrome

One of the craniofacial dysostoses in which there is multiple maxillofacial abnormalities, a small bird-like face, a hypoplastic nose, but a large cranial vault. There may be dwarfism, congenital cataracts, glaucoma, hyperextensible joints, and scoliosis. Difficult intubation may be compounded by the presence of brittle, deformed teeth, which are easily broken, and dislocation of the temporomandibular joint. Awake intubation under local anaesthesia was used in a patient requiring Caesarean section (Ravindran & Stoops 1979). A size 5.5-mm tracheal tube was the largest that would pass through the nose. Extradural anaesthesia for Caesarean section has also been performed (Hendrix & Sauer 1991). Anaesthesia may be required for ENT and eye surgery.

Hendrix S L, Sauer H J 1991 Successful pregnancy in Hallermann-Streiff syndrome. American Journal of Obstetrics and Gynecology 164: 1102–1104
Ravindran R, Stoops C M 1979 Anesthetic management of a patient with Hallermann–Streiff syndrome. Anesthesia and Analgesia 58: 254–255

Job's syndrome

High serum immunoglobulin E levels and a chemotactic defect in neutrophils, associated with recurrent skin and chronic upper and lower respiratory tract infections. Weeping eczematous skin lesions occur, with recurrent abscesses. Deep infections are, however, unusual (Donabedian & Gallin 1983). Patients present frequently for abscess drainage. The predominant organism is *Staphylococcus aureus*, although *Haemophilus influenzae* and *Streptococcus pneumoniae* may sometimes be responsible. A prolonged response to suxamethonium has been reported (Guzzi & Stamatos 1992). One patient required drainage of a hip abscess in late pregnancy. Extradural anaesthesia should not be performed (Miller & Mann 1990). Antibiotic prophylaxis helps to control infection.

Donabedian H, Gallin J I 1983 The hyperimmunoglobulin E recurrent-infection (Job's) syndrome. Medicine 62: 195–208
Guzzi L M, Stamatos J M 1992 Job's syndrome: an unusual response to a common drug. Anesthesia and Analgesia 75: 139–140
Miller F L, Mann D L 1990 Anesthetic management of a pregnant patient with the hyperimmunoglobulin E (Job's) syndrome. Anesthesia and Analgesia 70: 454–456

Joubert's syndrome

Agenesis of the cerebellar vermis with a cystic lesion in the brainstem, which results in respiratory abnormalities, especially panting with periods of apnoea, rigidity, and jerky eye movements. Congenital retinal blindness may also occur. A marked sensitivity to papaveretum was reported in an infant with an irreducible inguinal hernia (Matthews 1989). Apnoeic periods of up to 2 minutes occurred postoperatively. Intraoperative IPPV and subsequent close respiratory monitoring are advisable.

Matthews N C 1989 Anaesthesia in an infant with Joubert's syndrome. Anaesthesia 44: 920–921

Klippel–Trenaunay-Weber syndrome
Port-wine haemangiomas on the trunk or limbs are associated with spinal cord malformations, which may bleed spontaneously and result in paraplegia. Venous varicosities, A-V aneurysms, and hypertrophy of bone and soft tissues, usually unilateral, also occur secondary to increased blood supply. Anaesthesia is required for orthopaedic and vascular surgery of the limbs (Gloviczki et al 1983). If an A-V shunt is significant, high-output cardiac failure can occur. May be associated with Sturge–Weber disease. Careful control of blood pressure is required to prevent rupture of vessels in the spinal cord malformations and paralysis. Extradural and spinal techniques are contraindicated. A technique used during skin grafting to the leg has been described (de Leon-Casasola & Lema 1991).

de Leon-Casasola O A, Lema M J 1991 Anesthesia for patients with Sturge–Weber disease and Klippel–Trenaunay syndrome. Journal of Clinical Anesthesia 3: 409–413
de Leon-Casasola 0 A, Lema M J 1992 Epidural anesthesia in patients with Klippel–Trenaunay syndrome. Anesthesia and Analgesia 74: 470–471
Gloviczki P, Hollier L H, Telander R L 1983 Surgical implications of Klippel–Trenaunay syndrome. Annals of Surgery 197: 353–362

Leopard syndrome
Lentigines (multiple freckles), **E**CG conduction abnormalities, **O**cular hypertelorism, **P**ulmonary stenosis, **A**bnormal genitalia, **R**etardation of growth, and **D**eafness (sensorineural). Occasionally there is a hypertrophic cardiomyopathy, unilateral kidney and gonadal agenesis. Anaesthesia for dental treatment is recorded (Rodrigo et al 1990).

Rodrigo M R C, Cheng C H, Tai Y T et al 1990 'Leopard' syndrome. Anaesthesia 45: 30–33

Lipoid proteinosis (see Urbach–Wiethe disease)

Menkes' syndrome
An X-linked recessive disease in which there is defective collagen formation similar to that seen in Ehlers-Danlos syndrome, possibly secondary to abnormal copper transport. Mental and physical retardation, seizure disorders, gastro-oesophageal reflux, and airway complications may occur. Presents in the early months of life, with characteristic sparse, abnormally formed, kinky scalp hair, and

hypopigmentation. The infant has usually died by the age of 2 years. Anaesthesia for tracheostomy for acute stridor, secondary to subglottic stenosis, has been necessary (Tobias 1992). There is poor pharyngeal coordination and risk of gastro-oesophageal reflux.

Tobias J O 1992 Anaesthetic considerations in the child with Menkes' syndrome. Canadian Journal of Anaesthesia 39: 712–715

Proteus syndrome

A congenital hamartomatous disorder which may include scoliosis, cystic lung changes, macrodactyly, hemihypertrophy with gross asymmetry of the body, anomalous teeth, elongated neck with vertebral abnormalities, torticollis, pelvic lipomatosis, haemangiomas, and subcutaneous tumours (lipomas). A patient with severe deformities of the neck had a fibreoptic intubation under sedation (Pennant & Harris 1991). Laryngoscopy under anaesthesia did not allow visualization of any laryngeal structures, and intermittent upper airway obstruction occurred throughout his stay in hospital.

Pennant J H, Harris M F 1991 Anaesthesia for Proteus syndrome. Anaesthesia 46: 126–128
Tibbles J A R, Cohen M M Jr 1986 The Proteus syndrome: the Elephant Man diagnosed. British Medical Journal 293: 683–685

Saethre–Chotzen syndrome

Acrocephalosyndactyly. An autosomal dominant craniofacial dysostosis causing craniostenosis. A wide towering skull, flat forehead, squint and mild webbing of the neck. Inadvertent dural puncture occurred during caudal extradural anaesthesia in two brothers (Wrigley 1991). It was postulated that ballooning of the dura into the sacrum may have resulted from early closure of the coronal suture and intracranial hypertension.

Wrigley M W 1991 Inadvertent dural puncture during caudal anaesthesia for Saethre–Chotzen syndrome. Anaesthesia 46: 705

Soto's syndrome

Cerebral gigantism. An autosomal dominant condition with macrocephaly, mental retardation with skeletal growth acceleration in utero, followed by early pubertal development. There is an increased incidence of kyphoscoliosis. Other features have included hypotonia, a high-arched palate, and cardiac abnormalities. Problems encountered in anaesthesia for posterior spinal fusion in a 14-year-old, (height 170 cm, weight 90 kg), included a restrictive lung defect, obstructive sleep apnoea, a combative patient and the difficulties of performing wake-up tests (Suresh 1991). Somatosensory evoked potentials were monitored. Unusually, two hooks failed in the postoperative period.

Suresh D 1991 Posterior spinal fusion in Soto's syndrome. British Journal of Anaesthesia 6: 728–732

Spondyloepiphyseal dysplasia
A dwarfing syndrome involving the spine and epiphyses of long bones. Platyspondyly (flattened spine), odontoid hypoplasia with cervical spine instability, and thoracic dysplasia occur. There is a short xiphisternum to symphysis pubis distance and kyphoscoliosis. May be associated with a short trachea of 15 rings or less (Wells et al 1989). Two cases of laryngeal stenosis have been reported (Myer & Cotton 1991). In one there was circumferential stenosis from the cricoid cartilage to the third tracheal ring. The second had gradually increasing respiratory difficulty, followed by acute stridor requiring emergency tracheostomy. Laryngoscopy showed that the glottis was obliterated by thickened, supraglottic mucosal folds. A pregnant patient with C3–4 subluxation was managed for Caesarean section with extradural anaesthesia (Rodney et al 1991). Although the patient had pronounced kyphoscoliosis, the technique was performed without difficulty. However, the extradural space was shallow, located at 2.5 cm from the skin.

Myer G M, Cotton R T 1985 Laryngotracheal stenosis in spondyloepiphyseal dysplasia. Laryngoscope 95: 3–5
Rodney G E, Callander C C, Harmer M 1991 Spondyloepiphyseal dysplasia congenita. Caesarean section under epidural anaesthesia. Anaesthesia 46: 648–650
Wells A L, Wells T R, Landing B H et al 1989 Short trachea, a hazard in tracheal intubation of neonates and infants: syndromal association. Anesthesiology 71: 367–373

Swyer–James syndrome (MacLeod's syndrome)
Acquired unilateral pulmonary emphysema which follows an episode of viral necrotizing bronchiolitis in infancy. Obliteration of peripheral capillaries occurs. The contralateral side is usually normal, but may be affected. The abnormal side may only contribute 25% to the MVV (Avital et al 1989). Onset is in childhood or adolescence, with recurrent pulmonary infections, chronic respiratory distress secondary to reduced lung function, and failure to thrive. Hyperlucency of the lung with decreased markings is seen on CXR. Lung function tests show an obstructive pattern, but there may be no improvement with bronchodilators.

Avital A Shulman D L, Bar-Yishay E et al 1989 Differential lung function in an infant with Swyer-James syndrome. Thorax 44: 298–302

Tumour lysis syndrome
Associated with chemotherapy in children with advanced lymphomas or leukaemias. Breakdown of tumour cells results in the release of intracellular constituents such as potassium, uric acid, and phosphate. Cardiac arrest from hyperkalaemia, and acute respiratory failure have been reported. The highest serum potassium occurs in the first 24 hours, and haemofiltration, glucose and insulin or IPPV may be required. Two patients developed pulmonary oedema in association with a fluid load aimed at producing an alkaline diuresis (Stokes 1989). Increasing

numbers of patients require intensive care during treatment for malignancies (Lloyd-Thomas et al 1988).

Lloyd-Thomas A R, Wright I, Lister T A et al 1988 Prognosis of patients receiving intensive care for lifethreatening medical complications of haematological malignancy. British Medical Journal 296: 1025–1029
Stokes D N 1989 The tumour lysis syndrome. Intensive care aspects of paediatric oncology. Anaesthesia 44: 133–136

Urbach-Wiethe disease (Lipoid proteinosis)

An autosomal recessive disorder, particularly involving skin and mucous membranes around the face and upper airway. Skin plaques, ulceration and scarring of the face resemble acne. The thickening of the skin is secondary to deposition of a hyaline material in capillary walls and basement membrane of the epithelium. Minor trauma predisposes to widespread scarring. Hoarseness, secondary to thickening of the vocal cords, develops in early childhood. In advanced disease there is a woody tongue, dysphagia, and problems with mouth opening. Intracranial calcification and epilepsy may occur. Anaesthesia was required for dental extraction in a young man with a hoarse voice. The vocal cords were viewed under inhalational anaesthesia to ascertain the feasibility of tracheal intubation, which was then performed following suxamethonium. Both cords were thick and pale, one being irregular.

Kelly J E, Simpson Jonathan D, Hollway T 1989 Lipoid proteinosis: Urbach–Wiethe disease. British Journal of Anaesthesia 63: 609–611

Wilson's disease

An autosomal recessive disorder of copper metabolism in which copper accumulates in the body, initially particularly in the brain and liver where it causes cerebral and hepatic damage. There is inhibition of biliary excretion. Cirrhosis and oesophageal varices may ensue. Presents in early adulthood. Features include hypoglycaemia, coagulopathy including prolonged prothrombin time and sometimes thrombocytopenia, haemolytic anaemia, incoordinated voluntary movements, dystonia, dysarthria, dysphagia, and dribbling. Keyser-Fleischer rings result from granular deposits in the cornea. Fever, renal dysfunction, sodium retention and hypoxia from pulmonary shunting may occur. Treatment involves reduction in copper intake and the use of chelating agents such as D-penicillamine and trientine. This may result in iron and zinc deficiencies. Anaesthesia may be required for liver transplantation (Gunning & Park 1992).

Gunning K E J, Park G R 1992 Liver transplantation. Current Opinion in Anaesthesiology 5: 431–435

5

Normal Values

BIOCHEMISTRY
Plasma or serum data

The biochemical normal values depend upon the techniques used and the individual laboratory. When the values are particularly variable, space has been left for insertion of the local range

Constituent	Normal or reference value
ACTH	
ADH	
adrenaline + noradrenaline	
adrenaline	
alanine aminotransferase	5–40 IU/l
albumin	35–52 g/l
alcohol legal limit	80 mg/dl (<17 mmol/l)
aldolase	
aldosterone	
alkaline phosphatase	
adult	30–130 u/l
child	30–300 u/l
pregnant	100–300 u/l
aluminium	
amino acid nitrogen, fasting	
amylase	70–300 u/l
angiotensin converting enzyme inhibitor	
angiotensin II	
anion gap $(Na + K) - (HCO_3 + Cl -)$	6–16 mmol/l
antidiuretic hormone	
aspartate aminotransferase	5–40 IU/l
bicarbonate	22–32 mmol/l
bilirubin	
total	5–20 µmol/l
conjugated	<3.0 µmol/l
caeruloplasm	
calcitonin	
calcium	
total	2.15–2.60 mmol/l
ionised	1.14–1.30 mmol/l
calcium corrected	2.20–2.55 mmol/l
carbonic acid	
carbon dioxide, whole blood	4.5–6.0 kPa
C1 esterase inhibitor	
chloride	98–108 mmol/l
cholesterol	
cholinesterase	0.81–1.2 U/ml
dibucaine number	normal approx 80 homozygous approx. 20 heterozygous approx. 60
fluoride number	57–63

Constituent	Normal or reference value
cortisol	165–715 nmol/l
8 a.m.–10 a.m.	165–715 nmol/l
9 p.m.–midnight	<330 nmol/l
creatinine	70–125 μmol/l
creatine kinase	
males	25–170 iu/l
females	25–150 iu/l
creatinine clearance	
gamma glutamyl transferase	7–50 U/l
gastrin	
glucagon	
glucose (plasma)	3.3–6.2 mmol/l
growth hormone	
hydrogen ion activity (pH)	36–44 nmol/l
	7.36–7.44
hydroxybutyrate	
dehyrogenase	
insulin (fasting)	
lactate	0.75–1.25 mmol/l
lactic acid dehydrogenase	
total	240–525 U/l
lipids (total)	
luteinising hormone	
magnesium	0.7–1.2 mmol/l
methionine	
noradrenaline	
osmolality	275–295 mOsm/kg
oxygen (whole blood)	11–15 kPa
pancreatic polypeptide	
parathyroid hormone	
phosphatases (acid)	
acid total	0–5 U/l
prostatic fraction	0–1 U/l
phosphate	0.7–1.4 mmol/l
phospholipids	
potassium	3.5–5.3 mmol/l
protein	
total	62–80 g/l
albumin	35–52 g/l
pyruvate	
renin	
sodium	135–145 mmol/l
sulphate	50–150 μmol/l
testosterone	
thyroid stimulating hormone	0.4–4.0 mU/l
thyroxine	
T4	50–150 nmol/l
pregnancy	117–258 nmol/l
T3	1–3 nmol/l

Section 5

Constituent	Normal or reference value
transferrin	
triglycerides (fasting)	
urate	
male	0.11–0.45 mmol/l
female	0.12–0.40 mmol/l
urea	2.5–7.5 mmol/l

Section 5

HAEMATOLOGICAL VALUES

Bleeding time (template)	2.5–9.5 min
Coagulation time	5–11 min
Prothrombin time	12–15 s
Partial thromboplastin time (KCCT)	35–42 s
Prothrombin consumption index	≤20%
Plasma fibrinogen	2.0–4.0 g/l
Euglobulin lysis time	90–240 min
Fibrin degradation products	absent or trace
Platelet count	150–450 × 10^9/l
ESR (Westergren 1h)	
male	≤10 mm
female	≤20 mm
Serum folate	3–20 µg/l
Red cell folate	160–640 µg/l
Haematocrit	
male	0.47 ± 0.07
female	0.42 ± 0.05
Serum B12	160–925 ng/l
Serum iron	13–32 µmol/l
Serum ferritin	
male	20–340 µg/l
female	15–40 µg/l
Haemoglobin	
male	155 ± 25 g/l
female	140 ± 25 g/l
Haematocrit	
male	0.47 ± 0.07
female	0.42 ± 0.05
Red cell count	
male	5.5 ± 1 × 10^{12}/l
female	4.8 ± 1 × 10^{12}/l
Mean corpuscular volume	86 ± 10 fl
Mean corpuscular haemoglobin	29.5 ± 2.5 pg
Mean corpuscular haemoglobin concentration	33 ± 2 g/dl
Red cell volume	
male	30 ± 5 ml/kg
female	25 ± 5 ml/kg
Plasma volume	40–50 ml/kg
Total blood volume	70 ± 10 ml/kg
Total leucocyte count	4–11 × 10^9/l

Neutrophils (40–75%)	$2.0–7.5 \times 10^9/l$
Lymphocytes (20–45%)	$1.5–4.0 \times 10^9/l$
Monocytes (2–10%)	$0.2–0.8 \times 10^9/l$
Eosinophils (1–6%)	$0.04–0.4 \times 10^9/l$
Basophils (≤%)	$≤0.1 \times 10^9/l$
Reticulocytes (0.2–2%)	$10–100 \times 10^9/l$
Serum haptoglobin	0.3–2.4 g/l
Haemoglobin A2	1.5–3.2%
Haemoglobin F	0.5–0.8%
Plasma viscosity	1.5–1.72 cp
Serum immunoglobins	
IgG	6–15 g/l
IgA	1.0–4.5 g/l
IgM	0.5–3.5 g/l

THERAPEUTIC BLOOD LEVELS

Digoxin	0.8–2 μg/l
Ethosuximide	40–100 mg/l
Gentamicin	
therapeutic peak	5–10 mg/l
therapeutic trough	0.5–2 mg/l
Lithium	0.8–1.2 mmol/l 12 h after last dose
Lignocaine	1–5 μg/ml
Phenobarbitone	15–30 mg/l
Phenytoin	10–20 mg/l
Primidone	5–12 mg/l
Salicylate	
analgesic	<20 mg/l
anti-inflammatory	<300 mg/l
Theophylline	10–20 mg/l

CARDIOLOGICAL NORMAL VALUES

1. ECG TIMES

Small squares = 0.04 s   Large squares = 0.2 s

P wave	atrial wave	<0.10 s
PR interval	AV conduction	0.12–0.20 s

(Measured from onset of p wave to onset of QRS.)

QRS time	rapid ventricular depolarisation	0.05–0.10 s
QT interval	length of ventricular complex	0.35–0.42 s

(Measured from beginning of Q to the end of the T wave. The QT interval decreases with increasing heart rate.)

QTc is the QT interval corrected for heart rate

$$QTc = \frac{\text{measured QT interval}}{\text{square root of cycle length}}$$

T wave	repolarisation	0.22 s

2. CARDIOVASCULAR PRESSURE

Pressure	Systolic (mmHg)	Diastolic (mmHg)	Mean (mmHg)
Peripheral venous			6–12
Right atrial pressure			0–7
Right venticular pressure	14–32	0–7	12–17
Pulmonary arterial pressure	14–32	2–13	8–19
Pulmonary wedge or left atrial			6–12
Left ventricular end diastolic	100–150	2–12	
Arterial pressure	100–150	60–90	80–100

Haemodynamic variables (70 kg)	
Cardiac output	5l.min^{-1}
Cardiac index	$3.2 \text{ l.min}^{-1}.\text{m}^{-2}$
Stroke volume	75 ml
Stroke volume index	50 ml.m^{-2}
Ejection fraction:	>0.60
Pulmonary vascular resistance	$50\text{–}140 \text{ dyn.s.cm}^{-5}$
Systemic vascular resistance	$90\text{–}1500 \text{ dyn.s.cm}^{-5}$

3. RESPIRATORY NORMAL VALUES

Predicted peak expiratory flow rate $(l.min^{-1})$: men

Age (yr)	Height				
	5ft 3in (160 cm)	5ft 6in (168 cm)	5ft 9in (175 cm)	6ft 0in (183 cm)	6ft 3in (190 cm)
20	570	600	625	655	680
25	575	600	625	655	680
30	560	585	610	640	665
35	545	570	600	625	650
40	535	560	585	610	635
45	525	550	570	600	625
50	510	535	560	585	610
55	500	525	550	575	595
60	490	510	535	560	580
65	475	500	520	545	565
70	465	485	505	530	550
75	450	470	495	515	535
80	440	460	485	505	525

Predicted peak expiratory flow rate $(l.min^{-1})$: women

Age (yr)	Height				
	4ft 9in (145 cm)	5ft 0in (152 cm)	5ft 3in (160 cm)	5ft 6in (168 cm)	5ft 9in (175 cm)
20	375	400	435	460	490
25	375	400	435	460	490
30	365	390	420	450	480
35	355	380	410	440	470
40	345	370	400	425	460
45	335	360	390	420	450
50	325	350	380	405	435
55	315	340	370	395	425
60	300	330	360	385	415
65	295	320	350	375	405
70	280	310	340	365	395
75	270	300	330	355	385
80	260	290	320	345	375

Forced vital capacity prediction table (in litres): men

Age (yr)	Height				
	5ft 3in (160 cm)	5ft 6in (168 cm)	5ft 9in (175 cm)	6ft 0in (183 cm)	6ft 3in (190 cm)
20	4.17	4.53	4.95	5.37	5.73
25	4.17	4.53	4.95	5.37	5.73
30	4.06	4.42	4.84	5.26	5.62
35	3.95	4.31	4.73	5.15	5.51
40	3.84	4.20	4.62	5.04	5.40
45	3.73	4.09	4.51	4.93	5.29
50	3.62	3.98	4.40	4.82	5.18
55	3.51	3.87	4.29	4.71	5.07
60	3.40	3.76	4.18	4.60	4.96
65	3.29	3.65	4.07	4.49	4.85
70	3.18	3.54	3.96	4.38	4.74
75	3.07	3.43	3.85	4.27	4.63

Forced vital capacity prediction table (in litres): women

Age (yr)	Height				
	4ft 9in (145 cm)	5ft 0in (152 cm)	5ft 3in (160 cm)	5ft 6in (168 cm)	5ft 9in (175 cm)
20	3.13	3.45	3.83	4.20	4.53
25	3.13	3.45	3.38	4.20	4.53
30	2.98	3.30	3.68	4.05	4.38
35	2.83	3.15	3.53	3.90	4.23
40	2.68	3.00	3.38	3.75	4.08
45	2.53	2.85	3.23	3.60	3.93
50	2.38	2.70	3.08	3.45	3.78
55	2.23	2.55	2.93	3.30	3.63
60	2.08	2.40	2.78	3.15	3.48
65	1.93	2.25	2.63	3.00	3.33
70	1.78	2.10	2.48	2.85	3.18
75	1.63	1.95	2.33	2.70	3.03

Forced expiratory volume prediction table (at 1 s in litres): men

Age (yr)	Height 5ft 3in (160 cm)	5ft 6in (168 cm)	5ft 9in (175 cm)	6ft 0in (183 cm)	6ft 3in (190 cm)
20	3.61	3.86	4.15	4.44	4.69
25	3.61	3.86	4.15	4.44	4.69
30	3.45	3.71	4.00	4.28	4.54
35	3.30	3.55	3.84	4.13	4.38
40	3.14	3.40	3.69	3.97	4.23
45	2.99	3.24	3.53	3.82	4.07
50	2.83	3.09	3.38	3.66	3.92
55	2.68	2.93	3.22	3.51	3.76
60	2.52	2.78	3.06	3.35	3.61
65	2.37	2.62	2.91	3.20	3.45
70	2.21	2.47	2.75	3.04	3.30
75	2.06	2.31	2.60	2.89	3.14

Section 5

Forced expiratory volume prediction table (at 1 s in litres): women

Age (yr)	Height 4ft 9in (145 cm)	5ft 0in (152 cm)	5ft 3in (160 cm)	5ft 6in (168 cm)	5ft 9in (175 cm)
20	2.60	2.83	3.09	3.36	3.59
25	2.60	2.83	3.09	3.36	3.59
30	2.45	2.68	2.94	3.21	3.44
35	2.30	2.53	2.79	3.06	3.29
40	2.15	2.38	2.64	2.91	3.14
45	2.00	2.23	2.49	2.76	2.99
50	1.85	2.08	2.34	2.61	2.84
55	1.70	1.93	2.19	2.46	2.69
60	1.55	1.78	2.04	2.31	2.54
65	1.40	1.63	1.89	2.16	2.39
70	1.25	1.48	1.74	2.01	2.24
75	1.10	1.33	1.59	1.86	2.09

PAEDIATRIC VALUES

Tracheal tube sizes

Age	Internal diameter (mm)	Length (cm)	
		Oral	Nasal
Premature	2.5–3.0	11	13.5
Neonate	3.5	12	14
1 year	4.0	13	15
2 years	4.5	14	16
4 years	5.0	15	17
6 years	5.5	17	19
8 years	6.0	19	21
10 years	6.5	20	22
12 years	7.0	21	22
14 years	7.5	22	23
16 years	8.0	23	24

Paediatric haemoglobin levels

Newborn	20 g/dl (range 18–22 g/dl)
Second week	17 g/dl
3 months	10–11 g/dl
2 years	11 g/dl
3–5 years	12/5–13.0 g/dl
5–10 years	13.0–13.5 g/dl
>10 years	14.5 g/dl

Paediatric blood volumes and blood pressure

Age	Weight	Blood volume	Blood pressure (mmHg)	
	(kg)	(l)	Systolic	Diastolic
Newborn	3.5	0.2	70	45
3 months	5.0	0.4		
6 months	7.0	0.52		
9 months	8.5	0.65		
1 year	10	0.75	80	60
2 years	13	0.9	80	60
3 years	15	1.05	85	60
4 years	17	1.22	87	60
5 years	19	1.37	90	60
6 years	21	1.52	90	60
7 years	23	1.7	92	62
8 years	25	1.9	95	62
9 years	28	2.06	98	64
10 years	32	2.4	100	65
11 years			100	65
12 years			108	67

Paediatric respiratory parameters

| Body weight (kg) | MV (ml) | TV (ml) | RR/min | FGF with 'T' piece to prevent rebreathing | |
				Mask	ETT
2	480	14–16	30–45		
3	600	17–24	25–40		
5				8	6
10	1680	80	21	8	6
15				10	7.5
20	3040	160	19	12	9
25				14	10.5
30	4080	240	17	14	10.5
35				15	11.5
40	4800	320	15	16	12.0
45				17	12.5

Section 5

Paediatric weight conversion chart

st	lb	kg	st	lb	kg	st	lb	kg
	3	1.6	1	0	6.35	1	11	11.34
	4	1.81	1	1	6.80	1	12	11.79
	5	2.27	1	2	7.26	1	13	12.24
	6	2.72	1	3	7.71	2	0	12.7
	7	3.18	1	4	8.16	2	4	14.5
	8	3.63	1	5	8.62	2	8	16.3
	9	4.08	1	6	9.07	2	12	18.1
	10	4.54	1	7	9.53	3	0	19.1
	11	4.99	1	8	9.98	3	4	20.9
	12	5.44	1	9	10.43	3	8	22.7
	13	5.9	1	10	10.89	3	12	24.5

SI FRACTIONS OR MULTIPLES

10^{-1}	deci	d	10^{1}	deca	da
10^{-3}	milli	m	10^{3}	kilo	k
10^{-6}	micro	μ	10^{6}	mega	M
10^{-9}	nano	n	10^{9}	giga	G
10^{-12}	pico	p	10^{12}	tera	T
10^{-15}	femto	f	10^{15}	peta	P
10^{-18}	atto	a	10^{18}	exa	E

GENERAL WEIGHT CONVERSION CHART

st	lb	kg	st	lb	kg	st	lb	kg
2	0	12.7	5	3	33.1	8	6	53.5
2	1	13.2	5	4	33.6	8	7	54.0
2	2	13.6	5	5	34.0	8	8	54.4
2	3	14.1	5	6	34.5	8	9	54.9
2	4	14.5	5	7	34.9	8	10	55.3
2	5	15.0	5	8	35.4	8	11	55.8
2	6	15.4	5	9	35.8	8	12	56.2
2	7	15.9	5	10	36.3	8	13	56.7
2	8	16.3	5	11	36.7	9	0	57.2
2	9	16.8	5	12	37.2	9	1	57.6
2	10	17.2	5	13	37.6	9	2	58.1
2	11	17.7	5	0	38.1	9	3	58.5
2	12	18.1	6	1	38.6	9	4	59.0
2	13	18.6	6	2	39.0	9	5	59.4
3	0	19.1	6	3	39.5	9	6	59.9
3	1	19.5	6	4	39.9	9	7	60.3
3	2	20.0	6	5	40.4	9	8	60.8
3	3	20.4	6	6	40.8	9	9	61.2
3	4	20.9	6	7	41.3	9	10	61.7
3	5	21.3	6	8	41.7	9	11	62.1
3	6	21.8	6	9	42.2	9	12	62.6
3	7	22.2	6	10	42.6	9	13	63.0
3	8	22.7	6	11	43.1	10	0	63.5
3	9	23.1	6	12	43.5	10	1	64.0
3	10	23.6	6	13	44.0	10	2	64.4
3	11	24.0	7	0	44.5	10	3	64.9
3	12	24.5	7	1	44.9	10	4	65.3
3	13	24.9	7	2	45.5	10	5	65.8
4	0	25.4	7	3	45.8	10	6	66.2
4	1	25.9	7	4	46.3	10	7	66.7
4	2	26.3	7	5	46.7	10	8	67.1
4	3	26.8	7	6	47.2	10	9	67.6
4	4	27.2	7	7	47.6	10	10	68.0
4	5	27.7	7	8	48.1	10	11	68.5
4	6	28.1	7	9	48.5	10	12	68.9
4	7	28.6	7	10	49.0	10	13	69.4
4	8	29.0	7	11	49.4	11	0	69.9
4	9	29.5	7	12	49.9	11	1	70.3
4	10	29.9	7	13	50.3	11	2	70.8
4	11	30.4	8	0	50.8	11	3	71.2
4	12	30.8	8	1	51.3	11	4	71.7
4	13	31.3	8	2	51.7	11	5	72.2
5	0	31.8	8	3	52.2	11	6	72.6
5	1	32.2	8	4	52.6	11	7	73.0
5	2	32.7	8	5	53.1	11	8	73.5

st	lb	kg	st	lb	kg	st	lb	kg
11	9	73.9	14	6	91.6	17	3	109.3
11	10	74.4	14	7	92.1	17	4	109.8
11	11	74.8	14	8	92.5	17	5	110.2
11	12	75.3	14	9	93.0	17	6	110.7
11	13	75.8	14	10	93.4	17	7	111.1
12	0	76.2	14	11	93.9	17	8	111.6
12	1	77.1	14	12	94.3	17	9	112.0
12	2	77.2	14	13	94.8	17	10	112.5
12	3	77.6	15	0	95.2	17	11	112.9
12	4	78.0	15	1	95.7	17	12	113.4
12	5	78.5	15	2	96.2	17	13	113.9
12	6	78.9	15	3	96.6	18	0	114.3
12	7	79.4	15	4	97.0	18	1	114.8
12	8	79.8	15	5	97.5	18	2	115.2
12	9	80.1	15	6	98.0	18	3	115.7
12	10	80.7	15	7	98.4	18	4	116.1
12	11	81.2	15	8	98.9	18	5	116.6
12	12	81.6	15	9	99.3	18	6	117.0
12	13	82.1	15	10	99.8	18	7	117.5
12	0	82.6	15	11	100.2	18	8	117.9
12	1	83.0	15	12	100.7	18	9	118.4
12	2	83.5	15	13	101.2	18	10	118.8
12	3	83.9	16	0	101.6	18	11	119.3
12	4	84.4	16	1	102.1	18	12	119.7
12	5	84.8	16	2	102.5	18	13	120.2
12	6	85.3	16	3	103.0	19	0	120.7
12	7	85.7	16	4	103.4	19	1	121.1
12	8	86.2	16	5	103.9	19	2	121.1
13	9	86.6	16	6	104.3	19	3	122.0
13	10	87.1	16	7	104.8	19	4	122.5
13	11	87.5	16	8	105.2	19	5	122.9
13	12	88.0	16	9	105.7	19	6	123.4
13	13	88.5	16	10	106.1	19	7	123.8
14	0	88.9	16	11	106.6	19	8	124.3
14	1	89.4	16	12	107.0	19	9	124.7
14	2	89.4	16	13	107.5	19	10	125.2
14	3	90.3	17	0	107.9	19	11	125.6
14	4	90.7	17	1	108.4	19	12	126.1
14	5	91.2	17	2	108.9	19	13	126.6
						20	00	127.0

Section 5

PRESSURE CONVERSION CHART

1 mmHg = 1.36 cmH$_2$O = 133.3 N/m^2 = 0.0194 psi
1 mmHg = 0.133 kPa
1 cmH$_2$O = 0.098 kPa = 98.06 N/m^2
1 bar = 760 mmHg = 29.9 inHg = 1 atmosphere absolute
1 kPa = 1 × 10^3 N/m^2 = 7.5 mmHg = 0.146 psi
1 psi = 6.895 kPa = 51.7 mmHg

Appendix

Useful addresses and telephone numbers

Association of Anaesthetists
9 Bedford Square
London WC1B 3RA
071 631 1650

British Medical Association
BMA House
Tavistock Square
London WC1H 9JP
071 387 4499

British Postgraduate Medical Federation
33 Millman Street
London WC1N 3EJ
071 831 6222

Cholinesterase Research Unit
Hammersmith Hospital
Du Cane Road
London W12 0HS
081 743 2030

Committee on Safety of Medicines
Marker Tower
1 Nine Elms Lane
London SW8 5NQ
071 720 2188

Department of Health
Quary House
Quarry Hill
Leeds LS2 7UE
0532 545000

General Medical Council
14 Hallam Street
London W1N 6AE
071 580 7642

Health and Safety Executive:

Medical Division
Baynard's House
1 Chepstow Place
Westbourne Grove
London W2 4TF
071 229 3456

Home Office
50 Queen Anne's Gate
London SW1H 9AT
071 273 3000

Malignant Hyperthermia Unit
St James' University Hospital
Leeds LS9 7TF
0532 433144

Medical Defence Union
3 Devonshire Place
London W1N 2EA
071 486 6181

Medical Protection Society
50 Hallam Street
London W1
071 637 0541

**Medical Research Council
20 Park Crescent
London W1N 4AL
071 636 5422**

POISONS CENTERS

Belfast
Royal Victoria Hospital
Grosvenor Road
Belfast BT12 6BA
0232 240503

Birmingham
West Midlands Poisons Unit
Dudley Road Hospital
Birmingham B18 7QH
021 554 3801 ext. 4109

Cardiff
Llangdough Hospital
Penarth
South Glamorgan
0222 709901

Dublin
Jervis Street Hospital
Jervis Street
Dublin 1
0001 745588

Edinburgh
The Royal Infirmary of
Edinburgh
Edinburgh EH3 9YW
031 229 2477 ext. 2233

London
New Cross Hospital
Avonley
London SE14 5ER
071 635 9191

Newcastle
Royal Victoria Infirmary
Newcastle upon Tyne NE1 4LP
091 232 5131

Royal College of Anaesthetists
48–49 Russell Square
London WC1B 4JP
071 813 1900

**Royal College of Surgeons of
England**
35–43 Lincoln's Inn Fields
London WC2A 3PN
071 405 3474

**Royal College of Surgeons of
Edinburgh**
Nicholson Street
Edinburgh EH8 9DW
031 556 6206

Royal Society of Medicine
1 Wimpole Street
London W1M 8AE
071 408 2119

**Scottish National Blood
Transfusion Service**
Ellen's Glen Road
Edinburgh EH17 7QT
031 664 2317

**Welsh Office Health and Social
Services Groups**
New Crown Buildings
Cathays Park
Cardiff CF1 3NQ
0222 825111

Index